O9-AHV-872

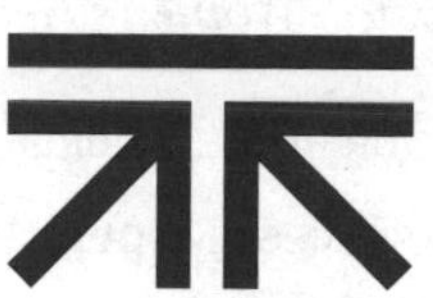

Books by the Boston Women's Health Book Collective

OUR BODIES, OURSELVES

OURSELVES AND OUR CHILDREN

THE NEW OUR BODIES, OURSELVES

Books by members of the Boston Women's Health Book Collective

CHANGING BODIES, CHANGING LIVES: A BOOK FOR TEENS

TALKING WITH YOUR TEENAGER: A BOOK FOR PARENTS

THE NEW OURSELVES, GROWING OLDER

WOMEN

AGING

WITH

KNOWLEDGE

AND

POWER

PAULA B. DORESS-WORTERS
AND DIANA LASKIN SIEGAL

IN COOPERATION WITH THE
BOSTON WOMEN'S HEALTH BOOK COLLECTIVE

ILLUSTRATIONS BY ROSELAINE PERKIS

A TOUCHSTONE BOOK

PUBLISHED BY
SIMON & SCHUSTER

New York London Toronto
Sydney Tokyo Singapore

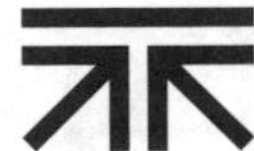

TOUCHSTONE
Rockefeller Center
1230 Avenue of the Americas
New York, New York 10020

DESIGNED BY BARBARA MARKS
Manufactured in the United States of America

5 7 9 10 8 6

Library of Congress Cataloging-in-Publication Data
Doress-Worters, Paula B. (Paula Brown)
The new ourselves, growing older : women aging with knowledge and power / Paula B. Doress-Worters and Diana Laskin Siegal, in cooperation with the Boston Women's Health Book Collective ; illustrations by Roselaine Perkis.
p. cm.
Rev. ed. of: Ourselves, growing older. © 1987.
Includes bibliographical references and index.
1. Aged women—United States–Psychology. 2. Aged women—Health and hygiene—United States. I. Siegal, Diana Laskin. II. Doress-Worters, Paula B. (Paula Brown). Ourselves, growing older.
III. Boston Women's Health Book Collective. IV. Title.
HQ1064.U5D669 1994
305.4–dc20 93-48494
CIP

ISBN: 0-671-87297-4

DISCOUNTS FOR LOW-INCOME, OLDER WOMEN'S GROUPS:

The New Ourselves, Growing Older is available at $5.40 per paperback copy (plus $2.00 shipping) to organizations and groups that are licensed by a state to operate as either a clinic, a health-counseling service, or a service center for older, low-income women. Orders must be for ten or more copies with payment, a document verifying health or social-service status, and your IRS number for tax exemption enclosed. The document must be a copy of a statement filed with a state or federal agency indicating health or social services as a primary purpose of your group. Make your check payable to Simon & Schuster and send to: Special Sales Department, Simon & Schuster, 15 Columbus Circle, New York, NY 10023.

COPIES SO PURCHASED MAY NOT BE OFFERED FOR RESALE.

DEDICATION

✦

To my husband, Allen J. Worters. Finding one another and falling in love at midlife provided one of the delightful surprises of my midlife years. Our relationship of the last ten years flies in the face of two persistent myths: that there are no good men out there for older women, and that women at menopause are not fit to live with. I am grateful to Allen for his unfailing support and generosity through a variety of personal, work, and family changes, a doctoral dissertion, and two editions of *Ourselves, Growing Older*.

To my friends and colleagues on the board and staff of the Boston Women's Health Book Collective who gave so generously of their time and resources to read and comment on chapters, to locate documentation material, and most important to simply be there for me personally, and as friends and supporters of this project.

To the memory of my parents, Ethel and Abraham J. Brown.

Like so many older women, my mother, Ethel, deserved a much better old age than she got. Despite the ravages of Parkinson's disease, until her death at the age of eighty-two she never allowed pain or difficult travel accommodations to keep her away from a family celebration. It was a great personal sadness that her death came just after Diana and I signed the contract for the first edition of this book and that she was not able to participate, yet her spirit inspires me daily.

My father Abraham—or Abe, as he preferred to be called—was one of the small but growing minority of caregiving husbands. He cared for my mother with unstinting devotion, risking his own health in doing so. Despite the many strains of caregiving, he was never too burdened to be supportive to his children and grandchildren. From my dad, I learned the importance of commitment and steadiness in accomplishing my goals.

P.B. D.-W.

To my mother, Ann Laskin, and my father, the late George Laskin.

Though very different from one another, my parents' outlooks combined to inspire me with the desire and the zeal to produce this book. My mother, Ann, ever the idealist who believes that the world should be a better place for everyone, is the inspiration for the reformer in me. She exemplifies the strength of older women in the way she has continued to grow and rise to new challenges. At age eighty-five she is still vital and learning. From the beginning, my mother gave her wholehearted support to the book project, including reading chapters, contributing experiences, and providing contacts and clippings.

My father, George, started his own business at midlife, demonstrating that one's earlier, seemingly unrelated work may be the necessary preparation for later accomplishment. His sense of humor, and his attitude that "of course" I can do anything I set my mind to, gave me the permission and confidence to do the things I wanted to do.

To my older, loving, enthusiastic women friends (you know who you are) who kept me going with laughs, parties, meals, movies, and hugs. I am grateful to all my friends for the support, understanding, and wisdom they have generously given me.

To Dick, whose memory will always be with me.

D.L.S.

To our respective children and stepchildren:

Diana's: Naomi Siegal and daughter-in-love Diane Benjamin; John Siegal, daughter-in-law Shelley English-Siegal, and grandchild, Joseph George Siegal

Paula's: Hannah Doress, Benjamin Doress, David Worters, and Susan Worters

with our support for the goals and paths they choose for their lives, and with the hope that in their older years they will see the results of our efforts

P.B.D.-W. AND D.L.S.

ACKNOWLEDGMENTS

✦

Ruby Abrahams
Alice Adams
Marie Adams
Rita Addison
Jeffrey Ahlin
John Albright
Anna C. Alden
Susan Allein
Kathleen Allen
Anne Alpert
Mark D. Altschule
Alzheimer's Disease and Related Disorders Association, Boston and Chicago
Alzheimer's Disease Support Group, Eliot Mental Health Center, Concord, Massachusetts
Donna Ambrogi
Leslie Antokolsky
Arthritis and Health Resource Centres, Inc., Wellesley, Massachusetts
Esther Atlas
Ellie Atlee
Abigail Avery
Byllye Y. Avery
Elizabeth Badger
Mildred L. Badnek
Agnes Barr
Lorraine Baugh
Connie Bean
Otilia Bengsston
Irma Sue Berkelhammer
Peg Bevins
Catherine M. Bishop
Mary Blackburn
Lillian Blacker
Robin Blatt
Joanne Baxter Bluestone
Barbara Bolduc
Louise Bonar
Christine Bond
Alice Bonis
Deanne Bonnar
Joan Borysenko
Boston Public Library, General and Humanities Reference Services
Miriam Pass Botnick
Stamata Bouloukes
Ursula Bowring-Trenn
Arminta Bradley
Barbara Bradley
Lydia Bragger
Elizabeth Bredin
Mimi Breed
Brookline Public Library, Main Reference Department
Kathy Brooks
Kay Brooks
Susan Brown
Vivienne Brown
Suzanne Butterfield
Yetta Butters
Cathy Cade
Blake Cady
Jessica Callahan
Susan Calloway
Peg Cameron
Caroline Campanella
Cancer Information Service, Dana-Farber Cancer Center
Norma Canner
Gloria Cartwright
Florence Charlton
Otta Chase
Aparna Chattoraj
Joyce Betries Chediac
Helen Cheeks
Eleanor Chilson
Bunny Clapper
Thelma Clapper
Mary Clark
Vidal Clay
Nora Coffey
Mabel Cohen
Michael David Cohen
Carola Cohn
Stuart Cohn
Louise Collier
Eleanor Collins
Mimi Conklin
Thelma Cooper
Louise Corbett
Sarah Corman
Naomi Cotter
Hildreth Coulter
Countway Library
Selma L. Crevoshay
Rosamund Critchley
Mary Ann Cromer
Sue Crook
Linda Crossman
Thelma Crowley
Cornelia Curtis
Jaffray Cuyler
Dorothy Dana
Jessica Daniels
Pamela Daniels
Elizabeth Deady
Hadwig Dertouzos
Tobey Deutsch
Lena DeVincent
Miriam Diamond
Bruce Ditzion
William Docken
Lorraine C. Doherty
Caroline Jo Dorr
Mildred Dreeszen
Buffy Dunker
Hannah Dupasse
Tess Durfee
Rosalind Durham
Frances M. Dwyer
Naomi Emmerling
Carol Englender
Johanna Erickson
Frederica Erlenmeyer
Chavela Esparza
Nancy Eustis
Kathy Fabiszewski
Jean Fairfax
Sally Feather
Stephen Feldman
Marie Feltin
Libby Fennel
Judith Ferber
Cindy Ferguson
Mary Ann Ferguson
Paul Ferguson
Norma Finkelstein
Judy Fischbach
Anne Fishbain
Libby Fishbane
Mary Flaherty
Jean Fleming
Edith Fletcher
Carmen Flores
George Foord
Inge Fowlie
Robin Ann Fradkin
Denise Frangules
Elsie Frank
Elizabeth Freeman
Roberta Freeman
Jeanette French
Kathie French
Mary French
Mike Friedman
Stella Friml
Mary Gaffney
Lillian Gallivan
Sally Gardner
Patricia Loring Garrity
Penny Gay
Ruth Gay
Natalie Gelbert
Tobin Gerhart
Jean Gilfillan
Frances Gill
Luke Gillespie
Sofia Gitter
Leonard Glantz
Pat Glasgow
Susan Glick
Gena S. Glicklich
Janet Goldberg
Barbara Goldmuntz
Lillian Golovin

Joan Kendall Gordon
Priscilla Grace
Linda Graham
Tova Green
Harriet Ford Griswold
Vera Gropper
Sarah Grosberg
Teri Guido
Lee Hadley
Pearle Hadley
Jane Halliburton
Christina Halkett
Eleanor Hamilton
Helen Hanchett
Elizabeth Harris
Marian Harris
Susan Harris
Ruth Haugen
Faith Hawkins
Alice Ryerson Hayes
Leonard Hayflick
Margaret Healy
Regina Healy
Renée Hecht
I. Craig Henderson
Jeanne Henderson
Charles H. Hennekens
Eileen Henry
Jan Keil Hernandez
Ruth Edmonds Hill
Lillian Holcomb
Tippie Holmes
Norma Holt
Charlotte Horblit
Betty Hoskins
Wanda Howard
Gudrun Howe
Constance Hsia
Jeanne Hubbuch
Joan Hughes
Virginia Huhndorf
Demetria Iazzeto
Ann Irwin
Beryl Jackson
Bill Jackson
Ellen Jackson
Margie Dixon Jackson
Celia Jacobs
Celene Jacobson
Claradine Moore James
Patricia Jean
Judith S. Jenkins
Janyce Jennings
Pat Jerabek
Judy Johannet
Anna Johnson
Alice Jones
Helen Makie Jones
Janet Jones
Sallie M. Jones
Jini Jordan
Hilda Kahne
Barbara Kahwaty
Gertrude Kaplan
Helen Kaplan
Liselotte Karplus-Wissing
Judith N. M. Kass
Seymour Kass
Geri Kassirer
Cynthia P. Keefe
Janet Keep
Monika Kehoe
Justine Kelliher
Dorothy Kemp
JoAnn Kerrick-Mack
Elana Klugman
Edna Knox
Richard A. Knox
Hazel Krantz
Gisela Krause
Maggy Krebs
Maggie Kuhn
Mildred Kuusisto
Anita Landa
Frances Landry
Joseph Lane
Virginia Lanzkron
Barbara M. LaRoche
Phyllis Larrabee
Patricia LaRue
Lorraine Laverriere
Marie Lavine
Rosemary Lawson
Mabel G. Leavitt
Marie T. Lee
Ruth Lee
Delores LeGrand
Teresa Leitner
Eleanor Lenke
Mary Leno
Clare Lesser
Rhoda Levinson
Roberta Levinson
Bess Levitt
Mary A. Lewis
Myrna Lewis
Frederic Li
Debbie Lieberson
Midge Lillis
Sophie Linkin
Deborah Little
Patricia Lockwood
Lucile Shuck Longview
Susan M. Love
Ethel McFerson
Sonja M. McKinlay
Elizabeth MacMahon
Isabel MacMahon
Diane Mahoney
Annette Maleson
Mary Jane Maloof
Laura E. Manning
Phyllis Mansfield
Thomas Manzelli
Julie V. Marsteller
Nancy H. Martin
Massachusetts College of
Pharmacy, Drug
Information Line
Massachusetts Nutrition
Resource Center
Carol Mathieson
Arthur Mazer
Kathleen Harrington Mazer
Janet Meacham
Margaret Vance Hay Means
Cathy Meecham
Jean Meggison
Nellie Kenick Meras
Barbara Merchant
Lucy Metting
Thelma Miles
Priscilla Mitchell
Fran Moira
Michael Moore
Anna Morgan
Susanne Morgan
Amadea Morningstar
Marion Morra
Winn Morrell
Ruth Moy
Freda Mulkern
Agnes Murphy
Dorothy Murphy
Alf Nachemson
Eva Naiherseg
Anita Nardini
Helen Nearing
Janet Neuman
Sue Newell
Margaret S. Nichols
Peggy Nickman
Elizabeth Noble
Agnes Norsigian
Loraine Obler
Judy Olmstead
Frances Olrich
Gloria C. Ortiz
Annabelle Osterberg
Elizabeth T. Palmunen
Florence Parker
Gloria J. Parker
Urada Parnell
Ginger Parsons
Dorothy Patten
Bradford Patterson
Cicely Payne
Roselaine Perkis
Helen Perry
Marguerite Pfeiffer
Robbie Pfeufer-Kahn
Minna Plotkin
Alonzo Plough
Mary Pogoryiliki
Elinor Polansky
Fran Pollner
Judith G. Poole
Mary Pratt
Gena Prenowitz
Helane Press
Avis Pretzler
Joanne Prince
Alice Quinlan
Agnes V. Quinn
Marguerite Ramedell
Myra Ramos
Tania Rash
Eloise Rathbone-McCuan
Shirley Renfrew
Neil M. Resnick
Beth E. Rhude
Miriam Rice
Sharon Rich
Janet Richards
Aldean Richardson
Joyce Richardson
Doris Richman
Georgie Ridlon
Martha Robbins
Harriet Robey
Virginia Robinson
Gregorita Rodriguez
Judy Rogers
Annette Rosen
Sandra Rosenthal
Alice Rossi
Anita Rossien
Grace Rossien
Mary Rovner
Lydia Roy
Jane Royse
Thelma Rutherford
Sally Rynne
Florence Sacarob
Dorothy Saccoccia
Rose Safran
Miriam Salomé-Haven
Judy Salzman
Dorothy Sanborn
Ethel Sanders
Shirley Sartori
Norma Satten
Christine Saulnier
Marian Saunders
Marnette Saz
Loretta Schalk
Jane Schaller
Toni Schiff
Irene A. Schmeid
Mildred Schuckstes

Hilda Schwartz
Hilda Scott
Mary Scott
Judith Seixas
Sarah Semerjian
Annie Senhouse
E. Mary Shannon
Jody Shaw
Beth Sheffel
Barbara Sher
Susan Sherry
Louise B. Shrieves
Rose L. Sidman
Naomi Siegal
Winifred Siegel
Irene Siegler
Phyllis Rolfe Silverman
Ethan A. H. Sims
Geraldine Sindut
Gladys Singman
Claudia M. Sisson
Lucy Skinner
Connie Slater
Joanne Small
Nancy Smart
Pearl Smith
Louise Snipes
Muriel Snowden
Jan Solet
Mickey Spencer
Ellen Sue Spivack
Erna Sporer
Betty Stanco
Marie Steinmeyer
Arlene Stern
Betsy Steven
Irene Stewart
Larry Stiffler
Greta Stone
Marian G. Stoodley
Janet Stout
Julia Sutton
Lillian R. Suvalle
Karyl Sweeney
Sharon E. Sweet
Carolyn Ruth Swift
Pauline Swift
Lois Swingler
Doris Tanner
Mary Taschner
Louise Taub
James Taylor
Jo Tempesto
Toni Tenette
Richard Thal
Elizabeth Theriault
Wendy Thurber
Olive Tiffany
Ruth M. Tinsley
Thelma Tisdale
Jean Tock
Frances Toy
Dorothy Tollifson
Anne Tremearne
Rona Troderman-King
Lonie Troub
Suzanne Tufts
Eleanore Tupper
Blanche Aurora Turner
Gladys Vanderbelt
VISION, Inc.
Joy Vronsky
Mary Waggener
Nancy Wagman
Judith S. Wallerstein
Lila Wallis
Janet M. Walther
Adeline Wanatee
Deborah Ward
Marjorie Waters
Liz Watson
Cassandra Batson Way
Ursula Weimersheimer
Ira Weinberg
Marlena Weinstein
Marya Weinstock
Sandra Weintraub
Fran Weisse
Rosemary Whiting
Sally Wilkins
Esther Wilson
Mollie Wilson
Gertrude Winchell
Bernice Winer
Richard Wolff
Bruce Wood
Irene Wood
Josephine Worrell
Frances Worters
Peggy Ann Wright
Sarah Yarrington
Marilyn M. Young
Aileen Zahn
J. Carolyn Zavarine
Geraldine Zetzel
Irving Kenneth Zola
Michael Zucker
Cecile Zunner

ACKNOWLEDGMENTS FOR THE 1994 EDITION

✦

Nancy E. Avis
Alan Balsam
Marybeth Barker
Lise Beane
Helene Bednarsh
Tia Bentley
Edna Biddy
Eleanor Bonsaint
Abigail Bottome
Carolyn Bottum
Judith Bowman
Claudia Costa Bowser
Gilda Brickman
Christie Burke
Barbara Cohen
Sandra Coleman
Sue Crawford
Rosalind Dépas
Adela Dolney
Kevin C. Donahue
Jen Douglas
Susannah Cooper Doyle
Peggy Edson
Ellen Feingold
Julie Flood-Page
Maxine Forman
Mindy Fried
Pat Gilbert
Dan Gillis
Leona Greenhill
Muriel Heiberger
Mike Heichman
Carolyn Helwig
Judith E. Heumann
Michael F. Holick
Cindy Hounsell
Ruth Housman
Betty Hudson
Naomi Isler
Barbara Laurie
Beth Levesque
Joanne Levesque
Liz Manion
Phyllis Kernoff Mansfield
José Marçal
Massachusetts Department of Public Health
Sonja M. McKinlay
Caroline McNeil
Members of the Saturday Discussion Series
Sylvia L. Memolo
Bruce H. Mitlak
Pamela Morgan
Denise L. Page
Ruth Palombo
Sarah F. Pearlman
Grace Petot
Roger Platt
Jane Porcino
Donald Putney
Paula Rayman
Sharon Rich
Alice Rothschild
Carole Roy
David Schardt
Tricia Selby
Rosemary Gladstone Strick
Daniel Swerdlow
Laurie A. Thompsen
James Trussell
Joanne Tuller
Ellen Valko
Patricia Vancil
Alice Welch
Julie Wendrich
Pat Williams
Sidney M. Wolfe
Helen Wood
Ann Voda
Irving Kenneth Zola
Marilyn Zuckerman

CONTENTS

✦

UNDERSTANDING, PREVENTING, AND MANAGING MEDICAL PROBLEMS

RESOURCES

FOREWORD TO THE 1987 EDITION

✦

We are all aging. The pioneers of the second wave of feminism are advancing into middle age or beyond. In fact, the whole postwar baby-boom generation is moving into midlife, which means that this will be an age group to reckon-with in every sense.

Yet the specific concerns of older women are just coming to the fore. There were so many women's issues to be dealt with, and in the 1970s, most of the women of the new wave of feminists were quite young. In the area of health, reproductive rights and childbirth issues understandably took precedence. While these remain important to all women because they deal so basically with control of our bodies, there are other concerns that can no longer be ignored.

This book examines the neglected health concerns of middle-aged and older women. The basic principle—that we must know our own bodies and ourselves in order to be free from mistaken notions, the legacy of the patriarchal culture in which we live—continues after reproductive functions have ended. We remain females to the end of our days, and our status as women affects us as long as we live.

Like its predecessor, *Our Bodies, Ourselves*, this book is a collaborative effort. Many women have participated in its writing, and it is based on common experience. It reveals the impact of ageism, compounded with sexism, on all of us. It opens up new ways to free ourselves of both of these, not only in our own minds but also in the society around us. Insights both from the older women's advocacy movement and the women's health movement are encompassed within it. For older women it is a milestone.

Some of us who have been advocates for older women's issues for a long time are delighted to observe this spread of consciousness. The circle of concern is widening; there are now many approaches, not one; and there is greater organizational and personal interest in the problems of the growing-older female. This book should be a landmark in speeding up that process of consciousness-raising.

A work like this encourages confidence and creativity and the acceptance of self-worth at any age. It should help women release the internal brakes we have applied so long and help us take off in any direction we would like to go. The idea is to enjoy life in our later years, to make the most of this most precious season of our lives. This health and living handbook will also increase women's ability to stay well, thereby expanding the growing force of active middle-aged and older women. More women will participate in the Older Women's League and other advocacy organizations to make things easier for the next generation coming along. For older women *can* change the circumstances of aging for all women, and men as well.

Such efforts expand the concept of sisterhood across generations, with women in midlife providing a crucial bridge. Together we are building a new road to aging, and at the same time that road is building us. Young women have as great a stake in our efforts as older women do, for their turn is coming.

When we finally bridge the generation gap, women will be a magnificent force for positive change in society. For we are the compassion experts—we've been socialized in that direction. Humanizing the social fabric is our special domain. We're the nurturers and informal healers, even though professionals of both sexes have medicalized the process, leaving only the unpaid part for us.

At present we're caught within the confines of an impossible health-care system, filled with absurdities and based upon an economic underpinning that distorts it into grotesque shapes. But given a long view, and our involvement, that too can be changed. Knowledge is the first step. The second is taking more control over whatever aspects of our own health that we can. From dependency on "experts" we must move toward greater independence, which means taking on a greater degree of responsibility for our own bodies, as well as for the policies that affect us.

I do believe that women will take the lead in remodeling the health-care system of the future, and those of us in midlife or older will play an important part of that eventual transformation. Why? Not only because we are the compassion experts—and healing is intimately connected with compassion—but also because we have the least to lose and the most to gain by that transformation. Women of all ages, by changing their own health habits and affecting others around them, by speaking up and then becoming involved with all aspects of health-care delivery, will, I predict, have far greater influence than we now can imagine in redesigning the whole system. But first we must start with ourselves. Then we should move on to try to understand the forces that drive the present system: its costs, its distribution of services, and where we fit in—or don't fit in. Then we will be able to join with others to create a health-care system worthy of the name.

Taking control of our own lives and of our bodies is the most basic feminist principle there is. This book moves us in that direction, for it breaks down that formidable barrier in our minds—the fear of growing old. It helps us to see that midlife and old age are stages of life, as important as any other. Since we cannot beat aging, we had better learn how to join it. That is what this book is about. I'm very glad to have been a part of it.

Tish Sommers
September 1985

FOREWORD TO THE 1994 EDITION

✦

We in the Boston Women's Health Book Collective are delighted to welcome this update of *Ourselves, Growing Older.* This book is like a beloved sister of *The New Our Bodies, Ourselves*—one look, and you know we're from the same family. Most of us in the Collective were in our twenties and thirties when we met in a circle of women talking together—haltingly at first, then with increasing candor, vigor, and excitement—about the pressing health issues of our lives. Childbirth, abortion, birth control, sexuality—those were the issues of our early years. And now, as a host of journalists have observed, we baby boomers are heading into the second half of life. As our menstrual cycles come to an end, we join our mothers, our grandmothers, and the growing number of postmenopausal women. While this marks the end of our reproductive years, it is only the midpoint of our productive lives.

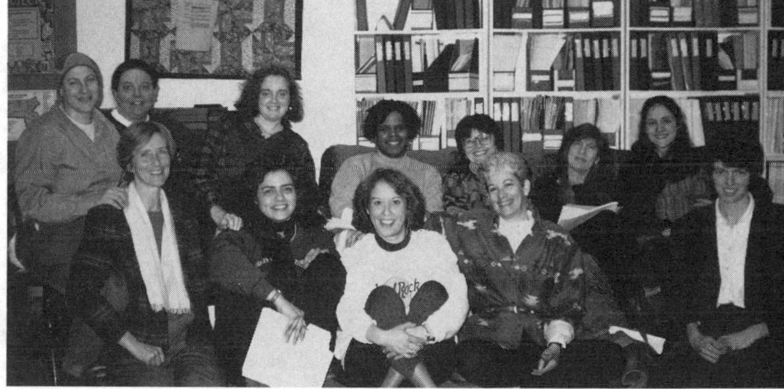

Some members of the Boston Women's Health Book Collective. Boston Women's Health Book Collective

What hasn't changed is the connection between the personal and the political, the ways that oppressions in our culture imprint themselves onto women's minds and bodies. As a Collective, we have fought the medicalization of childbirth; now we move to questioning the unnecessary medicalization of menopause. As before, we assert women's right to express our sexuality free of coercion or stigma, whatever our age. We challenge the notion that disability comes inevitably with aging, and decry the increasingly toxic air, water, and food that poison women's bodies and create disease. Aware of the role of poverty and racial injustice in undermining the health that should be every woman's birthright, we continue to work for a better life for all people. We celebrate *The New Ourselves, Growing Older* as a partner in this ongoing work.

WENDY SANFORD for the
Boston Women's Health Book Collective

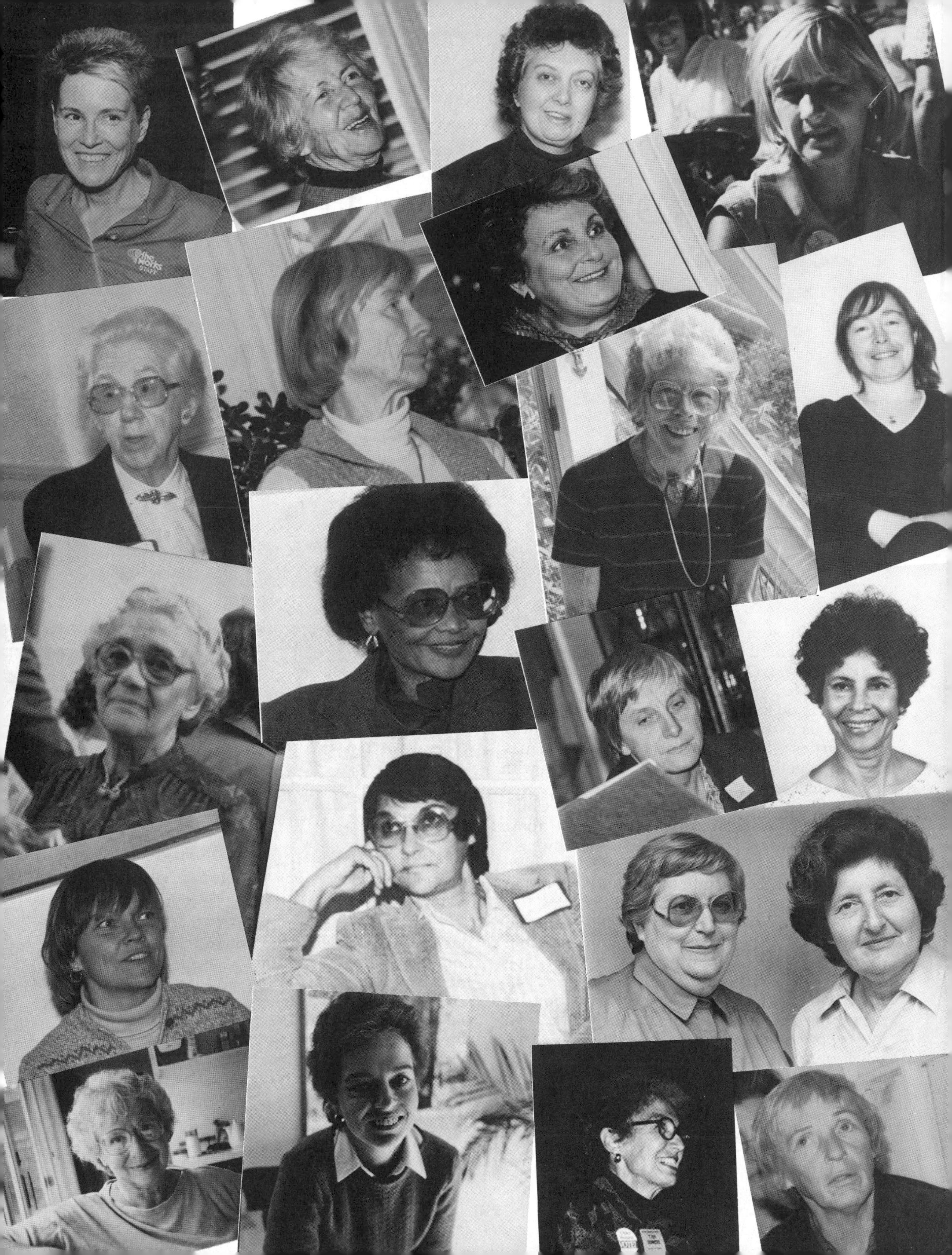
the Works
STAFF

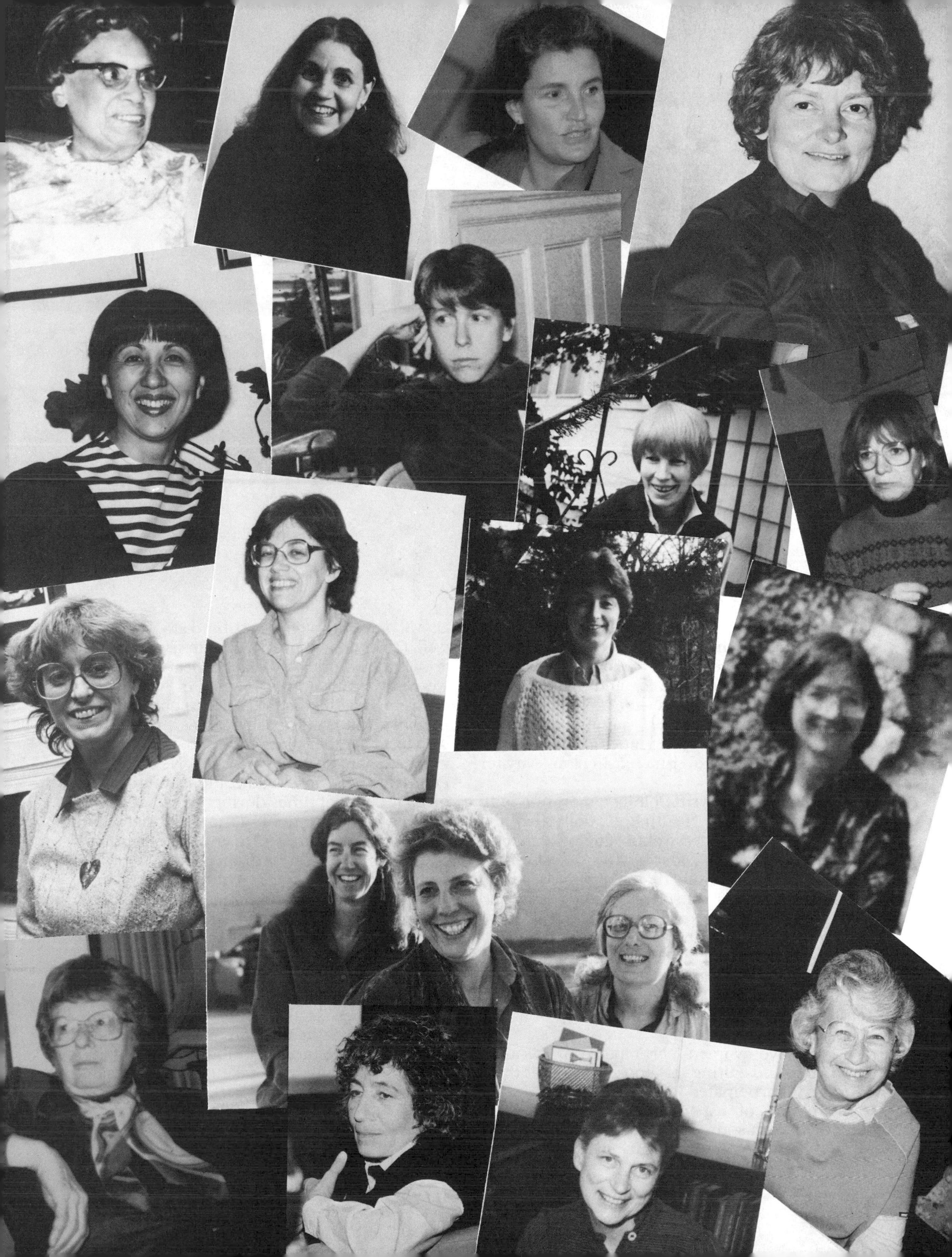

PROJECT COORDINATORS' PREFACE

✦

The contributors of this book constitute a rich mosaic of women whose life experiences span the length of the century, who come from a variety of religious, economic, and ethnic backgrounds, and who live in a wide range of housing and living situations. We came together to address the special opportunities and challenges of living in a time of ever-increasing longevity for women.

This book was written in collaboration with the Boston Women's Health Book Collective, and began out of the process of producing a chapter on Women Growing Older for *The New Our Bodies, Ourselves*. Writing that chapter presented challenges; the task of squeezing the health and living issues of four or five decades of life into one chapter seemed insurmountable. In a meeting, the coordinator of that chapter exclaimed, "Do you realize that we are trying to write a mini–*Our Bodies, Ourselves* for the second half of life?" With that awareness the idea of a new book was born.

Forty-five women participated in writing, rewriting, and editing this book, while over three hundred participated as readers, consultants, contributors of experiences and information, and links with sources of new information. Several of the women who contributed to *The New Our Bodies, Ourselves* contributed to this book as well. Other contributors came to us through the growing network of women's health and older women's organizations. Most of the project writers were based in the Boston area and rural New England, but a number of women participated who lived in other parts of the country—California, the Southwest, the Midwest, New York, and Pennsylvania. Those who could travel to Boston met a number of times during the life of the project to exchange mutual support and ideas about writing our chapters and to enjoy good company and delicious potluck dinners. Our more far-flung writers had to be content with coming together in spirit, communicating by mail and telephone, with occasional lucky opportunities to meet while someone was traveling. Networks were created and firm friendships forged, which we know will continue beyond the life of the project.

While most of the writers who coordinated chapters ranged in age from their mid-forties to early seventies, none of the most long-lived women were willing to take on such a task. As one woman put it:

I enjoy contributing my ideas to an intellectual discussion, but I find in my eighties that I no longer have the energy to coordinate a project. The time for that is past. Yet I enjoy putting my ideas into the pot with everyone else's. I continue to feel a valued part of many organizations and projects by participating in this way.

Special thanks are due to the oldest women who did contribute to the book project through sharing their experiences, attending group discussions, interviewing friends, and reviewing chapters, often while fighting increasing physical limitations. We especially want to thank the following women who contributed so much to the book: Lois Harris (age eighty-two), Lucy Mitchell (eighty-five), Faire Edwards (seventy-nine), Elsie Reethof (ninety), and Beth Rosenbaum (eighty). Their spirit, wisdom, and breadth of life experience enriched this book in so many ways. Their courage and optimism inspire us to carry on.

As project coordinators, we cannot possibly give adequate acknowledgment to the writers of the chapters for the hard work, maturity, and cooperation that the task we undertook together required. Many of the women who worked on the project donated hours of labor beyond what we were able to compensate. We hope they will enjoy the satisfaction of seeing the book in print.

We would especially like to thank Mary C. Allen, our project editor, who carefully and painstakingly edited each chapter and contributed immeasurably to the complex task of weaving them into a coherent whole. Our thanks to Barbara Williams, Henry Ferris, and the many others at Simon & Schuster who contributed to the editing, design, and production of this book.

Special thanks are also due to the members of the Boston Women's Health Book Collective for their collaboration and support in carrying out this project. Judy Norsigian, Esther Rome, Pamela Morgan, Sally Whelan, Norma Swenson, and Jan Brin constantly fed us information from the files of the Collective's Women's Health Information Center. Jane Pincus and Norma Swenson between them read and critiqued the entire book and Judy and Esther read substantial sections. Wendy Sanford and Nancy Hawley read and commented on important chapters. Special appreciation goes to Vilunya Diskin, whose support was critical at an early stage.

Many lesbians participated actively in this book from the very beginning as writers, readers, and consultants, as contributors of experiences, photographs, and poems. Some attended small discussion groups to share their concerns about their lives and relationships. We especially appreciate their openness in view of the homophobic pressures that make it risky for lesbians to reveal their sexual preference.

We are grateful to the secretaries and office workers who typed the manuscript, kept our files

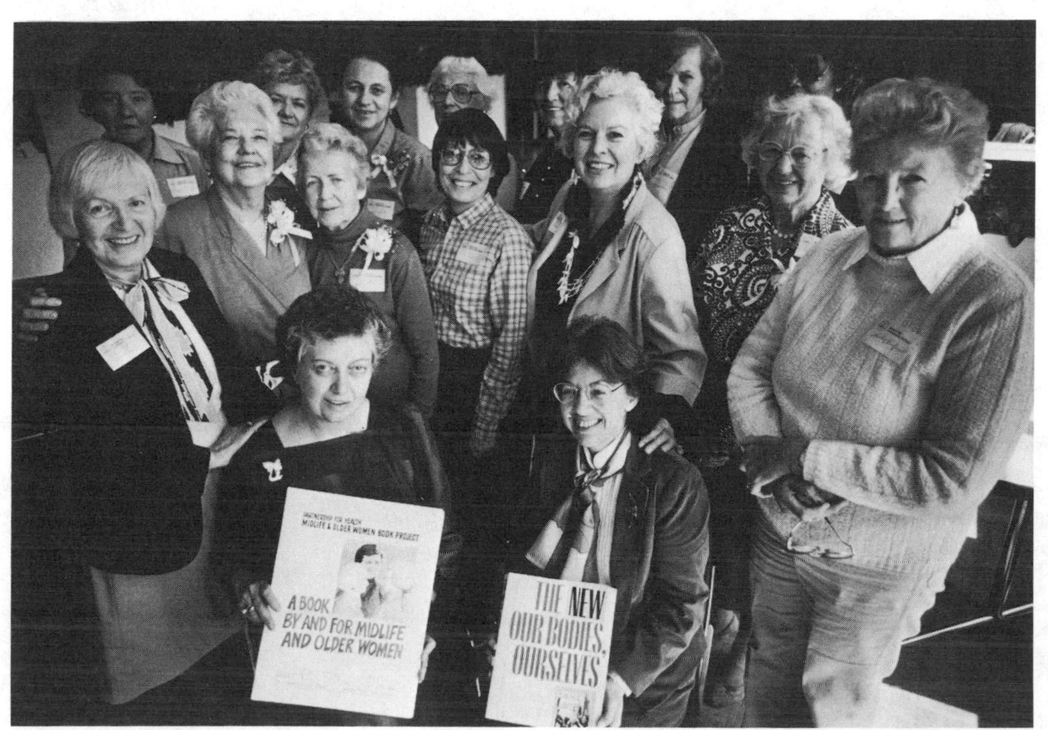

Janet Knott/The Boston Globe

Project coordinators (seated) with some of the project participants at a meeting of the Greater Boston Older Women's League.

organized, and often were our first critics: Mary Ann McCarthy, Carola Cohn, Chris Crandall, Barbara Connell, Laura Last, Felice Katz, Jasmine Loisell, Wendy Levine, and Bill Russell. While typing our manuscript, one woman stopped smoking and another reevaluated her eating patterns. We hope the book will have a similar effect on our readers.

A book such as this one would not be possible without the help of many women sending experiences, information, poetry, photos, and drawings, and women and men reading chapters and offering comments. The names of all those who helped are listed in the Acknowledgments. Many of those listed offered constructive criticism, and inclusion of their names does not mean that they agreed with the final product.

This book is not an anthology of individual statements, but a compilation of many women's ideas from a feminist perspective. To achieve this end, the project coordinators in dialogue with the writers deleted material that repeated other chapters, worked on contradictions between chapters, and moved material from one writer's chapter to another when that seemed to improve the flow of the book. The project coordinators retained and exercised final editorial control and thus are responsible for omissions, errors, and inclusion of controversial material. We hope others, women and men, will write more about the experience of growing older. We want this book to have plenty of company.

The death of Tish Sommers, author of the Foreword to the First Edition and the concluding chapter, in October 1985 was one of the saddest events that occurred during the writing of this book. She and her colleague and close friend Laurie Shields, cofounders of the Older Women's League, were among the first to urge us to expand *The New Our Bodies, Ourselves* chapter on Women Growing Older into a book of its own, and both generously encouraged the project. We felt privileged to work with Tish, to have the benefit of her empowering vision of older women's political potential. In her last years she accomplished what many would be proud to accomplish in a lifetime. Tish undertook the task of writing a chapter and a foreword for this book, making it clear that she would work as long as she was able, but that when her condition worsened she would bow out and trust us to do the final editing and provide the resource list for her chapter. Indeed, that is just what happened. Tish met all of her deadlines with characteristic optimism, directness, and flair. When she was no longer able to work, she let us know without delay. Her clarity, courage, and honesty with herself and others continue to inspire us.

PAULA B. DORESS-WORTERS
DIANA LASKIN SIEGAL
January 1987

PREFACE TO THE 1994 EDITION

✦

Since first publication of *Ourselves, Growing Older,* over 100,000 books have been sold. Often women buy our book for an older family member, but go on to read it themselves. Many of you have told us that the intergenerational focus of this book has helped you work out issues relating to planning for your own and your family members' health care, housing, and caregiving needs.

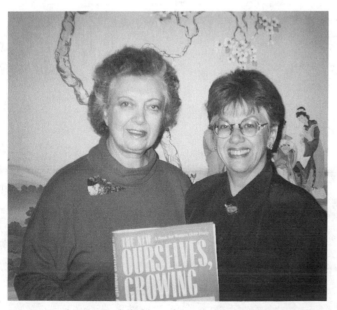

Diana Laskin Siegal (left) and Paula B. Doress-Worters
Allen Worters

We encourage everyone to let go of fears of aging and of the old. It does no good for one generation to blame another for its economic woes. We all need one another. When we unite across generations we can question business as usual and fight the true causes of social and economic inequality.

Cynics enjoy pointing out that the "youth generation"—whose battle cry had been "never trust anyone over thirty"—is now pushing fifty. Those of us past fifty, including the authors of this book, welcome the energy, creativity, and commitment of the generation that cut its teeth on the fight for racial equality, that ended an immoral war, and that gave birth to a second wave of feminism. We welcome the baby boomers to the promise of many more fulfilling decades ahead, and urge you to turn your generation's discerning lens on the double standard of aging for women.

We have updated this edition of *Ourselves, Growing Older* with the needs and questions of the baby-boomer generation in mind, based on readers' letters and a series of discussions with midlife women. We hope the new Menopause chapter will help with the often daunting task of making sense of the growing body of research on menopause, and the faster-growing body of popular writing that is misinformed or frequently uncritical of research reports. We have included extensive resources for all the chapters so that women can expand their access to information and participate in decisions about their lives and their health.

Creating a revised edition of *Ourselves, Growing Older* for the 1990s would not have been possible without the contributions of many women. We are grateful to authors of the original chapters who were available to update their chapters, and to new participants who were willing to step in and update other chapters, doing so with great thoroughness and dedication.

We are especially grateful to members of the Boston Women's Health Book Collective for thoughtful reading and comments on many chapters, and to the staff of the Collective's Women's Health Information Center (WHIC) for their assistance in retrieving information from the Collective's archives, and for many small favors.

Special thanks to Alice Welch for obtaining references and to Leona Greenhill for updating the organizational information in the Resources section.

Our thanks to Sheila Curry, our editor at Simon & Schuster, her cheerful assistant, Laurie Munroe Abkemeier, for their attention and commitment to this project and for keeping us on schedule, and the many others who contributed to the design and production of this book. We appreciate especially the responsiveness of Toni Rachiele, the copy-editing supervisor, and Gail Bradney, an exceptionally enthusiastic and well-informed copy editor who contributed beyond her job description.

Finally, we are especially inspired by the women who shared their experiences with us. In the chapters of this book women of all ages will hear the voices of hundreds of middle-aged and older women as they struggle with the challenges, and savor the triumphs of "aging with knowledge and power."

PAULA B. DORESS-WORTERS
and DIANA LASKIN SIEGAL

THE POTENTIAL OF THE SECOND HALF OF LIFE

✦

BY PAULA B. DORESS-WORTERS AND DIANA LASKIN SIEGAL WITH HELP FROM CAROLINE T. CHAUNCEY, ROBIN COHEN, MARILYN BENTOV, AND LOIS HARRIS

1994 UPDATE BY PAULA B. DORESS-WORTERS

SEE GENERAL RESOURCES ON PAGES 441–47

This book grows out of our conviction that the decades after forty can be rich and fulfilling, a time when we as women can come into our own. One in eight Americans is now over sixty-five. Older women are survivors, living an average of eight years longer than men, enjoying longer life spans than we might as young women have expected to or planned for. Life expectancy at birth for women is seventy-nine years. Those already over sixty-five can expect to live twenty years more. We can and do use our added years in ways that please us—learning new skills, traveling, and living out long-delayed dreams. Yet, as survivors, women are also likely to face more of the challenges of aging: chronic health conditions; inadequate income; caregiving responsibilities; lack of care when we need it;* and perhaps most devastating of all, the deaths of family members and friends. In this book, we have tried to give equal attention to both the promise and the challenge of the later years.

*We cannot rely on family ties for care. By the age at which most women need care the majority of those who had married are widowed; many others have never married; and 25 percent of women over seventy have no living children.

WHY A BOOK ABOUT BOTH MIDDLE-AGED AND OLDER WOMEN?

The economic problems of older women grow out of women's early experiences of sex discrimination in the workplace and the prejudicial belief that women do not need to earn enough money to support themselves. The two poorest groups in the United States today are women raising children alone and women over sixty-five living alone. Whether we have been poor all our lives or have experienced downward mobility in our middle or later years, many of us find that we do not have adequate financial resources for the second half of our lives. A feminist analysis is an important tool to help us become aware of the ways that we women are programmed from our earliest years for financial and emotional dependency. At midlife, we can begin to make changes in order to avoid the isolation, poverty, and ill health that mar the later years of so many older women.

In the role of traditional caregivers, women at midlife are in closer contact than any other group, except for the aging themselves, with the problems that arise when public policy fails to meet needs such as elder housing, long-term care, and in-home care. When such needs go unmet by public services, it is middle-aged women who are expected to give their unpaid labor to provide the services required. Frequently, our personal aspirations and careers suffer when we do so. Also, our future security suffers if we fail to earn pension and Social Security credits in those crucial middle years. Policies that require women to care for the elderly for free at home are short-sighted. Such policies sow the seeds for another generation of impoverished older women. We must demand the resources for at-home respite care, long-term care, and housing and support services that will provide alternatives to the limited choices of unsupported independent living versus a nursing home.[1]

Many of us become so habituated to caring for others and helping others achieve that we lose sight of our own goals or never get around to formulating any. In the second half of life, many of us have an opportunity to pay attention to ourselves and our own needs and aspirations, perhaps for the first time. The added years we gain with increased longevity can be ours to grow spiritually and intellectually. Midlife is often spoken of by women in metaphors of birth and rebirth, a time to nurture our own talents, casting off the external criteria by which we may have devalued ourselves and blossoming in new ways.

If we think of our future years as providing an opportunity to develop our creativity, our passions, and our activism, we can look forward to our older years with confidence and enthusiasm.

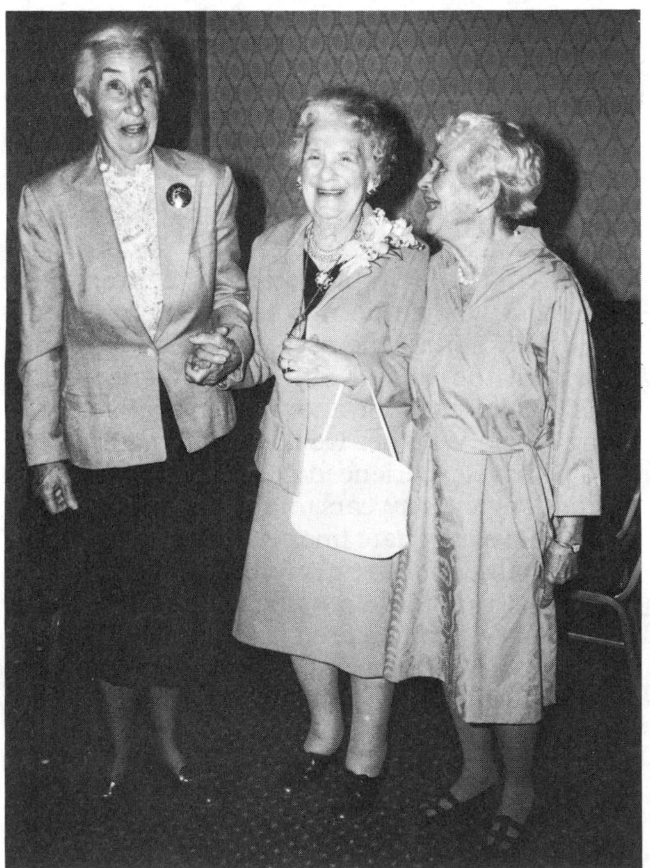

Ellen Shub

Aging and Ageism

Whole
Woman of the ^ Year

Have you ever known a woman named "November"?
Neither have I.
Now "May" and "June" and "April" have their
  namesakes—
Ever ask why?

We rarely picture woman as autumnal;
Female is spring.
Please, someone, name a newborn girl "October"
And hear her sing

Of harvest cut and growth complete and fruit mature,
Not just of birth.
Oh, let a woman age as seasons do;
Love each time's worth!

Miriam Corcoran

Ageism—the belief that a person's worth and abilities are determined solely by chronological age—is the enemy that threatens the creative, growing future we envision for ourselves. Research shows that intellectual capacity remains stable throughout life—the ability to learn new things continues unabated and, when actively exercised, enhances our well-being.[2] Yet ageism declares us obsolete at a socially defined deadline. At age sixty we find ourselves on our community's senior-citizen list, and at sixty-five many companies expect us to retire even though mandatory retirement has been abolished by federal law.

In a youth-oriented society, both middle-aged and older women struggle with ageism. Because of the double standard, women are labeled "old" at an earlier age than men are.[3] The sexist beliefs that relegate women to child rear-

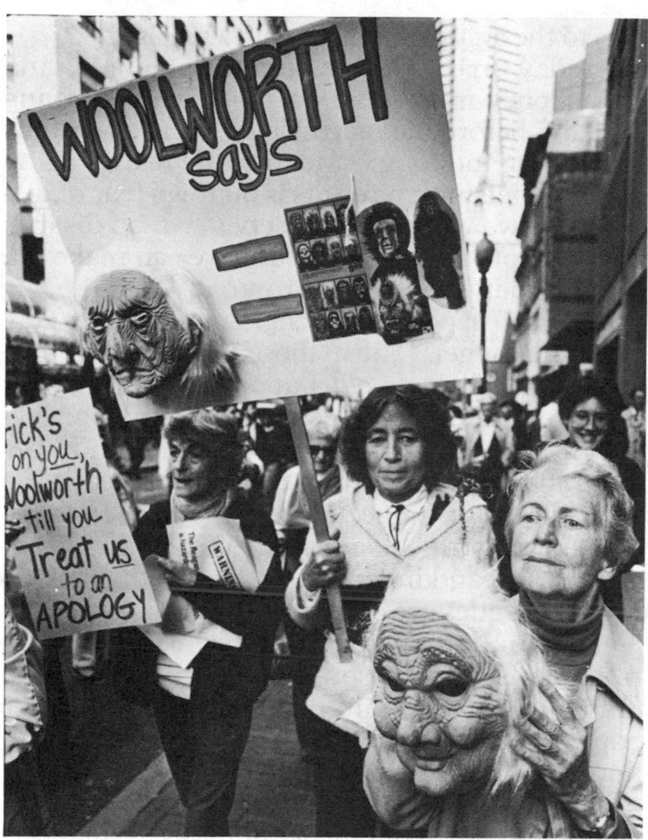
WOOLWORTH
says
rick's
on you,
Woolworth
till you
Treat us
to an
APOLOGY

The Boston Globe

ing and domestic work exclusively seem to mark us as obsolete when children leave home and our childbearing potential is at an end. Such archaic beliefs are irrelevant to most contemporary women, yet we continue to suffer the discrimination that is their legacy, especially when we enter or reenter the work force or change jobs in our middle years.

We live in a society that values the quick fix and the slick package. As one woman put it, "I'm a lot more interesting than I was at twenty-five or thirty-five, but it's a lot harder to get anyone to pay attention." We can fight such attitudes by actively reaching out and valuing one another. At a social or community gathering, if you seek out one of the oldest women and get acquainted with her, you will be amply rewarded.

I went to a women's brunch where most of the women ranged from the mid-thirties to the mid-fifties. I was curious about one much older woman who turned out to be a sculptor in her seventies. She invited me to visit her at her studio near the shore. I drove down with a photographer friend, bringing a picnic lunch, and enjoyed a delightful afternoon viewing her recent work, each of us sharing her experiences as a woman trying to do creative work at different times in the life cycle. [a forty-four-year-old woman]

At a wedding where I did not know many people I noticed an older woman in her seventies who seemed to have a visual disability. No one was speaking with her, so I struck up a conversation. I found out she was a founding member of a self-help organization for people with low vision and did counseling on the telephone from her home for others with low vision. It was fun to meet and talk with such a gutsy lady. [a forty-eight-year-old woman]

Unity and Difference Among Women

When you read the experiences of the women quoted in this book, do not automatically picture a white, middle-class, heterosexual, able-bodied woman. We reached out to and heard from a great variety of women—white women and women of color, middle-aged and old women, heterosexual and lesbian and bisexual women, able-bodied women and women with disabilities. Because the book is primarily about aging, we identified the speakers by age alone unless another characteristic was significant to her story and not apparent in what she said.

Sexual Preference

At least 10 percent of women, perhaps more, are lesbian. It is sad that homophobia, the irrational fear and hatred of homosexuality and bisexuality, is still so prevalent that many lesbian women are reluctant to openly acknowledge their preference. Many women who have found a way to survive and thrive in a woman-centered community still hide this important part of themselves from their heterosexual friends and colleagues.

In gathering personal experiences for this book, we found that the lesbians (mostly middle-aged) who are part of an organization or network with other lesbians welcomed an opportunity to discuss the satisfactions of living a woman-centered way of life. We were less successful in reaching the oldest and most isolated lesbians who grew up and lived in even more repressive circumstances. Their fear of exposure and learned discomfort with openness has rendered them understandably reluctant to share their experiences and keeps them isolated from all but a few of their lesbian sisters. This is a loss to all of us who could learn from their life experiences as women surviving on their own.

We must unite as women to fight against the ageism, sexism, racism, homophobia, and discrimination against persons with disabilities that blight all our lives, especially in our later years. Our unity will be more powerful and effective if we can honor our differences and work toward inclusiveness of all groups. Each of us, whether heterosexual, lesbian, or bisexual, can examine our own attitudes and practices. We may be able in our own social circles to build a climate of inclusiveness and openness that will make every woman feel accepted and affirmed for who she is.

Aging and Disability

It is a mistake to equate disability with a particular age. Some women have lived with severe limitations from birth or an early age, while others become disabled later in life as a result of an accident or disease. Even the longest-lived women may remain free of limiting disabilities, but a number of women must learn to manage a disability in the middle and later years. If that happens to us, we may have to learn about adapting our living space, demanding access to buildings, and coping with a whole host of other situations we may never have had to deal with before. In so doing, there is much we can learn from other women with disabilities and from the disabled people's movement. A 1986 conference on aging and disability marked the beginning of dialogue and cooperation between the disability-rights and aging advocacy organizations.[4] In 1992, the American Association of Retired Persons (AARP) formed a Disability Initiative (see General Resources, page 441) to serve the needs of older persons with a disability. Their staff and volunteers are trained to be knowledgeable about the Americans with Disabilities Act (ADA).* At the same time, organizations with a disability focus are starting to pay more attention to the aging of their constituencies.

Today, many people fear pain, illness, and dependency more than death—a fear of "dying socially" before biological death occurs—or they fear "living too long."[5] Much of the fear of aging and the ageism that results is our own fear of disability. If we work for a society in which disability does not mean social death, we can make it a better society in which to grow old.

As life expectancy lengthens, people stay youthful longer. Thus, those over seventy-five used to be called *old-old,* but now this term refers to those over eighty-five, as the group from seventy-five to eighty-four stays healthier and lives more independently than before. Some use the term *old-old* or *frail elderly* to refer only to those who are ill or disabled, while those who are in good health and independent even in their eighties and nineties are counted as young-old.

A recent study found a surprising drop in rates of disability among the elderly despite the dramatic increase in the eighty-five-and-over population. This was attributed to higher education and income among elders, and the success of cataract and joint-replacement surgery to correct potentially disabling conditions.[6] While this is the good news about aging, advocates for those who are disabled or frail are concerned that studies such as this will be used to cut services for those who need them.

Health and Aging

Most of the health and medical problems we face in our later years are chronic rather than acute, and require innovative approaches to people's needs for personal support, caregiving, and housing. However, our health-care delivery system and health insurance specifically for the elderly—even Medicare—are geared to medical intervention for acute medical problems, and frequently don't cover the chronic conditions more common in our later years. We can learn from the independent living/disability rights movement about the importance of planning for a possible future disability by adapting our homes and fighting for home-care programs so we can remain a part of our communities as we age.[7] Aging is a part of the life span and should not be turned into a medical event. We can help ourselves and one another in maintaining our good health, and in other situations in which we have been taught to turn to professionals for answers.

*For retraining or making job changes, see your state vocational rehabilitation agency, which is charged with helping people with disabilities return to work. Though called by different names, each state has one and may have a hot line. Since the passage of the Americans with Disabilities Act (ADA) in 1990, it is against the law to discriminate against the disabled in job preference or public access. If you think you have been discriminated against because of your disability, contact an agency counselor or the Civil Rights Division of the U.S. Department of Justice charged with enforcing the ADA. The ADA hot line is (202) 514-0301.

Women and Policy for the Elderly

The younger baby boomers, aged thirty-five to forty-four, are now the largest age group in the population. Their concerns about menopause and aging will profoundly influence attitudes and policy about aging in the coming decades. By the second decade of the twenty-first century, the numbers of older women aged sixty-five to eighty-four will increase by nearly 70 percent, and those over eighty-five by nearly 30 percent. As women of color also live to older ages, we will see a more racially and culturally diverse population of elders in the twenty-first century.[8] Increasing longevity among the economically disadvantaged will increase elder poverty, and will require all of us to take a more activist approach in pushing government to respond to our growing needs.

Women make up the majority of the over-sixty-five population, and outnumber men in the over-eighty population by two to one. Therefore, the needs of older women should be central to public policy for the elderly. While poverty has been reduced in the overall elderly population to nearly the average for the population as a whole,* it continues to be higher for older women—15 percent, compared to 8 percent for men. Of older women living alone, nearly one fourth are poor. Women outlive men an average of seven years, so nearly all once-married women experience widowhood for some part of their later years. In fact, women are twice as likely as men to live alone, largely because women are almost three times as likely to lose a partner as are older men.[9] Once widowed, we are much less likely than men to remarry. Although nearly three quarters of older men over sixty-five are married, less than half of older women are.[10]

Not surprisingly, older women living alone are more likely to be poor than those living with a partner or others. The poverty rate of Hispanic women over sixty-five is 25 percent, and that of black women over sixty-five is 38 percent;[11] for women of color over eighty-five and living alone, it is 73 percent.[12] Black women now live nearly as long as white women, both reaching an average age of over seventy-five years, so the needs of the elderly must be an interracial issue. Though black women are socialized to be financially self-supporting, their earnings are the lowest of any group. Because of racism, black women often worked as laundry workers and domestics, where they were paid low wages and were not covered by Social Security. Thus, older women of color continue to have the most serious and devastating economic problems of all. While programs such as SSI have raised the income level of the lowest-income elders, they still do not pay enough to assure that all elders can live above the poverty line. It is important to keep these significant economic differences in mind when we hear pronouncements about how well older Americans today are doing. Single older women must have strong community ties and substantial family support just to maintain an adequate standard of living.

The growth in numbers of older women gives us greater political clout. We have a lot to con-

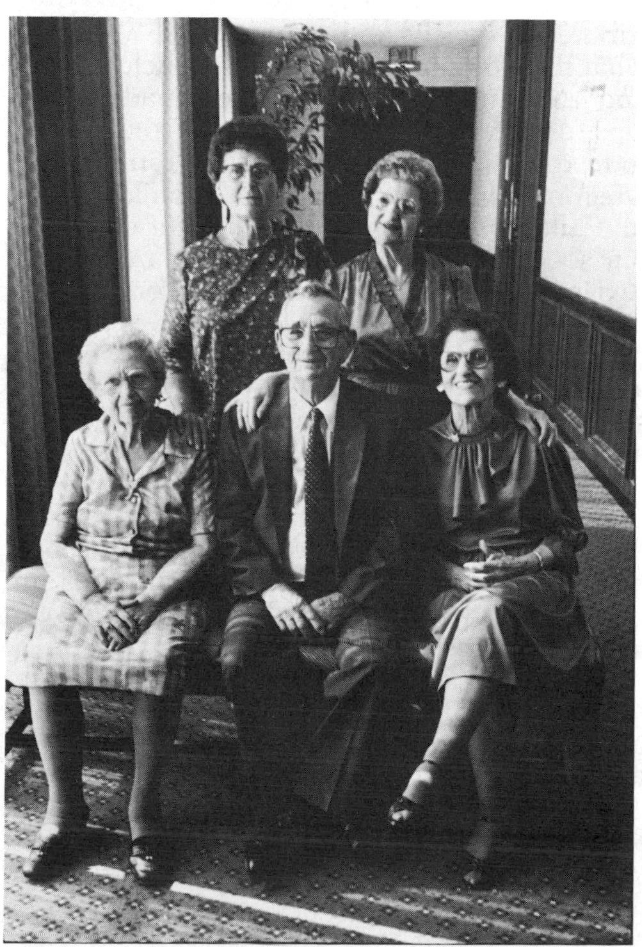

Jerry Howard/Positive Images

*An important statistical inconsistency makes it difficult for us to know just how many older people are poor. The Census Bureau applies a different poverty standard to elders than to other adult age groups on the assumption that an adult sixty-five years of age or older needs less income than an adult sixty-four or younger. Tacit acceptance of this double standard reinforces the inaccurate assumption that few older persons are poor.

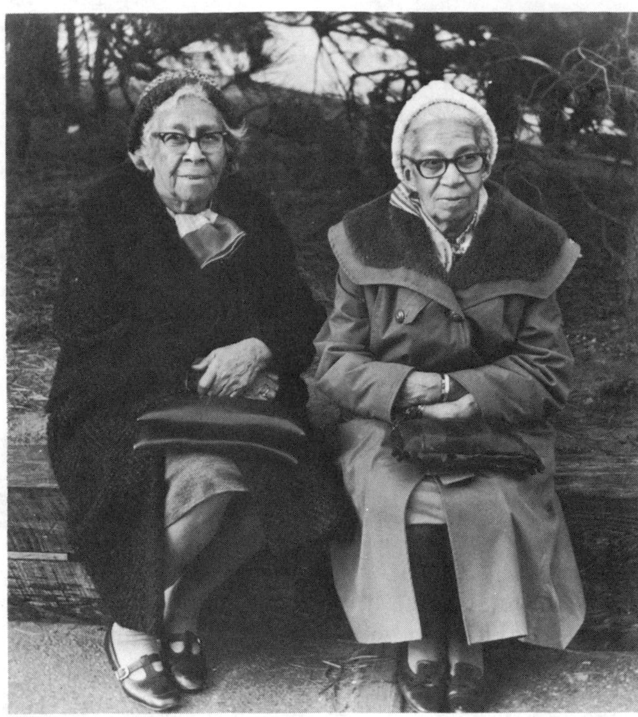

Jerry Howard/Positive Images

tribute to society and to ourselves. We know what the world felt like before the nuclear bomb and environmental deterioration made apocalypse a grim possibility. We won the vote, worked to feed families in the Depression, ran factories when men went off to war, raised children who in adulthood brought fresh winds of change to our society, and learned to confront racism and sexism. Now we are learning to confront ageism.

The supports we build for ourselves through organizing, community building, networking, and political activity can help change negative stereotypes of age, of women, of the powerless—and the negative concepts we have of ourselves. Our friendships with women can be lifelong relationships as important as family, often outlasting family ties. Being open to meeting new people and building on old and new friendships are important ways to counter the isolation that can occur as we sustain losses in our later years.

The Older Women's League, the Gray Panthers, the AARP, and other activist organizations provide plenty of opportunities on a local and on a national level to improve the status and image of older people. We can establish a safer, healthier environment for women in and through women's political organizations, in any way that opens—or resists the closing of—doors to more and better jobs, pay, education, and status for all women. We can band together, we middle-aged and older women, as allies to agitate for social change and to improve the prospects for our own not-so-distant future. In doing this work, we fight for ourselves, our mothers, our grandmothers, and the well-being of the generations of women who will grow old after us.

Notes

1. Irving Kenneth Zola, "Living at Home—The Policy Convergence of Aging and Disability." In Joan Hyde and Susan Lanspery, eds., *Staying Put: Adapting the Places Instead of the People.* Amityville, NY: Baywood Publishing. In press, 1994.
2. K. Warner Schaie and Sherry Willis, "Can Decline in Adult Intellectual Functioning Be Reversed?" *Developmental Psychology,* Vol. 22, No. 2, 1986, pp. 223–32.
3. Susan Sontag, "The Double Standard of Aging." *Saturday Review,* Vol. 95, No. 39 (Sept. 23, 1972).
4. Irving Kenneth Zola, "Policies and Programs Concerning Aging and Disability: Toward a Unified Agenda." In Sean Sullivan and Marion Ein Lewin, eds., *The Economics and Ethics of Long-Term Care and Disability.* Washington, DC: American Enterprise Institute for Public Policy Research, 1988, pp. 90–130.
5. Matilda White Riley and John W. Riley, Jr., "Longevity and Social Structure: The Added Years." *Daedalus: Journal of the American Academy of Arts and Sciences,* Winter 1986, pp. 51–75.
6. Kenneth G. Manton, Larry S. Corder, and Eric Stallard, *Journal of Gerontology,* "Estimates of Change in Chronic Disability and Institutional Incidence and Prevalence Rates in the U.S. Elderly Population from the 1982, 1984, and 1989 National Long Term Care Survey." Vol. 48, No. 4 (July 1993), pp. S153–66.
7. Personal communication, Judith E. Heumann, Worldwide Institute on Disability, Berkeley, CA.
8. Cynthia M. Taeuber and Jessie Allen, "Women in Our Aging Society: The Demographic Outlook." In Jessie Allen and Alan Pifer, eds., *Women on the Front Lines: Meeting the Challenge of an Aging America.* Washington, DC: The Urban Institute Press, 1993.
9. Robyn I. Stone, "The Feminization of Poverty Among the Elderly." *Women's Studies Quarterly,* 1989, Nos. 1 and 2, pp. 20–34.
10. Taeuber and Allen, op. cit.
11. U.S. Bureau of the Census. Current Population Reports, Series P-60, No. 174. *Money Income of Households, Families, and Persons in the United States: 1990.* U.S. Government Printing Office, 1991.
12. Karen Davis, Paula Grant, and Diana Rowland, "Alone and Poor: The Plight of Elderly Women." *Generations,* Summer 1990, Special Issue on Gender and Aging, pp. 43–47.

Aging Well

✦

1

AGING AND WELL-BEING

✦

BY MARILYN BENTOV, DORI SMITH, DIANA LASKIN SIEGAL, AND PAULA B. DORESS-WORTERS, WITH HELP FROM EVE NICHOLS

SPECIAL THANKS TO JOLEEN BACHMAN, RUTH HUBBARD, JANE JEWELL, AND FAITH NOBUKO BARCUS

SHARING TOUCH—MASSAGE BY SYLVIA PIGORS, MARILYN BENTOV, AND DIANA LASKIN SIEGAL

1994 UPDATE BY DIANA LASKIN SIEGAL

RESOURCES FOR THIS CHAPTER ON PAGES 447–50

AT MY AGE

Last summer our vegetable garden yielded small bounty: round pink tennis ball tomatoes ripening among the marigolds in an inferno of sun, captives of ninety degree days, of unwavering heat, fitful squalls of rain that released, not a drenching cool, but drops of water that glanced off tight shiny skins the way globules hiss from a sizzling fry pan.

One day I looked into the patch and there was one tomato seamed and split, a deeper fruitier juicier red inside, but with a frayed and largely open look.

I wanted to cup it into my hands and not lose a drop.

Doris Panoff

A PLAN FOR AGING WELL

Many of us want to live long lives, but fear the infirmities or disabilities that may come with advancing age. In this chapter we will emphasize that aging well is more than the absence of disease. It is a harmony of mind, body, and spirit. Each of us can take an active role in our well-being as we age—a holistic approach that involves sharing with others, reducing stress, and participating in community, among other methods.

The reason wellness is so important to me is that I have so many things I want to do, and I have to be well to do them. I don't want to live to be eighty or ninety unless I am well enough to be active. I don't want quantity of life without quality. [a fifty-seven-year-old woman]

Whether I am healthy because I can be busy and happy or whether I am busy and happy because I am healthy is a question. I can do many things that I never had time to do before. Among my activities, I play the recorder in two groups, make ceramics, take part in a book group and a financial-planning group, go to concerts, plays and lectures, garden with the help of a young man, and volunteer at a food collection center. For the good of my somewhat achy leg, I swim three or four times a week, take a yoga class, and sometimes bicycle. Life gets somewhat hectic but there's nothing I want to stop because I really enjoy the things I do very much. [a seventy-four-year-old woman]

At any age, we may have disease or disability to contend with, but we also have resiliency and recovery. We can still be as healthy and active as possible.

I am multiply disabled—legally blind, with chronic pain syndrome from head and neck injuries. I am very sold on the pain program at my local hospital. Instead of drugs (I was using narcotics), much of my pain can be relieved by

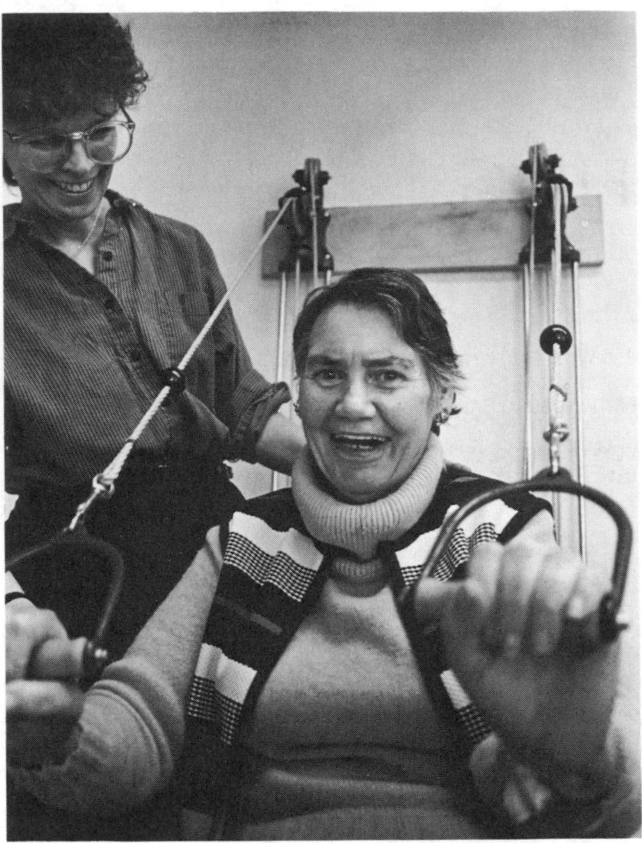

Randy Dean/VNA of San Francisco's Adult Day Health Care Center

physical therapy, particularly the aerobic treadmill, jogging, and the stationary-bicycle program. Every day, in addition to the aerobics, I do forty-five minutes or so of muscle stretching and isometrics, push-ups, sit-ups, etc. I am taught that these changes I am making in my lifestyle must be permanent, daily, lifelong. [a forty-one-year-old woman]

The self-care necessary to be well begins with self-value. *Deciding* on wellness reflects and fosters that self-value. We can prolong our healthy, active years by paying attention to good nutrition, activity and movement, solitude and rest, good relationships, and our links to the communities in which we live and work.

I'd been depressed and anxious and using sleeping pills for a number of years. With the help of a friend who was a therapist, I became aware of a lot of anger I'd been holding toward my mother and father—and toward my husband. I started adopting some new habits—like taking care of myself physically. I was all out of shape—I started jogging and I took yoga to learn to relax. Feeling better physically bolstered my self-esteem and gave me the courage to confront my husband about the inequities in our relationship and to push for changes. [a woman in her fifties]

Studies show that older people who give themselves a better health rating than their physician does frequently prove, in time, the greater accuracy of their own intuitive feelings about the state of their health.[1]

The best way I know to stay healthy and alive is to stay away from pills and out of the rocking chair. [a ninety-year-old woman]

To keep involved and growing, we must recognize and fight ageism in all of its manifestations. We can deal with ageism more effectively if we have energy and strength.

I realized that in another year I'll be on the senior citizens' list for my town, because once you turn sixty you automatically get the mailings. And you know, this is silly, but my mailman is someone I know personally, and I feel it's none of his business how old I am, but he would see those mailings.

Aging Is Not Old Age

There is a difference between "aging" and "geting old." Aging encompasses all the biological changes that occur over a lifetime—for example, increase and decrease in height, onset and cessation of menstruation, and shaping of the young-adult and middle-aged body. Changes in thymic hormones are sometimes used as a sign of the aging process because the thymus gland, a pyramid-shaped gland beneath the breastbone involved in regulation of the immune system, begins to shrink slowly after the age of two.[2] The pace of biological aging differs among individuals. In all people, some organs age faster than others. The impact of genetic and environmental factors on biological aging is just beginning to be understood.

Getting old, on the other hand, is a social concept, and our feelings about it may only be slightly related to the biological processes of aging.

It is not surprising that women have such strong feelings about being identified as aging; our culture has a strong prejudice against older women. Traditional cultures often hold their elders in high regard, seeing them as storehouses of wisdom to be transmitted to the next generation; older women, especially, are often seen as healers. The Pueblo Indians, for example, believe their elders' rituals help the sun to rise each morning. Imagine how it would feel to believe oneself so vital to life itself!

For as long as I can remember, I've cherished an image of my future self as a "wise old woman." I can see myself now—my silver hair provides softness around my face. I live in a log cabin by a stream, and my fireplace walls are decorated with well-used iron skillets and copper pots. I'm preparing to receive young guests who come regularly to visit me. I find my fulfillment in teaching them the wisdom gained over my lifetime. This image has sustained me through many dark hours in which I feared I would never make a contribution to life. [a forty-three-year-old woman]

It is especially important to distinguish physiological aging from the capacity for intellectual growth and social participation. Even very ill or frail old people can continue to learn and to be socially involved. If aging well is our goal, it is important to view health as the World Health Organization defined it in 1946: "A state of complete physical, mental, and social well-being, not just the absence of disease or infirmity."[3] Continued engagement and productivity is the best way of delaying the onset of frailty in the older years. Robert Butler argues that "health and productivity are interacting conditions: the unproductive human is at higher risk of illness and economic dependency and the sick person is limited in productivity and is, therefore, at higher risk of dependency."[4]

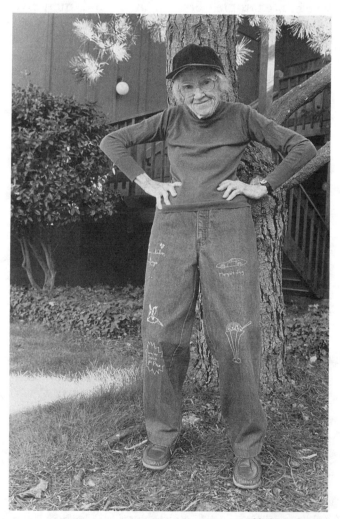

Marianne Gontarz

Scientists have learned a great deal about senescence, the biological changes that occur in different cells and tissues over time, but they still have fundamental questions about how and why these changes come about. Some think that aging is controlled by a genetically programmed "biological clock," but others think that aging results from cumulative damage to certain systems in the body. It may be many years before we know which theory or combination of theories explains biological aging.

Research is currently exploring factors that seem associated with longevity in the hope of finding a formula for extending human life or minimizing conditions associated with aging. We must be careful to differentiate between test results in the laboratory and what happens in our own bodies. For example, rats and mice placed on a diet containing 30 to 50 percent fewer calories than the normal diet for caged laboratory rodents but containing essential vitamins and minerals live longer than control animals.[5] But studies of the relationship between longevity and weight in humans have produced conflicting results.[6]

Commercial manufacturers sometimes take advantage of highly publicized laboratory results to promote products that have no proven value. Superoxide dismutase (SOD) supplements sold in stores are a good example of this. Research has discovered that SOD, an enzyme involved in the repair of cellular damage, is found at higher levels in animals with long life spans than in those with shorter ones. Advertisements touted SOD as an antiaging drug, but in fact, SOD is broken down during digestion and cannot be reassembled in the body.[7] Thus, these diet supplements have no effect on human longevity and are a waste of money.

Laboratory studies of the effects of vitamin and mineral supplements on the aging process also must be evaluated carefully. The possible anticancer action of vitamins E, C, and beta carotene, and the antiaging actions of the mineral selenium deserve further investigation, but the evidence does not support the contention that these supplements extend life.[8]

It is unlikely that researchers will find a single intervention to stop aging. Indeed, any promise of extraordinary benefit probably indicates something of which the buyer should beware. In the future, scientific advances in many areas may delay specific aging processes, such as the decline in immune function, but until then, caution should be used in assessing claims for the life-extending or rejuvenating properties of any antiaging agents or regimens.[9]

The term *life expectancy* refers to the average number of years of life expected for an individual in a given population. *Life span* is the maximum number of years of life possible for a species. Researchers involved in efforts to increase understanding of the aging process have found ways to increase both the life expectancy and the life spans of experimental animals.[10]

The average life expectancy in developed countries has increased steadily during the past two hundred years as a result of improvements in housing, nutrition, health care, and sanitation. In the United States today, the average life expectancy at birth is seventy-nine years for a girl; for a boy it is seventy-two years. More people are living to an old age than in past centuries, but the human life span has remained fixed at about 115 years for all of recorded history.

Although the prospect that the life span might be increased is exciting, we believe that the present focus of aging research should be to improve the quality of life for all members of society. The ways to do this are by perfecting techniques for the prevention and treatment of disease (including illnesses previously thought to be unavoidable signs of aging) and by changing the view that old age is a sure predictor of declining function.

Women and Research

The major problem with most clinical studies on aging is that until recently very few of them have involved women. For example, the Baltimore Longitudinal Study of Aging, which began in 1958, did not admit women volunteers until 1978. This omission was due to the traditional tendency to view males as the norm for the species. Processes that occur only in women have generally attracted less interest than male-related processes. In addition, studies focusing on one gender are less expensive, recruitment of subjects is easier, and data analysis is less complex.

Women are increasingly included in research and drug trials, but there are still not enough older people, women and men, included. Trials for drugs to treat arthritis, for example, rarely include people of the ages most likely to be using them. Recognizing that four fifths of persons over age seventy-five living at home disabled by physical frailty are women, the National Institute on Aging did start the Women's Aging Study in 1991 to assess the conditions and diseases responsible for frailty.[11] In 1995 look for results that, for the first time, will include minority women. We must continue to monitor proposed research both for its attention to older women's priorities and for inclusion of women from diverse groups.

Health statistics indicate that life expectancy at birth is greater for women than for men in most parts of the world, but that the length of time varies significantly depending on the country. For example, both women and men live longer in Sweden than they do in the United States, but the longevity gap between the genders is much smaller in Sweden. Research designed to help us understand the reasons for these differences could help improve the quality of life for all people.

Changing Health Habits

Science is developing information about the aging process that strongly suggests that our health choices—positive or negative—greatly affect how we age. Growing old well—maintaining, even improving, physical and emotional health—is something over which today's women in midlife and beyond have more control than ever before.

There are no magic wands or potions for good health, no fountains of youth, no products that cure all ills, no vitamins that prevent all ailments. A wellness program requires effort, planning, and persistence, but it is an investment that pays back with unbelievably high interest. When we feel good we are more likely to exercise, eat well, and take care of ourselves, all of which in turn are likely to make us feel better. Thus we create a "virtuous cycle."

Habits are like the backbones of our lives—the firm structures upon which we can rely. It helps not to have to think about every step we take—to have comfortable routines in our lives.

But as we grow older, some habits may no longer serve us well. The morning mad rush routine that helped us get ourselves and a whole family off to school and work may no longer be necessary. We may be happier and calmer with fifteen minutes of quiet meditation before starting our day. Illness may require us to change from a vigorous exercise program to a more gentle one. Or we may be inspired by new information or changes in our lives to pay better attention to ourselves, to pursue renewed health and vitality by dramatically altering our pattern of health habits.

It is not true that as we grow older, we become less flexible, less able to change. Change and renewal are possible at any age.

In my later years, my concept of time has changed, as has my use of it. In my late sixties, I was pleased that I was active and showed no sign of slowing down. I thought that slowing down was something to be avoided; it would show that I was getting old. While I had never aspired to fourteen-thousand-foot mountains, I had hiked up medium-sized peaks. Then in my seventies I went with the Appalachian Mountain Club on a week's camping and hiking trip. That summer, I found I was going up more modest elevations and enjoying them and my companions on the way thoroughly. As I left to come back to civilization, I heard a voice (and it was very distinct) saying, "Today you can stop running and start walking."

So I began to go slower. Because I have considerable vitality, I am far from stopping. In fact, I sometimes still rush but the overall result has been freeing, there's less reason to have to redo or undo mistakes caused by dashing. As I go slower, I am more aware of my companions. I can look at situations with greater calm. I am becoming more interested in the quality of time rather than the quantity of it. [a woman in her seventies]

Learning Kung Fu [a martial art] has really made a dramatic change in my life. During the two months I was away from home learning it, my life-style was markedly different—I ate only fresh fruits, vegetables, and grains—no sugar, dairy products, or meat. I was walking nearly ten miles a day and spending one to two hours a day on Kung Fu. The extra pounds fell away, my body became

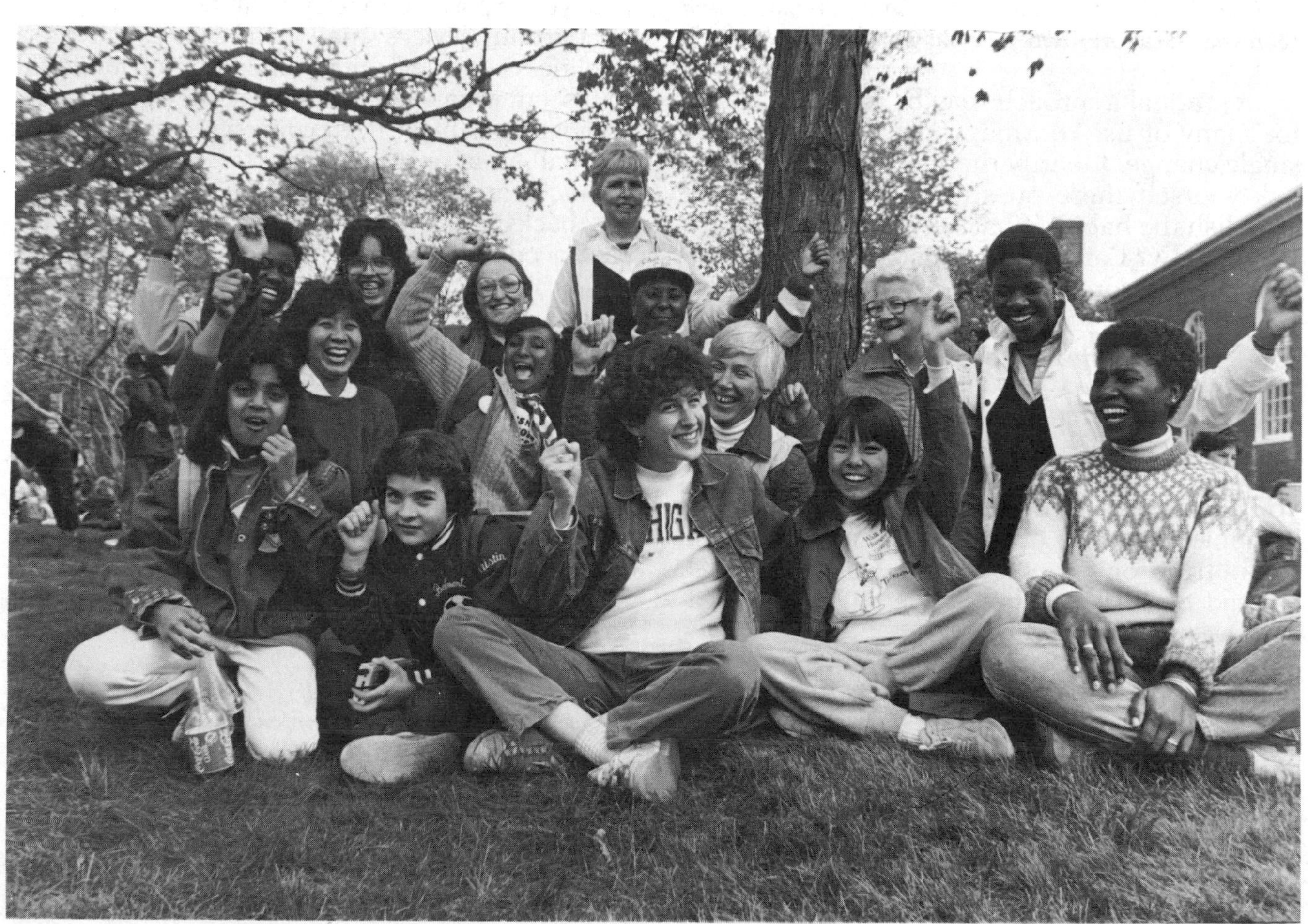

Gaye Hilsenrath with Julie Durlester

lithe, and my overall health was the best of my life. Now I can easily recognize problems immediately if I neglect my diet or cut back on my walking. When I stay very physically active and eat right, I always feel happy, ambitious, and have lots of energy. [a fifty-year-old woman]

A "clean slate" approach may be your style of change, and can be very helpful when you're ready.

I got in the habit, over a number of years, of "needing" a variety of legal drugs: coffee, six to eight cups a day, to keep my spirits up; alcohol before bedtime to calm me down; a couple of aspirin to make sure I didn't wake up with a headache; then in the morning I really needed that coffee to get going. Eventually, I was exhausted all the time and prone to illnesses. My doctor suggested that all these bad habits supported each other, and she was right. I was able to quit after some good introspection about getting my real needs met. I went on a one-week "cleansing fast" of fruit juices and spring water. I rested, walked, and watched clouds. Two months later, I had dropped all my unhealthful habits and I began to know what my own energy feels like—and I like it! It feels great to depend on myself, not on all those stimulants and depressants.* [a forty-two-year-old woman]

A gradual approach may be more successful for many of us. You may want to begin with a single change. Identify the roots of the problem. Ask yourself these questions: When did I first establish the habit? What need did it serve then? Does it now? Can other habits provide more satisfaction? Become aware of your *real* needs—for example, when you reach for a cigarette or coffee, you may be looking for a relaxing break or sociability. Fulfill them directly and in healthier ways.

Make changes in small, manageable steps. Many habits interact, so changing one may help you change others that are harder to break. For example, if you are trying to quit smoking, drink milk, fruit or vegetable juice, or herbal tea instead of coffee to break the coffee-and-cigarette association.

No matter which approach you choose, take on changing a habit when you feel strong and have no other major issues pressing on you. But watch out for procrastination. When you feel overwhelmed, call a friend, change environments if possible, or vary your activity. Get support from others to help you in your new behavior. Form a partnership with a friend to support each other's new habits.

I spent a vacation at a lake with my college roommate swimming, canoeing, and eating the macrobiotic style of food combinations and preparation which she has studied. I knew I didn't want to change my meals so drastically but enjoyed sampling her cooking. I also realized I felt better with more activity. A year later I am still following the changes I made. I am walking more, eating more whole grains and less fat in my meals than before the visit. [a fifty-four-year-old woman]

If your budget allows, find a supportive retreat or spa, and change attitudes, diet, and exercise all at once. These are more common in Europe, where they are less expensive. The best ones take into consideration all aspects of health—physical, emotional, and spiritual—to help you experience a deep change.

Certain devices may help you, such as a "wellness contract" with yourself or a friend that spells out what you want to achieve, and how you plan to achieve it. Keeping a record such as a journal or a progress report may help. Note obstacles and triumphs, but don't blame yourself for backsliding. Instead, reward yourself for each accomplishment.

As we become older, it is vital not only to break harmful habits but to develop new activities and establish new habits of living.

Mental-health researchers recommend that elders "flex their mental as well as physical muscles for better health" and offer suggestions such as working crossword puzzles or playing word games for inductive reasoning, or doing woodworking, assembling objects, reading maps, or doing needlework for spatial orientation. Most important is to do something you really like and are interested in.[12]

At sixty, I used to say to myself, "Whatever you were supposed to do in this world you've already done. There's nothing more." But at sixty-eight I discovered drawing and a whole new world opened up. [a seventy-five-year-old woman]

Flexibility ranks high with me as an important quality to cultivate throughout the life span. I feel that there are three characteristics important to flexible personality: the

*Some holistic health practitioners believe that fasting—going without food and taking only water and juices for a very brief time—is helpful in making the transition to a natural diet. See, for example, Dori Smith, "Guidelines for a Cleansing Fast" in Shepard Bliss, ed., *The New Holistic Health Handbook*. New York: Viking Penguin, 1985, pp. 144–45. Get guidance from a health practitioner, especially if you are older or have physical problems.

ENJOYING LIFE WITH LESS ENERGY

by Paula B. Doress-Worters, Lois Harris, Jane Hyman, and Dori Smith. Special thanks to Lucy Mitchell, Beth Rosenbaum, and Elsie Reethof.

Finding ourselves with physical limitations can bring frustration, sadness, and a strong sense of loss. We miss the things we are no longer able to do.

If you have anything wrong with you it makes all the difference in the world. Six years ago I was trying out lots of new things and the world was more or less my oyster. I had fun with music, I had fun with painting, and I was having fun with poetry. Anything seemed possible to me. Then I got rheumatoid arthritis, and I got it badly. I had three major operations in five months, and two new shoulders and one new knee. And at age seventy-three, three major operations take a lot of getting over. I still have the disease and feel lousy a great deal of the time. I don't quite feel that the world is my oyster anymore. [a seventy-nine-year-old woman]

We resent health problems when they are painful, make us feel weak and tired, and restrict our movements and our lives. We get angry with our bodies because we want to do everything the way we used to and we can't.

When joints ache, I calculate each step. I don't automatically get up to get a drink of water, or to put something away . . . I wait and take these steps in conjunction with some other necessary steps. I don't do things on the spur of the moment anymore. . . . Will our eyesight grow worse? Will we become increasingly hard of hearing? Will the arthritis be harder to control? and so on. . . . It makes no sense to let our thoughts wander in this direction, but inevitably they do. [a woman in her late eighties][1]

We have to deal with many losses.

I've had to give up many favorite activities—walks on the beach, sewing, reading. Now my eyesight is so bad that I decided to give up driving and use the senior van service. I found the inner resources to enjoy life in spite of each loss so I'll cope with this one also. [an eighty-nine-year-old woman who prefers to live alone]

Usually, the first change we make is to reorganize our environment as much as possible to accommodate our conditions. Basically, this means keeping all regularly used objects in the same place and within easy reach, and finding new ways to accomplish daily chores.

I always put my glasses and keys on a very attractive plate that I keep in the center of my apartment so I'm not always hunting for them. This is a way I conserve my energy. [an eighty-two-year-old woman]

Learn about ways you can adapt your environment to make the most of your abilities and reduce the impact of physical changes (see Housing Alternatives and Living Arrangements chapter, page 163). The disability rights movement is redefining the term *disability* as an improper fit between a person and an environment rather than a fault of the person.[2] In other words, if you can no longer get out of a chair by yourself, you get a chair that helps you get up. Social-service agencies and medical-supply companies have catalogs with helpful gadgets and appliances.

Support from others becomes a necessity. We may need the help of friends and family as everyday activities we took for granted—fixing a meal, doing the laundry, shopping—become difficult. We also need moral support. We want others to believe in us, that we can do it, that we can fight weaknesses. We need to believe it too.

The mind is terribly important. If I really believed I was ninety, I would think I couldn't do anything. But I'm still interested in many things and can make people happy. [a woman who maintains a high level of involvement living in a continuing-care community]

For most women, energy eventually becomes an issue, whether they have health problems or not. If, through most of our sixties and seventies, we have been "the marvelous old woman" whose vitality everyone admired, we may feel we are letting people

(continued)

Enjoying Life with Less Energy

(continued)

down as well as letting go of a valued image of ourselves.

I have reached a stage in my life that I had not given much thought to. Somehow I had thought that I would continue as active as I had been in the past. This is not so. I am now eighty-one and I think something is happening to me that may happen at an earlier or a later age for many women. It's a new stage—one that can be looked upon as negative, or it can be looked at simply as a continuation of the life span. [a woman in her eighties]

The first step in self-help is what many women with illnesses and disabilities had to learn earlier in life—to stop blaming themselves for limited energy and to plan realistically for it. If you have been very active on a professional or volunteer basis it may be necessary to reassess your activities and cut out those that tax your strength too much or are no longer personally rewarding.

After I retired, I was often asked to serve on committees. After a while, I learned to refuse to be a token old person on a committee and accepted only those appointments which seemed to value what I uniquely had to offer. I do not feel that I can continue attending as many meetings as I have in the past. There are other aspects in my life now to which I need to give more time and attention. [an eighty-two-year-old woman]

Look at your assumptions about what you *have* to do, and see how much isn't essential. You will feel better if you can pare down obligations while keeping up the pleasurable part of your commitments.

Everything I do takes so much longer—just getting dressed—I have to choose how to spend my time. I choose not to cook anymore because my back won't take it; all our family celebrations are now in my children's homes. My grandchildren have to accept that when they visit me they won't get chicken soup and potato pancakes anymore. [a seventy-nine-year-old woman]

When I think about packing and moving I feel overwhelmed. I can't do at seventy-eight what I could do at seventy-two. For the first time I am considering letting my son help me or paying the movers to do the packing.

Think of energy-conserving ways in which you can handle your needs.

The grocery store is about fifteen or twenty minutes away. I wouldn't think of going out to shop without my cart. I am experimenting with taking along a small folding chair and a book, so I'll sit down and rest when I get tired and also have a chance to read something. [an eighty-one-year-old woman]

Regular physical activity and exercise help improve energy and increase stamina and endurance, but don't assume that you have to continue your leisure activities at the same pace, or give them up entirely. Try walking, gardening, swimming, and exercising at a slower pace, or for shorter periods of time. Women often find they enjoy these activities more when they ignore any feelings of haste or need for achievement.

Thinking, meditating, watching, and listening are as worthwhile as more strenuous activities. In our younger years, we were often too busy and rushed for reflection. Now that we cannot rush, we can turn to these quieter pursuits if we wish.

I wonder if sometimes we who are concerned about stereotypes don't fall into the trap of using one ourselves, and that is talking about "getting out of the rocking chair" and looking askance at a person sitting in one. I don't know what we can do about the impression that when you sit in a rocking chair, you are really not "doing" anything. I want to save time for meditation, reflection, and just some plain ordinary thinking. In protecting our free time, we will be free to use it, not to think we have to be physically active. I hope that we can reinstitute a rocking chair as a valuable complement to our other activities. [an eighty-one-year-old woman]

Life Review

Reflecting on the past is a natural process that helps us to gain perspective on our lives and to count our contributions and our blessings. We can also look at our mistakes and disappointments, but it is vital to do this in a positive framework, letting go of guilt or sense of loss. We can arrive at a conviction of the utter rightness of our lives.[3]

I've had a wonderful life. Tell me, what could I have changed? There's nothing I could have made any different. Everything was the way it had to be. [a ninety-eight-year-old woman]

This is the time of life to write about your life's journeys, share experiences with others, and do the work of integrating past, present, and future. Your children or other loved ones will appreciate the legacy of your autobiography. Writing it—or tape-recording it—can motivate you to reflect on your life, and on the events you've witnessed or taken part in. Be sure to include rich detail to bring the picture to life—what you wore, what the furniture looked like, the sounds and smells. This can be a way of maintaining links between generations, needed so much in our life today.

One custom worth adapting for the twentieth century is the "ethical will." In medieval times, parents wrote extensive letters to their children and grandchildren advising them on the morals and values that had given meaning to their own lives.[4] You may wish to look back on your life, and write about the most important thing about you that you'd like your friends and family to remember after you're gone. What about you has made a difference in the world?[5] What are you most satisfied and proud of?

You can also relive the high points of your life. Think back to a peak experience—a time when you were in love, or viewing a beautiful sunset, or had a creative insight. Relive that experience. Then ask yourself, what are the essential qualities of that experience? How can you give that to yourself in your life *now?*[6]

There are many ways to reflect on your experiences. One is called the "Steppingstones" process.[7] In it, you review your life and identify specific events that stand out as signposts. Reflect and write about each one, using these words: "It was a time when . . ." If you read what you've written out loud in a group of friends or write letters to family members, you may find added significance. Courses in autobiography or life review are sometimes offered in senior centers or adult-education programs. If you can't find one, get together with your friends and create your own.

CRAFTSWOMAN

See, she threads with bleeding feelings
The jagged shards of her shattered past.

From that which was tragedy
Or at best, a grim joke

Will she, can she weave
A design of grace?

Gittel Simon[8]

1. Janet Neuman, "Old Age: It's Not Funny." *Perspective on Aging,* November/December 1982, published by the National Council on Aging.
2. Irving Kenneth Zola, "The Medicalization of Aging and Disability: Problems and Prospects," in C. W. Mahoney, C. L. Estes, and J. E. Heumann, eds., *Toward a Unified Agenda: Proceedings of a National Conference on Disability and Aging.* San Francisco: Institute for Health and Aging, University of California, 1986.
3. Based on Erik Erikson's theory of adult development, in Erik H. Erikson, "Eight Ages of Man." *Childhood in Society,* New York: W. W. Norton & Co., 1963, pp. 268–69.
4. "Ethical Wills: Twelfth and Fourteenth Centuries," in Jacob R. Marcus, ed., *The Jew in the Medieval World,* New York: Atheneum, 1974, pp. 311–16.
5. Adapted from Janette Rainwater, *You're in Charge: A Guide to Becoming Your Own Therapist.* Marina del Rey, CA: De Vorss and Co., 1985, p. 203.
6. Ibid., p. 44.
7. Ira Progoff, *At a Journal Workshop.* New York: Dialogue House Library, 1975, pp. 119–30.
8. In *Late Harvest: Poems from Lifetime Learning of Newton.* The Coalition for Newton Community Education, Inc., of Newton Community Schools, 360 Lowell Ave., Newton, MA 02160, 1982.

first is capacity for learning and interest in pursuing it; the second is imagination; the third is a realistic working philosophy of life. Since I have turned eighty I have had to slow down physically so I have developed new interests and taken more time for old ones. I write more poetry. I reread more books and seek out new ones. I have seen a therapist for the first time in my life to help me through some temporary difficulties. I tried massage and liked it. I plan to keep on growing. [an eighty-two-year-old woman]

Disarming Stress

Old Age Must Be Like This

Alone and sick at three in the morning
She relives each mistake
wonders if there's enough money in the bank
But it's her life that's overdue
She's made too many plans
Who did she think she was
in those hectic days of health—
magic legs moving from sink to stove
from barn to the woodpile
—and the telephone lifting itself so easily
off the hook
the throat making all those intricate movements
in order to speak
Now simple tasks
laundry
dinner
fetching the mail—
can't be done
Dishes pile up in the sink
wood stays in the barn
She turns the electric blanket higher
wonders who will feed her birds—

*Marilyn Zuckerman**

How we manage the stress in our lives is an important component of whatever disease-prevention and health-promotion regimen we undertake. In a dangerous situation, our bodies go "on alert," ready to take immediate action—to fight the threat, or to run away. This is called the "stress response" and is normal and evolutionarily significant in humans as in other animals. However, in modern society the threats we experience are not often direct physical dangers, but are more generalized and ongoing, such as the pressures of a job, or the lack of one, sex and age discrimination, losses of relationships, and global dangers. The threat of nuclear war has diminished but the threat of the depletion of the ozone layer and of global warming has increased. Sometimes, stress occurs when we feel emotionally threatened—such as when we perceive a neutral event or situation as threatening, or exaggerate a danger in our minds. There is a profound connection between thoughts, feelings, behavior, and what happens inside our bodies.

*Marilyn Zuckerman, *Poems of the Sixth Decade,* 1993. Garden Street Press, P.O. Box 380055, Cambridge, MA 02238.

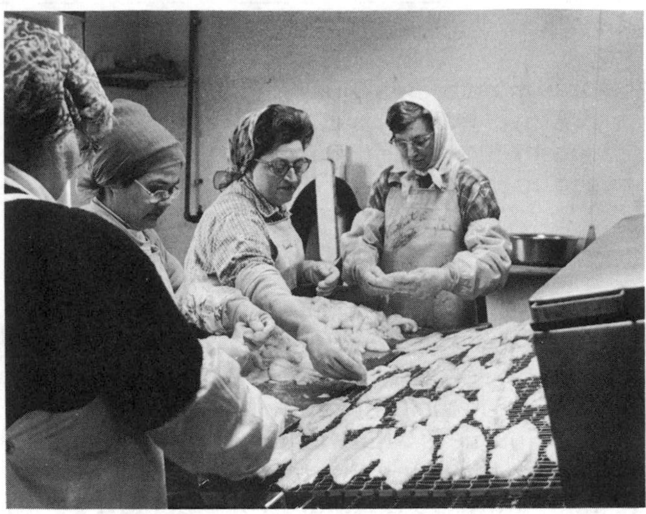

Cathy Cade

Stress can become a problem when it is continuous or ongoing, because the body does not return to its normal, nonaroused state. Chronic triggering of the fight-or-flight response has been shown to lead to many health problems, including hypertension,[13] elevated sugar levels, weakened immune system,[14] an overworked endocrine system, and possibly brain-cell loss.[15] By adopting new habits to reduce stress and reverse its harmful effects, we can prevent the damage that can result from continual or chronic exposure.

Signs of Stress

How can you tell that you are under stress? Our bodies usually send us warning signals, but we may ignore them or cover them up with pills or minimize their importance. Sometimes we are not even aware that we are under stress.

The first time I realized that feelings affect my health was during a routine physical exam. I was worrying, just a lit-

tle, about a decision I'd made. But my blood pressure was up—so much higher than usual that I knew I was anxious, terribly so, more than I wanted to believe. [a fifty-six-year-old woman]

Signs of stress that we all experience include muscle tightening, clenching, shallow breathing, headaches, and digestive disturbances. We may feel driven to compulsive behavior such as excessive eating, drinking, smoking, or talking. We may turn to alcohol, drugs, caffeine, or tranquilizers. Depression, difficulty in sleeping, sleeping too much, lack of concentration, or irritability—even getting a fair number of irritable responses from other people—are all signs that we are not handling stress effectively.

Special Stresses of Middle-aged and Older Women

As middle-aged and older women, we face special stresses caused by sexism and ageism. We women face sexism throughout our lives. But we face ageism earlier than men do, sometimes even before forty, because of the double standard of aging. This compounding of ageism and sexism brings with it added stresses. Each experience of prejudice—each rebuff, dismissal, act of condescension—is new and painful. Poverty and inadequate funds deepen all other stresses and contribute to a feeling of despair. All this has the effect of chipping away at our self-esteem. Growing older in a society that has few respected roles for elders can bring a multiplicity of stressful experiences.

Caregiving is a role that frequently falls to women in the midlife and older years and can be extremely exhausting, isolating, and stressful. Bereavement, one of life's most painful experiences, occurs most often in the second half of life. Sometimes we face a series of losses in quick succession.

It seems like everything happened at once. I had to put my mother in a nursing home, where she suddenly died. I didn't have time to grieve, because I had to work for weeks to settle her affairs. About then, my seventeen-year-old daughter was preparing to leave home. I now had the freedom to move where I wanted to but I had a hard time leaving my home. What could I let go of? Every little thing had meaning for me. I had to go slow in packing—I kept injuring myself and my skin kept breaking out. I'm still grieving, months later. Healing from my mother's death will take a long time. [a forty-nine-year-old woman]

Life Events Rated for Stressfulness[16]	**Stress Rating***
Death of a spouse	100
Divorce	73
Death of a close family member	63
Personal injury or illness	53
Marriage	50
Retirement	45
Change in financial status	38
Death of a close friend	37
Children leaving home	29
Beginning or finishing school	26
Christmas	12

*Participants were asked to rate each life event on a scale of 0 to 100, where marriage was rated 50.

In the above scale, among the life events ranked most stressful are those that are frequently faced by middle-aged and older women, sometimes in close succession. Women feel stressed about what happens to them and what is happening to their loved ones. Poor health and accumulated daily hassles and frustrations also contribute to women's stress levels.[17]

As older women, our lifelong socialization as nurturers can contribute to our feeling stressed. When we allow ourselves to be too generous to others with our time and energy, we risk overextending ourselves with too many commitments, some of which are neither vital nor beneficial. Thus we may damage our own well-being.

We are taught from early childhood to control our aggressiveness and suppress our anger. In fact, most of us don't even admit having aggressive feelings. Behind the mask of "being nice" often lurk anger, lack of self-esteem, and a frustrated sense of entitlement. When we repeatedly suppress our negative feelings out of fear or concern for others, we turn our accumulated anger and frustration against ourselves, and the chronic stress can damage our health.

I tried meditation, but my suppressed rage was so intense that nothing seemed to alleviate my health problems. When I was forty-seven, I finally woke up to the fact that I had been a doormat. I read that Tae Kwon Do [a Korean martial art] was good for assertiveness training for submissive women. To my surprise, yelling, hitting, and kicking at an imaginary opponent for an hour did wonders for my mind and body. My stress-related health problems began to disappear one by one. Today, at age fifty-nine, I have no pills in my medicine cabinet.

Learning to use our anger in appropriate and constructive ways helps us preserve ourselves, prevent stress, and make needed changes. Organizing to change society's laws and attitudes as

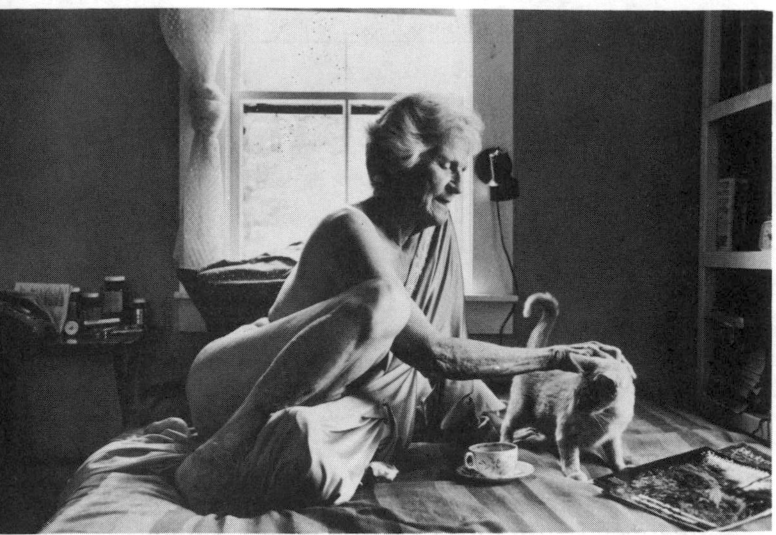
Norma Holt

well as making use of organizational resources can help us counteract the stress that comes from feeling powerless and anxious.

Most of the time we react automatically to stressors with feelings, words, thoughts, behaviors, and attitudes that we learned a long time ago—things that worsen the stress. An important part of coping with stress is learning to become less automatic in our responses. "Rule No. 1 is, don't sweat the small stuff. Rule No. 2 is, it's all small stuff. And if you can't fight and you can't flee, flow."[18] Some people find that sharpening their conscious awareness of stress and how it affects them helps them interrupt harmful patterns and adopt more constructive ways of coping. You can learn about your patterns through keeping a journal, talking with your friends, or seeing a psychotherapist. You can achieve a sense of *real* control by understanding what makes you tense, knowing what you can and cannot do to change or avoid these things, and knowing you can discharge the tension in various short-term and long-term ways.

- Paying attention to yourself, your desires, aspirations, and needs is a first step toward identifying who or what might be causing stress.
- Elicit the help of the people around you. Develop, cherish, and nurture friendships. Take care to maintain multiple friendships and roles. These can be a buffer when one relationship or role is in conflict. In times of stress, friendships are especially important.
- When the cause of your stress is too big and powerful to tackle alone, you can join together with friends, coworkers, neighbors, and others to work for change in movements and organizations.
- Laughter actually has stress-reducing effects on the body. Read funny stories and watch comedies on TV.[19]
- Catch yourself when you notice you are dwelling on negative thoughts without working toward problem solving. Concentrate on your strengths and accomplishments.
- In many situations, you can clearly express your dissatisfaction and work out a mutually satisfactory solution. For example, people respond better to "I" statements than to "you" statements. Don't say, "*You* are giving me a headache with that darn radio." Instead, say, "*I* can't think when the radio is so loud."[20] The idea is to clearly express your own discomfort and to avoid blaming anyone for it. Thus you enlist cooperation in solving a problem. Blaming passes your stress on to others—and it may bounce back.
- Scientists have proved what pet lovers already know—pets can be very beneficial to human health. Pets give and receive affection and touch.
- Eating well, especially foods that are high in vitamin B complex and vitamin C, can help you manage stress better. Avoid beverages containing caffeine (coffee, chocolate, tea, and carbonated soft drinks) because too much caffeine can cause nervousness, irritability, and problems with digestion and sleep.
- Getting enough sleep is very important. Many people report needing less sleep as they age, so if this is true for you, allow time for rest and quiet instead. Don't try to solve problems at night or when you are tired.
- Exercise helps reduce the effects of stress by bringing blood to the muscles and brain, and by stimulating production of chemicals called endorphins and enkephalins that give you a sense of well-being. Any expressive body movement can help make creative use of the pain of anger, fear, grief, or depression. Try dancing to a favorite record and using rhythm and strong movement to say what you feel. Any prolonged regular movement will loosen you up, such as a fast walk, a long swim, jumping rope, or simply stretching hard while doing rhythmic breathing.
- Have fun. Develop hobbies that you enjoy. Gardening, photography, amateur theater, and pottery all provide many hours of pleasure. Take advantage of adult-education programs,

in which you can learn and meet people at the same time.

I draw and paint. It gives me a sense of accomplishment. When you are all alone and living on a fixed income like I am, you have to find things to keep you occupied without spending a lot of money. I go to public auctions, local fairs, museums, or I window shop. I also like to keep my mind stimulated and work crossword puzzles and read novels, mysteries, and history. I watch basketball games on TV. I do sitting-in-the-chair exercises while watching TV. [a sixty-three-year-old woman]

The Relaxation Response

The Relaxation Response[21] is a simple meditation technique that synthesizes Eastern teachings with Western knowledge. The basic components are:

- A quiet environment and uninterrupted time
- A sound, word, or short phrase of your own choosing repeated silently. The word *one* is suggested—or a word from a prayer or meditation that is consistent with your culture or belief system.[22]
- A receptive attitude (the most important element). Clear your mind and visualize nothing. Keep your palms up as if you were open to whatever would happen.

Follow these simple steps:

1. Sit or kneel quietly in a comfortable position.
2. Close your eyes.
3. Deeply relax all your muscles, beginning with your feet and progressing up to your face. Keep them relaxed.
4. Breathe through the nose. Become aware of your breathing. As you breathe out, silently say the word or phrase you have selected. Breathe slowly and naturally.
5. Continue for ten to twenty minutes. When you finish, sit quietly for several minutes with your eyes closed and then for a few more with them open. (It is better to open your eyes when you feel the need to check the time than to use an alarm.)
6. Do not worry about whether you are successful in achieving a deep level of relaxation. *Permit relaxation to occur at its own pace.* If distracting thoughts occur, acknowledge them and let them go. Return to repeating your word or phrase.

Practice the technique once or twice daily, but not within two hours after any meal. Once you are comfortable with it, you can utilize the technique in a waiting room, in an empty classroom, or almost any place you wish. You will feel quiet inside, mentally clear, alert, and in charge.

A second relaxation method is Progressive Relaxation:[23]

1. Lie comfortably on your back in a quiet place. Allow yourself to relax.
2. Begin by taking a few deep breaths and then relaxing into your natural breathing rhythm.
3. Tense and release groups of muscles, one group at a time, beginning with your toes. Tense the muscles; hold for a count of five and then release. Do this same thing to each group of muscles until you reach the top of your head.
4. Notice what the tension feels like as you contract each muscle group. Focus on the experience of *letting go* of this tension as you progressively relax parts of your body. You might imagine the letting go as a warm sun that's melting your icy body, or as water flowing around whatever part of your body you're relaxing. Allow the tension to float out of your muscles as you let them go as limp as you can. You are gradually relaxing yourself into a state that is almost bodiless until you feel that you are floating in space.

Music and Imagery

Music and imagery can help you reach either a relaxed or an energized state, and can even help heal stress-related illnesses.[24] Try various kinds of music to see what states of awareness or mental pictures they encourage.

I put on Beethoven's Pastorale Symphony, lie down and imagine myself in my favorite spot—a high mountain meadow. I notice the freshness of the air, the light on the peaks. Sometimes I invite an imaginary friend. As the music progresses, I move through its moods. Birds sing as I frolic in a cool pond, then warm myself in the sun. I run through wildflowers, enjoy a glorious thunderstorm, then rest as a rainbow arches across the sky. When the music is over, I feel as refreshed as if I'd spent a week in the Rockies. [a forty-three-year-old woman]

I put on Dixieland jazz or Chopin for energy to start the day. There's a reggae [Jamaican] music program on the radio at 5:30 P.M. that freshens me when I'm tired. [a fifty-four-year-old woman]

Self-Hypnosis or Self-Talk

After you master deep breathing and relaxation, you can learn to achieve a meditative state using self-hypnosis, sometimes called *autogenesis*. With self-hypnosis you can suggest relaxation (or other desired states such as alertness or joy) to your unconscious mind, which then causes your body to respond appropriately. You can practice it in any environment—at your desk, waiting in line, or trying to fall asleep at night. To practice, sit or lie down. Loosen clothing (ties, belts); become comfortable. Allow gentle concentration. Let your day's experiences pass through and out of you. Concentrate on a sensation and suggest it to yourself. Repeat it three times and take it to each part of your body as you say it; for example, if you say, "I am at peace," imagine an area of tension and fill it with peace; peace may be a color, sensation, image, or something that conveys deep serenity to you.

To relieve a migraine, try decreasing blood flow in the head by saying to yourself, "Blood is flowing away from my head and down through my body." Concentrate on making that happen. Imagine a cool breeze going through your head; imagine the vessels dilating, expanding, and letting the blood flow rapidly.

I could not sleep because of all the noise outside. I decided that there was nothing I could do except not make it worse. If I couldn't sleep, I would rest. I just told myself things that would relax me. "I am healing. I will be better tomorrow. This rest is worth more than sleep." I relaxed each part of my body, thinking, "I am sinking into a profound state of rest that is even deeper than sleep." I told myself that if the noise stopped I might doze off for only a few minutes before being awakened again but in those few moments I would have several hours of rest and would feel refreshed. The next day I felt fine and gave one of the best classes I have ever given. [a fifty-five-year-old woman]

Prayer and Meditation

As we grow older, many of us find the spiritual aspects of our lives becoming more important. As our consciousness of our own mortality increases, we ask ourselves the meaning of our lives and of our places in the world. This can be especially true for women with physical limitations. As energy wanes and our movements are restricted, the pleasures of the mind and the spirit grow stronger. Some women continue an earlier bent for religion, philosophy, science, or literature, finding that their lives' experiences make study richer and more meaningful than ever before; some develop new interests.

Meditation and prayer can help you find spiritual strength and achieve a state of physical and emotional calm. Whether you choose meditation or prayer or a combination of the two will depend on your beliefs.

Some women find that, as they grow older, their religious beliefs and practices change. Some leave established religious groups, others renew their faith or find a new spiritual community. A growing body of literature on spirituality and its relation to well-being, healing,[25] and feminism[26] is available in libraries and bookstores.

Sharing Touch—Massage

As we get older, some of us fear that if we are not in a sexual relationship we may never be touched or held. We touch to express nonsexual tenderness and affection, to acknowledge each other's presence nonverbally, to comfort, to support, and to soothe. The misconception that touching always involves sex and is only appropriate in a sexual context causes real deprivation. People need to touch and be touched throughout their lives.

Some of us worry about touching or hugging others, especially other women, and so deny ourselves pleasure, comfort, and closeness. Some of us come from families where touching is limited to ritual holiday kisses. Intergenerational or homophobic taboos may make it hard to exchange hugs with friends or family members. But if we are able to free ourselves of these constrictions, we open ourselves to a whole array of rich experience.

Those of us who are disabled or very ill continue to need touching. Family members, friends, and staff members must recognize that patients in hospitals and residents in nursing homes need friendly touching every day. The wish for emotional intimacy and physical touching of another caring person is inseparable from other needs. Providing massage, allowing and encouraging patients to touch one another, and affectionate hugs and nonsexual touching on the part of staff members should all be part of the life of nursing-home residents. Staff members must be sensitive to individual and cultural differences in residents' acceptance of touch.

Since we never outgrow the need for warm physical touch, we may experience "skin hunger"[27] if we rarely touch or are touched. One way to meet this need is through giving and receiving massage.

Massage has had a bad reputation in the United States because of the tendency to equate pleasurable touching with genital sexual arousal and the association of massage parlors with prostitution. Yet most massage is not sexual. Massage has a respected history in both the East and West as a form of physical therapy. Massage offers many physical benefits, such as decreasing muscle tension and stiffness, lowering blood pressure, and stimulating circulation. In addition to its physical benefits, massage is one of the most pleasurable ways to relax. It is energizing yet relaxing to both the giver and the receiver.

Connecting with each other through caring touch is deeply affirming and fun. We can form "touch partnerships" with one or more friends and exchange massages regularly.

I enjoy sensuality. I gathered a group of women with whom I could do massage. Our group members would call each other up and exchange massages—twenty minutes each. We took lessons and learned techniques. We became fast friends. [a sixty-five-year-old woman]

Giving and receiving warmth and caring is healthy and imparts a sense of being connected with your own body. The message given by caring massage is, "I care about you just as you are."

Massage makes me feel re-created; it's so pleasant. When I look in the mirror, I'm lean and gaunt-looking, but I don't feel like that when I'm being massaged. [a seventy-seven-year-old woman]

It is also possible to use similar techniques to massage yourself, communicating your caring for your own body.

Keep conversation to a minimum during the massage. Silence deepens the experience, allowing both giver and receiver to pay more attention to what's happening. It is important for the person receiving massage to give feedback on what feels good and what doesn't. Often the clearest feedback comes without words in a sigh of relaxation or in a slight contraction against pressure that's too hard or too sudden.

Before starting a massage, be sure to ask about injured areas to be avoided. Do not massage varicose veins, a blood clot, or areas that are swollen, inflamed, or tender.

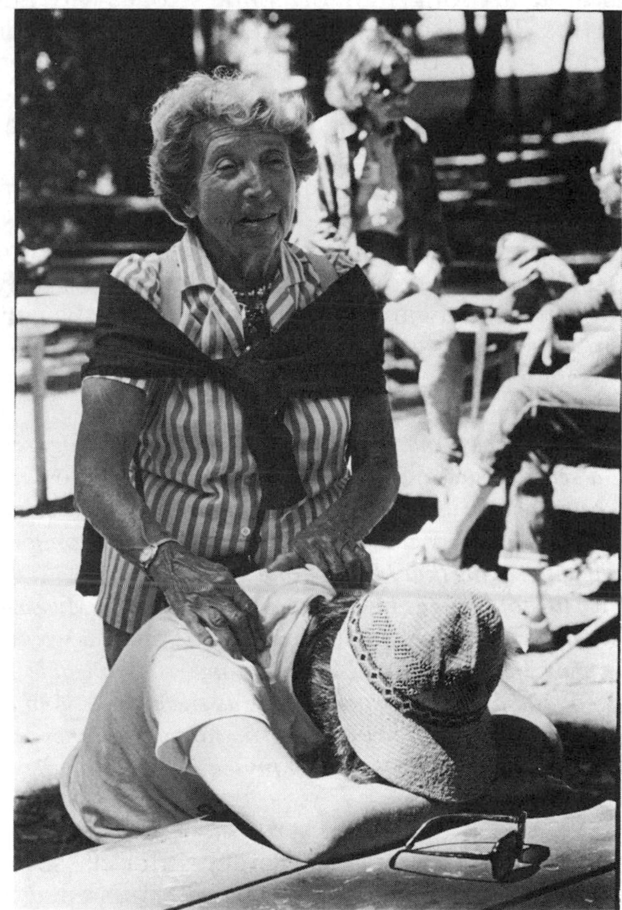

Marianne Gontarz

If you or the person you are massaging feels shy, start with foot and hand rubs, or head, neck, and face. A rapping motion with sides of hand, cupped palms, or loosely closed fists feels great on the arms, legs, back, and shoulders—try it on yourself first, then with each other. Finger tapping feels good on the head and face. Kneading, squeezing, and rolling or rocking can be done over loose clothing. In order to glide smoothly over skin, use a lubricant such as light vegetable oil with or without perfume, or a bar of cocoa butter. Do not use mineral oil or products that contain it, such as baby oil. Hand lotions and creams are too quickly absorbed and do not provide enough lubrication, but cream may work well for facial massage.

The person receiving the massage will be most relaxed if she lies on a firm, comfortable surface, but you can also work on her as she sits. The person giving the massage should always work in a comfortable position. Take slow deep breaths as you remind the person you are massaging to do the same. When finishing a particular area, use long, light brushing strokes with fingertips. To finish the massage session, place your hands gently on the head or feet for a long moment, visualizing the person as healed and perfect. See Resources, page 448, for books that illustrate various massage techniques.

Technique is less important than transmitting a sense of caring through your hands. Remember that you are touching a person, not just skin. As you touch, allow yourself to be fully attentive and aware of the uniqueness of the person you are massaging. The experience of giving massage is as heartwarming as receiving it.

I learned to be a massage therapist at the age of fifty-six, as a second career. Conditioned as a "proper Bostonian" to be extremely cautious and doubtful of my own sensuality and sexuality, it took me a long time to feel comfortable with saying that I like to touch people.

This touching is inward as well as outward. Massage deepens my connections with people. It offers a way to drop my judgments and expectations so I am able to accept and affirm someone exactly as she or he is. And in creating that acceptance and affirmation of the other person, I am creating the same for myself. [a fifty-nine-year-old woman]

Many adult-education centers offer classes in massage. There you can find people interested in massage and find out about the different techniques. There are several: Swedish massage, Heller work, Soma, Rolfing, myotherapy, and Trigger Point therapy deeply penetrate muscles and joints. Polarity therapy, Acupressure, Shiatsu, Trager, reflexology, Jin Shin Jitsu, Therapeutic Touch, and Reiki concentrate on energy balancing. Aston-patterning and Rolf movement combine massage and movement reeducation.

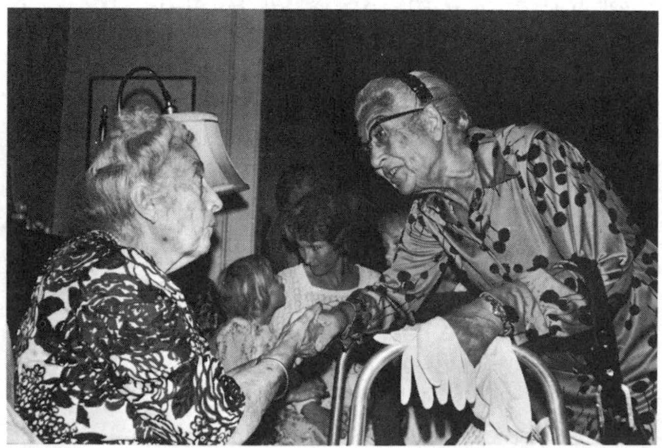

Jerry Howard/Positive Images

There are also techniques specifically tailored for athletes, infants, and pregnant women. A woman experiencing Therapeutic Touch for the first time described it this way:

I had driven over 2,000 miles in three days, and my head was tight and buzzing. The therapist had me sit in a chair, fully clothed, telling me to close my eyes and deepen my breathing. She kept her hands for several minutes, motionless, on different parts of my body; sometimes she'd make long sweeps downwards, either not touching me, or only very lightly. "How can this help?" I thought. But 45 minutes later, all the tightness had gone out of my head. I felt calm and ready to deal with the world again. [a fifty-two-year-old woman]

I worked with a client for two years when she was ninety-one through ninety-three years old. Her doctors were amazed at how massage helped her regain her range of motion after a car accident in which several of her bones were broken and her muscles were in spasm. Numbness in her feet and hands also cleared up and she was always more clear mentally and invigorated after massage. [a certified massage therapist]

You may, as you are being massaged, feel an opening awareness of emotion, as massage is more than just physical manipulation. It is your decision whether the person giving the massage is the person with whom to discuss the feelings that come up during a massage. Alternatively, you may want to think through these issues yourself, write in a journal, talk with a friend, or discuss them with a psychotherapist.

Getting in Touch with Others—Friends and Support Groups

We have the power to enrich our lives and those of others through our personal relationships. Research has shown that those who maintain strong bonds with family, friends, or neighbors actually have lower death and illness rates. When we feel isolated, it takes courage and initiative on our part to reach out to make new friends. A ten-year study of seven thousand people across the nation found that the mortality rate among people with poor social bonds was 2.5 times higher than among people with a good support system of friends and relatives.[28]

One thing that American society lacks, from my point of view, is that people don't have groups of friends. You have

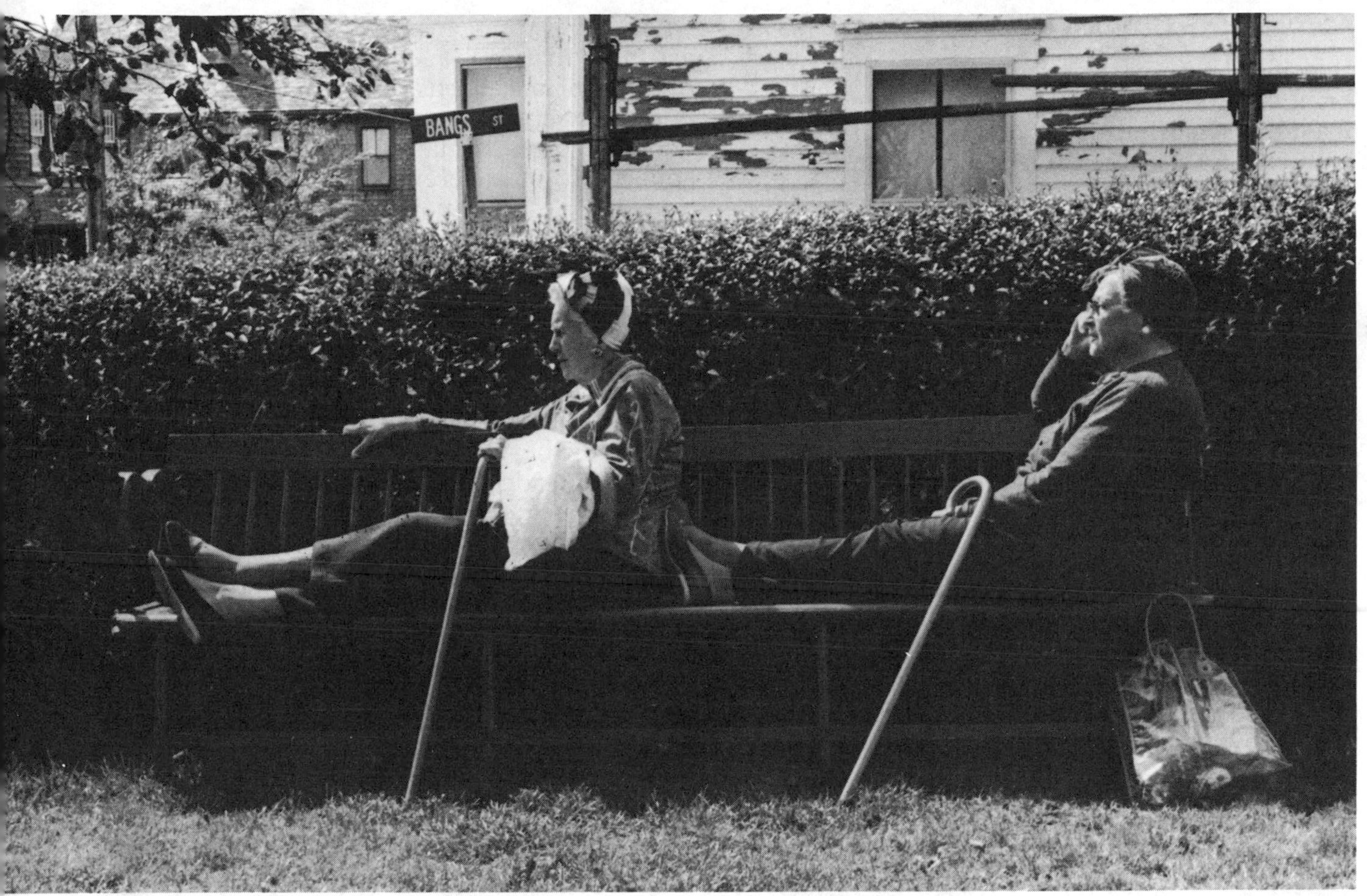

Norma Holt

one individual friend. And if something happens to him or her, you have no one to talk to. And you wind up at the psychiatrist. . . . I have friends who let me talk things out. Through the talking, I realize what I must do. [a Chinese-American woman, age eighty][29]

When we were younger, neighborhood women often gathered to talk over coffee, discussing child rearing, sharing homemaking tips, and enjoying the pleasure of conversation. At work, coworkers band together to help each other survive the pressures of the job. Now that we are older, these natural groups may have fallen away. And as society becomes more mobile and fragmented, with family members often far away, there's a vital social gap to be filled. Friends become our family of choice on whom we depend.[30]

Though many groups meet for specific purposes, simple friendship can be a sufficient reason for gathering. One group of women of all ages, fearing a future alone, call themselves "Just Friends." They meet not only for the enjoyment of being in a group with women of diverse ages, but also to help each other. Another group who talk together while working on handcrafts call themselves "The Stitch and Bitch Club."

THE STREAM

bubbles
below the falls
rush complete small circles
most float on like raindrops each one
alone

many
dash from side to
side striking out hectic
until they disappear from sight
dissolved

there are
a few that move
toward some others
they touch they blend then they go on
growing

Lois Harris

Mutual-Help Groups

Specific shared issues can be a good catalyst for bringing people together. You, perhaps with a friend, may wish to form a mutual-help group of women who share a common problem, such as a troubled relationship with an adult child, arthritis, allergies, or urinary incontinence. You can also join a short-term group such as Widow-to-Widow, or a hospice group that supports you after the death of a loved one.

Mutual-help groups often have practical results. A good example is the effect an older-women's group had in helping older people stay in their homes. The group organized a pool of younger volunteer and paid workers who helped with housekeeping, repairs, transportation, companionship, and a variety of other personal services.[31]

Mutual-help groups are different from old-style authoritarian groups, and it takes some adjusting and patience to get one working well. Here are some pointers:

A mutual-help group sets its own goals. Begin by discussing, in democratic fashion, what the group members' needs are. It is assumed that each member is an expert on her own problems, needs, and goals. Avoid letting one member take over; encourage those members with professional expertise to participate as equals, without reference to credentials.

Leaderless mutual-help groups ensure that each woman's needs, goals, and experiences are equally respected. The results are well worth the time and trouble. Another approach is to rotate leadership among group members, or to appoint one member as a facilitator to keep the group focused. Whoever leads the group has the same needs as the other members and must be given time to air her concerns while another member fills in as leader. In such groups, we learn new skills of openness and flexibility, and develop our natural leadership and communication abilities.

I was a member of a support group that had started off with a leader. When we became independent, I sometimes felt frustrated, so I thought, "What would Ann [the former leader] say if she were here?" and then I would try it. Now we all share the responsibility of keeping the group moving. [a woman in her fifties]

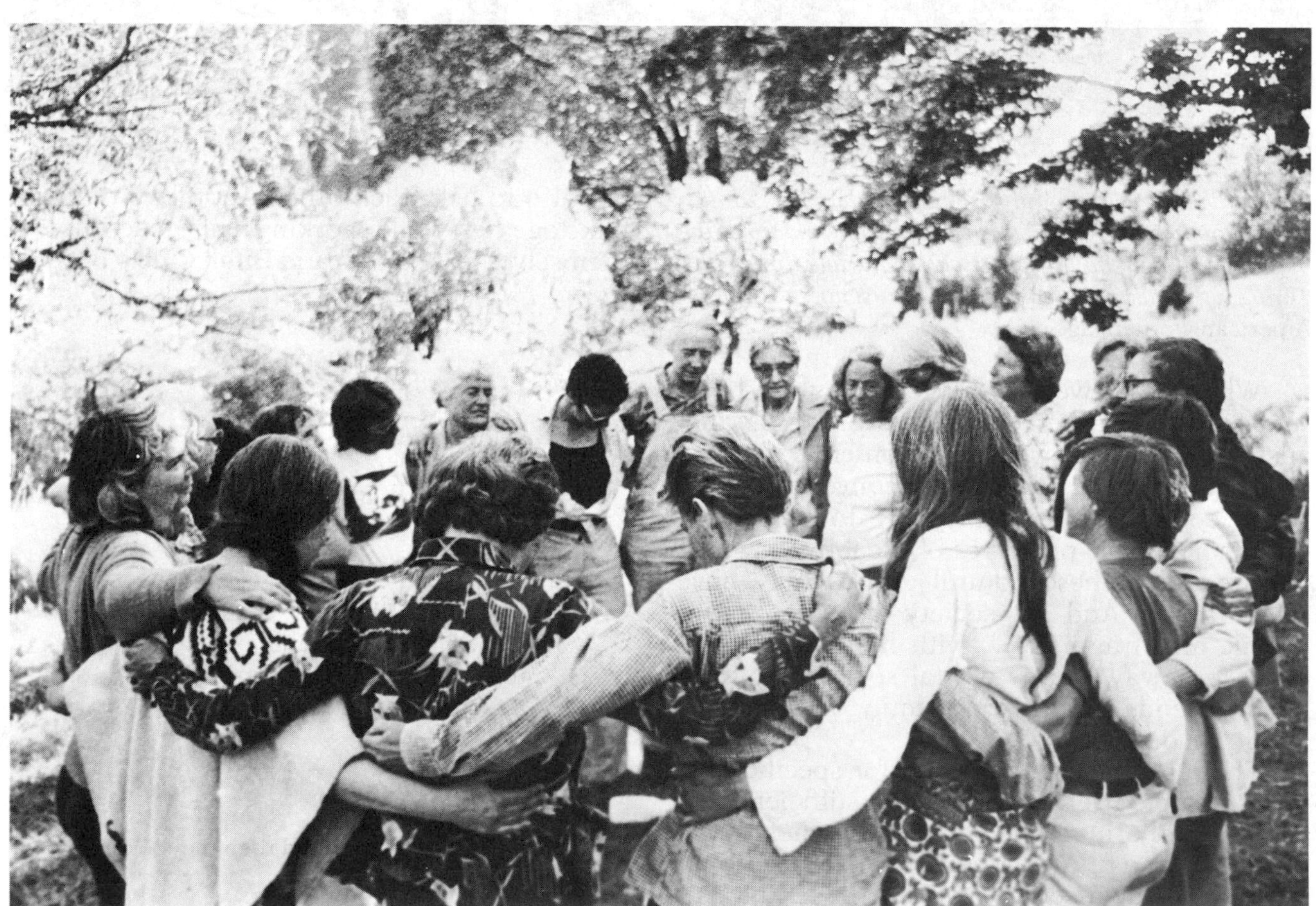

Cathy Cade

In my women's group we divide up the tasks of leadership and take turns doing them. At each meeting one woman is "watch witch," keeping track of the time allowed for each person to speak. Another woman is responsible for keeping the discussion on track, so that as each woman speaks she is free to concentrate solely on what she is saying. [a forty-seven-year-old woman]

NOTES

1. Asenath LaRue, et al., "Health in Old Age: How Do Physicians' Ratings and Self-ratings Compare?" *Journal of Gerontology,* Vol. 34, No. 5 (1979), pp. 687–91.

2. Marc E. Weksler, "Genetic and Immunologic Determinants of Aging." In *Proceedings of the Second Conference on the Epidemiology of Aging.* Bethesda, MD: U.S. Department of Health and Human Services, National Institutes of Health, 1980, pp. 15–22.

3. Robert N. Butler, "Health Productivity and Aging: An Overview." In Robert N. Butler and Herbert P. Gleason, eds., *Productive Aging: Enhancing Vitality in Later Life.* New York: Springer, 1985, p. 8.

4. Ibid., p. 12.

5. Mary Anne Kurz, "Theories of Aging and Popular Claims of Extending Life." *News and Features from NIH,* Vol. 85, No. 4 (1985), pp. 8–10.

6. Edward L. Schneider and John D. Reed, Jr., "Life Extension." *New England Journal of Medicine,* Vol. 312, No. 18 (May 2, 1985), pp. 1159–68.

7. Kurz, op. cit.

8. Jeffrey B. Blumberg, "Dietary Antioxidants and Aging." *Contemporary Nutrition,* Vol. 17, No. 3 (1992); Meir J. Stampfer, et al., "Vitamin E Consumption and the Risk of Coronary Heart Disease in Women." *New England Journal of Medicine,* Vol. 328, No. 20 (May 20, 1993), pp. 1444–49; "Editorials," same issue, pp. 1487–89.

9. *In Search of the Secrets of Aging.* U.S. Department of Health and Human Services, Public Health Service, NIH Pub. No. 93-2756, May 1993.

10. Ibid.

11. *Physical Frailty: A Reducible Barrier to Independence for Older Americans.* U.S. Department of Health and Human Services, Public Health Service, NIH Pub. No. 91-397, September 1991.

12. K. Warner Schaie and Sherry Willis, "Can Decline in Adult Intellectual Functioning Be Reversed?" *Developmental Psychology,* Vol. 22, No. 2 (1986), pp. 223–32.

13. Herbert Benson, *The Relaxation Response.* New York: Avon Books, 1976, p. 70.

14. Daniel Goleman, "New Light on How Stress Erodes Health." *The New York Times,* Dec. 15, 1992.

15. R. M. Sapolsy, et al., "Hippocampal Neuronal Loss During Aging: Role of Glucocorticoids." Paper given at Conference on Aging and the Dementias, Montefiore Centennial Series, Rockefeller University, New York, October 24, 1984.

16. Excerpted from T. H. Holmes and R. H. Rahe, "The Social Readjustment Rating Scale." *Journal of Psychosomatic Research,* Vol. 11 (1967), p. 213.

17. Sandra P. Thomas, "Predictors of Health Status of Mid-Life Women: Implications for Later Adulthood." *Journal of Women & Aging,* Vol. 2, No. 1 (1990), pp. 49–77.

18. Robert Eliot, a Nebraska cardiologist, quoted in Claudia Wallis, "Stress: Can We Cope?" *Time,* June 6, 1983, p. 48.

19. Norman Cousins, *Anatomy of an Illness.* New York: W. W. Norton and Co., 1979.

20. Thomas Gordon, *Parent Effectiveness Training.* New York: P. H. Wyden, 1970.

21. Benson, op. cit.

22. Herbert Benson, *Beyond the Relaxation Response.* New York: Times Books, 1984. How to harness the power of faith and personal belief in the healing process.

23. Steve Kravette, *Complete Relaxation.* Rockport, MA: Para Research, 1979, pp. 21–37.

24. Carolyn Latteier, "Music as Medicine." *Medical Self Care,* Issue No. 31 (November/December 1985), pp. 48–52.

25. Benson, *Beyond the Relaxation Response.* op. cit.

26. *Ms.,* December 1985, special issue on women and spirituality; and Charlene Spretnak, "Essay: Wholly Writ." *Ms.,* Vol. 3, No. 5 (March/April 1993), pp. 60–62. See also Resources, Spirituality, pages 449–50.

27. Flora Davis, "Skin Hunger—An American Disease." *Woman's Day,* Sept. 27, 1978, p. 156.

28. Leonard S. Syme and Lisa Berkman, "Social Class, Susceptibility, and Sickness." In Peter Conrad and Rochelle Kern, eds., *The Sociology of Health and Illness: Critical Perspectives.* New York: St. Martin's Press, 1990.

29. Grace Chu, in Jane Seskin, ed., *More Than Mere Survival: Conversations with Women Over 65.* New York: Newsweek, 1980, p. 223.

30. Karen Lindsey, *Friends as Family.* Boston: Beacon Press, 1982.

31. Mike Samuels and Nancy Samuels, *Seeing with the Mind's Eye.* New York: Random House, 1975, pp. 56–64.

2

HABITS WORTH CHANGING

✦

BY DORI SMITH, DIANA LASKIN SIEGAL, AND PAULA B. DORESS-WORTERS.

1994 UPDATE BY DIANA LASKIN SIEGAL.

1994 UPDATE ON *SMOKING* BY MARTHA C. WOOD

ALCOHOL BY SANDRA T. BIERIG AND RUTH L. FISHEL

1994 UPDATE ON *ALCOHOL* BY ANITA H. SHIPMAN

DEALING WITH PAIN WITH SPECIAL THANKS TO SYLVIA PIGORS

RESOURCES FOR THIS CHAPTER ON PAGES 450–53

We live in a substance-abusing society. We are surrounded by billboards, store displays, and ads in all the media touting alcohol, over-the-counter drugs, cigarettes, soft drinks, coffee—all promoting a glamorous and happy life. The message is, "Reach for a [whatever it is] and all your problems will be solved." Physicians are also bombarded by drug-company salespeople and medical-journal ads offering drugs for every symptom. But these substances—tobacco, caffeine, alcohol, and drugs—when turned into habits are so common and damaging that they warrant special attention. They also interact with each other in ways that increase their dangers.

SMOKING

Cigarette smoking is the chief avoidable cause of death in our society, and the most important health issue of our time.[1] Smoking is on the rise for women. Since World War II, women have been smoking in large numbers and now our smoking-related disease patterns are beginning to resemble men's. In fact, our favorable advantage in life expectancy over men (seventy-nine years to men's seventy-two years, as of 1991) may change for the worse as a result.[2] Lung cancer is now the number one cancer killer of women, exceeding both breast cancer and colorectal cancer.[3]

The dangers of "passive smoking"—smoke inhaled from other people's cigarettes—are also very high. "Secondhand smoke" contains thousands of chemical compounds, including some deadly ones. It contains fifty times more ammonia, five times more carbon monoxide, and *twice as much tar* as the smoker inhales.[4] Passive smoking causes cancer, heart disease, respiratory illnesses, headaches, and allergies. Children are more harmed by passive smoking than adults. Groups such as ASH (Action on Smoking and Health) and GASP (Group Against Smoking Pollution) support efforts to create no-smoking areas in public places and the workplace and to prohibit the easy access of cigarettes for minors.

The risks of smoking increase with age and with the number of years you've smoked. These risks include osteoporosis, glaucoma, a full range of cardiovascular and respiratory diseases, and many more kinds of cancer than the obvious lung cancer. Smoking accounts for about 30 percent of all cancer deaths.[5] There is an increased danger of cardiovascular disease among users of oral contraceptives who smoke, and an increased risk of cancer of the mouth, pharynx, larynx, and esophagus among people who both drink and smoke. Smoking also increases wrinkles.

Nicotine is by no means the only dangerous ingredient in cigarettes. We must also count carbon monoxide (in an amount eight times greater than the amount industry is allowed to release into the air), tars, and even the heat itself. Chemical additives and modern tobacco-curing processes apparently add to cigarette smoking's deadly results.

The good news is that smoking is avoidable. The highest mortality rates are among current

HOW TO CELEBRATE A TWENTY-FIFTH SMOKELESS ANNIVERSARY

by Beth Rosenbaum

It is now twenty-five years since I smoked my last cigarette. In 1960 I inhaled the last nicotine-laden draft into my then fifty-four-year-old lungs. For thirty-four years a cigarette had been my constant companion, my picker-upper, my relaxer, and my security blanket. "Put me in a padded cell," I told my family, "if you want me to stop smoking."

In the Roaring Twenties the cigarette was the flapper's logo of sophistication. "Cigarette me, big boy," said Joan Crawford, and we all bought carved ivory holders. "Be nonchalant, light a Murad," said the elegant smokers on the billboards.

Now the government, doctors, and health organizations warn, cajole, raise consciousness, modify behavior, hypnotize, segregate, and abuse smokers—with questionable success.

But in my twenty-fifth Smokeless Anniversary year, I offer my method free to all nicotine addicts. No coupons to clip. No salesperson will call. No obligations.

First: Build up a strong guilt feeling. Guilt can be very productive if used constructively. How can one feel guilty about smoking? Many ways. You don't want to give your children and grandchildren unhealthy habits, do you? More children of smoking parents become smokers than the lucky offspring of nonsmoking parents. No children? Think of all the money you could give to your favorite charity—at today's cigarette prices, many hundreds of dollars a year. Besides, don't you feel uneasy about all the air you're polluting? Your loved ones are breathing it, not to mention innocent strangers. So, pick the guilt that suits your situation and dwell on it.

Second: Choose a day with a spiritual, mystical, or sentimental association for you. I chose Yom Kippur—the Jewish Day of Atonement—after reading in the service: "This day . . . I have set before you life and death, blessing and curse; therefore choose life, that you and your descendants may live" (Deuteronomy 30:19). Good advice, I decided, from an authorized source. Or choose your birthday, surely a symbolic day. You came into this world with clean, rosy-pink lungs. Do you really want to go out with dirty black lungs? Don't choose New Year's Eve. Decades of bad jokes about New Year's resolutions have conditioned us to break the ones we make.

Third: Think upbeat. Make a little ceremony around smoking that last cigarette. Tell yourself, out loud: "This is the last time in my life I'll smoke. I am not giving anything up. I'm starting something new." You, yourself, built the habit of smoking. You can build a new habit. After you eat anything, even a snack, use a toothpick vigorously. Keep that toothpick in your mouth or put it in an ashtray. You'll find your own substitute habit. Sweets and coffee won't help. They tend to make you want to eat and smoke . . . a never-ending cycle. Concentrate on something—like a crossword puzzle. Occupy your mind and hands. It works.

Fourth: Enjoy. It's a great ego booster. Feel superior to all those lily-livered, black-lunged weaklings who think their very lives depend on a tiny, dangerous, expensive paper tube stuffed with straw.

Fifth: Declare a victory. A poet and soldier described the First World War as "damned dirty, damned dull, and damned dangerous." *You* have just won a war, also dirty, dull, and dangerous. Congratulations. You deserve a medal to pin on your healthier chest.

smokers, and quitting *at any age* causes the mortality rate to drop. In the case of coronary heart disease, quitting causes a 50 percent drop in death rate within twelve months, and after a decade or more of not smoking the mortality rate from coronary heart disease approaches that of nonsmokers.[6] Smokers who quit, even after age sixty, have better lung function than continuing smokers.[7]

Take heart in knowing that a high percentage of those who try to quit succeed, even if it takes several attempts. The "frontal attack" on the smoking habit—going "cold turkey"—may work. But there's a risk: if you slip—take one cigarette—you may feel like a failure and go into a full-scale relapse. The motto of Alcoholics Anonymous, "One day at a time," can be helpful to anyone trying to quit. Many quit on their own, assisted by self-help literature. For others, mutual-help groups and cessation programs (the cost of which may be covered by insurance if prescribed by a doctor) are essential.

Smokers reach for cigarettes to relieve boredom, to fill time, to do something when feeling tense or anxious. One reaction to tension is to hold your breath or to take little, shallow breaths. If you smoke, inhaling a cigarette may be your own way to take a full, deep breath. Try taking three deep breaths when you crave a cigarette. You may actually crave oxygen.

Smoking a cigarette may be the only socially accepted way of taking a break at your workplace. You may have to fight for acceptance of a more healthful break, like going for a short walk, or just to the door or window for air, or getting up to stretch.

Some women are working to create a smoke-free environment where they are employed. One woman wrote to tell us how she fought and won such a struggle:

Over the past eight years I have worked in an office with no ventilation system, no windows that opened, and no source of fresh air except the front door. I got so angry about having to endure all the smoke that I even filed a union grievance and went through all the steps. The union said that I was the problem and that perhaps I should just get another job.

I tried the fire department. The chief inspected and, though sympathetic, said that he could not ban smoking since there were no volatile gases or inflammable materials in the worksite.

I started going to GASP meetings, and I read and brought their literature to the office. I decided that I was willing to sue for a smoke-free work environment. After being turned down by many law firms that would not take the case on a pro bono basis, we finally found a lawyer whose wife was an oncologist (a physician who specializes in treating cancer).*

I was jubilant when the judge issued a ten-day restraining order against smoking in the office. The office was divided on the issue. A few people said the air was better after the smoking stopped. Others were angry and sarcastic. People told me I would never be promoted and might even lose my job.

The case went on for a year. The hardest thing was being portrayed in court as a maladjusted woman. I was indignant because there was plenty of evidence available about the hazards of smoking. I felt it was a public health issue, just like having a clean water supply.

The outcome was that when our office moved into new space it was divided up. Four addicted smokers chose a room with a separate ventilation system; the rest of the space is smoke-free. The other smokers chose to work in a smoke-free environment and do not smoke at their desks.

Three years later, the tension has subsided and some of my coworkers have even thanked me. Finally, the agency ruled that smoke-free offices must be provided at every site. [a fifty-eight-year-old woman]

Smoking is an addiction, and for various reasons women have a harder time quitting than men. Stopping smoking often requires that we confront these obstacles:

- Tobacco manufacturers spend millions on special advertising efforts to expand their markets among women. The financial clout of the tobacco industry inhibits the flow of antismoking information while assuring that the pro-smoking messages remain in the media—a serious infringement of freedom of the press. Earlier advertising attempted to link smoking with sexiness. Now the ads play on a caricature of feminism that links smoking to women's struggles for equality and feeling "tough" and "cool." The only way smoking helps you to "come a long way, baby" is by catching up to men's lung-cancer rates.
- Nicotine is a physiological addictor. When you smoke, you reward yourself for smoking, and when you try to quit, it feels as though you are punishing yourself. You can reverse this by developing a reward system for every cigarette you do *not* smoke. One suggestion is to set

*From *pro bono publico,* a Latin phrase meaning "for the public good." In English usage, this means legal work done for free or at reduced rates in order to bring certain issues before the courts.

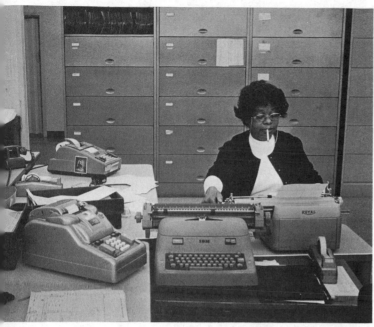

Cathy Cade

aside the money you spend on cigarettes for a present for yourself. By *not* smoking you can spend the money on something you will enjoy longer than a cigarette.

- Smoking is higher among groups stressed by job pressures and economic concerns—women (especially very young women), people of color, blue-collar workers.* Much of the material on the dangers of smoking is in publications that reach high-income persons; much of the advertising promoting smoking is in media reaching lower-income persons.
- Women learn to suppress anger, and some of us tend to reach for a cigarette when feeling angry.

It took me eight years to stop smoking completely. The last cigarettes I gave up were the ones I "bummed" at work when I didn't feel free to say what I really thought. My close coworkers would ask me after the meeting, "What didn't you like?" [a fifty-four-year-old woman]

- Many women use cigarette smoking to reduce calorie intake, picking up a cigarette instead of a dessert. We fear gaining weight if we quit. Cigarette manufacturers play on such fears through advertising and use of such names as Virginia Slims. Food will taste and smell better without cigarettes, but major weight gain is not inevitable. Research shows the average weight gain in women is only eight pounds.[8] Try noncaloric or low-calorie substitutes like gum or carrot sticks rather than resorting to high-calorie foods to sate your reawakened appetite. Try chewy, satisfying whole grains like brown rice to restore the B vitamins lost in smoking. Drink extra fruit and vegetable juices to speed elimination of nicotine from your system. Increase your walks or other exercise. Try swimming; nobody smokes in a swimming pool.

*Even among health professionals, smoking continues to be a problem when job pressures go hand in hand with the lack of authority to make changes in the workplace. Doctors and nurses are equally aware of the health risks of smoking, but approximately 19 percent of nurses still smoke, whereas less than 10 percent of doctors smoke.

When you resolve to quit, prepare for your new adventure. You can expect to feel rocky for a period of time, so get support from family and friends. Other helpful supports are self-help manuals and "stop smoking" groups. A good "stop smoking" program will help you confront your individual smoking patterns.

Smokers need a doctor's prescription for nicotine patches or gum that can be used over a period of months to gradually reduce the amount of nicotine released to the body. **Persons could receive a fatal level of nicotine if they smoke while wearing the patch.** New shipments of other over-the-counter smoking cessation products in gum, pill, or lozenge form were banned as of December 1, 1993, because they are not effective.

Some immediate rewards of quitting smoking are an increase in endurance, an end to "smoker's cough," and a regaining of your senses of taste and smell. Some long-term rewards are better health, longer life, and the pride of being in control.

CAFFEINE

Coffee is the "drug of choice" for millions of Americans. We use coffee as fuel for our industry and business, making typists type faster and executives work longer hours.

Caffeine and related compounds are found in coffee, colas, caffeinated teas, and chocolate. Partly as a result of public awareness, coffee consumption is slipping, and caffeine-free colas are now available. The coffee industry has gone on the offensive, asking us to become "coffee achievers" again.

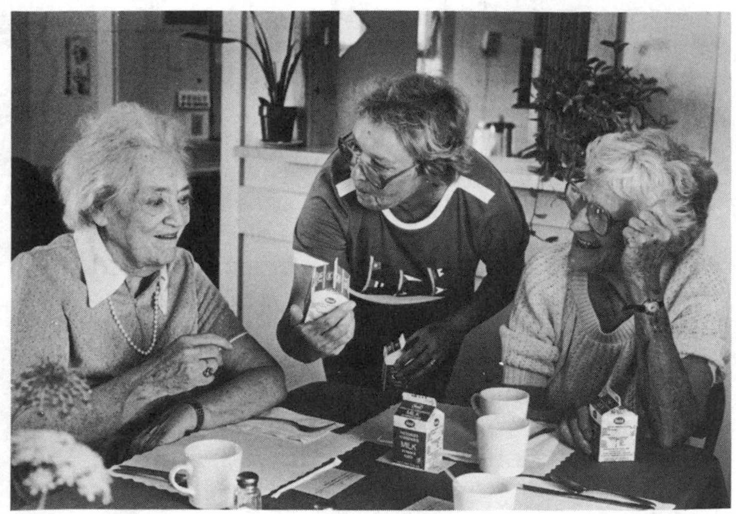

Norma Holt

What caffeine in fact achieves is partial responsibility for a wide range of disorders: panic attacks,[9] chronic nervousness, and irritability; digestive difficulties, including heartburn, indigestion, and ulcers; urinary incontinence; migraine headaches; and low blood sugar. Some women find that eliminating caffeine can ease their fibrocystic breast lumps. Caffeine can lead to increased risk of pancreatic and bladder cancers,[10] and, as a heart stimulant, is linked to blood-pressure abnormalities and myocardial infarction. In a 1973 study of 440 patients with acute myocardial infarction, the disease was seen 60 percent to 120 percent more frequently in coffee drinkers.[11]

"Decaffeinated" coffee varies in caffeine content. Some is only half decaffeinated! It still contains about 3 percent caffeine, compared to regular coffee's 6 percent, as well as other harmful substances such as tars, acids, and oils. If you drink several cups of decaf, you may still get a lot of caffeine. The safest way to remove caffeine from coffee is the water-processed method. Chemically processed decaf has been specifically implicated in pancreatic cancer.[12]

The "coffee klatsch," which developed among neighborhood women to inject a little sociability in a day filled with chores and isolation, is often just an excuse to sit down together. You can still have the sociability without the dangers of caffeine.

What can you do if you want to switch? Cut down gradually. When you feel like having a cup of coffee, find other ways to increase circulation and oxygen to the brain, such as aerobic exercise. Drinking milk, vegetable juices, unsweetened fruit juices, herbal beverages, grain-based coffee substitutes (iced or hot) may add a new flavor dimension to your life. Don't forget your need for water. Evaluate your priorities, and see if you are pushing yourself harder than necessary using coffee as a whip.

Alcohol

During their middle and later years, women undergo significant life changes and cultural pressures. Trying to cope with these changes and pressures is very difficult, and a drink or a tranquilizer may seem like an easy way to cope. Women can often trace changes in their drinking habits to upsetting events in their lives. But drinking opens a door to a nightmare of alcohol abuse and possible addiction.

If we are having trouble sleeping, we may be tempted to have a drink before bed to encourage sleep. To add to this danger, physicians may prescribe drugs that can eventually control us physically, mentally, and spiritually, and can interact dangerously with alcohol.[13]

If we have been social drinkers, it is difficult to imagine that alcohol can become a problem as we age. Yet it can do just that!

When I was living alone with no car, I felt really alone. I had a morbid fear: suppose I lost my mind or something? I'd open a can of beer and make a gin and tonic, and have a sip of one and then a sip of the other. It was so warm and soothing. But it was dangerous. [an eighty-eight-year-old woman]

Are we overstating the case, being alarmist? After all, most Americans drink. It is a customary part of our social life. Sometimes there is social pressure to drink. We are more apt to drink, or to drink more than we usually do, in a group for the sake of sociability. It is important to remember that we have the right to abstain.

When I was going through menopause I found that any alcohol triggered severe hot flashes and so asked for seltzer water or juice. I was amazed at the pressure from people (not from my close friends) who were unrelenting in trying to get me to drink alcohol. I finally started to lie and told them I was taking medication that could not be taken with alcohol. Then they were sympathetic and stopped pressuring—until the next time. [a fifty-five-year-old woman]

Recent studies show that we are more likely than men to develop problems with alcohol in later life.[14] Our average body weights are lower than men's, so the same quantity of alcohol hits us harder. Even at the same weight, alcohol enters our bloodstreams faster because of our higher proportion of body fat, which doesn't absorb alcohol. Twenty-five percent of women who become alcoholics do so between the ages of forty and fifty-five,[15] and anywhere from 1 to 5 percent succumb to the disease after age sixty.[16]

My family and friends knew there was something wrong with me, but they just couldn't put a finger on it. The changes had been too subtle. They could see that I was drinking a little too much, now and again. What they did not know, because I went to great pains to hide it from them, was that the times I drank had become more and more frequent, and the times between shorter. [a woman in her fifties]

Many women fall prey to problem drinking without realizing it is happening. They may experience pressure to keep up with men on the job including drinking at lunch or after work.[17] Some women take a drink to get a lift when they feel down or blue or tired without realizing that alcohol is actually a depressant. If alcohol becomes a problem for you, will you realize it? Will you know how to handle it? Will you want to do so? We owe it to ourselves to be aware of certain telltale signs of problem drinking in ourselves or in others close to us.

No one starts life with the goal of becoming an alcoholic. There are no sure ways to predict who will or will not become one. The onset of alcohol abuse is usually very slow and insidious.

My tolerance to alcohol grew so that I had to drink more to achieve the same effect. My daily activities began to be planned around my drinking time, and more and more often, drinking became my main activity. I could manage to rationalize anything if it meant defending my right to drink. At that point, of course, my "right" was a synonym for my physical and emotional need. [a fifty-one-year-old woman]

While it is not possible to predict exactly who will or will not become an alcoholic, the following questions can provide some early clues. Are you, for example:

- Minimizing or making excuses for your drinking?
- Drinking faster or more frequently? Are you gulping your drinks or trying to maintain the feeling drinking gives you, while looking for more opportunities to drink and feel okay about it?
- Changing your daily pattern of drinking? Has a glass of wine with dinner expanded to include a drink before or after dinner or a nightcap?
- Changing companions? Are you breaking dates with old friends and trying to find new ones who drink as you do?
- Having trouble maintaining your activity level at work or at home? Do lunches include an alcoholic beverage? Is it increasingly difficult to return to work afterward? Have you lost interest in activities that used to make you happy but did not include drinking?
- Becoming unable to resist when you want to drink, even at times you would normally consider inappropriate? Are you planning ahead to ensure your supply? Are you finding reasons to justify drinking? Can you rationalize almost anything if it means you can drink when you want to do so?
- Denying that anything has changed? Are you lying to yourself and others about the frequency of your drinking and your need to continue it? Are your friends and family members

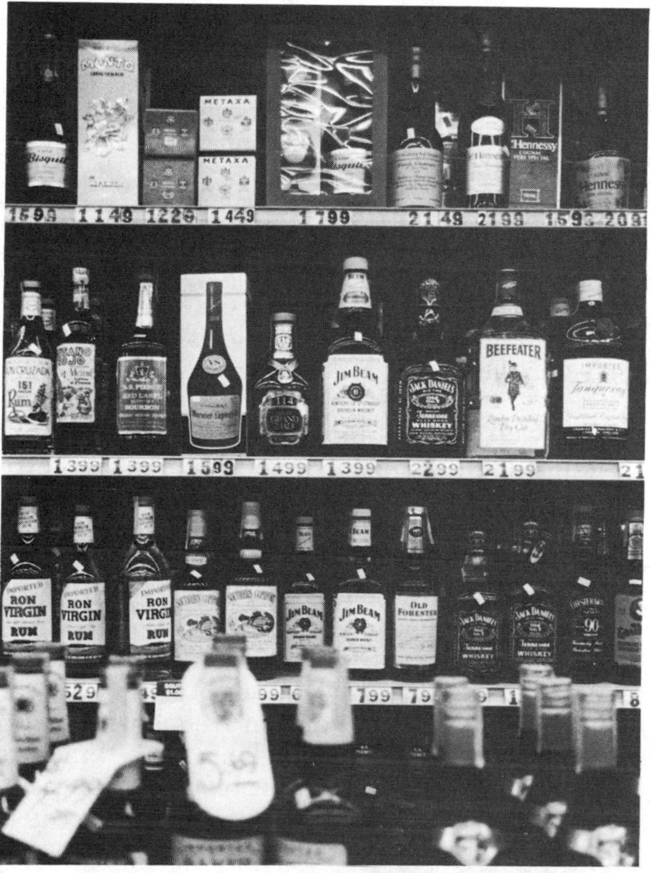

Ellen Shub

making excuses for you? Is your relationship with them changing for the worse?
- Experiencing blackouts? Are you beginning to have times when you cannot remember things you did while drinking?

"The quality of life returns as we learn a day at a time how not to drink." As these words were spoken at an A.A. meeting recently, there flashed before me the scene of a Christmas morning in my living room—and the faces of my husband and son—as I stood shakily before them following what I hope is my last drunken blackout, seven years ago. [a seventy-two-year-old woman]

- Having more accidents? Are you falling more, or getting burns or cuts without being able to explain how?

Until I almost fall down, or become ill, or wake up the next day with a massive hangover, I don't truly recognize how drunk I am. [a fifty-year-old woman]

FACING PROBLEM DRINKING

Drinking is considered to be inappropriate behavior for women, especially for older women. Women who drink to excess are judged harshly, their value as people and women challenged. Those of us who grew up during times when women were more restricted socially may feel this prejudice more keenly, but few of us are free of it entirely.

I called A.A. at least three times over my last five years of heavy drinking. Each time I called with a different story, a different lie! Once I said I was calling because my son drank too much. I don't remember the other lies. I even disguised my voice because I felt so ashamed. [a forty-nine-year-old woman]

As well as robbing women who drink too much of their self-esteem and security, this attitude keeps many from getting help. Most women are reluctant to seek treatment, even privately, because of the stigma attached. Seventy percent of women who drink to excess hide their drinking for as long as possible.[18] Some women can hide the extent of their drinking or drug abuse better than others. Women who live by themselves or with partners who are absent frequently can do so more easily. Women in higher income brackets may also be able to hide problems more easily because expense is less of an issue and because they rarely come to the attention of social workers or the criminal justice system.

However, no one is exempt from addiction. Although it often seems as if no one wants to admit it, the woman alcoholic or problem drinker can be anyone—a next-door neighbor, a coworker, or a close relative. She can be a lesbian, a member of an ethnic minority, a strict churchgoer, a professional, an eighty-five-year-old great-grandmother, or you.

ALCOHOL AND THE LESBIAN

Most lesbians over thirty-five experienced more pressure to remain "in the closet" about their sexual orientation while growing up than their younger sisters do today. The experiences of older lesbians involved the painful conflict of fear of being found out versus a deep need to socialize. The situation was made more complex by the fact that social life in past years centered around bars.

Too many older lesbians still feel isolated, guilty, ashamed, and have low self-esteem because of society's homophobia. Alcohol, first used as a temporary relief from those pressures, grew to be a constant need for almost one third of all lesbians.[19]

I so deeply suppressed my homosexual feelings that I was no longer aware that they existed. Married at twenty-three, I lived the role of a traditional mom and wife. I had always felt different from my friends, and I thought that something must really be wrong with me. Having a drink before supper was a nightly event for my husband and me. Gradually, however, this one drink became two or three for me. I really looked forward to those drinks because they were the only times that I felt able to relax. Gradually, over the years, I lost control of my drinking and became an alcoholic.

Fortunately, at forty-two, I found A.A. and began my road to recovery. In the process, my old feelings began to resurface and I could no longer deny that I was both emotionally and sexually attracted to other women. While these feelings frightened me, I could no longer suppress them. Instead, I began to actively seek out other women like me. While I had been afraid that going to bars would be my only way to find them, I discovered that the A.A. meeting book actually listed several gay meetings.

Nervous and frightened, I went to my first meeting. I was so paranoid that I thought everyone from my small town had followed me. I sat in a chair close to the door so I could make a quick escape if necessary. But when I heard an attractive young woman on the podium say, "Welcome. My name is Kathy and I am an alcoholic and a lesbian," tears of relief streamed down my face. [a forty-nine-year-old woman]

New organizations for older lesbians provide opportunities for socializing in an alcohol-free environment.

I was in A.A. and alcohol-free for some years when I found an older-lesbian group of more than two hundred women over the age of forty. The group sponsors an activity each month plus two weekends a year. All of the group's activities are alcohol-free. Our members have started small groups to read books, play cards, and other activities. Alcohol had been such an integral part of my life-style back in the 1940s and '50s, when the only place to socialize was the gay bars. Perhaps life would have unfolded differently for me if we had had other places then. How wonderful for all of us now, but especially for the younger women, to have sane and safe places free from the dangers of alcohol and police raids in the bars. [a sixty-two-year-old woman]

SOCIAL EFFECTS OF ALCOHOL ABUSE

A long list of troubles can be the outcome of problem drinking and alcoholism. Choosing to take a mood- or mind-altering substance instead of dealing with issues that come up in daily life also causes problems. We can lose friends and lovers, see our marriages break up, lose jobs, run up debts by spending money to ensure our supply rather than paying our bills, be picked up for drunk driving violations, and so on.

As I began to drink more, I began to be late to work. At first it was just once in a while, and then more frequently. Finally I started missing days completely. When I was at work, the quality of my work was becoming more uneven. At first my friends covered up for me, but eventually they were less and less willing to do so. Finally my boss began to notice. I was warned a number of times, and people bent over backward to help me. When I lost that job I rationalized that it hadn't been much of a job anyway, and I would be happier without it. [a fifty-one-year-old woman]

Alcohol can cloud our judgment and lower inhibitions, leaving us vulnerable to sexually transmitted diseases including HIV infection.

HEALTH HAZARDS OF ALCOHOL ABUSE

Heavy alcoholism over a period of years adversely affects every organ and system of the body. There is help available. A thorough medical examination can reveal health problems caused or masked by the use of alcohol. Some of these damaging effects can be reversed, but many cannot. When we drink, we might like to think that any long-term effects will happen only to others, but they can happen to us. The possibilities include:

- Memory loss caused by the effects of alcohol on the brain.
- Digestive problems, including inflammation of the pancreas, gastritis, fatty liver, hepatitis, and cirrhosis. Heavy drinking can impair the absorption of vitamin B_1 (thiamine), which can contribute to both brain damage and many problems of the intestinal system.
- High blood pressure and cardiac arrhythmia (irregular heartbeat), coronary artery disease and alcohol cardiomyopathy (heart-muscle damage)
- Nerve and muscle disorders resulting in weakness, the gradual wasting of muscles, and even paralysis
- An increased susceptibility to infection. Alcohol suppresses the production of white blood cells and impairs their ability to get to the site of an infection quickly.
- An increase in the effect of carcinogens (cancer-causing substances) such as tobacco. Alcoholics with cancer have a poorer chance of survival and a greater chance of developing another primary tumor than do nonalcoholics with the same cancer.
- Malnutrition. Alcoholics often neglect their nutrition, leading to anemia and increased tendency to bleed.
- An increased potential for urinary incontinence and diarrhea, since alcohol causes the body to lose water.

It cannot be overstated that, in addition to the above, there can be severe, sometimes fatal, effects as a result of combining alcohol with other drugs, even those drugs that are necessary for various health problems.

My friend Margo had a serious thyroid problem which was controllable with medication. She was also one of those unfortunate people who suffered from long- and short-term memory loss related to alcohol use. Over the years of heavy drinking, her thyroid condition worsened because she would forget to take her medication, increasing the burden on her overworked heart. Ultimately her heart did give out and Margo died when she was just fifty-two years old. The death certificate stated that she died of heart failure, but it was her alcoholism which was the real cause.

GETTING HELP

If you cannot stop drinking when you want to; if, on any given occasion, you find you are taking drugs more than you want to; or if you know deep inside that drinking or drugs are affecting any part of your life in a negative way, help is as close as your telephone. Even if you are only beginning to wonder if you have a problem, it is never too early to seek help, nor is it ever too late.

Finally, after twenty years of drinking, I went to a psychiatrist to whom I confessed out loud for the first time that I couldn't stop drinking. In his ignorance of the disease of alcoholism, he said, "There, there, dear. You are just a little neurotic. A few pills and a few more visits and you should be all right in a few months." In my own ignorance and desperation, I actually believed this man. He started me on Librium and then when that didn't work, Valium. And then Elavil and then lithium. Two and one-half years later he had tried thirty-one different drugs on me, including Artane because I shook so much from the combination of all these drugs. I now know that Artane is particularly dangerous when used in combination with alcohol. When he gave it to me, this doctor knew that I had not stopped drinking. I had always told the truth about that.

At last I told this doctor that I felt I was wasting my money, and that I planned to go to A.A. Though he had been unable to help me, he did not encourage me to go. He subscribed to the stereotype that A.A. is only for people who are down and out and he told me that I would never find a group in which I could be comfortable. Instead, I found hope and love and warmth from my first A.A. meeting. I have been sober for several years now, and my life has changed dramatically for the better. [a forty-nine-year-old woman]

You no longer have to be alone, feel guilty, or hide. Help and support are available in every state, town, and neighborhood. Your anonymity will be protected.

You must get sober and stay sober. You may need a detoxification program* to get sober, and A.A. to keep sober.† Once you are sober, you may want to work on your problems. If you choose to work with a therapist, it is important to find someone who has a clear understanding of A.A. and can help you to use both systems effectively.[20] Many therapists will urge an alcoholic to go to A.A. if she is not already doing so. Most important is that with help there is hope.

HELPING SOMEONE WE CARE ABOUT

When someone we care about has a drinking or drug problem, it is not easy to find the best way to help. Helping a friend or family member acknowledge that she or he has a problem can be one way to make a difference.

My best friend became an alcoholic and was progressively getting worse. She was raised in a teetotaling family, and I knew how the dichotomy between her upbringing and her secretive drinking was tearing her apart, in addition to the physical destruction of alcoholism. I assumed she would deny any accusation with vigor, and was very fearful that she might be so angry she would terminate our friendship, an outcome I would find intolerable. So time dripped by and I did nothing. After three years, I knew that I could no longer call myself a friend if I continued to ignore what she was doing. I arranged a day's outing and confronted her. She was so relieved! Nobody in her family had acknowledged what she was doing and she had concealed it from her therapist. As always, with confrontation, my only regret was that it took me so long to be able to do it. [a fifty-seven-year-old woman]

When we are closely involved with alcoholics—whether our spouses, lovers, parents, or children—we tend to become caught up in the illness as well. We spend prolonged periods of time trying to change our loved ones and convince them that they are destroying themselves by continuing to drink. We find ourselves fighting a losing battle to maintain some semblance of normalcy. The effects of being in a relationship with someone who is alcohol or drug dependent can be serious. We may need counseling to help us unravel how we feel and what is happening to us. Al-Anon for us and Alateen for our teenaged children can also help us to live our own lives, and teach us how to put the responsibility on the alcoholic for her or his own behavior, and not shoulder the blame ourselves.

We women are such good nurturers that we are usually loyal to our relationships even when we suffer as a result. Alcoholism is one disease in which the effort to smooth over and solve prob-

*There is a serious shortage of treatment programs for alcoholic women throughout the country. However, you may be able to find one suitable to your needs through one of the organizations listed in the Resources section, pages 451–52.

†If the A.A. group in your community is "too religious" for your comfort, you can write to Women for Sobriety (see Resources, p. 452) for information on whether more secular practices are available in your community.

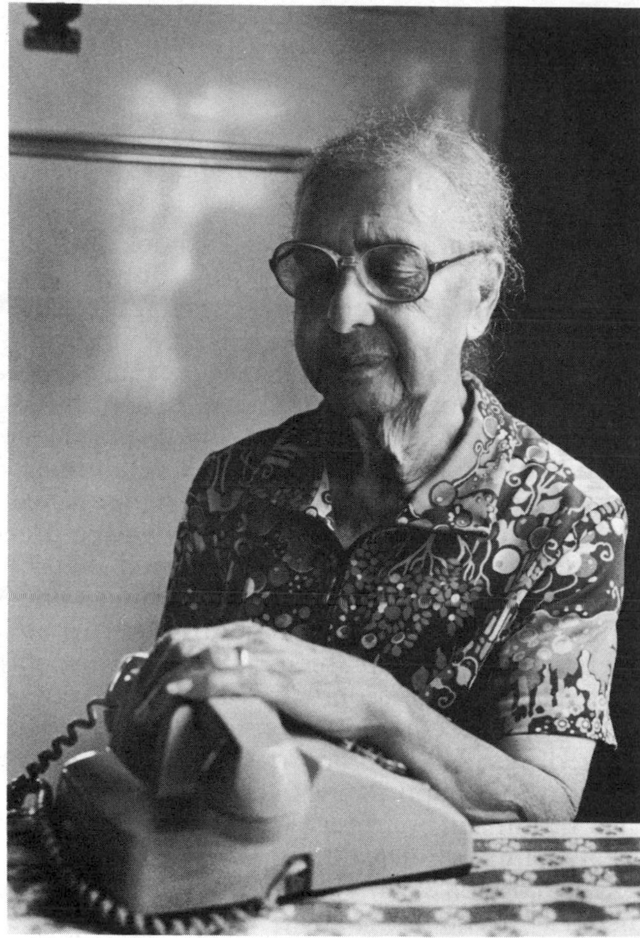

Norma Holt

lems all by ourselves is misplaced. We can become what has been called a coalcoholic or para-alcoholic, exhibiting the same denial, guilt, and blame as the alcoholic. The responsibility for alcoholism should rest squarely on the alcoholic—where it belongs. Even after many years of unhappy marriages and other close relationships with alcoholics, women have been able, through Al-Anon and other organizations, to reconstruct their own lives.

Over-the-Counter and Prescription Drugs

Though persons over the age of sixty-five constitute 13 percent of the total population, they take 30 percent of all the prescription drugs dispensed in the United States.[21] More than 240,000 people ages sixty and over are admitted to hospitals yearly because of adverse reactions to prescription and over-the-counter (OTC) drugs. This is 50 percent more than the number of emergency-room visits caused by street drugs.[22] In the United States in 1992, consumers spent an estimated $50.5 billion on prescription drugs and more than $12.8 billion on over-the-counter products.[23] Many of these drugs may be needed, even lifesaving, but many are not. Often old prescriptions are not reevaluated for continued need and for interactions with new prescriptions and with OTC preparations. *Polypharmacy* is the term used to describe taking too many, or excessive amounts of, drugs at a time. It is common among older women who may be given prescriptions by several physicians for different conditions.

Drug companies, in business for profit, have offered new drugs to the market while sometimes failing to report adverse and life-threatening reactions to these drugs.[24] The U.S. Food and Drug Administration continues to permit drugs on the market that later prove harmful and have to be withdrawn. Do not agree to use a drug that has been on the market for less than four years unless you are willing to be part of an experiment.

Harmful effects from drug interactions are too numerous to list here, so always inform your physician of everything you are using (prescriptions, OTC drugs, and vitamin supplements) and always double-check with your pharmacist. OTC drugs and vitamins, herbs, and supplements from health-food stores can be just as potent and dangerous as prescription drugs. Do not take leftover or other people's medicines.

Most drug dosages should be adjusted to the size and age of the person taking the drug. Women at any age may require lower drug dosages than men because of women's lower body weight and mass. We become even more sensitive to drugs over time because, as we age, drugs are metabolized more slowly, the kidneys and the liver excrete them more slowly, and so they remain in the body longer. Also as we age, some muscle mass turns to fat, so many drugs that can be stored in fat tissue, such as Valium, stay in the body a longer time, increasing the likelihood of harmful effects or addiction even from low, infrequent doses. Drug companies have started testing the effects of drugs on older people but still do not always distinguish the more severe effects of drugs on people over the age of seventy from the effects on the whole group over fifty. Drugs may be harmful or may be taken in too high doses if individual adjustments and frequent reevaluations are not made.

One study of older persons admitted to a state mental hospital found that 15 percent were actually suffering from drug toxicities rather than from dementia or other mental illness.[25]

Over half the adult women in this country have used tranquilizers, sedatives, and amphetamines (stimulants often used in "diet pills"). These drugs are legally available and are the most commonly abused classes of drugs among older women. The practice of some physicians freely to write prescriptions for these types of controlled drugs has declined in those states that require monitoring of physicians' prescription-writing habits. This policy of monitoring, with the penalty of withdrawing medical licensure for physicians who overprescribe these drugs, should be adopted in all states.

Since these drugs tend to be chemically and emotionally addictive and don't cure anything by themselves, they seem to be a nonproductive treatment for stress or fatigue. Their use is an attempt to treat medically what is really a social problem—the stress and isolation of many older women's lives. Taken in combination with alcohol, they can cause permanent damage, even death. Still, millions of dollars are devoted to promoting tranquilizers as the solution to women's depression and anxiety; and too many doctors who recommend exercise for men under stress prescribe drugs to their female patients with the same symptoms.

We do not know the long-term effects of illegal recreational drugs. We do know that sharing needles can lead to HIV infection. We know that marijuana can damage the respiratory system and that cocaine is addictive and can cause sudden death through its action on the heart. The continued use of such substances will compound the health problems of future generations of older women who started using such drugs when they were young.

Some physicians do not realize how they help to create drug problems. When women ask them for help with complaints, many doctors are apt to treat the symptom rather than to probe a little deeper to find the source of the complaint.

On my frequent trips to my family doctor for treatment of recurring bouts of bronchitis, he did not seem to attach significance to the facts that I was putting on weight, that my blood pressure had begun to rise, and that I was generally sluggish. I told the doctor that I was having trouble sleeping so he gave me a prescription for some sleeping pills, and told me to cut back on my activities a little. He knew I had an alcohol problem but he never asked if I was drinking more than usual. He never asked me to check back with him after I had tried the pills. [a fifty-one-year-old woman]

This woman might have died from the combination of pills and alcohol in her system.

It is imperative that medical schools include more courses on alcohol, drug abuse, and related illnesses. Pharmacists need more legal power to write warnings on bottles and to caution their customers. Despite the fact that these addictions are national problems with enormous impact on the public, only a few medical schools teach their students anything at all about them. Physicians often assume we do not feel satisfied with our visit unless we come away with a prescription. One study, however, showed that 72 percent of the patients surveyed preferred a non-drug remedy when it and a drug were both offered and fully explained.[26] We might benefit more from explanations, answers to our questions, support, and sound practical advice than from drugs. Unfortunately, training of physicians in these approaches is even weaker than their training in pharmacology.

It is important to know what the drugs we take can do for us and to us. Antihistamines, for instance, frequently cause drowsiness. Some other cold medicines contain drugs to clear stuffy noses (vasoconstrictors), which may make you feel jumpy, and caffeine to keep you active when you probably should be resting in bed. Most liquid cold preparations and mouthwashes contain alcohol; many preparations and vitamins contain sugar. Be forewarned: the advertising for many products never mentions that the drugs they contain could cause problems, dependency, or undesirable interactions with other drugs.

When considering any medication, consult your health-care provider and your pharmacist. Bring a list of all the prescription and nonprescription preparations you are using. Report any allergies or reactions to medications you have suffered in the past. Seek the answers to the following questions.[27]

1. What are the brand name and the scientific (generic) name of the medication and what is it supposed to do?
2. How do I store it and take it, and for how long? What should I do if I miss a dose?
3. What foods, drinks, other medicines, and activities should I avoid while taking this medicine? What do I especially need?

4. What other effects might I have while taking this drug, and what should I do if they occur?
5. Is there any written information available about this medicine?

If you decide to take a medication, save money by requesting the generic drug. Find out as much as you can so you can take the medication in the most beneficial way. Do not, for example, crush a coated tablet, for the coating has been put on to protect you or to improve the drug's absorption.

Two common problems for which too many women habitually use harmful drugs are insomnia and constipation. Both are better dealt with by nonpharmaceutical methods.

DEALING WITH INSOMNIA

Some changes in sleep patterns may occur as we get older but at any age we need adequate, deep sleep for good health. Do not assume you have a problem just because you get less sleep than you used to. Judge by how you feel, not just by the number of hours you sleep. Some women have problems falling asleep; others may readily fall asleep, but wake up after only a few hours and have trouble going back to sleep. There are many things we can do to sleep better.

Worries and depression can cause sleeplessness. Many women will focus on the sleeplessness rather than on the causes of the worries and depression. If you seek and find the right kind of help for the underlying cause of the problem, you may be able to sleep better. Labeling the problems as insomnia will not solve either the problems or the insomnia, and may make it worse by starting a cycle in which you go to bed each night worrying about whether your "insomnia" will keep you awake.

Many activities can interfere with sleep. Among them are eating late at night (especially sugar); having unsuspected caffeine in soft drinks, cocoa and chocolate, and tea; taking vitamin B or C before bed; not getting enough protein in your diet.

Drugs are a common cause of sleep problems. Caffeine is not the only one. The complete list of prescription and over-the-counter drugs that interfere with sleep is too long to include here. Just a few are: nicotine in cigarettes; pain relievers and cold remedies that contain caffeine or antihistamines; appetite suppressants; decongestants; drugs for asthma, high blood pressure, and heart rhythm and thyroid problems; and many others. Antihistamines (contained in cold remedies and over-the-counter sleeping pills) and alcohol cause drowsiness initially but interfere with later sleep and can cause early awakening. The insomnia caused by certain conditions such as an overactive thyroid will be relieved when treated appropriately—not by sleeping pills.

Changes in our internal clocks may affect our sleep patterns as we age but can be readjusted. If you fall asleep at 8 or 9 P.M. and wake up at 3 or 4 A.M., try to increase your exposure to very bright light in the early evening. If you can't get to sleep until late at night, you may benefit by exposure to light in the morning.[28]

Medications formulated to help you sleep, including sleeping pills, tranquilizers, and antianxiety drugs, can cause sleeplessness after their use is discontinued. They can also be addictive. Sleeping pills may make older people less alert, aggravate memory loss, and have other adverse effects, all of which may be confused with dementia. Their use increases the likelihood of falls, and resultant broken hips or other broken bones. Chloral hydrate, commonly prescribed, interferes with rapid eye movement sleep (REM, the time when we dream), which is vital for mental health. While you might choose to use sleeping pills for a few nights in some special situation, you should be especially cautious as you get older. Smaller-than-usual doses will probably suffice.

Sleeping pills slow down respiratory function in some people and are particularly dangerous for people with sleep apnea (the sudden cessation of breathing during sleep) or heavy snoring. Sleep apnea may occur from a few times to several hundred times a night with or without heavy snoring. If your bed partner or roommate tells you that your breathing seems to stop during sleep, you should seek medical advice, preferably at a hospital sleep center, because this behavior often signals a more serious problem.

To deal with sleeplessness:

- Try to go to sleep and arise at regular hours in whatever pattern suits you best. You may want to avoid daytime naps in order to sleep more hours at night, or you may feel better sleeping fewer hours at night and taking a daytime nap.
- Exercise during the day, not just before bed.
- Soak in a hot tub before bed. Our skin gets drier as we age. After the bath, lubricate your

skin. People with diabetes should use powder rather than lotion after drying well between the toes.

- Don't go to bed hungry but avoid eating a huge meal before bed. Being too full may disturb sleep. Try milk before bed, warm if you like, or soporific herbal teas.
- Try relaxation techniques. If something is on your mind, make a note to deal with the problem the next day and then try to forget it.
- Make your surroundings as comfortable as possible, including the bed, temperature and humidity, sound and light.
- Develop the association between bed and sleep. Follow the same rituals every night before going to bed. Do not read or write in bed. If you cannot sleep, get out of bed and go back later.
- Keep a journal of your sleep patterns to help you identify problems and the success of changes you try.

I have a tape of the sound of ocean waves on a cassette by my bed. If I wake up in the middle of the night, I reach over and turn on the tape. It seems to crowd out distracting thoughts and lulls me back to sleep. [a fifty-five-year-old woman]

Dealing with Constipation

Laxatives are another commonly overused medication. Many of us were taught that we were supposed to have a bowel movement each and every day. In fact, though two thirds of the women in a survey claimed one bowel movement per day, the normal variation was between three times a day and twice a week.[29] Consider yourself constipated only if your customary pattern changes or if you have hard, difficult-to-pass stools.

Changes in diet can alleviate constipation. White flour products with or without sugar are the most common culprit. Add more natural fiber by eating plenty of vegetables, fruit, and whole grains as well as breads and cereals that contain bran. Drink six to eight glasses of fluid each day, more on very hot days or if you are sweating heavily from work or exercise. Fresh fruit and fruit juices, especially prune juice, can have a laxative effect. Additional fluids are necessary if you add bran to your diet in order to prevent the stool from becoming too bulky and hard. Large amounts of caffeine usually cause diarrhea, but in some women may cause constipation. Withdrawing from coffee may also cause constipation temporarily.

Activity is needed to keep the bowels active. A little exercise each day, especially walking, does wonders. Exercise also alleviates stress, anxiety, and depression, which can all cause constipation. Strengthening weak abdominal and pelvic muscles can help elimination. It is particularly important to keep the stool soft if you have a weakening in the wall of the rectum (a rectocele) in which the feces can collect.

Many women become constipated because they are too busy to take time in the bathroom. They may "hold it" too long, just as they hold urine too long, losing awareness of their need to "go." (See Urinary Incontinence chapter.) Go to the toilet at regular times but do not strain. Holding the breath while pushing can raise blood pressure. If you can't move your bowels, relax and try later.

Common medications and vitamins can affect bowel movements. For example, magnesium-aluminum antacids are the most effective for persons who suffer from gas and other problems that might be relieved by an antacid. However, milk of magnesia can cause diarrhea, so the aluminum is added to counteract it.[30] Aluminum antacids interfere with the absorption of calcium. Iron supplements often cause constipation. Taking vitamin C increases the absorption of the iron and also helps alleviate the constipation. Many other drugs, especially painkillers, slow down the bowels.

One of the most common causes of chronic constipation is the use of laxatives. The body can become habituated to the laxatives and lose the ability to function normally without them. Laxatives also interfere with the body's absorption of vitamins, minerals, and many medications. If you are used to laxatives, try tapering off gradually while improving your eating habits and exercising regularly.

While you are tapering off, use the type of laxative most suitable for your problems. Read the labels so you will know what you are taking. Bulk laxatives (such as psyllium seed) add bulk to the stool. Lubricants (such as docusate sodium) encourage water to enter the stool, thereby increasing its bulk and softness. Salt laxatives (such as milk of magnesia) also hold water, making the stool softer and bulkier, but are not recommended for those on low-salt diets. Irritant drugs (such as castor oil or senna) stimulate the intestinal nerves, thus increasing bowel activity. Glycerin suppositories stimulate the bowel muscle and lubricate the stool already in the rectum. Mineral oil helps lubricate stools higher in the intestines but prevents absorption of many needed nutrients. If it is necessary to use mineral oil, take it at 6 A.M. and take a supplement of fat-soluble vitamins (vitamins A, D, E, and K) at 6 P.M. A combination of unsweetened applesauce, bran, and prune juice might be just as effective as, and less harmful than, commercial laxatives.[31]

Dealing with Pain

Many people overuse and misuse pain medication. They may become addicted to pain medication and continue its use long after the pain has stopped. Others suffer needlessly from pain because they fear reliance on medication, or addiction. Our instinct to pull away from something painful—such as a hot stove—has great survival value. Pain can be a signal to protect ourselves or a warning for us to pay attention. Ignoring pain can put us in great danger, and even cause death. People vary in how they interpret and tolerate pain signals, and there are as yet few ways to measure how much pain people feel. Understanding our bodies will help us know when to seek help.

We have to cope not only with pain, but with what the pain means to us—usually our fear of what we think might be causing the pain, or fear that the pain will not end. Sometimes we ignore pain that could easily be helped because we fear a more serious cause. Stress and pain have a close relationship. It's easy to understand that being in pain stresses us. But stress can also cause or intensify pain. When pain does not have a clear-cut cause or, worse, is interpreted as signaling a dangerous illness, it can feel more intense. Factors such as tension or tightening up, anxiety, depression, and fatigue can modulate the pain threshold.

There are many pains for which no specific cause can be found, or for which there is no single effective cure. That does not mean that our pain is imaginary or should be dismissed. Unfortunately, many doctors believe that much of women's pain is imaginary or a device for getting attention. All pain is real. We should not be told that we must just learn to live with pain; we should be given specific suggestions.

Traditional healing methods, many from Eastern medicine and philosophy, approach pain as if it were blocked energy. The practitioner of such methods should be our partner in exploring the possible connections between our present pain and our entire life-style—day-to-day habits of eating, exercise, emotional patterns, social relationships, occupation, creative and spiritual connections—as well as possible disease. We can learn to use deep breathing and relaxation exercises to control and manage pain. Some of us have used the techniques learned in childbirth classes throughout our lives. Techniques such as relaxation, meditation, massage, yoga, and acupuncture are helpful for managing pain. Although these techniques seem to work particularly well with chronic pain (pain lasting more than six months), they can also help us with acute pain. In a situation of acute, even life-threatening, pain that requires immediate emergency medical care, such as a heart attack, techniques learned from relaxation, meditation, and self-hypnosis can help us avoid panic and cope with pain.

Physicians need to be reminded that to manage pain and relieve suffering is at the core of a health-care provider's commitment. Yet many of them believe the myths that pain is part of normal aging and that old people don't feel pain as much as young people. As usual, most studies of painkillers have excluded anyone over the age of sixty-five.[32]

But Western medicine is beginning to combine Eastern mind-body concepts with modern technology to develop techniques—such as biofeedback—that can be useful in pain control. Other new methods include TENS and PCA. TENS (transcutaneous electrical nerve stimulation) sends measured pulses of electric current to the pain sites through electrodes attached to the skin, providing significant but temporary relief for up to 70 percent of the users. Some researchers think TENS causes the body to release natural opiates called endorphins; others think it interferes with the transmission of pain signals. Patient-controlled analgesia (PCA) is an innovation that provides individualized pain control. This technique utilizes a device that permits the intravenous self-administration of narcotic drugs within limits of dose and frequency established with the physician.

Pain clinics, which now exist in many cities, focus on the whole person and may use both Western and traditional techniques appropriate to the individual. As one client in a pain-relief clinic said, "It's a relief to be treated as a person, instead of as a hip problem." This approach, which should be used by all health-care providers, invites us to be more active on our own behalf, befriending those parts of us that have hurt for so long that we may have given up on them—our bum knees, miserable back, aching head.

I've changed my attitude toward pain. I don't think of my foot that's hurting as a separate, bad part of me—something to be angry at. I now try to take a more caregiving approach, to see what kind of special attention it wants. I massage my feet and calves every night. The trouble with having the doctor be the only one who can fix you is that, if he can't do it, then you're a goner. It's good I've found some things I can do for myself to help myself feel better. [a thirty-five-year-old woman]

Once we adopt a body-befriending approach to pain management, we can create many self-help techniques. There are many things that alleviate pain, such as exhaling or panting rather than holding the breath while we do physical work, thinking about something else more pleasant while the dentist drills, stopping negative self-talk, soothing painful areas with Therapeutic Touch (see *Sharing Touch—Massage,* p. 16). Many others are well known: taking a hot bath or a cold shower, taking a walk, distracting ourselves by doing some favorite thing. It's difficult to feel depressed when we are singing or to feel anxious while we are taking slow, deep breaths.

There are many painkilling drugs, including aspirin, acetaminophen, acetophenetidin, codeine, and morphine. All pain-relieving drugs have undesirable and potentially harmful effects. They may cloud our consciousness at the very time when we might wish to get as much out of life as possible.

On the other hand, many of us are so fearful of pain medication that we deprive ourselves of comfort and help when we could most use it. Pain is very tiring; pain can use up the energy we need for caring for ourselves and managing the condition causing the pain. Many times a moderate and careful use of pain medication can help us have the strength we need for dealing with the cause. Using the nondrug pain-relief methods already described can reduce our need for medication. Smaller, more frequent doses of pain medication may keep us comfortable and result in the use of less medication than if we wait until the pain becomes so severe that we need massive doses to feel relief. Avoid drugs or combinations of pain-relieving drugs that make you sleepy without reducing pain.[33]

When faced with severe pain, we should be able to choose the extent of pain relief that suits us. Each woman has her own level of pain tolerance. When death is imminent, we need not fear addiction. Especially at that time we should be able to remain in control and be able to choose among all options.

Notes

1. U.S. Office of the Assistant Secretary for Health and Surgeon General, *The Health Consequences of Smoking: The Changing Cigarette. A Report of the Surgeon General.* Rockville, MD: U.S. Department of Health and Human Services, Public Health Service, 1981.
2. G. H. Miller and D. R. Gerstein, "The Life Expectancy of Nonsmoking Men and Women." *Public Health Reports,* Vol. 98, 1983, pp. 343–49, quoted in Jonathan E. Fielding, "Smoking: Health Effects and Control," *The New England Journal of Medicine,* Vol. 313, No. 8 (Aug. 22, 1985), p. 491.
3. American Cancer Society, *1985 Cancer Facts and Figures,* p. 9. Still true in 1992.
4. Massachusetts Department of Public Health/ Massachusetts Hospital Association brochure, "Are You Really a Non-Smoker?"
5. American Cancer Society, op. cit., p. 17.
6. Miller and Gerstein, op. cit.
7. Millicent W. Higgins, et al., "Smoking and Lung Function in Elderly Men and Women: The Cardiovascular Health Study." *Journal of the American Medical Association,* Vol. 269, No. 21 (June 2, 1993), pp. 2741–48; Thomas L. Petty, "Editorial," same issue, p. 2785.
8. David F. Williamson, et al., "Smoking Cessation and Severity of Weight Gain in a National Cohort." *The New England Journal of Medicine,* Vol. 324, No. 11 (Mar. 4, 1991), pp. 739–45; "Editorial," same issue, pp. 768–69.
9. Paul Raeburn, "Caffeine Tied to Panic Attacks in Over 2 Million People." Associated Press, printed in *The Boston Globe,* Oct. 19, 1986, p. 23.
10. Frances Sheridan Goulart, *The Caffeine Book: A User's and Abuser's Guide.* New York: Dodd, Mead and Co., 1984. Thorough coverage of health effects of caffeine-containing foods and beverages.
11. Hershel Jick, et al., "Coffee and Myocardial Infarction: A Report from the Boston Collaborative Drug Surveillance Project." *The New England Journal of Medicine,* Vol. 289, No. 2 (July 12, 1973), pp. 63–67.
12. Goulart, op. cit.
13. Barbara Gordon, *I'm Dancing as Fast as I Can.* New York: Harper & Row, 1979, pp. 304–5.
14. *Alcohol Abuse and Misuse Among the Elderly.* Select Committee on Aging. U.S. House of Representatives, February 1992. Comm. Pub. No. 102-852, available from the U.S. Government Printing Office, Washington, DC.
15. *Report on the White House Mini-Conference on Older Women,* Alcoholism and Drug Abuse Section, 1980, p. 36.
16. Jacob A. Brody, "Aging and Alcohol Abuse," in *Nature and Extent of Alcohol Problems Among the Elderly.*

Presented at the White House Conference on Aging, Washington, DC, 1981, p. 305.

17. Norma Finkelstein, et al., *Getting Sober, Getting Well: A Treatment Guide for Caregivers Who Work with Women.* Available from The Women's Program of CASPAR, Inc., 6 Camelia Ave., Cambridge, MA 02139. Tel. (617) 661-1316.

18. Jonica D. Homiller, *Women and Alcohol: A Guide for State and Local Decision Makers.* Washington, DC: The Council of State Authorities, Alcohol and Drug Problems Association of North America, 1977, p. 15.

19. Nancy Taylor, *Alcohol Abuse Prevention Among Women: A Community Approach.* Presented at the National Council on Alcoholism, Washington, DC, 1982, p. 1.

20. Alvin Rosen, "Psychotherapy and Alcoholics Anonymous. Can They Be Coordinated?" *Bulletin of the Menninger Clinic,* Vol. 45, No. 3 (1981), pp. 229–46.

21. "Treatment of Sleep Disorders." NIH Consensus Development Conference *Consensus Statement,* Vol. 8, No. 3 (Mar. 26–29, 1990), p. 2.

22. Judy Foreman, "The 'Other' Drug Problem in Our Society." *The Boston Globe,* Dec. 28, 1992, pp. 25–26.

23. Figures from the Pharmaceutical Manufacturers Association and the Nonprescription Drug Manufacturers Association.

24. "Prescription Drug Pushers" and "Five Dangerous Drugs." *Health Letter,* Vol. 3 (July–August 1986), pp. 1, 12.

25. "Report of the Public Health Service Task Force on Women's Health Issues." *Public Health Reports,* Vol. 100, No. 1 (January–February 1985), p. 96.

26. Gail Povar, et al., "Patients' Therapeutic Preferences in an Ambulatory Care Setting." *American Journal of Public Health,* Vol. 74, No. 12 (December 1984), pp. 1395–97.

27. Adapted from the National Council on Patient Information and Education.

28. Judy Foreman, "Trouble Sleeping? In Later Years Our Internal Clocks Change." *The Boston Globe,* Apr. 26, 1993, pp. 39, 44.

29. Marie Feltin, *A Woman's Guide to Good Health After 50.* An AARP Book. Glenview, IL: Scott, Foresman and Company, 1987, p. 174.

30. "Gas, Heartburn and Antacids." *Living Healthy,* Vol. 3, No. 3 (August 1980), pp. 1–12.

31. Combine 1 cup unsweetened applesauce, 1 cup unprocessed wheat bran, and ½ cup prune juice (100 percent juice). Mix into a pasty consistency and refrigerate in a covered container. Take 2 tablespoons at bedtime with a glass of water or juice. If constipation is severe, increase gradually up to 3 tablespoons twice a day, morning and evening. Be patient. It may take six weeks to reestablish good bowel function. From R. Behm, "A Special Recipe to Banish Constipation," *Geriatric Nursing,* Vol. 6, No. 4 (1985), pp. 216–17. Quoted in Diana A. Smith and Diane K. Newman, "Beating the Cycle of Constipation, Laxative Abuse, and Fecal Incontinence." *TNH,* September 1989, pp. 12–13.

32. *Acute Pain Management: Operative or Medical Procedures and Trauma. Clinical Practice Guideline.* AHCPR Pub. No. 92-0032. See Agency for Health Care Policy and Research on page 482.

33. Kathleen M. Foley, "The Treatment of Cancer Pain." *The New England Journal of Medicine,* Vol. 313, No. 2 (July 11, 1985), pp. 84–95.

3

OUR LOOKS AND OUR LIVES

✦

BY JANE HYMAN

1994 UPDATE OF *COSMETIC SURGERY* BY PAULA B. DORESS-WORTERS WITH SPECIAL THANKS TO JANE SPRAGUE ZONES

RESOURCES FOR THIS CHAPTER ON PAGE 454

HERSTORY—IN A PLATE

Her face reminds me of my
grandmother's antique plate—
cracked with fine-lined patterns
of living.
I can see either the beauty or the imperfection—
Usually I see the beauty,
except when she irritates me, or my
fears of my own mortality block my vision.
We are both—mortal and perfect—
beautiful and imperfect—
a crazed pattern of sanity
in a cracked world—
a throwback to another time,
and a vision yet
to be.

Molly Smith Strong

As we get older, we have to come to terms with our changing appearance and others' reactions to it. We wrinkle, our hair turns gray, and our body weight changes and is redistributed. Chronic diseases or disabling conditions can also affect the way we see our bodies. Such challenges require fresh sources of strength and a reassessment of our interests, abilities, and needs.

LOOKING OLDER—WHAT IT MEANS TO US

Those of us who grew up knowing and loving our grandparents or other older people probably remember loving their wrinkled faces. In the years before we learned to think of the signs of aging as "unattractive," a wrinkled face was often the most loving and the most beloved face we knew. However, as adults, we live in an environment in which standards of beauty are important, narrow, and restricted to the young.

I have no passion to look eighteen forever, but I still have vanity. I rather hate looking at that reticulated network of wrinkles that looks like downtown Schenectady traffic—but there it is! What can you do about it? [a sixty-nine-year-old woman]

Looking older can be hard on us, since as women we are raised to please others rather than ourselves, and to value ourselves by how pleasing we are to others. This makes us especially vulnerable to the idea that through makeup, hair dyes, face lifts, diets, and clothes we can—and must—live up to a certain ideal of beauty. Many of us were very hard on ourselves in our younger years, not beginning to accept or like

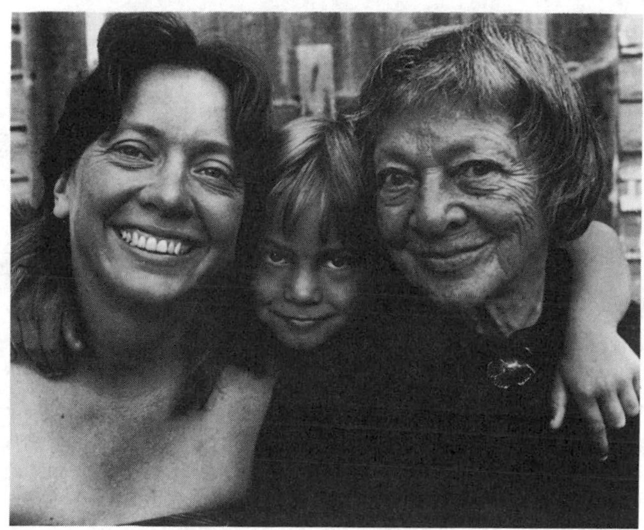

Marianne Gontarz

our faces or bodies until we were in our late thirties or early forties. We may have hardly overcome early prejudices against ourselves—hips too large, nose too small—when we are faced with another: ageism.

When I was thirty-eight I looked at my naked body in the mirror, and for the first time in my life thought, "Gee, nice!" And then I started aging. [a fifty-two-year-old woman]

The quest for physical perfection may be taken more seriously by women in the United States than by women in other countries. America is a young and powerful country and it admires the young and powerful. The message is that we only count if we are white, slender, attractive, able-bodied—and young. For some women, especially in midlife, this narrow standard of acceptability leads to a period of grieving over the loss of "peak" years. Barbara Macdonald, at age sixty-nine, coauthor of a book on ageism, reflects on her own aging:

Sometimes lately . . . I see my arm with the skin hanging loosely from my forearm and cannot believe that it is really my own. It seems disconnected from me; it is someone else's. It is the arm of an old woman. It is the arm of such old women as I myself have seen, sitting on benches in the sun with their hands folded in their laps; old women I have turned away from. I wonder now how and when these arms I see came to be my own—arms I cannot turn away from.[1]

Middle-aged men are a possible exception to the generally narrow standard of looks. According to one study, they are considered even more attractive than young men. This same study showed that middle-aged women are considered less attractive than young women, and that old men and women are both considered less attractive than the young or middle-aged. Some researchers think that middle-aged men gain in attractiveness because others see them as being at the peak of success in their social roles. Conversely, middle-aged women, seen primarily as mothers, are considered to be past their social usefulness because they are no longer bearers of children.[2] If looks are associated with usefulness and power, it may be that the looks of old age are considered unattractive because the elderly are seen as useless and powerless. As middle-aged and older women become more powerful, others may see them as more attractive. We may see ourselves as more attractive as well.

Sometimes I think of the alternatives to looking older, and I wonder what it would be like to have my face frozen the way it was in my thirties, and I think—that would be ridiculous! That's not me, that doesn't reflect the years I've lived and all the things I've experienced. I don't want to deny my experiences and I feel that if I dislike my aging looks I'm denying all the wonderful parts of my life. I don't want to do that. [a forty-eight-year-old woman]

Women's responses to looking older vary greatly. Women who grew up in warmly affectionate families where they were hugged, kissed, and cuddled, for example, tend to accept their bodies as they are. There are indications that women whose families provided opportunities for physical activity or who were athletes in high school and college feel more positive about their looks than women without such experiences.[3] In general, warm, close family relationships and physical activity foster self-confidence and high self-esteem. When self-esteem is high, body image is often positive. Considering the importance of athletics and self-esteem, it is no surprise that studies show that men (always encouraged to participate in sports) *over*rate their body image, thinking that others have a higher opinion of their looks than they actually do, while women *under*rate their body image, thinking others have a lower opinion of their looks than they do.[4]

If you were considered unusually attractive as a younger woman, looking older may be more difficult for you than for a woman who never set great store by her looks. A woman who is constantly praised for being pretty may come to

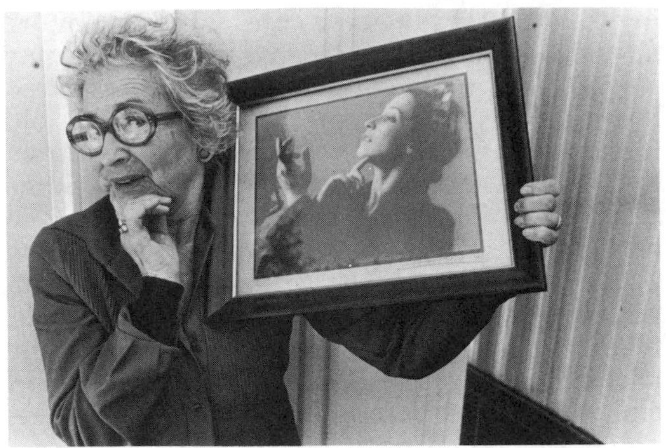

Marianne Gontarz

believe that her worth as a person depends on her looks. A woman who never considered herself pretty, however, has already dealt with that issue and gone beyond it.

Women who are concerned about looking older seem to experience this concern during midlife up to their middle or late sixties. In fact, many women in midlife like *getting* older; they feel freer and more confident. What they don't like is *looking* older.[5]

I'm forty-three now and this whole past year I've felt a sense of getting older which I never did before. When I look in the mirror, I don't like what I see, so I don't look at myself. When I go someplace I try to forget about what I look like, and that isn't the way it used to be. I used to think, "Today I look good!"

In later years, this concern tends to disappear. It seems that the anticipation of looking older is more distressing than the actual experience. Perhaps with the years we learn to place greater value on our inner qualities. Also our own or our partner's health and energy become more important, and losses or other concerns can become paramount.[6]

Body changes as a result of health problems can also cause a temporary or permanent difference in the way we see ourselves. Skin diseases, scaly dryness or chapping of the skin, a stoop due to osteoporosis, and swelling of the joints as a result of arthritis are all visible changes.

I am trying to recognize that my hands are indeed a part of me, and a part of me that I love. Because I do a great deal with my hands, of course, and they are very capable despite the fact that they have these configurations [arthritic swelling]. And I realize that I have indeed been taken in by what a woman's hands should look like, and mostly they're supposed to look pretty useless. My hands don't look useless at all. In fact they look as though they've been used a great deal. [a sixty-four-year-old woman]

Appliances such as a hearing aid, pacemaker, cane, or walker can change our body image, especially when we first begin to wear or use them. They often seem much larger and more conspicuous to us than to anyone else. The effects of drugs, scars or a limp from operations or accidents, and amputated limbs or organs can profoundly influence our body image. Integrating such changes into our self-image is an important factor in feeling whole again despite the loss.

In a bathing suit I'm not so hot because there is a huge gouge where one hip was taken out, and the incision got infected. That is hard for small children to have to look at so I wear very matronly bathing suits. So my image of myself as a sexy-looking woman went, and I decided to be quaint—a quaint old lady. [a sixty-nine-year-old woman]

As we grow older we may become slightly shorter due to the gradual drying of the discs of the spine or compression fractures caused by osteoporosis. Otherwise, most of the visible changes associated with age occur in the skin, hair, and underlying muscles and fatty tissue.

Since the skin is susceptible to influences from inside and outside the body, it is hard to distinguish between "normal" signs of aging and those caused by unhealthful habits such as smoking, and environmental damage such as overexposure to sunlight. Skin changes that normally occur with time can be accelerated by smoking and by exposure to the elements, especially radiation from the sun. Black and olive-skinned women experience a slower rate of change with age, partly because of the larger amounts of melanin (pigment) in their skin. All women can protect themselves against skin damage and skin cancer by avoiding tanning and sunburning.*

Skin cells grow more slowly with age, and the outer layer of skin is not shed and replaced at the same rate as in younger years. Changes in a protein called collagen make the skin stiffer and less pliable, and some sebaceous glands that provide oil for the hair and skin become less active.

*See pages 61–62 and 283 on need for obtaining vitamin D from sunlight.

With age, cells lose some of their ability to retain water, causing dryness. Some women relieve dryness and itching by patting themselves dry after washing, and applying cream or oil while the skin is still moist. It can also help to bathe less often and to use only a mild or creamy soap or no soap at all on trouble areas.

As the skin loses tone and elasticity it sags and wrinkles, especially in areas where there is frequent movement, such as the face, neck, and joints. Sagging is also caused by the pull of gravity over the years. The underlying muscles and fatty tissue undergo similar changes. Small blood vessels become more fragile due to thinning of the vessel walls, and can cause frequent black-and-blue marks. "Age spots" (also called "liver spots") may appear. They would be more appropriately called sun spots, since they are caused by exposure to sunlight over the years. Hair becomes thinner as hair follicles decrease their activity, and grayer as cells stop producing a color-determining pigment. These gradual changes are a part of the cycle of life, and everyone who lives long enough will experience some of them.

How Weight Influences the Way We See Ourselves

As we grow older, many of us tend to gain weight. Since our metabolism slows down, our bodies need fewer calories, yet we often consume the same amount of food as in our younger years (see Weighty Issues chapter). Many of us get less exercise or have disabling conditions that keep us sedentary. Weight gain in our older years can be particularly hard to accept because we are also trying to come to terms with other changes in our bodies.

I went to Weight Watchers and lost eight pounds. But I gained them right back. Then last summer I fractured my shoulder. I was home a lot. It was a terribly hot summer. The only exercise I got was a little walk every day. That walk always included a stop at the ice cream parlor. Now I look in the mirror and I say: "You are fat!" and I don't like it. [a seventy-three-year-old woman]

Studies have shown that the value placed on thinness in advertising has a strong impact on us. Many women live in constant fear of gaining

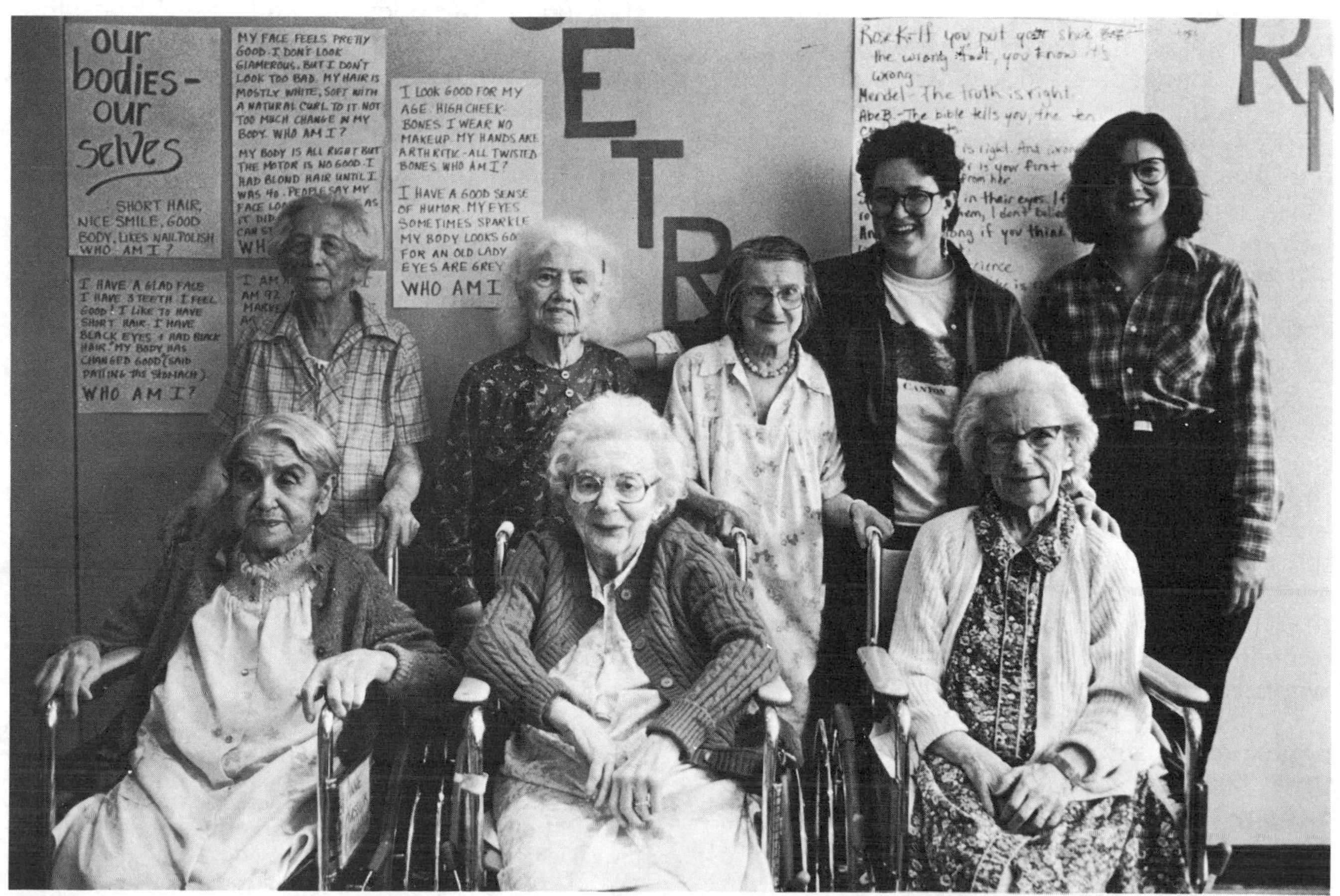
our bodies - our selves
SHORT HAIR, NICE SMILE, GOOD BODY, LIKES NAIL POLISH WHO AM I?
MY FACE FEELS PRETTY GOOD. I DON'T LOOK GLAMEROUS. BUT I DON'T LOOK TOO BAD. MY HAIR IS MOSTLY WHITE, SOFT WITH A NATURAL CURL TO IT. NOT TOO MUCH CHANGE IN MY BODY. WHO AM I?
I LOOK GOOD FOR MY AGE. HIGH CHEEK BONES. I WEAR NO MAKEUP. MY HANDS ARE ARTHRITIC - ALL TWISTED BONES. WHO AM I?
I HAVE A GOOD SENSE OF HUMOR. MY EYES SOMETIMES SPARKLE
WHO AM I
I HAVE A GLAD FACE I HAVE 3 TEETH. I FEEL GOOD! I LIKE TO HAVE SHORT HAIR. I HAVE BLACK EYES + HAD BLACK HAIR. "MY BODY HAS CHANGED GOOD" (SAID PATTING THE STOMACH).
WHO AM I?

Marianne Gontarz with Sandra Hassett, Recreational Therapist/Hebrew Rehabilitation Center for Aged

another pound. We tend to see ourselves as overweight even when we are within what is generally considered a desirable weight range. Women want to be even thinner than men want them to be.[7] The influence of advertising is also evident in the growing incidence of eating disorders such as anorexia and bulimia in middle-aged women.[8]

It isn't easy to fight the effects of advertising single-handedly. Through body-image workshops, reading, or exercise, we can make our image of ourselves more positive. It is worth trying to accept our size rather than using our energy disliking our bodies and going on unnecessary diets.

When I swim or walk regularly I feel stronger and more energetic and my body is more limber. My weight stays the same but people say to me, "You've lost weight!" as if only pounds mattered. [a fifty-three-year-old woman]

Some women think that if they learn to accept and love their bodies they will just eat everything and gain more weight. Only punishment through diet can work, they believe. But, in fact, many women have found that if you punish your body you cannot lead it to a positive, healthy state. "You have to love your body *before* you can change it—if indeed you wish to change it once you love it."[9]

Belly dancing is an example of an exercise only weighty women can do well. The movements make you feel sensuous, not heavy. Belly dancers love their bellies, have fun "throwing their weight around," and benefit from the exercise.

The "Beauty" Business

As they grow older, many women attempt to mask or alter their physical appearance. Even the poorest women spend money on cosmetics and beauty parlors. Some of us wear makeup, or more of it, and dye our hair. According to one survey, most women who color their hair do so to cover the gray. This is most common among women in their forties and fifties, 45 percent of whom dye their hair.[10]

It is hard to resist the temptation to alter our appearances, since in every store we see bottles, tubes, and jars containing cosmetics advertised to make us more attractive and younger-looking. The cosmetics industry makes millions of dollars by reinforcing the message that we need not, dare not, look older. As the population ages, advertisements abound for products that are said to prevent or hide wrinkles.

Advertisements for skin care preparations and advice columns in the women's magazines spell out an impossible prescription: clear, fresh, firm, and youthful [skin] . . . in short, a skin that shows no sign of physical maturity, hard work, aggravation, exhaustion, hormonal changes, the effects of pregnancy, or the normal wear and tear of daily living.[11]

Cosmetics manufacturers are not required to obtain FDA approval before putting their products on the market. Responsible manufacturers test their products for safety before marketing. Still, many cosmetics contain dangerous substances.* One hundred cosmetic ingredients are suspected chemical hazards, according to the National Institute of Occupational Safety and Health.[12] Many of these hazardous substances can be absorbed through the skin, including the scalp. Be wary of cosmetics that list hormones in the ingredients. They usually contain estrogen, which can affect the body's hormonal balance. Reported effects of hormonal cosmetics include vaginal bleeding in women over sixty-five.[13] Lipstick enters the body through the throat along with food and drink. Many lipsticks and other cosmetics contain color additives that cause cancer in laboratory animals. These colors include reds 3, 8, 9, 19, and 37, and orange 17.[14] Petroleum-based hair dyes, most in dark shades, cause cancer in laboratory animals. If you do color your hair, a hair crayon, available from a beauty-supply store, can help you use less hair dye by extending the time between hair-dyeing applications.

For a small but growing number of women, the need to look young or thin may be so strong that they choose to undergo surgical procedures such as face or eyelid lifts, or surgery that slenderizes the abdomen, thighs, or buttocks, or dewrinkles hands.† Some women hope that plastic surgery will lead to a major life change, but surgery is no guarantee that a woman will get or keep a partner or a job, nor is it a cure for low self-esteem.

*Write your representative in Congress to get up-to-date information. The Food, Drug, and Cosmetics Act of 1938 should be amended to include required testing and FDA approval of cosmetics *before* marketing. See Resources, page 454, for 1990 Report on Cosmetics Regulation.

†Wrinkles, sags, and fat deposits are called "deformities" in medical literature on cosmetic surgery.

The number of plastic surgeons has nearly quadrupled since 1960, increasing at more than twice the rate of physicians generally.[15] Almost one third of physicians who practice plastic surgery are board certified in another specialty, or are not board certified at all.[16] To determine whether a surgeon is board certified in plastic surgery, call the American Society of Plastic and Reconstructive Surgeons of America at (800) 635-0635.

The risks of plastic surgery include scarring, severing of a facial nerve, infection, hemorrhage, and blockage of a blood vessel in the lung or brain. The latter three risks can cause severe impairment and, in rare cases, even death.[17] Other complications include blindness caused by bleeding behind the eyes. High blood pressure can cause excessive bleeding during surgery. Women who take large amounts of aspirin should stop five to seven days prior to surgery, since the drug interferes with clotting. A recent study shows that 10 percent of people who had face lifts experienced skin slough, the death of skin from inadequate blood supply, after surgery. The majority of those who experienced skin slough smoked more than one pack of cigarettes a day.

At a time in life when our risks of medical complications are going up, why expose ourselves to the additional hazards of unnecessary surgery and anesthesia?

The Social Impact of Looking Older

Relationships with Men

Many women fear that looking older means losing the power to attract men. This can mean losing the excitement of sexual attraction and the warmth of physical intimacy. For many women, men have played the role of the great critics of their lives. Men's opinions of our outward appearances, their acceptance or rejection of us based on our looks, have strongly influenced the way we see ourselves.

Last year when a much younger man I was very attracted to told me that what he really wanted was friendship, I felt shattered. I assumed that he rejected me sexually because of my age, and that started a whole train of bad feelings about myself—about growing older and not having anybody love me anymore—especially men. That blow has been repaired by the love and attention of another man, which is wonderful. Yet it bothers me that I seem to be so reliant on the opinions of men, as though I didn't have it within me just to care about myself. It's amazing—since I met this other man I feel much, much better about myself. It's as though I look in the mirror and see a different person—as though my whole outward appearance changes in my own eyes, to be built up or torn down by someone else. [a forty-five-year-old woman]

Unattached women seeking a sexual partner are often more concerned with signs of age than those who feel secure in a marriage or relationship.[18] Midlife divorce can heighten a woman's sense of competition, throwing her back into the "dating game."

Women who feel sexually dissatisfied in longstanding marriages or relationships may be frustrated because they believe that their age makes it impossible to have new sexual experiences.

I have tried to talk about sexuality with my husband but it's been a long time, a long marriage, and it's very hard to change things. Then when I read The Hite Report *I suddenly found myself validated. I hadn't known that I had any sexual rights and that the desires that I had were normal desires of a so-called normal woman. It made me feel a lot better, but also it made me feel that I'd been cheated. I was fifty or so and I felt that I could not retrieve some of these things or start over again because I was not sexually attractive enough anymore. I thought that these are privileges of the young. You have to have a smooth body, no wrinkles—be "juicy," as I call it. This voice kept telling me, "You're too old for that; who would want you?" And I was angry, at being "too old."* [a sixty-year-old woman]

Some women who are in generally unsatisfactory marriages or relationships may stay in the relationship, afraid that they are too old to find another partner.[19]

With the years we may feel that our partners turn away from us, and this can cause or reinforce negative feelings about our looks. It helps to realize that low self-esteem can cause us to perceive rejection when none was intended.[20] Finding a new relationship or a new source of self-esteem can help us overcome negative feelings.

It's nice to be appreciated. I can tell by the way he looks at me that he loves my face and my body, as old as it is. [a sixty-eight-year-old woman, remarried five years]

Now, I feel I have to press ahead in the world out of some inner sense of myself rather than with the help of my looks. And that's exciting because it makes me more adventur-

ous. I'm working on my Ph.D. and preparing for a life of teaching and scholarly writing. As a younger woman I wouldn't have had the courage to embark on such a challenging career. [a forty-three-year-old woman]

I'm no longer the completely lonely person I was before because I have established an inner strength. I find new patience and compassion with others. I had always thought that the emptiness in me could only be filled by someone else. I'm finally discovering that I can be a complete and happy person through my own inner resources. [a sixty-eight-year-old woman]

Some women have found their relationships unsatisfactory and burdensome, and are not concerned about looking young for men.

Now that I'm fifty-two—who needs an old man around! And he'll be retired pretty soon and sitting around all day. It's different when a woman retires because she has friends and can get around with other women. But when a man retires you've still got to cook for him and wash. He doesn't have any friends—he just sits there, in the way.

Relationships with Women

Some lesbian women may be less concerned with weight gain and aging than heterosexual women. Loving another woman can change the way a woman sees her body.

When I came out as a lesbian at thirty-seven, my body image changed. My lover's body was like mine, with breasts and curves, yet different. Our love was based on mutual respect and caring, bodies came second. I remember looking in the mirror a couple of years after we met and noting that my body seemed to have changed. My breasts hung lower, were less prominent. But mostly it was the feeling inside me that had changed. My breasts were part of a whole, not something to be leered at or mauled. I found myself looking at my breasts and body with pleasure. I liked what I saw. I claimed my body. [a forty-two-year-old woman]

Although I do have difficulty with aging, I believe that it is easier as a lesbian. I am less self-conscious about cosmetic perfection, about weight gain and wrinkles—and feel that I have more sexual/romantic opportunities than a straight woman of my age. I cannot say that I love getting older. However, I am more comfortable with myself than I have ever been before. And peaceful. I feel confident, for the most part, attractive and assured. My life is rich, full, adventurous and really quite wonderful. [a fifty-year-old woman]

But many lesbian women feel a strong pressure to look young and see themselves at a disadvantage in finding partners.

I cannot say that I am unself-conscious or not preoccupied at times with aging. Most of my self-esteem as a young woman was based on my looks and it has been a shock and an adjustment to have wrinkles and look older, especially when I feel so young inside. I am self-conscious about approaching younger women, worry about being inappropriate and question what younger women see in me in terms of my looks. My lovers have all been much younger than me, which is a concern. I worry that I will not remain attractive to them and what their reactions will be to my aging and possibly declining health. [a fifty-year-old woman]

Work

For many of us, our main concerns about looking older center on our power to earn money and to be valued as workers. As we look for jobs, or want to change from an unsatisfactory job, we become aware that looking older can mean being unemployable.

I do free-lance work in a young business. All the people I deal with are my age or younger, and each time I have a new project interview I go thinking, "Do I look young enough, do I look young?" I'm afraid people will stop hiring me, because you don't hire fifty-year-old women to do this kind of stuff. I'm scared about what it means for me professionally. [a thirty-nine-year-old woman]

Sometimes we can counteract employers' or colleagues' ageist attitudes with the help of our own strong self-esteem and/or the support of other older workers.

At first it seemed strange to me that everyone in the department is about thirty-five years younger than I am. But then I thought, if they have trouble dealing with a colleague old enough to be their mother, that's their problem! [a sixty-nine-year-old woman]

If you use your beauty to get a job, a man, then you are always indebted to it. You're always chasing it, looking in the mirror to see if it is still there. Once you stop that and realize you can use your head, *your whole person, nobody can take that from you! You are* powerful *if you realize you have a brain and can use it. Society says: "You are no longer valuable because you aren't gorgeous." We say we are valuable, because we* think *and* do. [a sixty-five-year-old woman]

Some women find that being older brings more respect and power on the job. Looking older increases our credibility and authority. Being older brings better judgment and wisdom. We can speak more freely and be listened to. These advantages depend on the kind of work we do, and seem to be greater in the professional world.[21]

As a therapist, my age really is an advantage. I have a much larger store of experiences and understanding of what makes people tick and of what kinds of things happen to people, just because I've lived so much longer. [a seventy-nine-year-old woman]

Being older has helped me in my profession. I have much more authority: the fact that I'm known, that I've published, my experience in running a department. With my students I don't have to prove that I know something; they take that for granted. Certainly it would be much more difficult at twenty-five to be the authority I am. It would be impossible! Whatever my fears may be, whatever my private problems, what my students see is a woman of power. [a fifty-six-year-old woman]

Age and Identity

We live in a culture that rejects us for our looks just when we have the most to offer. Some women feel betrayed by such a society. Some of us, however, feel sorry for those who cannot see through our wrinkles and gray hair to our talents and abilities.

When I was younger I was considered more attractive than I am now. I no longer feel as though people look at me and say, "Oh, wow, what an attractive woman," which they did when I was younger. And I feel sorry for them because I am really a much more interesting person now than I was then. But that's their problem. [a sixty-five-year-old woman]

Our culture's view of how older women should look and behave is constricting to them and detrimental to society as a whole. Many women refuse to be confined by set images of what they should look like, be, and do. We dress and move according to our tastes and our personalities. We are as emotionally and physically involved with life as our wishes and our health allow. We see aging as a new experience for which we are setting the pace.

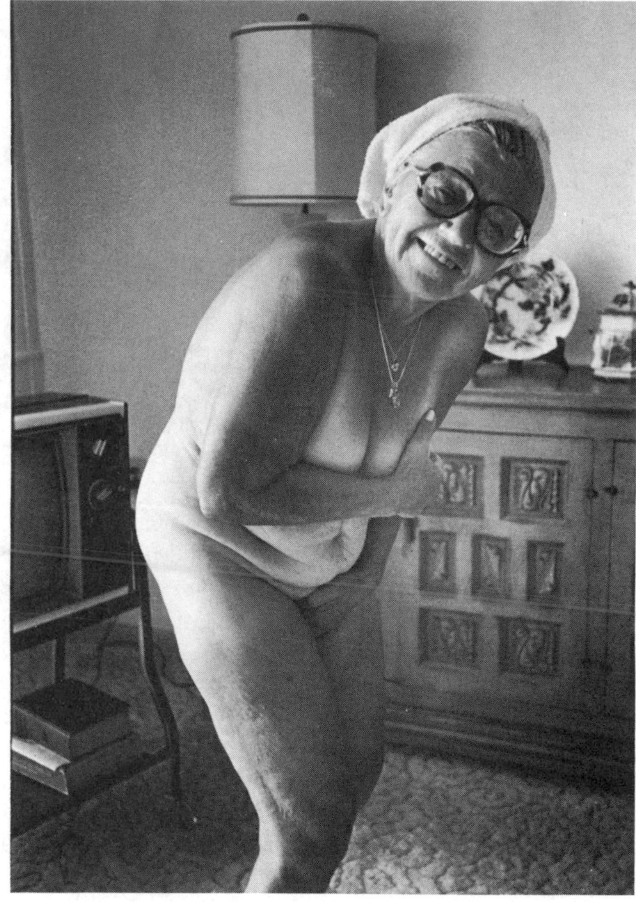

Mikki Ansin

Getting old can be wonderful if you're not imposed on by other people's rules about how you should be when you're old. I consciously break as many as I can because then I'm breaking through oppression. [a sixty-five-year-old woman]

Life's less confining for me now, things are falling into place. In a way I feel happier than I did at thirty—I like myself much better. And I think that's a key point—to like oneself, to be your own best friend. [a fifty-seven-year-old woman]

We can choose whether or not to use the technology—cosmetics, plastic surgery—offered us to look younger. And, in fact, many women find that instead of wanting to look different they see an inner and outer beauty in themselves and other older women that they didn't see before. Some of us find that we like signs of aging and that they make a face more interesting than the smoothness of youth. We respond to other, lasting qualities of appearance, such as bone structure, or an alert, lively expression.

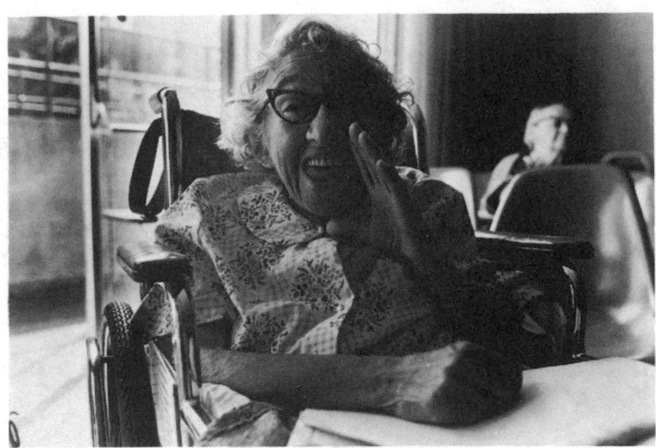

Marianne Gontarz

I know a lot of handsome older women. They have character! They're people! They've lived! One friend my age has the most animated, humorous, charming face. She would really beguile anybody! [a seventy-nine-year-old woman]

Self-confidence brings us a freedom many of us never felt in our younger years; we no longer feel obliged to be youthfully "feminine" sex objects. We feel free to be ourselves, to be honest and outspoken, and are relieved and relaxed with this freedom.

You can make conscious efforts to change your own and others' ideas of beauty. Older women can learn, from the impact of the phrase "Black is beautiful," how to raise self-esteem. One way to do so is to tell your older friends how good they look, how alive and interesting. Tell them how fine and handsome are the visible signs of years, experiences, and characer. This is an important way women can help each other deal with our culture's negative attitude toward age.

Notes

1. Barbara Macdonald and Cynthia Rich, *Look Me in the Eye.* San Francisco: Spinsters, Ink., 1983, p. 14.
2. Gwendolyn T. Sorell and Carol A. Nowak, "The Role of Physical Attractiveness as a Contributor to Individual Development." In Richard M. Lerner and Nancy A. Busch Rossnagel, eds., *Individuals as Producers of Their Own Development: A Life-Span Perspective.* New York: Academic Press, 1981, pp. 389–446.
3. Jan Benowitz Eigner, "Interaction and Building of Body Concept and Self Concept Over the Lifespan: A Study of 20 Women Age 40 to 60." Unpublished dissertation, Saint Louis University, 1984.
4. Daniel Goleman, "Dislike of Own Body Found Common Among Women." *The New York Times,* Mar. 19, 1985, pp. C1, C5.
5. Diane White, "An Age-Old Problem." *The Boston Globe,* Oct. 26, 1983.
6. Carol A. Nowak, "Does Youthfulness Equal Attractiveness?" In Lillian E. Troll, Joan Israel, and Kenneth Israel, eds., *Looking Ahead: A Woman's Guide to the Problems and Joys of Growing Older.* New York: Prentice-Hall, 1977.
7. Jennifer Robinson, "Body Image in Women over Forty." *The Melpomene Report,* Melpomene Institute for Women's Health Research, 316 University Ave., St. Paul, MN 55103, October 1983, pp. 12–14.
8. While eating disorders are epidemic among adolescent women, their incidence, although small, is growing alarmingly among middle-aged women.
9. Marcia Germaine Hutchinson, author of *Transforming Body Image,* quoted in "Body Hatred." *McCall's,* April 1985, p. 136.
10. Clairol, 1983, as cited in Robin Marantz Henig, *How a Woman Ages.* New York: Ballantine Books, 1985, p. 61.
11. Susan Brownmiller, *Femininity.* New York: Fawcett, 1985.
12. Jane E. Brody, "Personal Health." *The New York Times,* Sept. 19, 1984.
13. *The Medical Letter on Drugs and Therapeutics,* June 21, 1985.
14. *Health Facts,* Center for Medical Consumers, Inc., New York, October 1985.
15. Gene Roback, Lillian Randolph, and Bradley Seidman. *Physician Characteristics and Distribution in the US.* Chicago: Physician Data Services, Division of Survey and Data Resources (annual publication), American Medical Association, 1993.
16. Ibid.
17. Robin Marantz Henig and the editors of *Esquire, How a Woman Ages—Growing Older: What to Expect and What You Can Do About It.* New York: Ballantine Books, 1985, p. 28.
18. Cleo S. Berkun, "Changing Appearances for Women in the Middle Years of Life." In Elizabeth W. Markson, ed., *Older Women.* Lexington, MA: D. C. Heath/Lexington Books, 1983, p. 24.
19. Berkun, op. cit., p. 28.
20. Troll, Israel, and Israel, op. cit., p. 51.
21. Berkun, op. cit., p. 24.

4

WEIGHTY ISSUES

✦

BY JANE HYMAN, DIANA LASKIN SIEGAL, AND ELIZABETH VOLZ

SPECIAL THANKS TO ESTHER ROME, ROBIN COHEN, AND MARY P. CLARKE

1994 UPDATE BY PAULA B. DORESS-WORTERS WITH SPECIAL THANKS TO ESTHER ROME

RESOURCES FOR THIS CHAPTER ON PAGES 454–56

In this country we are preoccupied with weight. Every women's magazine has articles on diets and "fitness." Many of us think we are overweight when we really are not. It may be that the biggest problem facing weighty women is outright discrimination due to stigmatization of obesity.[1]

Many women avoid healthful foods they think are fattening and skip meals in an effort to lose weight. "Fat phobia"—the fear of being fat—can interfere with proper nutrition. We can feel well and strong without being exploited by the multimillion-dollar weight-loss industry. Our money is better spent on healthful foods and activities that are fun, sociable, and cause no injury.

ANOTHER LOOK AT DIETING AND WEIGHT

Each of us has a unique size, shape, and body chemistry strongly determined by heredity.[2] How much we weigh is a function of energy input (food), energy used (activity), our own body's rate of using energy (metabolism), and other factors that are not well understood. The amount of energy we use to perform tasks, including sedentary activities such as office work and reading, can vary from woman to woman.[3]

Because of the constant pressure to be thin, many women try sporadically or constantly to lose weight by reducing the calories they consume. This is so common that to most of us the term *diet,* which in its original meaning simply refers to what we eat, has come to mean a plan to lose weight. Dieting to lose weight can become a way of life. Most dieters never learn healthful food habits. When you go on a low-calorie diet, your body reacts as if it were being starved and tries to preserve as much energy as possible by decreasing its rate of metabolism. Your rate of metabolism may slow down more with each diet and remain slower once you return to your usual eating habits. Ironically, this means that after each diet, unless you drastically increase your exercise, you may gain weight more easily than before, since your body adds more fat to protect itself in case you deprive it of food again. This partially explains why 90 to 99 percent of dieters regain their weight within five years, or even regain more than they lost.[4] It also explains why some researchers say that repeated low-calorie dieting may be a major cause of weight gain.[5]

Women are frequently encouraged to lose weight not only because "thin is in" but because

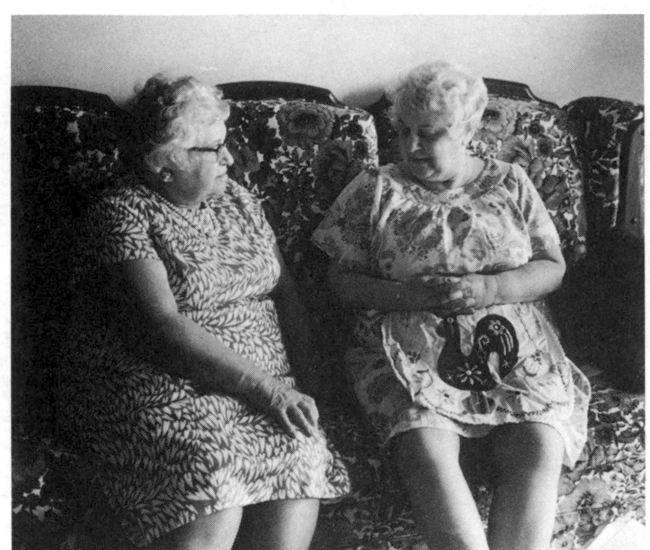

Rachel Perkis Durland

medical authorities believe that being "overweight" puts us at risk for a variety of diseases and even death. But studies done on weight and health contradict each other, and many are faulty. Some studies find a relationship between high weight and early death, and others do not. Many studies do not take into account other known health risks such as cigarette smoking, repeated dieting, or hereditary factors, and most studies do not include women. One study that included women (but did not ask if they repeatedly dieted) did find an increase in death rates among women who for many years were 55 percent to 65 percent over the average weight charts.[6]

We tend to read weight charts with the assumption that "overweight" is bad no matter how old we are, what kind of body tissue we have, and where it is located on the body. Increasingly, body mass index (BMI) rather than weight is used in health-education and research literature. Body mass is a better measure than weight because your BMI number takes both your height and weight into account. Poundage by itself is not a measure of fat; skin-fold measurements and water-immersion tests are better indicators. The weight we add as a result of exercise and body conditioning is not a hazard to our health. Increasing our weight by increasing our muscle mass will strengthen our bones and help prevent osteoporosis.

In addition, recent research shows that when studying the association between weight and disease, not only fat mass but the distribution of fat has to be considered. Women aged forty to fifty-nine with fat distribution predominantly on their waists and upper bodies have significantly more hypertension, diabetes, and gallbladder disease than women with fat predominantly on their lower bodies. Relatively more fat from the waist up (as compared to hips) is associated with higher rates of these diseases even among women with comparable total body fat. Arthritis is associated with fat on the hips in some women.[7] Thin women who jog may be stressing their joints as much as fat women who walk.

Healthy people should not be concerned if they gain some weight as they move from early adult years to late middle age. As menopause approaches, the midlife woman's body undergoes typical changes: breasts enlarge, the waistline thickens, and fat is deposited on the upper back. Yet women are falsely encouraged to believe that through dieting and use of hormones we can maintain the body of a thirty-five-year-old woman throughout the second half of life.[8] The weights in the often-quoted Metropolitan Life Insurance Height and Weight Chart were increased in 1983 but are still too restrictive for women in their fifties and sixties. There are advantages for women in being a little heavier than previously thought—gaining a pound a year is apparently healthy.[9]

As we grow older, some lean muscle tissue is replaced with fatty tissue. Even if we stay the same weight, we will have more fat proportionately at eighty than we did at forty. Since it takes less energy to maintain fat tissue than to maintain muscle tissue, we would have to cut our calories* by 10 to 15 percent from age twenty to age sixty just to maintain the same weight.[10] But if we cut our intake, we may not get adequate nutrition.

Emphasis on "ideal" weight dictated by weight charts masks the damage caused by the constant pressure on women to be thin. Fat women suffer more from discrimination against fat than from any weight-related health problems. Many dieters experience emotional disturbances due to the effects of starvation on the body. Studies show that weight-related emotional disturbances are related to overeating, disparagement of body image, and the complications of dieting. Eating at night, insomnia, and skipping morning meals are associated with stressful life circumstances and often related to depression,[11] perhaps made worse by fruitless dieting attempts.

*A calorie is simply a way of estimating the energy available in a particular food.

The following "diets" have dangers in addition to the general hazards mentioned above.

- The use of "diet pills." Just because a drug is prescribed by a doctor doesn't mean that it is either effective or safe. Many prescription "diet pills" contain amphetamine, a stimulant that speeds up the body's processes and can cause insomnia and diarrhea. It is addictive, toxic, and can even cause violent behavior and death. Also, don't assume that, because something is sold over the counter (OTC) without a prescription, it is harmless. Most OTC diet pills contain phenylpropanolamine (PPA), which is chemically similar to amphetamine. PPA raises blood pressure and alters brain function, but is not a proven aid to weight loss. It is also used as a nasal decongestant and is found in many cold remedies. Many diet pills and cold remedies also contain caffeine, which heightens the effect of PPA. Even recommended doses can cause confusion and hallucinations; high doses can cause heart damage, seizures, strokes, and even death. **A person can easily overdose by combining diet pills and cold remedies.**
- High-protein/low-carbohydrate, and sometimes high-fat diets. These raise triglycerides (fats) in the blood, promote dangerously high levels of ketones* in the blood, increase calcium loss, and trigger carbohydrate "binges." Very low carbohydrate intake can cause fainting spells and depression.
- Grapefruit, banana, egg, or other limited-food diets. No single food is a "magic" way to reduce weight. No enzymes in them melt away or otherwise remove fat from our bodies. High-egg diets are also high in cholesterol. These diets lack the nutrients you can obtain only by eating a variety of foods.
- Powdered-protein or high-protein liquid diets. These products (also called protein-sparing) are supposed to protect the lean body mass. They have many adverse effects, such as causing irregular heartbeats and even sudden death.[12] They should be used only under the close supervision of a research physician skilled in weight loss.
- Special supplement combinations, such as vinegar, lecithin, kelp, and vitamin B_6. These substances by themselves do not cause weight loss. Rather, weight loss is achieved through the limited-calorie diet that is supposed to accompany the supplements.

*Ketones are the end product of fat metabolism. Abnormally high levels are found in people with conditions of impaired metabolism.

An increase in two severe eating problems that primarily affect women, anorexia nervosa and bulimia, reflects the general tendency in society to promote thinness at all costs. Anorexia is a form of severe and initially deliberate self-starvation; bulimia is an eating pattern of bingeing and then purging, usually by vomiting or laxative usage. Anorexia is more common among young women, but may be increasing among older women.* Bulimia seems to be found among all age groups. Anorexia and bulimia can result from severe psychological distress as well as cause it. Both create many physical problems, including loss of tooth enamel (from regurgitated stomach acid), loss of ability to absorb food properly, loss of the gag reflex, and imbalances in the body's fluids severe enough to cause death. Even some best-seller diets encourage these methods as ways to lose weight.[13]

Therapists who treat people with eating problems agree with the feminist critics who first pointed out that anorexia and bulimia affect women more than men because of women's lack of power in society and because of the constant messages that women should be thin.

I felt out of control in my life. This was the one place where I could exert control—over my eating—and I did. Ultimately, however, I didn't have control of it—it had control of me. I could not stop when I wanted to. [a forty-five-year-old woman]

BEING THIN

With all the emphasis on thinness, we may be so proud of ourselves if our weight is low that we do not realize when we are malnourished. Thin people are more susceptible to certain diseases, including lung diseases, fatal infections, ulcers, and anemia.[14] Studies show that older people who are "significantly underweight" die sooner than those who are not.[15] But the term *underweight* is just as controversial as the term *overweight*.† Many weight studies do not take into account smoking and preexisting diseases that

*We do not know the extent of eating disorders among middle-aged and older women. Funding for this research has been cut.

†Underweight is usually defined as 10 to 15 percent below the Metropolitan Life Insurance weight-for-height charts.

might have caused both the thinness and the early death.

Being thin is just as natural for some women as being heavy is for others. However, as older women, we frequently lose weight simply because we fail to eat enough. This may be a consequence of depression or loneliness, lack of interest in preparing or eating food, physical conditions that make preparing food or chewing difficult, not being able to afford enough to eat, and changes in the ability to taste food as we age. Certain drugs and certain illnesses, such as Type I diabetes, overactive thyroid, and cancer, can also cause weight loss. If you lose weight and are not sure why, or if you have no appetite, you should see your health-care provider to make sure there is not an underlying problem.

Feeling Well: Achieving a Healthful Food/Activity Balance

The entire concept of an "ideal" weight for any woman or group of women should be abandoned.[16] Instead, we should focus on getting plenty of good food and exercise. We need to create new patterns for dealing with food and activity if old patterns are not serving us well. Here are some suggestions.

- *Listen to your own body's feelings of hunger and fullness.* Years of dieting and bingeing can cause us to lose awareness of our body's signals. Eat when you are hungry and stop when you are full.
- *Learn good nutrition.* Basically, this means cutting down on high-fat foods and replacing them with whole grains, vegetables, fruits, and legumes.* If you ate four candy bars a day you would get 1,600 calories but you wouldn't be feeding your body what it needs.
- *Increase physical activity.* Begin slowly. Don't do more than feels comfortable, or you won't keep it up. Statistics from many studies show that if you use 300 to 350 calories a day in exercise (2,100 to 2,500 per week), you will feel happier, more energetic, and stronger. Some people take two or more years to work up to that level. In twenty minutes you consume about 90 calories in light housework, 100 calories in brisk walking, and 240 calories in swimming.

*Examples of legumes are peas, beans, and lentils.

I didn't lose weight in my exercise program. Rather, I stayed the same but built muscle and lost fat. Now I look better and I feel better too. [a woman in her fifties]

Months of pain and inactivity had seriously limited my ability to move. I love to swim, but at first I could only walk the length of the pool, though the support of the water made it easier. When I felt well enough to swim one length, I had to rest until my heart stopped pounding. It took twenty months, with setbacks from illnesses which meant I had to work up slowly again, for me to be able to do thirty lengths in one hour. Now with swimming, some walking, and stair-climbing, I've reached my goal of 2,000 calories of exercise a week. [a sixty-one-year-old woman]

- *If your caloric intake is too low, try to eat more.* This is usually best accomplished by eating small, frequent snacks that are high in nutrition and calories, such as ice cream, puddings, milk shakes, cheese, nuts, nut butters, and whole-grain cookies, crackers, and muffins. Choose the vegetables and fruits that have the most calories. Use the fortified instant breakfast drinks and meal-in-a-can drinks *in addition* to your regular foods. Flavor your food with herbs and spices. Arrange to eat with others when you do not feel like eating.
- *Keep records.* Keep daily records of exercise, and of what and how much you eat (written within fifteen minutes of eating). If you discover you are gaining or losing more weight than you wish, a review of accurately kept records can be enlightening. One woman thought she could cut calories by giving up bread. Keeping a record showed her that eating bread helped her avoid overeating. Consider the records over a period of a week rather than for each day.
- *Set goals for success.* Unrealistic food and exercise goals set you up to fail. Sometimes the only achievable goal seems small (one day a week I'll carry a piece of fruit to work instead of cookies), but the fact that you *do* achieve it helps you take the next step.
- *Control your environment.* Make your meals as attractive, tasty, and fun as possible. Try moving your TV into the bedroom and take your planned snack with you to enjoy during late-night watching. Don't skip parties and celebrations because you want to avoid food. Enjoy yourself and choose nutritious food—or bring your own.
- *Enjoy what you choose to do or to eat.* For example, when choosing among several kinds

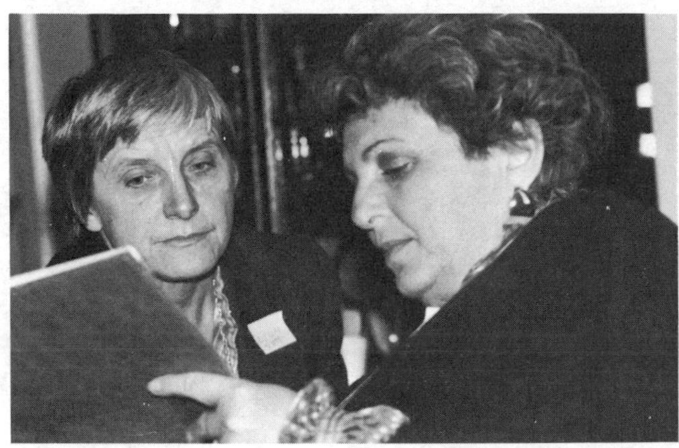

Jane Jewell

of cookies, remember that an oatmeal-raisin cookie gives you more nutrients than a chocolate cookie. A glass of skim milk and a potato have approximately the same number of calories as the same size glass of Coke and ten to fifteen potato chips. But the first two provide protein, calcium, vitamins A and D, and other nutrients while the latter provide calories and little else. If you decide on the chocolate cookie or the potato chips, enjoy them. When you decide to treat yourself to a favorite food, whatever it may be, this is an informed choice, not a "failure."

Last night at a restaurant I chose fried shrimp and french fried potatoes because I wanted them. I didn't fool myself by ordering broiled fish and a baked potato which I really didn't want and then pretending I wasn't adding extra butter. I felt satisfied and know I won't binge the way I used to when I felt deprived. [a fifty-eight-year-old woman]

I have developed such a sweet tooth in my old age. I just can't resist candy or sweets when I have them in the house. My neighbor told me about a wonderful substitute: frozen banana slices. You freeze the banana peeled and wrapped in foil, then slice as many slices as you want with a sharp knife and rewrap the rest. It's amazing how much a banana tastes like candy when it is frozen. [a seventy-five-year-old woman]

NOTES

1. Albert Stunkard and Thorkild Sorensen, "Obesity and Socioeconomic Status—A Complex Relation." Editorial, *The New England Journal of Medicine,* Vol. 329, No. 14 (Sept. 30, 1993), pp. 1036–37.

2. Albert J. Stunkard, et al., "An Adoption Study of Human Obesity." *The New England Journal of Medicine,* Vol. 314, No. 4 (Jan. 23, 1986), pp. 193–98. Though the title mentions only obesity, the study showed that the relationship between biological parents and adoptees was not confined to the obesity weight group but was present across the whole range of fatness—from very thin to very fat. The conclusion was that family environment alone has no apparent effect. Obesity is usually defined as at least 20 percent over the "ideal weight" according to life insurance weight tables.

3. Susan C. Wooley, O. W. Wooley, and Susan R. Dyrenforth, "Theoretical, Practical, and Social Issues in Behavioral Treatments of Obesity." *Journal of Applied Behavior Analysis,* Vol. 1 (Spring 1979), p. 8.

4. W. Bennett and J. Gurin, "Do Diets Really Work?" *Science,* Vol. 82 (March 1983), p. 43.

5. Susan C. Wooley and O. W. Wooley, "Obesity and Women—I. A Closer Look at the Facts." *Women's Studies International Quarterly,* Vol. 2 (1979), pp. 69–79.

6. Artemis Simopoulos and T. Van Itallie, "Body Weight, Health, and Longevity." *Annals of Internal Medicine,* Vol. 100, No. 2 (February 1984), pp. 285–95.

7. Arthur J. Hartz, David C. Rupley, and Alfred A. Rimm, "The Association of Girth Measurements with Disease in 32,856 Women." *American Journal of Epidemiology,* Vol. 119, No. 1 (1984), pp. 71–80.

8. Ann M. Voda, et al., "Body Composition Changes in Menopausal Women." *Women and Therapy,* Vol. 11, No. 2 (1991), pp. 71–96.

9. Reubin Andres, "Impact of Age on Weight Goals." *Health Implications of Obesity,* Program and Abstracts, National Institutes of Health Consensus Development Conference, February 11–13, 1985, pp. 77–80. More complete information is available in Reubin Andres, et al., eds., *Principles of Geriatric Medicine.* New York: McGraw-Hill, 1985, pp. 311–18.

10. Daphne A. Roe, *Geriatric Nutrition.* Englewood Cliffs, NJ: Prentice-Hall, 1983, p. 64.

11. Albert Stunkard and Thomas A. Wadden, "The Adverse Psychological Effects of Obesity." *Health Implications of Obesity,* NIH Consensus Development Conference, February 11–13, 1985, pp. 59–62.

12. Rafael A. Lantigua, et al., "Cardiac Arrhythmias Associated with a Liquid Protein Diet for the Treatment of Obesity." *The New England Journal of Medicine,* Vol. 303, No. 13 (Sept. 25, 1980), pp. 735–38.

13. O. Wayne Wooley and Susan Wooley, "The Beverly Hills Eating Disorders: The Mass Marketing of Anorexia Nervosa." *International Journal of Eating Disorders,* Vol. 1, No. 3 (1982), pp. 57–69.

14. Paul Ensberger, "Fat and Thin Not Black and White." *Radiance,* Vol. III (Spring 1986), pp. 21–22.

15. Simopoulos and Van Itallie, op. cit.

16. T. R. Knapp, "A Methodological Critique of the 'Ideal Weight' Concept." *Journal of the American Medical Association,* Vol. 250 (1983), pp. 505–10.

5

EATING WELL

✦

BY ELIZABETH VOLZ AND DIANA LASKIN SIEGAL WITH HELP FROM MARY P. CLARKE

SPECIAL THANKS TO KATHLEEN I. MACPHERSON

1994 UPDATE BY DIANA LASKIN SIEGAL AND NANCY JAGODNIK WITH SPECIAL THANKS TO ESTHER ROME AND RUTH PALOMBO

RESOURCES FOR THIS CHAPTER ON PAGES 456–58

Food is important to us on many levels. What we eat is connected to our health, our feelings about ourselves, our social and family ties, our ethnic backgrounds, and our roles as women.

When I was sick with the flu as a little girl, my mother would fix me chicken soup. To this day I never smell chicken soup but what I don't remember how much better it made me feel then. Even now when I'm feeling bad, I'll want some soup like my mother made for me. This canned stuff is not a good substitute. [a sixty-eight-year-old woman]

Many of us are experienced in meal planning and preparing food. We may have spent many hours clipping and trying out new recipes or preparing our family's favorites over and over again. Being responsible for one to three meals a day, seven days a week, however, can sometimes dampen our enthusiasm for cooking. Many of us are more familiar with taking care of others than taking care of ourselves. It may be hard to prepare a nice meal for ourselves when we feel lonely. Or we may enjoy the freedom from fixed schedules and complicated meals but fail to pay attention to our nutritional needs.

Since my husband died and my youngest daughter left home, I find it hard to prepare meals for myself. If I haven't planned ahead, I'll stand at the refrigerator and eat whatever is handy—pickles, ice cream, cold hot dogs, whatever. [a fifty-five-year-old woman]

I gained ten pounds after my husband died. I like sweets, but he had so many restrictions on what he could eat when he was ill, and I just ate what I prepared for him. When it was over, I felt a certain release and indulged myself in eating all those "forbidden" cookies.

Now I plan more what I am going to eat. I cook ahead and freeze small portions in packets that can be dropped into boiling water when I am ready to use them. I bake a large sheet cake, freeze half and keep half in the refrigerator, so it will be there when I want it, but I won't be tempted to eat it all at once. [a woman in her eighties]

Mass advertising promotes high-profit processed foods and soft drinks, promising fun and eternal youth but delivering only empty calories. Health-food stores and food co-ops are good sources of foods not easily found in supermarkets, but supermarket managers are responding to increased consumer sophistication about nutrition by stocking low-fat products, whole-grain breads and crackers, and a wider variety of fruits and vegetables. Stores now also contain a variety of ethnic and new foods that can improve our food selections and broaden our eating pleasures. A good tip for supermarket shopping is to begin by going around the edges of the market where the unprocessed food is—dairy, meat, fish, plain frozen foods, and produce. Use the center aisles mainly to restock staples and paper products.

Eating in healthier ways usually means deciding to change and then doing it slowly. One way to start is to learn more about what a healthy yet flavorful diet can be.

Making Eating Sociable and Easy

The company of others can seem particularly important at mealtime. Make eating a happy sociable event by sharing a meal or two a week with friends. Going out to lunch or to the "early bird" specials is generally cheaper than eating out at night. For people over sixty, most senior centers provide one hot meal a day. In some areas, nursing homes, schools, and churches serve as meal sites.

Though some women avoid the meal sites because they mistakenly perceive them as only for the economically needy or because they don't want to be associated with "old people," those who do go enjoy it a lot and frequently become "regulars."

I live alone but I am rarely by myself, due to a steady stream of family, friends, and international visitors, and many activities. I enjoy eating at the local senior meal site. This is how I solve my problem of thinking of a meal as a true communion. I urge others to try it. [an eighty-seven-year-old woman]

Not all of us are able to travel or live in a group setting, but we can certainly make our home or apartment a place where people want to be—and then ask them over! Potlucks are popular, economical, and fun.

You can eat well more easily if you simplify the storing and cooking of food. For example, if you have freezer space, cook food ahead of time, divide it into meal-size packages, and freeze it. You don't have to make a complicated meal to have nutritious food. Fresh or frozen vegetables can be cooked quickly in a steamer (for under five dollars you can buy one that fits any saucepan). A small, simple microwave oven is a useful investment. Small pieces of chicken, fish, or meat can be broiled or cooked in a microwave oven in a short amount of time. Low-fat dairy

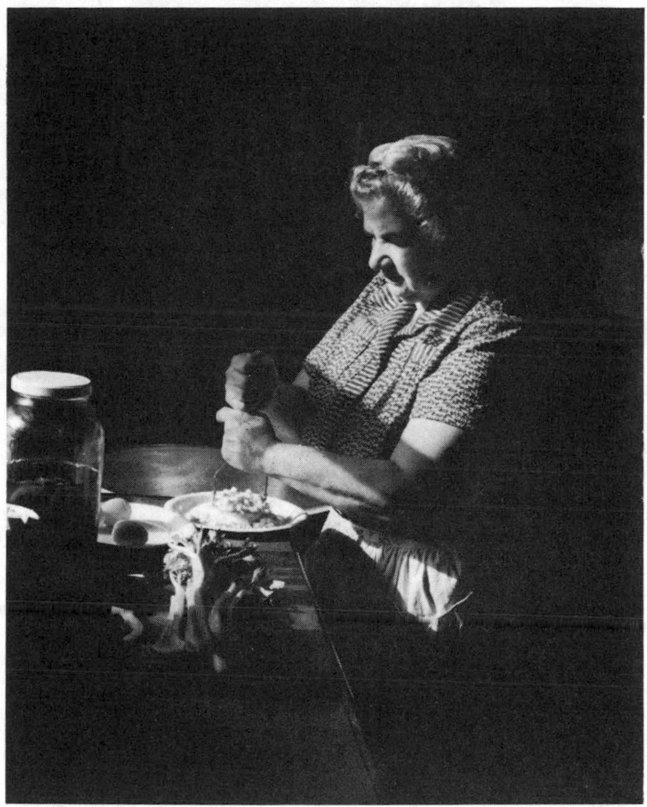

Norma Holt

products such as skim milk, cottage cheese, and yogurt can make convenient, nutritious snacks. Add meat or tofu and vegetables to cooked grains such as brown rice. Whole grains can also be eaten in cereals (shredded wheat, oatmeal, wheat germ, bran cereal) or in whole-grain bread, crackers, and pasta.

Other circumstances can affect how we eat. For instance, living too far from a market or having too many stairs to climb can limit the amount of food you can get into the house. Apartments or houses may have too little storage space, or refrigerators or stoves that don't function properly. Poorly fitting dentures can be an impediment to good nutrition. Sometimes help can be found in the form of a friend or neighbor to shop or eat with, a senior center that serves meals, a neighborhood health center that provides dental care or social services, or a legal-services agency for housing problems.

Eating Well for Less Money

For many of us, the kind and amount of food we eat is influenced by the cost. Most families spend an average of 15 to 20 percent of their income on food. Poor older women may have to spend 30 percent or more of their income on food.[1] For these women, the choice may come down to paying the rent or buying food.

Some suggestions that may help those on a limited budget are:

1. Buy only as much as you can use or store. Split cheaper "economy sizes" with a friend.
2. Buy foods that are "nutrient dense." Unprocessed foods give you the most nutrition per dollar. For instance, eggs, low-fat milk and cottage cheese, dried beans, whole chickens, protein-enriched spaghetti products, peanut butter, oatmeal, whole-grain cereal, inexpensive fish, and hamburger.
3. Avoid highly processed foods when possible. They seem economical but aren't. Although a bologna sandwich, canned beef-noodle soup, and a frozen creamed chicken dinner are in the same price range as the foods mentioned above, their percentage of protein and other beneficial nutrients is far less, and their percentage of unwanted additives such as salt, sugar, fat, and chemical preservatives is far more.
4. Fresh vegetables and fruits are cheapest in season. Frozen vegetables are often less expensive than fresh and have approximately the same nutritional value. Avoid frozen vegetables packed in sauces because they cost more and contain more salt and fat. Canned vegetables can be quite inexpensive although there is some nutritional loss. For instance, 4 ounces of canned green beans contain one third the amount of vitamin C of fresh or frozen beans.
5. Meals at a senior nutrition center or meal site are inexpensive. You can also save cooking time and meet new friends.
6. Don't hesitate to apply for food stamps at your local welfare office and use surplus foods. If you qualify, you are entitled to them.

FOOD IN INSTITUTIONS

People in nursing homes and hospitals often don't have much choice about what they eat. Institutional food is often inadequate. If you, a friend, or a relative is in this situation and finds the food lacking in nutrition or taste, one solution is to bring in or have brought in small amounts of food from the outside. Another is to put pressure on the institution to provide better food. Discuss this with your doctor or dietitian. If that doesn't improve the situation, talk with other residents informally, bring it up in the residents' council, if you have one, or contact an ombudsman (see Nursing Homes chapter) or one of the nursing-home reform organizations (see Nursing Homes in Resources, page 487).

WHAT IS A GOOD FOOD PLAN?

No single food program is right for everyone. We all have different nutritional needs as well as different physical and economic limitations. Advertisements, books, magazines, and television all present conflicting information on what to eat.

I still don't know what I should eat or how much. I try to keep up with nutrition through magazines and newspapers, but I am never sure I'm getting what I need. [a fifty-five-year-old woman].

The purpose of this chapter is to help us evaluate what we read and hear so that we can eat healthier food.

More research has been done in the area of nutrition for older women recently. The U.S. Department of Agriculture's (USDA) Human Research Center for Aging is currently studying the nutrition of healthy older people. We're beginning to get more information.

Nutrients—carbohydrates, fats, proteins, vitamins, and minerals—and water work together in our bodies to provide energy, regulate bodily processes, and provide material for repair and growth. Each nutrient has its own function, so the food we eat must contain all of the nutrients for our bodies to function really well.

Labels on food packaged in the United States used to contain information on the United States Recommended Daily Allowances (USRDA) for certain nutrients set by the Food and Drug Administration but derived from guidelines from the National Academy of Sciences. The academy sets its guidelines within a range from the minimum amount needed to prevent deficiencies (MDA) to the amount that would cause an overdose. The USRDA is usually close to the minimum amount. Also, the guidelines do not include all known essential nutrients. The USRDAs were standards to compare one product with another, not to judge the unique nutritional needs of each person.

New labels went into effect in spring 1994 for almost all foods. The new labels provide food facts so we will know more about what we are eating. Serving sizes will be standardized for almost two hundred categories. What must appear on every label are total calories, calories from fat, total fat, saturated fat, cholesterol, total carbohydrate, dietary fiber, sugars, protein, vitamin A, vitamin C, calcium, and iron.

The amount of grams of each component will appear along with their percentage of Daily Value (based on the USRDAs) for a daily diet of 2,000 calories. Terms used to describe the level of a nutrient in a food, such as *low, lite,* and *free* have been defined.* To help those with allergies and food preferences, a full list of ingredients on foods with more than one ingredient is required. You may have to carry a magnifying glass with you to read the labels.

The Senate Select Committee on Nutrition and Human Needs concluded in 1977 that we as a country are not particularly well nourished. We know that the poor of this country, a large proportion of whom are older women, have a hard time meeting their nutritional needs. A 1990 study found that at least 25 percent of the elderly living in the community and 40 percent of the elderly in nursing homes were malnourished.[2] Although we have far more than our share of agricultural resources, our nutrition has suffered because processed food has become an ever-increasing part of our diets.

*For new definitions of terms, call the American Dietetic Association, (800) 366-1655, and ask for their pamphlet *Understanding Food Labels.*

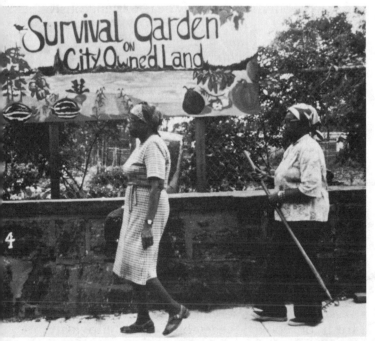

Ellen Shub

Our food supply has changed from reliance on whole, unrefined foods to highly processed, "fortified," preserved, synthetically manufactured "convenience" foods. The latter take up at least half the space in any supermarket and an even larger percentage of space in convenience stores. Our use of fats and oils increased by 50 percent from 1910 to 1980. Our use of sugar and other sweeteners has increased by one third since 1909, largely because of the use of hidden sugars in processed foods and beverages.[3]

The following suggestions, adapted from the goals set by the Senate Select Committee and from the 1985 *Dietary Guidelines for Americans,* are still valid.

1. *Increase consumption of complex carbohydrates.* This category includes legumes such as split peas, lentils, chick peas, lima, navy, and other beans; whole grains such as brown rice, bulgur, and buckwheat; and whole-grain products such as whole-wheat bread, whole-grain crackers, bran cereals, noninstant oatmeal, and shredded wheat.
2. *Reduce consumption of refined sugars.* This category includes processed foods that list sugars as first, second, or third ingredients. Sugars may have a variety of names, such as corn syrup or corn sweetener, sucrose, dextrose, maltose, lactose, fructose, or levulose. "Natural" sugars such as honey, barley malt, maple syrup, apple and grape juice concentrates, and molasses are only slightly better for you and should be eaten only in small quantities.
3. *Reduce overall fat consumption.* Foods to cut down on include fatty cuts of meat, processed meats (cold cuts, sausages), deep-fried foods, butter, margarine, mayonnaise, high-fat cheeses, pastries, chips, and other "snack" foods. Good substitutes for some of these foods are lower-fat animal products such as fish, poultry without the skin, low-fat dairy products, and vegetable proteins such as grains and beans. Unbuttered popcorn is a good snack.
4. *Change the ratio of saturated to unsaturated fats, reducing the use of all fats, especially saturated fats.* Saturated fats are generally solid at room temperature and include animal fats, hydrogenated (hardened) vegetable fats, and coconut and palm oils. Unsaturated fats are liquid at room temperature and include vegetable or nut oils such as safflower, sunflower, soy, corn, linseed, and walnut oils. Saturated fats raise LDL and total cholesterol levels

while unsaturated fats lower them. Monounsaturated fats, like peanut, canola (rapeseed), or olive oil, are liquid at room temperature but solidify easily with refrigeration. Monounsaturates may lower LDL and total cholesterol levels while raising HDL and can be used in cooking, as they remain stable* at high temperatures. (See pages 336 and 337 for definitions of these cholesterols.)

5. *Reduce sodium consumption.* Eat only small quantities of salt-cured foods, most condiments, salty snack foods, soy sauce, foods containing monosodium glutamate (MSG), most canned vegetables and soups, and any processed food in which salt or sodium is high on the list of ingredients. Keep track of your use of salt in cooking and at the table. Be aware that some water softeners work by adding salts. Avoid over-the-counter medications high in sodium, including many antacids. Some sodium, however, is essential for our well-being and cutting intake too low for our needs can result in weakness.

*Oils other than monounsaturated oils are undesirable to cook with because at high temperatures they form harmful substances.

CARBOHYDRATES

Carbohydrates should provide 50 percent or more of our energy needs and supply the glucose necessary for brain function. Adequate carbohydrate intake keeps the body from using protein as an energy source, so that protein can be conserved for body-building functions.

Carbohydrates are divided into two categories—simple and complex. Simple carbohydrates are sugars such as table sugar, honey, and the sugar in fruits (glucose and fructose). Complex carbohydrates are starches such as grains, pastas, breads, starchy vegetables, and beans. All sugars and starches are converted by digestion into a simple sugar called glucose, which is released into the bloodstream. However, the glucose from starches is digested and absorbed more slowly than that from sugar, avoiding the rapid rise and fall of blood sugar that can come from eating too many simple sugars at one time. Whole foods with complex carbohydrates such as grains also furnish essential nutrients and fiber, while simple carbohydrates such as sugar and refined flour tend to be "empty calorie" foods—they supply too many calories for the nutrients they provide. White flour loses most of twenty-three of its vitamins and minerals in the refining process and is then labeled "enriched" when only four are replaced.

CHOOSING OUR FOOD

What should we eat on a daily basis for the nutrition we need? The *Food Guide Pyramid* is the latest design for helping us understand what to eat. It was published by the U.S. Department of Agriculture in 1992 to offer guidance for what healthy Americans two years of age and older should eat. The pyramid visually illustrates the food groups in the proportion in which we should eat them for a balanced menu. Plan your daily meals to include at least the lowest number of suggested servings in each food group. The pyramid also reminds us that complex carbohydrates should be the basis of our menu and the largest amount of what we should eat.

Foods are now divided into five groups: (1) grains, breads, and cereals; (2) vegetables; (3) fruits; (4) dairy products; and (5) meats and other protein foods. Fats, oils, and sweets are to be used sparingly. They are a natural part of many of the foods in the main five groups. Herbs and spices (but not salt!) may be used generously to taste.

- *Whole grains, including bread and cereal*—6 to 11 servings (one serving is ½ cup grain or cereal, or one slice of bread). Includes all whole grains—rice, barley, millet, cracked wheat, corn, whole-grain breads and cereals—1 ounce of ready-to-eat or ½ cup cooked oatmeal, bran, shredded wheat; whole-grain crackers, pasta, and tortillas. If you are not used to whole grains, start gradually to substitute them for white-flour products and eat only as much as your digestive system can comfortably handle. For example, you can cook a combination of brown rice and enriched white rice, gradually shifting toward more of the whole grain. Starchy vegetables such as corn, peas, and potatoes are included in this group.
- *Vegetables*—3 to 5 servings (one serving is ½ cup fresh or cooked vegetables or 1 cup leafy greens). Includes all fresh, frozen, or canned

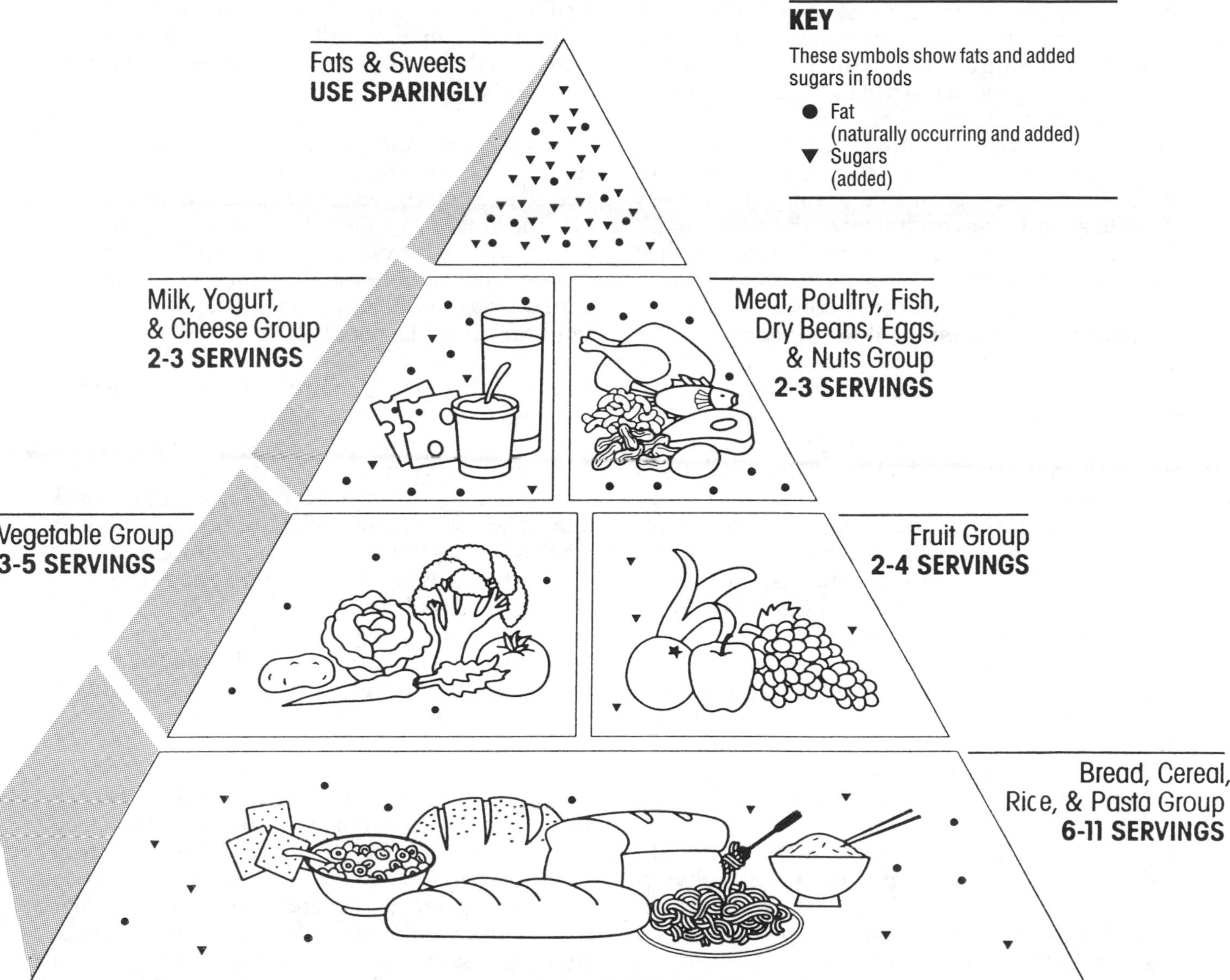

DAILY FOOD REQUIREMENTS

U.S. Department of Agriculture and U.S. Department of Health and Human Services

vegetables. Generally, the deeper the color of the vegetable, the more nutritious it is in vitamin A, so tip the balance in favor of dark green leafy and yellow/orange vegetables.

- *Fruit*—2 to 4 servings (one serving is one average-size fruit, or approximately ½ cup). Includes all unsweetened fruit—fresh, frozen, canned, dried, or ¾ cup juice. Whole, raw fruit is generally the most nutritious. Include a vitamin C fruit or vegetable source daily. Examples would be citrus fruits, strawberries, tomatoes, peppers, and broccoli.
- *Dairy products*—2 to 3 servings (one serving is approximately 1 cup liquid milk or yogurt, or 1 to 1½ ounces cheese). Includes milk, yogurt, all cheeses, or ½ cup ice milk. Be sure to use mostly low-fat dairy products such as skim milk, low-fat yogurt, and ½ cup low-fat cottage cheese.
- *Protein*—2 to 3 servings (one serving is 2 to 3 ounces cooked lean meat, chicken, or fish, 3 to 4 ounces tofu, 2 large eggs, 1 cup cooked beans, 4 tablespoons peanut butter, or combinations such as ⅓ cup beans with ⅔ cup rice). Many women over age seventy do not eat enough protein.

Protein is the second most plentiful substance in the body. It is important for the growth, development, and repair of all body tissues. Proteins are composed of units called amino acids. The body requires approximately twenty-two amino acids to make human protein. All but nine of these can be produced by the body. These nine are called "essential amino acids" and must come from the food we eat. Animal proteins from foods such as meat, poultry, fish, dairy products, and eggs contain all of the amino acids in adequate amounts and are therefore called "complete proteins." Many vegetables, grains, beans, nuts, seeds, and other complex carbohydrates contain proteins but are "incomplete" by themselves and have to be combined in order to have sufficient amounts of all of the amino acids. Combined vegetable proteins have the advantage of being lower in fat, higher in fiber and minerals, and generally lower in cost than complete proteins.

Many traditional food combinations yield complete protein—such combinations as grains and beans (Mexican rice and beans), beans and nuts or seeds (Middle Eastern hummus), grains and nuts or seeds (American peanut butter sandwich on whole-grain bread), and any vegetable protein with any animal protein such as potatoes with dairy products. For more information on combining foods to make complete protein, see *Diet for a Small Planet* by Frances Moore Lappé or other books in Resources, pages 456–58.

- *Essential fatty acids*—approximately 1 tablespoon per day in salad dressing or cooking. This is not really a food group, but we do need small amounts of oil and fat in our diet for good health. If you eat fatty fish, whole grains, seeds, and nuts, you may not have to add extra oil. Fats are part of the basic structure of every cell. Furnishing more than twice the number of calories per gram as carbohydrates and proteins, they provide the most concentrated form of energy in the diet. Fats act as carriers for fat-soluble vitamins (A, D, E, and K) and provide insulation and protection for our organs and the skeleton. Oils high in essential fatty acids (in descending order) are fish oils and linseed, walnut, soy, safflower, sunflower, and corn oils.
- *Water,* although it is not a nutrient, is the most important element for life and is frequently overlooked. Our bodies are made mostly of water, which is vital to maintain life and health. Water is essential for proper functioning of both the kidneys and the bowels, and is an important vehicle for disposing of poisonous substances. It is the basic transport system of the body, moving all nutrients, hormones, blood cells, waste products, and oxygen through the body.

As we age, our mechanisms for controlling fluid balance become less efficient. Most of us need 6 to 8 cups of water daily, and more in some circumstances. Water can also be obtained from soups, juices, beverages, fruits, and vegetables. Coffee and other beverages containing caffeine actually push fluids and minerals out of the system and should be avoided.

- *Fiber,* although not a nutrient, is nonetheless a necessary component of a well-balanced diet. Fiber serves primarily as a vehicle for holding water, binding both toxic and essential nutrients, and providing the soft bulk that absorbs body waste. Because of these properties, fiber helps our intestines work more smoothly. This is particularly important as we grow older and our intestines lose some of their elasticity and motility, increasing the tendency toward constipation. Adequate fiber intake may also help prevent such conditions and diseases as diverticulosis, gallbladder disease, colitis, colon cancer, and high cholesterol.[4]

Different forms of fiber have different functions; for instance, oat bran lowers cholesterol, whereas wheat bran does not. Pectins from foods such as apples and beans prevent diarrhea and help excrete cholesterol. Cellulose and other fibers from whole grains help prevent constipation and colon cancer. It is therefore important to eat a variety of fibrous foods, including whole grains, beans, fruits, vegetables, nuts, and seeds. Beware of fiber-enriched white breads. Some contain harsh sawdust products. Fiber has its negative side as well. Very high fiber intake can cause gas and bloating. More seriously, it can interfere significantly with calcium, iron, and zinc absorption.[5] The new labeling will help us obtain the suggested daily intake of 20 to 30 grams of fiber. A prudent course is to have enough fiber (and adequate fluid) to make our bowel movements soft and easily passed.

- *Vitamins* are organic compounds found in living things. Their function is to act as catalysts for chemical reaction. Some chemical processes require the presence of several vitamins simultaneously. Vitamins themselves do not furnish energy, as they have no calories, but they are necessary for metabolism.

Vitamins are soluble in either fat or water. The fat-soluble vitamins—A, D, E, and K—require fat in order for the body to absorb them from the intestinal tract. They are also easily stored in the body and can become toxic at high doses. This is particularly true for vitamins A and D. Water-soluble vitamins are the B complexes and vitamin C. Because they are water soluble, unneeded amounts can be disposed of easily in the urine. And because they are not stored easily in the body, we need to be more careful to get them on a daily basis. They are generally not toxic except at very high levels.

- *Minerals* are inorganic compounds that originate in soil, rocks, and water. Approximately seventeen minerals are necessary for human nutrition; several others are thought to have at least a minor role in body processes.

Like vitamins, minerals act as catalysts for many chemical reactions in the body. These include regulation of muscle contractions, transmission of messages through the nervous system, and aiding the digestion and metabolism of foods. Certain minerals also constantly adjust our internal water balance and regulate the flow of substances in and out of cells. They control the acid balance in our blood and tissues. The essential "macrominerals," those present in relatively high amounts in the body, are sodium, potassium, calcium, magnesium, and phosphorus. The essential "trace minerals," those present in only very small amounts, are iron, copper, zinc, manganese, chromium, selenium, vanadium, and molybdenum.

Should We Take Nutrient Supplements?

Unfortunately, there is no simple way to know how well nourished you are. Hair analysis does not give accurate information about the nutritional condition of the body. For example, zinc in hair can be low if a diet is deficient, but it can be normal if hair is slow growing because of semistarvation.[6]

There has been much in the news about the possible benefits of taking supplements, especially about beta carotene (which converts to vitamin A), vitamin C, and vitamin E to reduce the risks of heart disease[7] and cataracts.[8] Not everyone agrees that there is value in singling out a few nutrients from the number we know about and the ones we have still not identified. Beta carotene, for example, is just one of more than five hundred carotenoids, so many research nutritionists still urge eating a variety of foods from the food groups as the best assurance of adequate nutrition.[9]

There are some conditions under which you may want to consider taking a supplement: when you don't have control over the food you eat (for instance, in a nursing home); when you are on a medication that can interfere with absorption of nutrients; if you use cigarettes, alcohol, or caffeine; if you haven't yet changed to healthful food habits.

Remember that supplements are supposed to do just that—supplement your diet. You cannot use them to replace food or to make up for a nutritionally unsound diet. A good vitamin-mineral supplement is low in the fat-soluble vitamins A and D (A—5,000 IUs or less, D—400 IUs or less), contains a complete B complex (B_1, B_2, B_6, B_{12}, biotin, folic acid, niacin, pantothenic acid, choline, inositol, and PABA), vitamin C, vitamin E, and minerals such as copper, magnesium, iron, selenium, chromium (at least 50 mcg a day), manganese, and zinc. Compare before you buy—store brands are less expensive yet provide the same nutrients as the national brands. If you feel you need more than a general supplement or are confused about what to take, you can consult a nutritionist or dietitian or try to find one of the few medical professionals who have knowledge and experience in clinical nutrition.

SPECIAL NEEDS FOR WOMEN OVER FORTY

The specific nutritional needs of older women have not been determined. The nutritional levels of the healthiest of the elderly—those who are largely free of disease and are mobile—are remarkably similar to those of younger people. Unfortunately, what is clear is that as many as 50 percent of women over the age of sixty-five are malnourished because they consume too few calories, proteins, and essential vitamins and minerals for good health.[10] Specifically, many do not get enough thiamine (B_1), riboflavin (B_2), vitamins B_6, B_{12}, C, D, and K, folic acid, magnesium, zinc, and iron, as well as calcium.[11]

Adequate daily calcium intake is vital through-

out our life span. The USRDA for adult women remains at 800 mg per day, but surveys show that most women consume barely half that amount.[12] The 1984 Osteoporosis Consensus Conference recommended increases in calcium for women taking estrogens and for postmenopausal women. The 1989 revisions by the National Academy of Sciences did recognize that women need to develop strong bones early in life and so they increased the amount of calcium recommended for ages eleven to twenty-four to 1,200 mg per day. They left at 800 mg, however, the recommendation for women twenty-five years of age and older. The following chart, compiled from several sources, lists recommendations higher than 800 mg per day.

CALCIUM NEEDS OF WOMEN

Age	Milligrams per day
1–10	800
11–24	1,200
If pregnant	1,500–2,000
If breastfeeding	2,200
25–50 (premenopausal)	1,000
Postmenopausal or for early natural or surgical menopause	1,500

A thousand milligrams of calcium can be obtained in one day by eating all of the following: two ½-cup servings of cooked green vegetables, 1 ounce cheese, and 2 cups skim milk. Adding a corn muffin made with milk or a serving of sardines or yogurt and increasing the two green vegetables to 1-cup servings will increase the calcium to 1,500 mg for the day.

All dairy products are rich in calcium. Skim or fat-free or 1 percent milk is commonly recommended. You can add additional low-fat, fortified, powdered milk to muffins, pancakes, soups, custards, puddings, and casseroles.

You can still obtain calcium if you are lactose intolerant. Some people can tolerate half a glass of milk with each meal and can eat yogurt, cheese, and buttermilk without discomfort; but others are uncomfortable with even small amounts of milk. The most common signs of lactose intolerance (lack of the enzyme required to digest the lactose in milk) are gas, stomachaches, and intestinal cramps. Many have diarrhea but some people who tend toward constipation may not have diarrhea. Many people develop these signs as they age because their stomachs produce less of this enzyme. Eliminate all milk products for several days and see if the symptoms go away. Then try milk again and see what happens. If the discomforts return, you might have lactose intolerance. Enzyme drops to add to regular milk, tablets to take before eating something containing milk, and milk with the enzyme already added are now available in some grocery, drug, and health-food stores.

GOOD CALCIUM SOURCES

Food	Portion Size	Mg of Calcium
Whole milk	1 cup	290
Low-fat (2%) or skim milk	1 cup	300
Buttermilk	1 cup	285
Nonfat dry milk	¼ cup powder	377
	1 tablespoon	60
Cheddar cheese	1 ounce	205
Cottage cheese	½ cup	77
Parmesan cheese	1 ounce	320
American cheese	1 ounce	175
Yogurt, plain low-fat	1 cup	290
Ice cream	½ cup	90
Collard greens, cooked	1 cup	350
Parsley	3½ ounces	203
Kale, cooked	1 cup	200
Spinach, cooked	1 cup	150
Broccoli, cooked	1 cup	130
Sardines (with bones)	¼ pound	300
Salmon (canned with bones mashed in)	¼ pound	225
Oysters (fresh)	¼ pound	210
Shrimp	1 cup	147
Brazil nuts	¼ cup	140
Almonds	¼ cup	80
Tofu made with calcium sulfate	4 ounces	145
Corn tortilla	6″ diameter	60
Kelp	½ ounce	150
Blackstrap molasses	1 tablespoon	135

Many magazines now carry ads for calcium supplements, playing on our fears of bone fractures. Because of these ads, some women may now be adding *too much* calcium to their diets. This may interfere with the absorption of iron and other nutrients, and may cause imbalances in calcium metabolism. Adding a calcium supplement to bring the total daily intake from food and the supplement up to 800 mg on days when we can only eat less than 800 mg of calcium is certainly safe, but high-dose supplementation should probably be reserved for women with established osteoporosis or a high risk of osteoporosis. If you have a history of kidney stones, check with your physician about calcium levels that are safe for you. For most women, however, a maximum calcium intake from *food and supplements* of 1,500 mg a day is considered safe. Make sure to divide your intake throughout the day and save the final for bedtime, as the body tends to lose calcium during sleep. Calcium before bed may prevent leg cramps during the night. A glass of milk before bed also contains tryptophan (which will help you sleep), protein, and vitamins.

If calcium supplements are desirable for public health then they should be sold at reasonable prices. Instead, prices keep climbing. The labels on some calcium supplements now list the percentage of elemental calcium in the supplement based on the assumption that 1,000 mg per day is the recommended amount. If the label lists 200 mg of elemental calcium, then that is the actual amount in the supplement.

The question is not only how much calcium you are eating, but how your body is using it. It is doubtful that the calcium in these supplements is absorbed as well as the calcium in food. If a tablet dropped in vinegar doesn't dissolve in thirty minutes, it probably won't dissolve in your stomach. Calcium carbonate is not water soluble and is not absorbed well, especially as we get older. Water-soluble calcium in calcium citrate, gluconate, aspartate, and lactate is more readily absorbed. Do not use calcium lactate if you have lactose intolerance. Many women, nevertheless, prefer to use calcium carbonate, which can be purchased at drugstores in an inexpensive powdered form. Calcium carbonate is also found in antacid tablets such as Tums, which, however, also contain sugar. Be careful not to use an antacid containing aluminum as it can cause calcium to leave the bones. In addition, all calcium supplements are harder on the stomach than the calcium in food. For some women, calcium carbonate causes constipation, gas, or "acid rebound" with heartburn. If you have an insufficient amount of hydrochloric acid in your stomach, which is common in older people, these products may make digestion difficult and can interfere with the absorption of other nutrients.

Vitamin D and magnesium are two important nutrients necessary for calcium absorption and utilization. Because vitamin D is formed on the skin in the presence of light, vitamin D deficiency can occur when we are not often exposed to sunlight. Only one half hour of sunlight on 20 to 30 percent of the skin several times a week is needed. Sunscreens reduce the absorption of vitamin D, so get sun exposure early or late in the day, when you can use a sunscreen numbered 8 or lower or no sunscreen. Getting enough sunlight can be a problem for women who are housebound or institutionalized, or who spend the winter months in cold climates. Vitamin D is

HOW MUCH CALCIUM IS IN THE SUPPLEMENTS?

• Calcium carbonate*	40%
• Tricalcium phosphate	39%
• Calcium chloride	36%
• Calcium phosphate	29%
• Calcium citrate	21%
• Calcium aspartate	19%
• Calcium lactate	13%
• Calcium gluconate	9%
• Bone meal*	31%
• Dolomite*	22%

To find the actual amount of calcium contained in each tablet, multiply the percentage of calcium contained in that particular form by the number of milligrams of the entire tablet. For instance, a 500-mg calcium carbonate tablet actually contains only 200 mg of elemental calcium (500 mg of calcium carbonate x .40 = 200 mg of calcium).

*These products contain small amounts of toxic minerals, but it is the amount of lead they contain that is of most concern. Exposure to lead is undesirable at any age. The most recently reported analysis shows amounts of concern in bone meal, carbonate from oyster shells, and dolomite. Chelates had some, but laboratory-made carbonates had only minute amounts. Many older women who are taking large amounts of powdered bone meal because it is one of the cheapest sources of calcium may be accumulating too much lead in their bodies. Lead levels in products sold should be more carefully controlled. *Nutrition Action Healthletter,* Vol. 20, No. 10 (December 1993), p. 4.

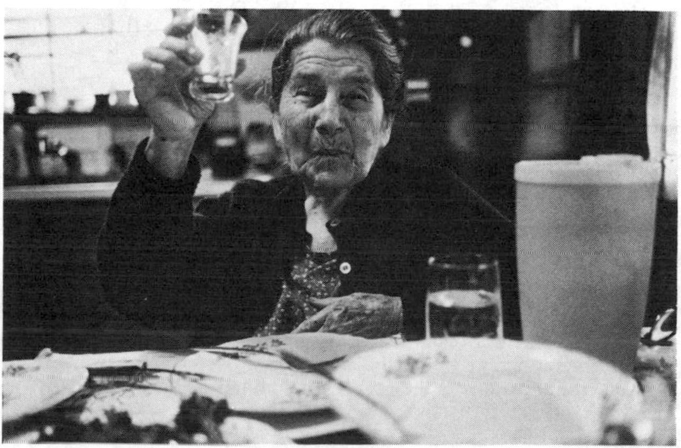

Marianne Gontarz

FACTORS THAT DECREASE CALCIUM ABSORPTION

- Foods containing oxalic acid in combination with calcium interfere with calcium absorption. These are spinach, rhubarb, Swiss chard, sorrel, parsley, beet greens, and unhulled sesame seeds. Collard greens are high in calcium and do not contain oxalic acid. None of these foods should be used as a main source of calcium, but can and should be added to a diet that is varied.
- Foods containing phytates (a substance found in the outer layers of grain seed, such as wheat bran) may also make calcium unavailable for absorption. Sprouted-grain breads contain no phytates, but unprocessed bran does. Phytates may be broken down more in breads baked with yeast than in unleavened breads and crackers. If your general calcium intake is varied, however, you do not need to worry about phytates.
- Exercise helps retain calcium. Sedentary and bedridden people tend to lose calcium.
- High stress levels decrease absorption.
- Calcium absorption tends to decrease with age in both women and men.
- Caffeine and alcohol act as diuretics and can cause loss of calcium in the urine. Alcohol also directly interferes with calcium absorption.
- Drugs that impede calcium absorption include tetracycline, laxatives, corticosteroids, Dilantin, diuretics, heparin, caffeine, antacids containing aluminum, and nicotine.
- There is a direct relationship between high salt intake and loss of calcium in the urine.
- Foods high in phosphorus (red meat, cola drinks, and processed foods that have phosphorus additives) prevent calcium absorption.

DRUG EFFECTS ON NUTRIENT ABSORPTION[13]

Drug	Effect
Over-the-Counter	
Aspirin	iron loss
Antacids	phosphate loss, thiamine deficiency
Laxatives	decrease in potassium, calcium, magnesium zinc, vitamins A, D, and E
Prescription	
Antibiotics	can decrease riboflavin, vitamin C, and calcium absorption and destroy the bacteria in the intestinal tract that produce vitamin K
Phenytoin (Dilantin)	decrease in vitamins D, K, and folic acid
Phenobarbital	decrease in vitamin D
Indomethacin (Indolin) and other anti-inflammatory drugs	iron loss
Chlorpromazine hydrochloride (Thorazine) and thioridazine (Mellaril)	decrease in riboflavin
Tricyclic antidepressants	weight gain or loss

And many others. Check with your pharmacist.

not found in many foods. Cod-liver oil and other fish oils contain the highest amounts. Milk is fortified with vitamin D but yogurt and cheeses are not. You may be vitamin D deficient if you have reduced your consumption of egg yolks, butter, liver, and vitamin D–fortified dairy products in order to reduce saturated fats and avoid lactose. If you need to supplement your diet with vitamin D, 400 IUs per day is a reasonable amount. Magnesium is plentiful in green leafy vegetables, whole grains, nuts, seeds, and fruits. If you take a dietary supplement with calcium, it is a good idea to increase magnesium intake to half the level of your calcium intake.

Chronic diseases as well as changes in cardiac, respiratory, liver, and kidney functions can affect our nutritional needs. In addition, many medications interfere with the absorption or utilization of nutrients. Eating well will help us stay healthy and resistant to disease.

NOTES

1. Agriculture Research Service, *Family Economics Review.* Washington, DC: U.S. Department of Agriculture, No. 1, 1983, p. 31.

2. From a survey done for the Nutrition Screening Initiative, a campaign to publicize ten warning signs of

poor nutritional health. One sponsor of the initiative is the National Council on the Aging. (See General Resources, page 000.)

3. Jeffrey Bland, *Nutraerobics*. San Francisco: Harper & Row, 1983, p. 59.

4. C. W. Suitor and M. F. Crowley, *Nutrition: Principles and Applications in Health Promotion*, 2nd ed. Philadelphia: J. B. Lippincott Co., 1984, p. 152.

5. Rudolph Ballantine, *Diet and Nutrition*. Honesdale, PA: Himalayan International Institute, 1978, p. 10.

6. K. M. Hambridge, "Hair Analysis: Worthless for Vitamins, Limited for Minerals." *American Journal of Clinical Nutrition*, Vol. 36 (November 1982), pp. 943–49.

7. *Harvard Health Letter*, Vol. 3, No. 7 (March 1993), pp. 1–5.

8. "Nutrition and Aging." *Nutrition Action Healthletter*, Vol. 19, No. 4 (May 1992), pp. 1, 5–7.

9. Marian Burros, "Eating Well: Supplements? Even Experts Can't Agree." *The New York Times*, Apr. 14, 1993.

10. Erik Eckholm, "Malnutrition in the Elderly: Widespread Health Threat." *The New York Times*, Aug. 13, 1985; and Felicia R. Lee, "Fear of Hunger Stalks Many Elderly." *The New York Times*, Nov. 16, 1993, p. B4.

11. Jeffrey B. Blumberg, "Nutrient Requirements for the Healthy Elderly." *Contemporary Nutrition*, Vol. 11, No. 6 (1986); Janet R. Mahalko et al., "Nutritional Adequacy in the Elderly." *The American Journal of Clinical Nutrition*, Vol. 42 (September 1985), pp. 542–53; Institute of Food Technologists' Expert Panel on Food Safety and Nutrition, "Nutrition and the Elderly." *Food Technology*, Vol. 40, No. 9 (September 1986), pp. 81–88; and Ronald R. Watson, *Handbook of Nutrition in the Aged*. Boca Raton, FL: CRC Press, 1989.

12. "Nutrition and Aging." *Nutrition Action Healthletter*, Vol. 19, No. 4 (May 1992), p. 6.

13. See also Daphne Roe, *Handbook of Drug and Nutrient Interactions*. Chicago: American Dietetic Association, 1982.

6

MOVING FOR HEALTH

✦

BY ELIZABETH DUBOIS, MARILYN BENTOV, DIANA LASKIN SIEGAL, AND DORI SMITH

1994 UPDATE BY DIANA LASKIN SIEGAL

RESOURCES FOR THIS CHAPTER ON PAGES 458–59

Many women walk, lift, bend, and stretch daily in their work. Increasingly, however, we are becoming more sedentary. Our desk jobs offer us little relief for the strain and inactivity imposed on our bodies. The washing machine and the car have replaced arm and leg power. Decreased energy, illness, age-related problems, and partial immobilization also make it easy to slip into sedentary habits.

There is strong evidence that appropriate levels of physical activity not only safeguard health, but improve it at any age, even if you have disabilities. In one exercise program sixty- and seventy-year-old women and men became as fit and energetic as people twenty to thirty years younger. The older people in that program who improved the most had been in the poorest shape![1] The increases possible in muscle strength even of people in their nineties are remarkable.[2]

I was having back pain, so I started to swim at the Y. When I began, I was forty-six. I thought twenty-five lengths a day was terrific for my age. Now I'm fifty-four and I swim almost a mile (seventy-two lengths). My resting heart rate is fifty-three. That's the rate for a young male athlete.

After stopping exercises for one year for personal reasons, I got stiff, sluggish, flabby, and had aches and pains. I felt old and tired all the time. My spirit was low, too. When I started a regular regime again three times a week, I improved after three months. I felt alive again, got my stamina and good spirits back. [a seventy-five-year-old woman]

People who are active and who exercise tend to suffer less from headaches, chronic back pain, stiffness, painful joints, irregularity, and insomnia. Women often report renewed sexual energy and enjoyment, and the alleviation of hot flashes. Inactivity causes depression, poor circulation, weak muscles, stiff joints, shortness of breath, loss of bone mass, and "that tired feeling."[3] It's hard to get started if you're tired all the time.

But where to begin? Fortunately, the societal prejudice against women being physically active, especially in their later years, has diminished.

When we exercise as hard as our bodies allow us to, we're actually being kind to ourselves. Joints develop or regain flexibility, muscles become strong, blood pressure lowers, bone density improves, our cardiovascular system becomes more efficient, and food digests better. We have more, rather than less, energy for every-

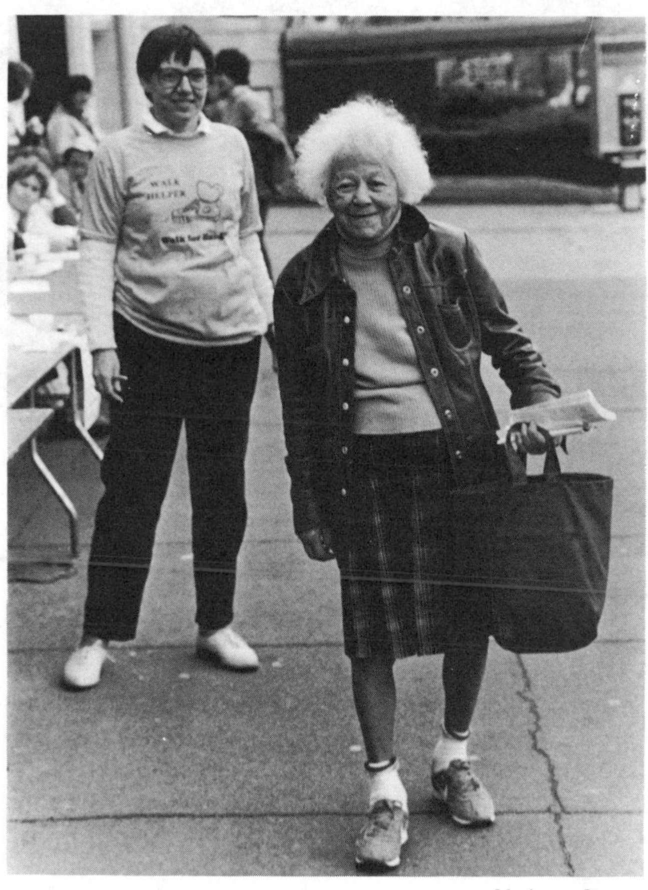

Marianne Gontarz

day living. Feelings of alertness, well-being, and energy from exercise provide us, in turn, with reasons to stay active.[4]

Age is not the crucial factor in determining and improving fitness. Patterns of activity adopted today will affect the strength and agility of our bodies tomorrow and in the years to come. Regardless of what we did in the past, today is the time to start living healthier, more active lives.

Just a year ago I was feeling slow with stiff, aching joints. I got that "What do you expect at your age?" comment from my doctor. Today I am stronger and move easily because I go to a cardiac fitness program designed for old people—most are women. I don't have cardiac problems but there I have a woman coach who plans and supervises my program—a mile walk, using various machines for building strength, flexibility, and endurance, and a weight-training program. I shocked my sister by reaching into the trunk of my car and lifting out the spare without any strain. I go for one and a half hours, three times a week. The $55-a-month cost is offset in my case by fewer visits to the doctor. Others have insurance coverage. [a seventy-four-year-old woman]

GETTING STARTED

SHEDDING

My skin scares me. It feels tight.
I envy the snake who sheds his. Mine
binds me in limited space.
I circle, move more slowly, less,
a running-down top.

taking three deep breaths I
soar   make
spirals that sweep
add more space
am alive

Lois Harris

Unless you've been consistently exercising, start your new activities slowly and gradually. For example, find ways to increase the amount of time you spend walking each day. Try parking a block or two away from your destination or getting off the bus a few stops from where you're going, and walking the rest of the way. Add a few stairs whenever possible. Find reasons to walk instead of using your car.

No matter where you are, you can begin moving by stretching your fingers and toes, rotating your ankles, wrists, and shoulders, stretching out your arms and legs, and breathing deeply.

My idea of a woman in motion is me: I walk instead of riding; I climb stairs instead of using the escalator or elevators. I do these in addition to normal lifting, bending, carrying, stretching. [a seventy-two-year-old woman]

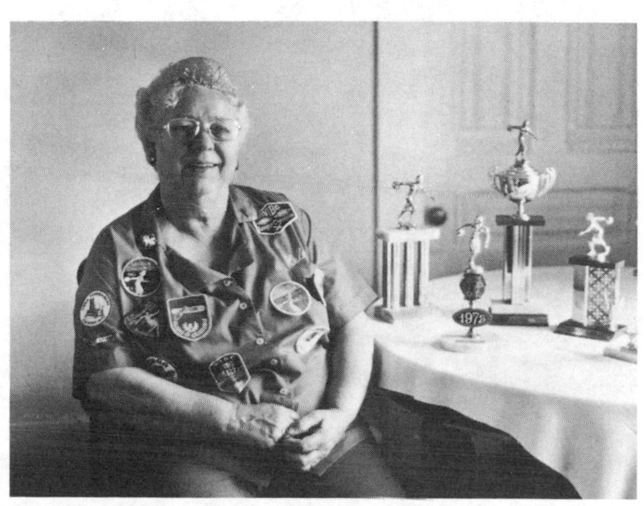

Cathy Cade

There are hundreds of daily opportunities to move—look for them! Try tightening abdominal and pelvic muscles while waiting for a bus, or swinging arms and legs while watching TV.

While daily activities keep us moving, they are usually not sufficient to promote and maintain the degree of fitness that promotes radiant health. Unless we do them correctly, many movements such as vacuuming, making beds, lifting, and even standing actually put added strain on the body, especially the lower back. To counteract inactivity or movements that potentially tire or strain our bodies, we need a complete exercise program that includes stretching, strengthening, corrective posture, and cardiovascular conditioning. Among the activities that help achieve these are folk dancing, ballroom dancing, ballet, belly dancing, walking, running, biking, camping, boating, yoga, Tai Chi, jogging, hiking, weight training, swimming, skating, skiing, tennis, bowling, racquetball, golf, squash, volleyball, and—you name it!

Some activities promote contact with other people. You can cultivate new friendships while you get fit at community and senior centers, parks, continuing-education centers, YW- and YMCAs, community schools, and colleges. Folk dancing and square dancing traditionally attract people of all ages. Hundreds of clubs exist for middle-aged and older people who like swimming, walking, bowling, golfing, bicycling, or cross-country skiing.

If you can't find the activity or kinds of people you enjoy, you can always start something yourself. Many older women are seeking adventurous outdoor activities such as hiking and backpacking, wilderness camping, and rafting.

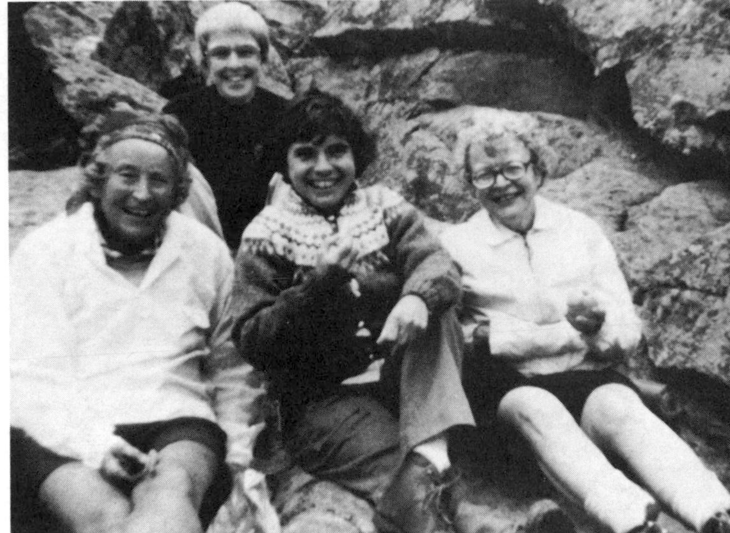

Anna Alden

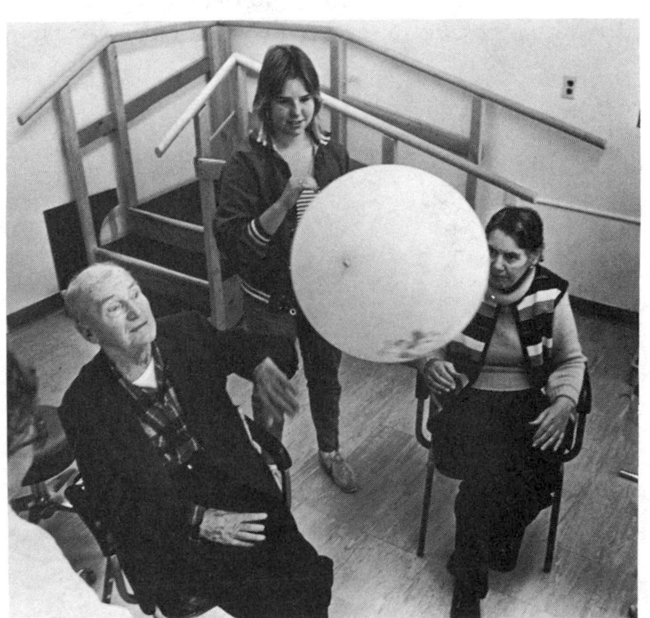

Randy Dean/VNA of San Francisco's Adult Day Health Care Center

I celebrated my fiftieth birthday by flying from Pennsylvania to Vermont to snowshoe ten miles to a campsite. I carried a fifty-pound backpack and learned how to pitch a tent at night in ten-degree temperatures and snow. Through the tent flap, I watched the sky at night, the moonlight on snow and ice covering the branches. This was a birthday I'll never forget!

For years I had been an active member of the Appalachian Mountain Club, hiking in this country and abroad. Then, at seventy-eight, came difficulties with walking. I had to carry a cane. Would I have to give up active interaction with nature? I needed to find out. I decided to try a two-week camping trip in the Virgin Islands. I learned that strolls on beaches and quiet rambles over other near-horizontal terrain will do nicely to keep me feeling connected with nature. [an eighty-two-year-old woman]

Your movement program should be varied and should be compatible with your preferences and physical limitations.

When my mother was in her seventies and wheelchair-bound with Parkinson's disease, she was very excited and proud of learning to play "basketball"—aiming the ball at a wastebasket in the center of a circle of fellow players in wheelchairs. My mother came from a very traditional community in Poland, where girls' sports were virtually nonexistent, so she was learning to play for the first time. [a forty-eight-year-old woman]

I am blessed with quite good health. I have arthritis, which I ignore. I have a bike and ride whenever I can, but every morning I take a standing-still ride on the contraption I have in my bedroom. I also have a series of exercises which I do each morning to get my bones moving. I live very close to the center of the city, and can walk practically anywhere I want to go.* [a seventy-five-year-old woman]

Finding time for exercise despite all the demands of jobs and a busy home life can be difficult but empowering.

A good plan of exercise will allow for improvement in the four areas that constitute total fitness: flexibility, cardiovascular endurance, muscular strength, and body composition (ratio of body fat to lean body mass). We can set realistic and achievable goals for ourselves.

KEEPING OUR JOINTS LIMBER

Flexibility is the ability of a joint to move freely about its axis. Chronic joint stiffness can lock us into painful fixed positions and keep us immobile and unable to do what we want to do. Gentle activity warms the gel that surrounds joints and that acts as a fluid lubricant. It's a good idea to exercise in the morning to liquefy the gel and lubricate the joints. Always warm up with about ten minutes of walking, light jogging, or marching in place, stationary biking, or any activity that gently accelerates heart rate, breathing, and circulation. Try gentle swinging motions of arms and legs, circling of the wrists and ankles, and shoulder shrugs.

When I wake up I take a warm shower, run up and down the stairs a few times, ride a stationary bike while my cereal is cooking, and then am "warmed up" enough to do my stretches before I eat. [a fifty-year-old woman]

Once the body is warmed up, do stretches by holding each one for ten to twenty seconds, letting gravity gently increase the stretch. Breathing should be continuous and normal. This is called static stretching, which helps increase the space between joints and keeps the spine flexible. Do not do the bouncing, pulsing kind of stretches (called ballistic stretching), which can tear connective tissue, and do not stretch "cold" muscles without sufficient warmup.

*In fact, she is not ignoring her arthritis but is helping it with exercise (see Joint and Muscle Pain, Arthritis and Rheumatic Disorders chapter).

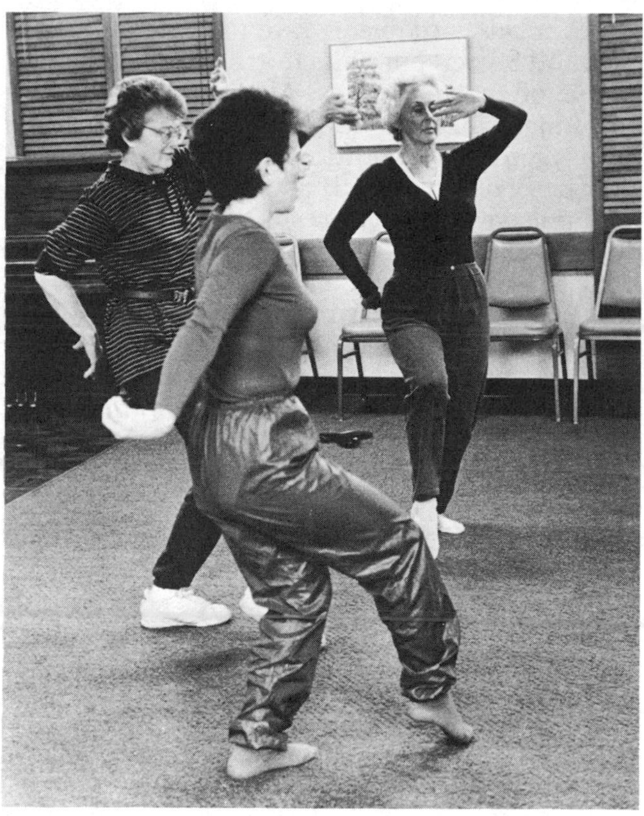

Pam White

Be *especially gentle* when doing the following: (1) bending or rotating the head (it is best to go forward and side to side—not back); (2) dropping the head and body over the legs from a standing position (don't lock your knees when doing this); (3) extending the legs (lift, don't kick); (4) standing knee bends (always keep the knees over the toes and do not bend lower than 90 degrees); (5) arching the lower back (always be cautious: don't do "donkey kicks" on your hands and knees, bringing the knee to the chest and then lifting the leg straight back, and don't do "fire hydrants" on hands and knees, lifting the leg like a dog peeing); (6) don't do forced two-person stretches or bouncing stretches.

PUTTING YOUR HEART INTO IT: AEROBIC EXERCISE

The lungs, heart, and blood vessels, working together to carry oxygen to every cell in the body by means of the blood, compose the cardiovascular system.

Aerobic (meaning "in the presence of oxygen") exercise is any physical activity that uses the major muscle groups of the body in a rhythmic manner and that is performed at an intensity that raises the heart rate to between 60 percent and 80 percent of its maximum capacity for twelve or more minutes. At this rate, the heart and lungs can keep up with the body's demand for oxygen and a conditioning effect takes place.

The benefits of such conditioning are a lowered pulse rate both at rest and during exercise, due to a larger and stronger heart muscle that allows more blood to be pumped with each beat, decreased blood pressure because of more elastic and stronger blood vessels, and more efficient removal of carbon dioxide—the end or waste product of breathing. Such conditioning can lengthen life.

Anaerobic exercise is any activity done so vigorously that the heart and lungs cannot keep up with the body's demand for oxygen and cannot carry away the chemical by-products of exercise. Anaerobic exercise cannot be done continuously for long periods of time. Examples are sprinting and weight lifting.

Naturally, a beginner must get into aerobic exercise gradually. Start with three to five minutes of stationary biking, walking, or simple dance steps. Take your pulse count for ten seconds at rest, and then several minutes into your exercise routine. A pulse count is the most accurate way of monitoring aerobic progress, but also pay attention to how you feel. In time, the aerobic portion of your exercise routine can last thirty minutes or longer, three times a week—or more. The safe way is to warm up, stretch, do your aerobic workout, then to cool down with slow walking or another gentle movement.

I have a series of yoga-type stretches I have done every morning for years that stretch every part of my body. They take ten minutes to do. Then I go out for a brisk thirty-minute walk. When I come in from my walk I am ready for my breakfast and feel energetic enough to face the day's work. [a sixty-year-old woman]

Since the first edition, the most remarkable advances in reducing physical frailty among old people have come from strength-building exercises. For example, strength and balance can often be restored in people with ankle and leg weakness, a major cause of falls and fractures. People have been able to walk away from wheelchairs and walkers, even people in their nineties. Some experts say to forget your age and weight and concentrate on improving aerobic capacity and muscle strength.[5] A well-designed aerobic-exercise and strength-training program com-

How to Determine Your Heart Rate

1. Resting Heart Rate: Take your pulse for sixty seconds. Most people will get a 60, 70, 80, or 90. Take your pulse several times during the day to determine your average.

2. Maximum Heart Rate: Subtract your age from 220. This is the fastest your heart can beat. DO NOT EXERCISE AT THIS RATE!!!

3. Training Heart Rate, or Target Zone: Subtract your resting heart rate from your maximum heart rate; multiply by .60 and by .80; add to each your resting heart rate; the result is your training heart rate, or target zone, per minute. To find the rate for ten seconds, divide by 6.

Example: A fifty-five-year-old woman has a resting heart rate of 85 beats per minute. To calculate the target zone (or range of heartbeats per minute within which she should carry on an aerobic activity):

220 - 55 (age) = 165 (Maximum Heart Rate)
165 - 85 (Resting Heart Rate) = 80
80 x .60 + 85 = 133 beats per minute
80 x .80 + 85 = 149 beats per minute
133 ÷ 6 = 22.2 (22 beats per ten seconds)
149 ÷ 6 = 24.8 (25 beats per ten seconds)

When this woman exercises, she should maintain a heart rate of 133 to 149 beats per minute (22 to 25 beats per ten seconds).

Those on beta blockers, blood-pressure medications, or other medications that may affect heart rate should check with their physician about computing their maximum heart rate and about the percentage they should use in calculating their target zone.

Once you have calculated your target zone, take ten-second pulse checks at regular intervals (every five or ten minutes) during aerobic activity. Keep moving as you count, as heart rate drops rapidly when exercise is stopped. All you have to remember are the two ten-second figures—don't go below or above those numbers. It's also best to work near the lower or middle end of your target zone. The beneficial results are the same, and you are running no risk of injury if you are in normal health.

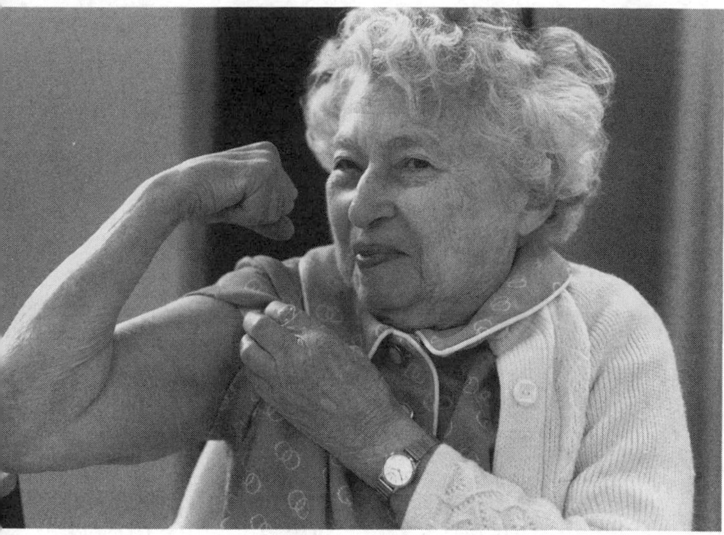

David Witbeck/Hebrew Rehabilitation Center for Aged

bined with proper eating may actually *increase weight* by increasing muscle and bone mass, but will *decrease fat*.

THE STRENGTH FACTOR

Results from a National Institute on Aging project called the FICSIT trials, started in 1990, should be available shortly. These trials are evaluating the benefits of various combinations of activities in reducing frailty and falls in old men and, at last, women too.[6] When a gradually increasing demand is placed upon muscles, they respond, given sufficient rest between exercise sessions (at least forty-eight hours), by becoming larger and stronger. Also, as muscles contract during exercise, they act beneficially on the bones, causing calcium to be properly deposited within them to make them dense and stronger.[7] This reduces chances of brittle, easily breakable bones—the condition known as osteoporosis.

Conventionally, girls and women have not been encouraged to be strong. Fortunately, that picture is changing.

I train people of all ages on Nautilus and on free weights. At least 50 percent are women and they love the results. They stand taller and are stronger and have more endurance and muscle strength for walking, dancing, aerobics, skiing, and swimming. [a fifty-one-year-old trainer]

Weights were once a man's domain. Though men tend to develop greater muscle mass than women do, this does not mean that women cannot or should not develop their muscular potential to the fullest. Society has stereotyped women as soft, round, weak, and submissive. We can and must break that image. Our very health and survival depend on it.

Gaining muscular strength need not be difficult. Each day find ways to use your leg, arm, chest, back, and buttock muscles to lift, carry, support, or move weight. When lifting, always bend your knees, use your leg not your back muscles, and keep objects close to your body. You can add weights to your home exercise program by holding objects such as small cans of food or by purchasing a set of light hand and ankle weights with instructions. Some women make weights from mattress ticking filled with sand.[8]

If you have experienced bone fractures because of osteoporosis, check with your physician before working out with weights. Other exercises to strengthen the muscles and bones should be done first.[9]

POSTURE: STANDING TALL

Posture? We'd all like it to be good; but aside from appearance, does it matter that much? Yes, it does, because posture profoundly affects physical and mental health.

Simply sitting for hours at a job, even slightly bent over, can induce high states of anxiety. The reason is that in this position the lungs are constricted, oxygen intake is reduced, and thus the amount of glucose (fuel for brain cells) that reaches the brain cells is greatly diminished. Sitting bent over can contribute to round shoulders, which can reduce breathing capacity, elevate blood pressure, and contribute to the formation of a dowager's hump.

Poor posture can affect digestion and elimination, contribute to hernias, hemorrhoids, intestinal diverticuli,[10] and bladder-control problems. With prolonged poor posture, some muscles shorten while others lengthen and weaken. A ripple effect takes place: one disturbed set of muscles, especially around a joint, affects others, and they, in turn, affect still others. Gradually, posture becomes increasingly faulty and injurious.

Good posture permits free movement and offers the best starting point for any physical work or exercise. Since posture affects us all the time, it is advisable to pay attention to body alignment and body coordination while walking, standing, sitting, stooping, lifting, or doing more complicated movements. You can begin to change poor postural habits by strengthening abdominal, back, and chest muscles.

As one whose posture was poor all of my life, I speak from experience. No amount of urging me to "stand up straight" on my mother's part or my own efforts to do so ever improved my posture one iota. At fifty-plus years of age I stand taller and prouder than ever before in my life. I owe it all *to weight training. We have to be aware of what is holding the body upright. It's not bone. It's not fat. It's not water or blood. It's* muscle*—the active tensing of moving muscle tissue pulling upwards against the downward pull of gravity.*

Designing Our Own Fitness Program

The major muscles of the body that we need to strengthen are the abdominal muscles, the chest and back muscles, and the muscles of the legs and arms. Without fancy equipment and expensive clubs, we can use the most effective method of strengthening muscles—moving against the force of gravity. Walking, swimming, bicycling, and dancing strengthen our muscles and improve the cardiovascular system. At any age, these are the most all-round beneficial, easily accessible, and least expensive kinds of activity.

In planning your activities, consider safety factors. Dress comfortably, wear proper shoes and a bicycle helmet when biking outdoors. Campaign with others for bike paths, safe streets, snow removal, and swimming lessons for the disabled and other adults in your community.

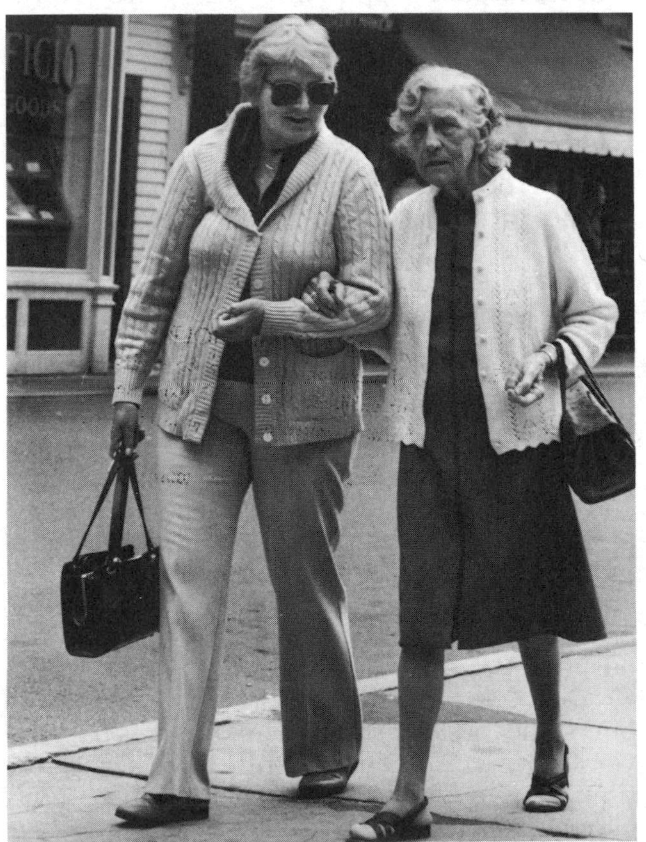

Norma Holt

Walking

Vigorous walking helps accelerate blood flow: the veins in the legs get squeezed with every step, sending the blood back to the heart. Brisk walking, including a few hills, can be an effective aerobic exercise. Keep your target zone in mind and calculate your pace. You might begin with one-quarter- to half-mile walks or even shorter ones daily. When that distance becomes easy, increase it gradually. When you can walk a mile without tiring, try walking that same distance a little faster. Then add a little more distance, then more speed, etc. Walking provides the same benefits as jogging without the extra stress on joints.

Swimming

Swimming sets off a reflex action that enlarges the heart, causing it to pump more blood than it does in land sports, and also increases flexibility. Swimming does increase bone density, especially in the upper body, which is not strengthened by walking.

In swimming, as in other aerobic activities, when you hit your stride, your mind is free to wander, plan, solve problems, imagine.

I've learned to keep my pencil and a pad of paper in my locker so I can write down all the solutions that come pouring into my head after I've done about a third of my laps in the pool. [a fifty-four-year-old woman]

Bicycling

Bicycling is an excellent exercise for the cardiovascular system. There are adult three-wheeled bicycles that are easier to balance than two-wheelers. Stationary bicycles are also convenient for those who never learned to ride and for exercising while watching television, reading, or listening to music.

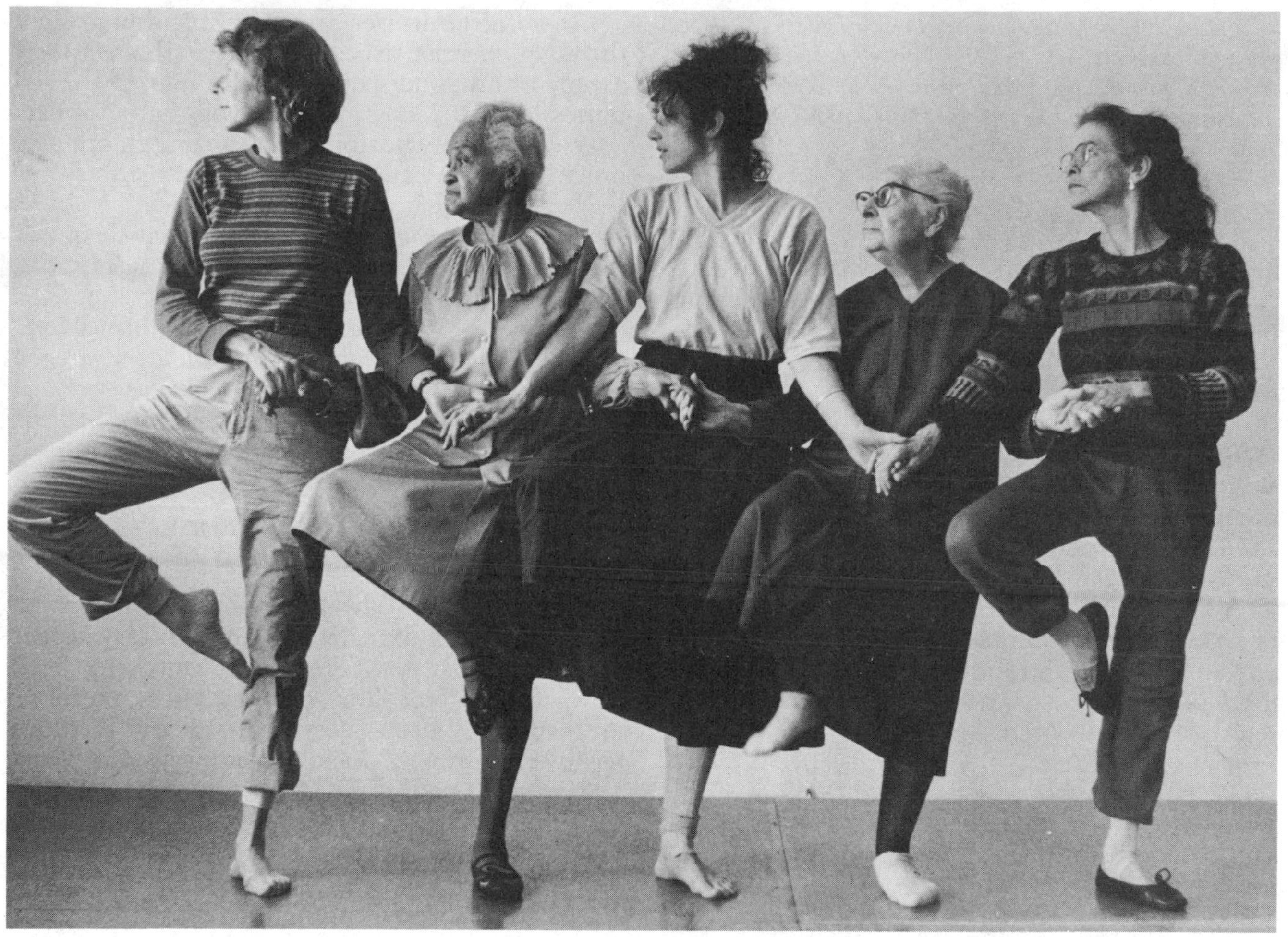

The Dance Exchange, Dancers of the Third Age/Dennis Deloria

DANCING

Dancing is perhaps second only to walking as the most beneficial form of exercise. Besides developing flexibility and strength, it gives a natural "high" and a feeling of well-being. Moving to a beat or to music is one of the oldest activities on earth.

*As I dance, I affirm the beauty of my rounded belly that birthed two babies who are now adults, of my heavy hips that carried them, the beauty of my breasts that nursed them, of my skin that is hard from years of heat and cold. As I dance, I affirm the strength of these legs that have labored up fifty-six years of steps. I insist that my asthmatic lungs still work for my pleasure, and my curved back still supports my desire. As I dance, I reach out to other women and say, "Look, we are beautiful; no one need tell us so; we know it; and we love each other."**

*Excerpted from an unpublished manuscript by Carolyn Ruth Swift.

Furthermore, you can dance alone in the privacy of your own home to a record or the radio, as well as socially at gatherings, clubs, dance groups, and parties.

I learned how important it was for me to do some kind of movement as I got older. I developed an exercise and yoga program for the elderly people who ate lunch at a nutrition site. Our movement leader was an enthusiastic fifty-nine-year-old dance therapist. At first, people were reluctant to get up from the lunch tables. But a seventy-eight-year-old Chinese woman got up, smiling and dancing, and gradually others joined her. (She told us later that old people in China are very active. She was feeling depressed about being old in America before she discovered us.)

People came regularly for about three months. We saw women begin to unbend locked elbows and to twist heads and torsos that had stiffened into one piece. Once after a two-hour session, they didn't want to leave. So we did circle dances with tambourines, castanets, drums, ribbons, and scarves for another half an hour. While we were dancing, one woman, in her late eighties, turned to me and said: "My husband would never believe this if he saw me." Another, who always carried a cane, left and forgot it. The therapist joked: "And the lame shall walk." But she had tears in her eyes. So did I. [a fifty-four-year-old woman]

Hatha Yoga

Hatha Yoga is one of the best exercises for attaining total body flexibility. Its fringe benefits can include inner peace, relaxation, help with insomnia, decreased blood pressure, and relief from anxiety and stress.

Hatha Yoga has a great calming effect. It's good for stress reduction and flexibility. I was immobilized at age fifty-two by an arthritis attack. My yoga exercises helped me return to being as flexible as anyone.

Yoga is particularly useful as we age because its stretches keep joints flexible. Yoga positions help strengthen abdominal muscles and foster good posture—both areas that are vital to the health of older women.

Tai Chi

Tai Chi is a beautiful exercise and "martial art" developed in ancient China. In modern China, it is considered especially appropriate for the old. Tai Chi is a continuous sequence of forms that includes gently moving all the joints and paying attention to the effect of breathing on the ebb and flow of energy. Tai Chi is becoming increasingly popular and available in this country because it has such positive effects on physical and emotional fitness.

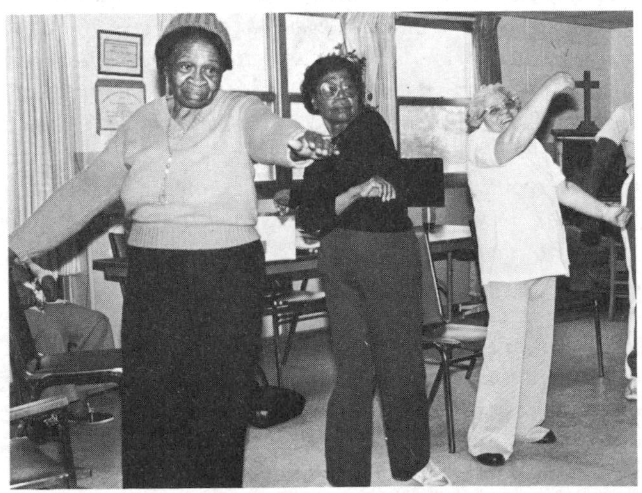

Elana Freedom

In some countries, inner or spiritual growth through exercise is considered to be a major aspect of an aging person's daily life. The disciplines from the East, such as yoga and Tai Chi, develop not only flexibility and strength, but also inner awareness and concentration.

I learned once, in a dance class, that it's important to talk to your body. It's like mothering a child. Instead of getting upset or angry because it isn't behaving the way you'd wish, you praise your body for small achievements, comfort it when it hurts, promise it pleasure, and encourage it to push just a little harder. In this way, I've learned that my body and I, though we feel separate, are different parts of the same being. [a fifty-four-year-old woman]

Methods to Change How We Move

Several movement/awareness approaches, such as the Feldenkrais method and the Alexander technique, use movement for improving both physical and emotional health. These methods are especially useful for learning how to move easily without pain despite disabilities and physical restrictions.

Some forms of psychotherapy also use the body to diagnose and treat emotional problems. The two best known, bioenergetics and psychomotor therapy, attempt to break through chronic muscle tensions developed early in life in response to emotionally disturbing situations. These methods can also improve coordination.

How Much of a Good Thing?

The average woman should start slowly and work up to one hour three to five times a week in a combination of flexibility, cardiovascular, and muscle-strengthening exercises to create and maintain fitness. Let your body be your guide. It helps to keep a journal for several months after starting a movement plan to clarify needs, expectations, and feelings about the program you've started.

When Movement Is Limited

There are times when we can't be active—during illness, or when recuperating from an illness or an operation. Some of us suffer from disabilities that greatly restrict movement. If you have a disability, you can still benefit from exercise. Even if you are bed- or wheelchair-bound, you can

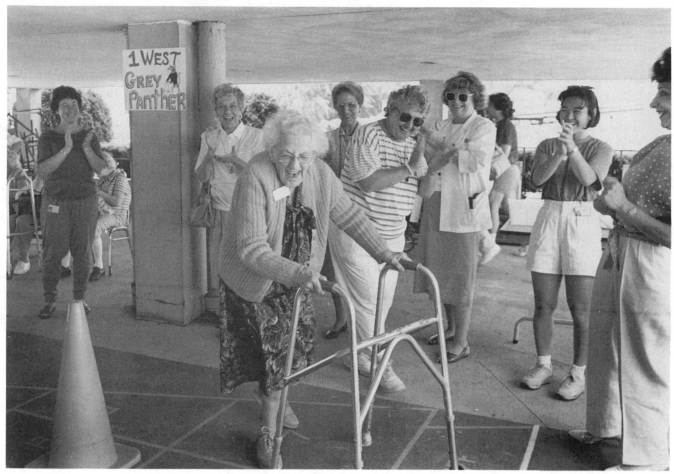

Gustav Freedman/Hebrew Rehabilitation Center for Aged

improve lung capacity, muscle strength, and flexibility with consistent daily exercise tailored for you. Few conditions require total rest or immobility. Encourage your health-care providers to guide you in designing a medically sound movement program.

It's difficult and discouraging to exercise when we're feeling weak or in pain. But there is no question about the importance of exercise in rehabilitation. A moderate and regular exercise program helps many problems.

A massive stroke impaired my ability to function independently. The effects seriously damaged my physical and emotional stability. Learning to swim was one of my most effective coping techniques. Two swimming sessions (forty-five minutes each) weekly increased my strength and endurance. The encouragement from the therapist and members of the group for even a small accomplishment was a tremendous morale booster. We adopted the motto "Press on regardless." The formation of new friendships was essential in helping to develop emotional security. [a thirty-eight-year-old woman]

Close to 100 percent of persons responding to a survey of women with arthritis mentioned that regular exercise decreased their pain.[11]

If you are confined to a chair or bed, exercise can help maintain strength and flexibility of joints and muscles, good digestion and bowel movements, good blood circulation, and a better mental outlook. It can prevent bedsores, and it makes things easier for the caregiver as well. Home health aides and nursing-home personnel should be trained to provide exercises for persons in beds or chairs.

Here is a list of things you can do at your own pace. Try them for a few days and experience the relaxation and the gentle glow of energy that simple movement can give you. Do the exercises with energy and concentration to enhance their effectiveness. Start slowly and do more each day. *Many of these exercises are the same ones that women in more fit condition will find useful also.*

1. Breathe deeply.
2. Contract and relax any muscle group you

can control. While breathing regularly, tighten the muscles for several seconds, and then slowly release. Be aware of the relaxation that follows.

3. Do Kegel exercises and "tummy blops" (see pages 75–77).
4. Exercise your face muscles by making "funny faces." Move your lower jaw from side to side and forward and back. Open eyes wide, then scrunch shut. Wiggle your ears if you can.
5. Stretch and limber the neck slowly, carefully. In bed your neck is protected from bending too far backward. Rotate the head in wide circles in both directions. Alternately, look slowly to the ceiling, stretching the front of the neck, then look slowly down, being aware of a stretch in the back of the neck ("Yes"). Then turn the head from side to side ("No").
6. Placing hands on shoulders or by your sides, rotate shoulders in both directions.
7. Stretching arms out to your sides, twist them in both directions. Make small circles with your hands and then with your arms. Then open and close fists. Alternately stretch each arm upward from the shoulder as if picking apples.
8. Circle wrists as far as they can go. Quickly open and close fists several times, stretching fingers. Circle your ankles in both directions. Flex feet backward and forward, then clench toes and release.
9. Tie a rope to the foot of your bed (or have someone do this for you) and slowly pull yourself to sitting position, then lower again.
10. "Walk" against the footboard of the bed.
11. If you can, pull one knee to your chest, then the other knee, then both.
12. If you can stand, hold on to the back of a chair while rotating your legs, one at a time, from the hip. Rotate in both directions. Then extend your leg forward and slowly swing your lower leg backward and forward.

Avoiding Injury

The best way to avoid injury is to get a medical checkup before you start an exercise program. The examination should make you aware of potential problem areas and possible limiting factors, and help you to set realistic goals. Particularly if you decide to undertake demanding movement programs like tennis, racquetball, cross-country skiing, use of Nautilus or other weight-lifting equipment, or if you have physical disabilities, it's best to get a medical evaluation to prevent injury, to get the maximum benefit from what you do, and to set realistic goals. Your physician may recommend a stress test, which monitors your heart while you are performing an ever-increasing work load on a treadmill, to discover and make you aware of any hidden heart disease. It isn't infallible, however, especially for women, and may be too stressful (see pages 339–40).

In the long run, only you can choose how much caution (or precaution) to use before starting your exercise plan. Most important, always pay close attention to how you feel.

Normal Reactions to Exercise:

Increased depth and rate of breathing
Increased heart rate
Feeling/hearing your heartbeat
Mild to moderate perspiration
Mild muscle aches and tenderness at first

Abnormal Reactions to Exercise—
STOP IMMEDIATELY:

Severe shortness of breath
Wheezing, coughing, difficulty in breathing
Chest pain, pressure, or tightness
Lightheadedness, dizziness, confusion, word slurring, fainting
Cramps, severe pain, severe muscle ache
Nausea
Severe, prolonged fatigue or exhaustion after exercising

If these symptoms recur with further exercise, check with your physician. You might need special guidance.

Some General Precautions

1. Lubricate *all* joints with gentle bending and swinging (shoulders, elbows, wrists, knees, ankles), contraction and release (fingers, toes, arches, spine), and stretches.
2. Don't hold your breath; coordinate full breathing with each movement.
3. Drink fluids before, during, and after exercising. It is common as we age not to feel thirsty, even when dehydrated.
4. When ill, do only mild stretches, joint lubrication, and deep breathing. Gentle movement that doesn't cause you to tire will allow your

MUSCLES OF THE PELVIC FLOOR

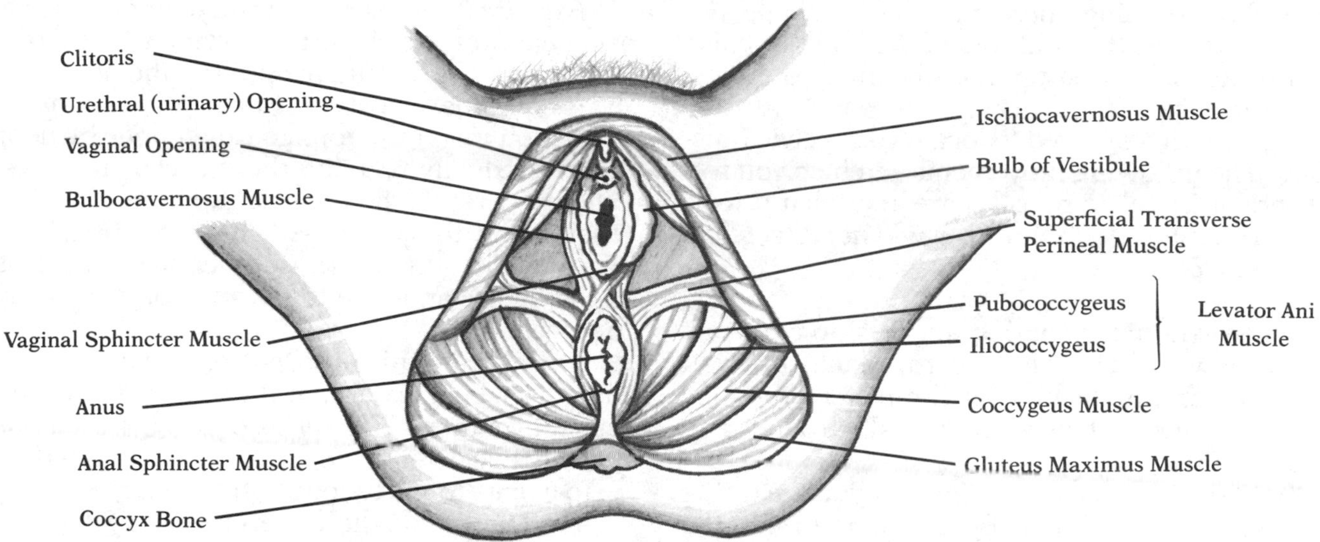

body to use its energy for rehabilitation. This is a good time to practice deep breathing and meditation.

5. No two bodies are alike. Achieve what is possible for yourself; do not compare yourself to others.
6. Wear any comfortable clothing that breathes (natural fibers like cotton are best), that doesn't bind in the crotch, around the shoulders, or at the waist. There's no need to spend money on expensive sportswear unless you want to. *Never* wear rubberized or plastic sweat suits. They can cause high internal temperatures (hyperthermia), dehydration, and even death. Supportive shoes with arches are necessary to soften impact on your organs and spine. If you decide to jog, buy running shoes; if you do aerobic dancing, buy aerobic shoes. They are not the same. Running shoes have more support in the heel and aerobic shoes have more support under the ball of the foot.

Exercises for All Women

Two problems that are special issues for women are very much affected by exercise. These are:

- Bladder control to prevent loss of urine, particularly when we cough, sneeze, or laugh. The strength of the muscles in the pelvic floor, abdomen, and back is very important.
- Loss of bone density and muscle strength due to inactivity, resulting in osteoporosis and bone fractures.

Kegel and Other Exercises to Develop Your Own "Girdle"[12]

Dr. Arnold Kegel, after whom this exercise is named, first began his pioneering research in the 1940s, in response to women's complaints of leaking urine.[13] He later demonstrated how strengthening the pubococcygeal muscle (also called the levator ani muscle) not only improves bladder control, but also contributes to increased sexual satisfaction and more comfortable childbirth.

When you exercise the pubococcygeal muscle you will become aware of your vagina. Many women have to be taught how to locate this muscle and how to exercise it; they have been living for years with a kind of inertness or numbness in this region. Others, even at an advanced age, still do not know that there are three separate openings in the pelvis of the female body. One woman in her seventies wanted to use tampons in her vagina to absorb urine leakage.

There are also several sets of muscles that run across the abdomen that act like a mat, keeping the internal organs in place and protecting and supporting the uterus and bladder, helping to maintain their correct position. When women use cloth and elastic girdles, they are trying to compensate for the loss of control over these muscles. Keeping these muscles in shape not only improves the contours of the body, but also contributes to the support of the internal organs and the back.

To begin, you need to locate your pelvic muscles. The following movements can help you feel where your pelvic muscles are and what it feels like to tighten them, but *they will not strengthen your muscles*.

- When you are urinating, try to stop and start the flow of urine. Afterward, make sure you always empty the bladder completely. You may need to wait a few seconds, walk around, and try again.
- Tighten your rectal muscles as if you are trying not to pass gas. Then, if you can, try to shift the tightness from the rear to the front of your bottom area.
- Tighten your vaginal muscles around an object such as one or two inserted fingers, a tampon inserted halfway, or a man's penis during intercourse.

Your ability to do these movements indicates how strong your muscles are. Do them periodically as a test of your increasing strength, but they are not adequate exercises. For strengthening, start the following exercises by lying down, as there will be less pressure from the abdominal organs on the pelvic muscles. Sometimes placing a pillow under your buttocks or your bent knees can be helpful, but always make sure you feel relaxed and comfortable. As you progress, you will also be able to do the exercises while sitting, standing, or bending.

Place your hand on your abdomen to make sure you do not contract your abdominal muscles while doing the exercises. Also, it is important to make sure you do not squeeze your buttock muscles or hold your breath while doing the exercises.

Exercise 1: Contract or draw up the pelvic floor, hold for two to four seconds, and relax for ten seconds. Repeat five times. Do this three times a day. Work up gradually until you can hold the contraction for eight seconds. If you find your muscles getting sore, do not stop doing the exercises but decrease the time you hold each contraction, and then gradually increase it again. Work up to sets of ten.

Exercise 2: When you are comfortably able to hold the contraction for eight seconds, add three to four short, fast, but strong twitches at the end of each long contraction.

Exercise 3: Think of your bladder and uterus as an elevator which you are trying to raise to a higher floor, and visualize pulling them up into the abdominal cavity toward your stomach. When you reach the top, go down floor by floor again, gradually relaxing the muscles in stages. When you reach the basement, let go of all the tension and think release. Then come back up again to the first floor, so the pelvic floor is slightly tense and able to hold the organs firmly in place.

Exercise 4: Raise the entire pelvic area, as though sucking water into the vagina. Relax and repeat five times. This series of five contractions may be repeated four to six times a day, building up to twenty to thirty contractions a day.

Find time to do these exercises every day. You can do them at any time that is convenient—for instance, while stopped at a red light, watching TV, or doing dishes.

Beware of spring-loaded gadgets to squeeze between the thighs that are now advertised as "Kegel" devices. They strengthen the inner thigh but not the pelvic muscles.

Be patient. Like any type of muscle training, pelvic muscle exercises take time to work, often several months. Over this time, you will be making progress. You will need to continue these exercises to keep the muscles strong. Many women find the effort to be worthwhile because of the improved bladder control they are able to achieve.

Since you can't see the pelvic muscles, the exercises can be hard to learn. If the exercises are not helping you, a physical therapist or nurse may be available in your area to assist you. They may also have special equipment for biofeedback training that can help you learn to do the exercises correctly and evaluate your progress.

The following exercises will strengthen the upper and lower abdominal muscles. In order to do them effectively and protect your back, tighten your abdominal muscles before you start rather than doing them with your abdomen sticking out.

For the upper abdominals, do modified bent-knee sit-ups. Lying on your back with knees bent and feet flat on a bed or the floor, lift the head and shoulders while reaching forward with the hands to touch the knees, then lie back again, keeping eyes looking up and shoulders off the

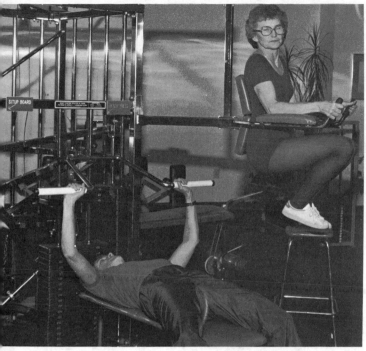

Candace Pratt/The Works Athletic Club

bed or floor. Reach for your left knee with your right hand as you twist your waist slightly, then do the same with the right knee and left hand. As you become stronger, you can do these sit-ups with your hands behind your head (do not pull up on your head—use hands only to support your head on the way down), reaching your elbows toward your knees. Do not do sit-ups with straight legs.

For the lower abdominals, lie on your back with legs extended straight up overhead. You may find this easier to do with your buttocks against a wall. "Walk" your feet in the air in place or toward your head. "Bicycling" with legs as high as possible also strengthens the lower abdominals.[14] Also while standing, tighten your abdominal muscles with tummy "blops." On an empty stomach only, inhale fully, exhale fully, then tighten and release stomach muscles three or four times. Another way is to lie on your side with your knees drawn up. Contract your belly muscles so that you pull your knees and head closer together.

Exercising for Strong Bones

Remember that when we are physically active, the body uses calcium efficiently for bone growth and maintenance. When we are inactive, calcium is not absorbed well into the bones but is "dumped" and excreted in the urine. The depletion of bone cells (osteoporosis) can lead to a dowager's hump and to bone fractures. Many physicians treat osteoporosis with special exercises.[15]

For older women, fast walking is the best exercise to increase bone density in the lower body. If you have no spinal or skeletal problems, jogging may be all right, but it is more stressful on the joints. Exercise the upper body as well so calcium will be deposited in all the bones. Weight training, which develops muscle, is especially beneficial because it also increases the strength of the connective tissues, tendons, and ligaments. Exercise also improves balance and coordination so we are less likely to fall or, if we do fall, more likely to fall safely.

"Going Formal": Choosing a Movement Facility

If you want to undertake a conditioning program that requires special facilities or instructions, take time to find the best place. Any facility or program should provide safety, well-trained instructors, and personal attention. It should be reasonably priced, easily accessible, and suited to your personal needs. In considering whether you can afford instruction, keep in mind the intangibles that aren't price-tagged: better health can give you time otherwise spent in illness; you will feel better about yourself and life; better fitness can bring down your medical costs.

What should you look for in a fitness center or program?[16] First, find the facilities that have the activities you want. Next, check further about each: Are their hours convenient? Can you get there easily? If you have special needs, will they be met there? Are the costs reasonable?

Then, arrange a tour of centers that meet your criteria, and ask questions. What credentials does the staff have? (Look for college degrees in and certification in applied anatomy and physiology, physical education, nutrition, and exercise physiology and current CPR certification.) Try to visit at the busiest time of day, or at a time you will want to use the center. Ask some of the clients how they like the center and what some of the problems are. Look to see whether equipment is in good condition and whether showers and other wet areas are clean. Beware of places that push "lifetime contracts." A life membership lasts only as long as the life of the facility or organization unless another facility or new management agrees to honor it. Buy the shortest-term package to try out before committing a lot of money. Does the center take a medical history? Do they take blood pressure and pulse rate before, during, and after exercise? Can you get personal guidance in the use of equipment? Some centers have special rates for club usage during the midday hours, when it is least busy. If those hours are convenient for you, this may be an ideal arrangement, as it benefits both you and the club.

Don't make a decision on your first visit. Beware of high-pressure salespeople who offer you bargains if you "make a decision today," or who refuse to allow you to take the contract home to review before signing. The right choice can make a big difference in whether you use the center regularly, consistently, and safely.

Finally, guard against giving up instead of accepting limits and going on.

I used to like to go mountain climbing. When I couldn't do that, I went hill climbing. Now I walk on more level ground. You don't have to give up your dream. You just shape it differently. [an eighty-two-year-old woman]

NOTES

1. Herbert A. deVries with Diane Hales, *Fitness After Fifty.* New York: Charles Scribner's Sons, 1974, pp. 9–11.

2. Maria A. Fiatarone, et al., "High-Intensity Strength Training in Nonagenarians: Effects of Skeletal Muscle." *Journal of the American Medical Association,* Vol. 263, No. 22 (June 13, 1990), pp. 3029–34.

3. James Blumenthal and R. Sanders Williams, Duke University Center for the Study of Aging. *Center Reports,* Vol. 6, No. 3 (December 1982), p. 4.

4. Robert S. Brown, et al., "The Prescription of Exercise for Depression." *The Physician and Sports Medicine,* Vol. 6, No. 12 (December 1978), pp. 52–58.

5. Judy Foreman, "Are You Younger Than You Think?" *The Boston Globe Magazine,* Apr. 25, 1993, pp. 14–19.

6. For an excellent discussion of overcoming frailty, see National Institute on Aging, *Physical Frailty: A Reducible Barrier to Independence for Older Americans.* NIH Publication No. 91-397. The entire Vol. 41, No. 3 (March 1993) issue of the *Journal of the American Geriatrics Society* is devoted to a description of the FICSIT trials including each of the eight projects.

7. A. Chamay and P. T. Schantz, "Mechanical Influences in Bone Remodeling: Experimental Research on Wolff's Law." *Journal of Biochemistry,* Vol. 5 (1972), pp. 173–80; and E. L. Smith, Jr., et al., "Bone Involution Decrease in Exercising Middle-Aged Women." *California Tissue International,* Vol. 36, Supplement 1 (1984), pp. 129–38.

8. Kay Flatten, Barbara Wilhite, Eleanor Reyes-Watson, *Exercise Activities for the Elderly.* New York: Springer Publishing Co., 1988.

9. Joseph Lane, "Post Menopausal Osteoporosis: The Orthopedic Approach." *The Female Patient,* Vol. 6 (November 1981), pp. 43–50, 54.

10. Gerda Hinrichsen, *Body Shop: Scandinavian Exercises for Relaxation.* New York: Taplinger Publishing Co., 1976, p. 46.

11. *Hot Flash,* Vol. 3, No. 2 (Winter 1984), p. 1.

12. With thanks to the Adelaide Women's Community Health Centre, North Adelaide, Australia, for their instructions, "Exercising and Strengthening the Pelvic Floor, Kegel Exercises"; Sheila Kitzinger, *Woman's Experience of Sex.* New York: Penguin Books, 1985, pp. 48–50; Elizabeth Noble, *Essential Exercises for the Childbearing Year,* 3rd ed. Boston: Houghton Mifflin, 1988; and Kari Bo et al., "Pelvic Floor Muscle Exercises for the Treatment of Female Stress Urinary Incontinence." *Neurology and Urodynamics*, Vol. 9 (1990), pp. 471–77, 479–87, 489–502.

13. Arnold Kegel, "The Physiologic Treatment of Poor Tone and Function of the Genital Muscles and of Urinary Stress Incontinence." *Western Journal of Surgery, Obstetrics, and Gynecology,* Vol. 57 (1949), pp. 527–35.

14. Personal communication from Maggie Lettvin, author of several useful books on women's health and fitness.

15. Lane, op. cit.

16. Adapted from Gretchen M. Von Mering, *The Fitness Directory: A Guide to Exercise, Nutrition, and Recreation Programs and Services in the Greater Boston Area.* Boston: The Medical Foundation, Inc., 1983, pp. 5–15.

Living with Ourselves and Others as We Age

✦

7

SEXUALITY IN THE SECOND HALF OF LIFE

✦

BY AURELIE JONES GOODWIN WITH LYNN SCOTT

SPECIAL THANKS TO MARY C. ALLEN, SARAH F. PEARLMAN, AND WENDY SANFORD

1994 UPDATE BY PAULA B. DORESS-WORTERS WITH HELP FROM AURELIE JONES GOODWIN

HIV AND SAFER SEX AND *SAFER SEX GUIDELINES* BY CHRISTIE BURKE AND WITH THANKS TO WENDY SANFORD, LIZ GALST, AND ALLISON MORRILL

RESOURCES FOR THIS CHAPTER ON PAGES 459–62

LETTER TO MY CHILDREN*

If we
could start again
You, newbegotten, I
A clean stick peeled
of twenty paper layers of years
I'd tell you only what you know,
Teach one commandment,
"Mind the senses and the soul
Will take care of itself
Being five times blessed."

Anne Wilkinson

We affirm ourselves as we experience pleasure through our senses. Now that we are older, if we attend to the wisdom of our minds and bodies, we can enhance our sexual pleasure. The pleasures of the body, and specifically sexual pleasures, provide us with release, shared intimacy, communion with our inner selves and with our partners, and a chance to express ourselves physically. We can give ourselves pleasure through masturbation, whether or not we are in a sexual relationship with another person. Sex allows us intimate connection with someone we love, or adventure with a new partner. Our senses provide us with pleasure and our thoughts and feelings give meaning to our experience.

Almost all of us who are middle-aged or older grew up in an environment where attitudes toward sexuality were more rigid than they are today. We may have learned that we should not talk about sex. People who do not talk about sex are less likely to practice safer sex (see pp. 96–97). We may have learned that women do not or should not enjoy sex as much as men, or that men should always initiate sex. Because of this early training, we may still feel embarrassed or ashamed over sexual issues. Paradoxically, we may believe that because of the "sexual revolution" we shouldn't be uncomfortable, or that we ought to have more sex than we do. A double standard of sexual behavior still exists, particularly among middle-aged and older people. This chapter is intended to affirm and support our sexuality and to help all of us enjoy our sexuality more fully and protect ourselves more effectively.

Two misconceptions occur when women are stereotyped by ageist thinking. Older women are considered neither sexually attractive nor sexually active. Those men who are available often choose as partners younger women or women

*From *Collected Poems of Anne Wilkinson*, A. Smith, ed., Macmillan Co. of Canada Ltd., 1968, p. 94.

who look young. As the baby boomers and some of their pop icons approach middle age, the trend toward an ever-younger age of peak desirability seems to have leveled off. Yet we are still expected to maintain the body image of a thirty-five- or forty-year-old for the rest of our lives, making it hard for us as we grow older to fully express our sexuality. Believing the stereotypes leads to fear and denial of aging, and takes a toll on our self-esteem when we see the signs of aging in ourselves and in those we love.

As we age, some physical changes occur that may affect our sexual activity. But there is no physical reason based on age alone why we cannot continue to enjoy sex for as long as we live. Despite social pressures, many of us are accepting and enjoying our sexuality more freely than ever. One way we can help ourselves in this respect is to break through the barrier of silence and talk with each other about sexuality. Although it may be hard to talk openly with other women about sex if you have never done so, it is such a positive experience that it is worth the effort. By listening to older women in our families or in women's groups, we can recognize negative messages about sex that we received as children, and then reevaluate our attitudes. Talking to family members about sex can be especially difficult; yet it is often liberating.

Women's groups in which we talk about sexual experiences and feelings have developed since the late 1960s as an outgrowth of the women's movement. There are women's groups at most women's centers and some churches and other community organizations. It is common to hear women exclaim, "I never knew anyone else felt the way I do!" One long-married woman, aged fifty, who had complained of lack of sexual interest, returned to a women's group to say, "After our discussion last week I went home and talked with my husband and we had an absolute orgy!"

MYTHS AND REALITIES ABOUT WOMEN, SEX, AND AGING

Sexism, ageism, homophobia, and Victorianism all interact to create a pervasive mythology about sex and the older person. These myths do the most damage when we ourselves accept and act on them, and in so doing give up pleasures that are an important and valuable part of our humanity. Consider the following:

Myth 1: Older people are no longer interested in sex and sexuality and no longer engage in sexual activity. Sex is for the young.

This myth has its roots in several notions that link sex and youthfulness. Since society equates attractiveness with youth, it follows that, according to the myth, when you are no longer young, you are no longer desirable.

This myth also connects sexuality with romantic love. In the media, in stories, songs, and the general folklore of our culture, romantic love is the exclusive province of young heterosexual women and men.

The reality is that if you are interested in sex and want to act on that interest, you are just like many other people your age. A study of people sixty to ninety-one years old revealed that 91 percent enjoyed sex for a variety of reasons: it reduces tension, makes women feel more feminine, helps people sleep, and provides a physical outlet for emotion. The people studied engaged in sexual relations an average of 1.4 times a week—about what they averaged when they were in their forties.[1] Both the Kinsey research and Masters and Johnson found that women and men continue their accustomed sexual patterns through their later years. If you led an active sexual life when you were younger, you can look forward to continuing to do so. If you found sex a burden, you may decide to cease sexual activity as you grow older. Masters and Johnson's research confirmed what many women have discovered for themselves: that there is no time limit on women's sexual capacity. Although our responses may slow down, we can continue to enjoy sex and orgasm throughout our lives.[2]

When older people are viewed as asexual, they are less likely to be offered safer-sex information (see pp. 96–97), and their risk of HIV infection increases.

Myth 2: Changes in hormone levels that occur during and after menopause create a "deficiency disease" that causes women to find sex uncomfortable and unpleasant.

Menopause has been the subject of many fallacies and myths, several created and perpetuated by physicians, psychiatrists, and drug companies. The notion that menopause is a deficiency disease[3] has, among other things, fostered widespread use of hormonal supplements. In fact, menopause is a normal life transition, not a disease. Women can continue to feel sexual and enjoy sex until very late in life.

Myth 3: Women who are beyond childbearing years lose their desire and their desirability.

Sexuality and sex appeal are not the same as

fertility. For many older women and men sex is actually *better* in the later years. Many women experience a reawakening of sexual interest when pregnancy is no longer a worry. Couples often have more time to relate to each other sexually after children are grown. A divorce or other life change that has nothing to do with fertility may also contribute to a reawakening of sexual interest.

Myth 4: In order to have a full and complete sex life, a woman must have a male partner.

Although the majority of women do have relationships with men, we can be sexual in a variety of ways—with a man or a woman or by pleasuring ourselves alone. The choice is ours to make.

Myth 5: The only truly satisfying and acceptable sex is through intercourse, culminating in mutual orgasm. All other sexual activity is "foreplay" and doesn't count.

While sex is sometimes defined in terms of intercourse, it is not true that intercourse is the only satisfying form of lovemaking. As we age, our experience of intercourse changes. Older women and men need more time for sexual stimulation before they are ready for intercourse. Once we learn that gratifying sexual experience without penetration is a possible choice, we can feel free to explore the variety of other caresses that can provide pleasure.

Older people report in several studies that oral sex is a favorite activity.[4] Cuddling, caressing, and manual stimulation are also satisfying. Lovemaking may continue to be satisfying whether one, both, or neither party has an orgasm.

SEX AND AGING: SOME WOMEN'S EXPERIENCES

People have this idea that sex is somehow naughty for older people. They picture serene and wise grandparents. Older people are not supposed to be feeling and passionate. But at fifty I thought, "Hey, I'm old enough to do as I damn well please."

There is a current of sexuality in everyday life. I find him a very attractive man and he finds me a desirable woman and we tell each other that without words all the time. There's a kind of flow. [a fifty-eight-year-old woman whose husband is seventy-five]

After I came out as a lesbian I danced more than I had in the previous thirty-five years. People ask if I feel foolish—not at all! It's good for the young to know you can keep right on doing, and not pay attention to the wrinkles. [a woman in her eighties]

When searching for a new partner, I often felt discouraged about looking older and worried that I would no longer be appealing to men. Once I was in a relationship, the years I've lived became a plus; I felt proud of my experience and skill as a lover, something I did not have as a younger woman. [a forty-eight-year-old divorced woman]

I've worked at learning to let go of rational thinking during sex. I say I'm going to experience the moment. Here is a wonderful experience I'm going to have, a dedicated time and place. I'm going to live it fully. I soak up the feelings, immerse myself in the sensation and pleasure. The more I do it, the better it gets, like turning a golden key. It is very beautiful to me. [a single woman in her late fifties]

At seventy-three, being sexual feels right, comfortable, and just plain satisfying, but it wasn't always like this. Growing up with Victorian spinster aunts, the family disgrace of a flapper cousin who "had to get married," and baffling warnings to always be careful *on infrequent dates left me with feelings of being ugly and unwanted. Where I am today is one stage in a constant process of growing. I learned to love and be loved, helped by friends and lovers. I bore a child at age thirty-eight and raised him, developing my own changing value system.*

When I was growing up women worried about being thought bossy or willful when we were outspoken or assertive. Now my husband has become more nurturing and accepting of my assertiveness. Our relationship is more balanced. [a woman in her sixties]

We could be equals. We could be friends. I didn't need anything from him and I was free to be me. We were like two kids playing in a sandbox. Oh Lord. A chance to play! [a divorced woman in her fifties]

Now I can just enjoy it. I don't have to be such a good citizen. When I was younger I worried so much for my partner that I never got much real pleasure for myself. [a woman in her fifties]

I have earned the right to express what I like and expect to get it. I want pleasure, joy, fun, and passion during sex for the rest of my life. My contribution to a partner is to give her the same. [a woman in her fifties]

I feel more accepting than I used to—if I don't have an orgasm, if he doesn't have an orgasm, if we stop in the middle, or if we just go to bed and hold each other—it's much more all right than it was when I was younger. [a fifty-five-year-old divorced woman]

Last year I spent several months without sex. I masturbated occasionally, but I even stopped that after a while. I simply didn't miss it; it didn't seem terribly important. I was working pretty hard. Now I'm enjoying it again, but I could do without it. I don't find myself with that rush about sex any more—that feeling of getting hit in the stomach—none of that passion. I still have orgasm, but I seem to have lost my passion, lust. In a way, that's restful. [a fifty-five-year-old woman]

I used to enjoy masturbation and orgasm. But now I don't have any desire for that or a sexual relationship. [an eighty-year-old woman]

Sex was fine but it was only a part of our marriage and I was happily married for thirty years. Since my husband died I've never looked at another man. I masturbate occasionally, but it's not important to me. Knowing another person—that is what matters. I get as much pleasure from my work as I might get from sex. [a sixty-year-old woman]

I miss the intimacy, the love letters, but I'm back solidly celibate. I never could masturbate. It's not the orgasm I crave, but the intimacy—the candles, the flowers, the feeling of another body. [a seventy-two-year-old woman commenting on the ending, several years ago, of a relationship with a woman]

Pleasuring Ourselves*

Self-stimulation is one way of giving ourselves pleasure. Most of us enjoy a variety of sensual pleasures and view pleasure as a good thing, yet many of us were taught to believe that giving ourselves *sexual* pleasure is bad. Whether we do so or not is our choice. Pleasuring ourselves can be a satisfying alternative to sex with a partner. If you have lost a partner with whom you enjoyed good lovemaking, you may not be ready to start over with someone new.

After my divorce masturbation was an important part of my life that made it very nice to go to bed. It's still a special occasion. [a seventy-eight-year-old woman]

If you do have a partner, pleasuring yourself can be a good way to learn about your own sexual responses—what fantasies you enjoy, what kinds of touch arouse you and please you—without having to worry about your partner's needs and opinions. Then, if and when you choose, you can tell or show your partner what you've learned. Some of us incorporate masturbation into our lovemaking with a partner as a way to enhance pleasure and to reduce pressure on both partners to "satisfy" the other.

If you have never masturbated but would like to try, it may take some time to adjust to the idea and to find the way that gives you the most pleasure. The Resources section for this chapter lists some excellent books that offer specific suggestions. Deliberately setting the mood in much the same way you would with a partner—candles, incense, and music—can enhance the experience. A soothing bath or a glass of wine may help you relax and focus on yourself for an interlude of personal sexual pleasure. You may enjoy the feelings of arousal whether or not you have an orgasm.

Those of us for whom self-stimulation is not an acceptable choice can still enjoy sensuality—luxuriating in a bubble bath, moving to music, exchanging a massage with a friend. These body experiences can enrich our lives and help us feel alive and vital.

Fantasies

Sexual fantasy can help arouse, maintain, and increase sexual excitement. It is particularly helpful to women who lose their concentration during sex. A fantasy can be a story or stories, or a series of erotic images. Sometimes partners share their fantasies.

We have a wide variety of scenes. I am the rampaging female who leaps into bed in a comical way. Or when I'm very tired he says, "You rest, I'll do all the work." Or we play who gets to be the baby—or other psychological conditions—we play with them and we don't feel threatened. [a woman in her late fifties]

We may feel disloyal to a partner if we fantasize while lovemaking, or worry that something we imagine is bad or "sick." Yet creating erotic images is just a way of allowing ourselves to experiment without risk. It may take a while to accept our fantasies and understand that we can enjoy them without having to act on them.

*The expression *pleasuring ourselves* as an alternative for the word *masturbation* was suggested to us by Eleanor Hamilton, a pioneer in sex education who has written a great deal about cultural biases against pleasure and sex. Hamilton objects to the word *masturbation,* which is derived from the Latin meaning "to pollute with the hand."

Sexuality and Relationships

During the second half of life, we often face major physical and emotional changes affecting our sexuality. Many longtime partners feel increasingly comfortable over time learning how to give sexual pleasure to each other.

In a long-term relationship, lovemaking provides a way to express our deepest feelings of tenderness and mutual caring. Lovemaking can also provide comfort during times of loss and change.

We were feeling so troubled and unhappy we just went to bed and made love to give each other some solace from this terrible sadness. [an eighty-two-year-old woman]

A loving partner who understands and accepts us and is willing to compromise is an important element in a satisfying sexual relationship.

We have a generalized sexual relationship. We're very sexy with each other in a continuous way. It doesn't show a lot . . . just through little things like touching fingers in the movies. [a fifty-eight-year-old woman]

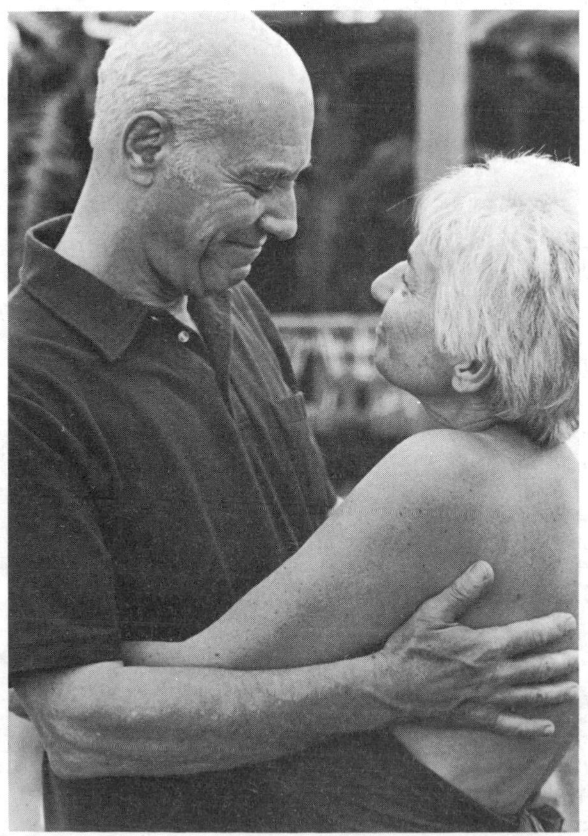

Marianne Gontarz

There are several factors that can diminish interest in sexual activity between long-term partners. The sexual activity of married women seventy or older is directly influenced by physical disability, illness, or loss of their male partners.[5] In many instances, when a male partner loses his interest in sex, his self-confidence, or his ability to have an erection, all sexual activity ends. Sometimes when both partners retire they feel they are spending too much time together; each person feels emotionally crowded. Women in long-term lesbian relationships often share the same activities and friends; they may be even more likely to find themselves struggling with this problem. For all couples, having some separate interests, activities, and friends can help keep each partner and their mutual relationship vital and interesting.

Sometimes sadness, unresolved anger, or disappointment with a partner can block sexual feeling. Allowing your feelings to surface, acknowledging them, and discussing them with your partner may renew sexual desire.

A number of studies suggest that in marriage, satisfaction increases after child rearing is finished and children leave home.[6]

We didn't have the choice of time when the kids were young. Now we have time during the day. We seldom make love at nighttime. Now we can choose. It might be 10 A.M. or 2 P.M.—whenever we're feeling turned on. [a sixty-five-year-old woman]

Because of the double standard in aging, some women as they grow older worry about losing their partner to a younger woman.

My husband is going through some kind of change—he's on a strict diet and runs several miles a day. I have to admit to myself he looks fifty. Me, I look my age. He's got this young woman at work—says she's like a daughter and he's helping her—she keeps calling for this and that. Joe wants me to invite her to dinner but I'm not fooled by this daughter business. I think he's trying to hold on to youth. I keep suggesting things we can do together. We joined a theater group and sometimes we go out dancing with another couple. [a sixty-five-year-old woman, married forty years]

Because women on average have a longer life expectancy than men, most of us will experience the loss of a partner through death. If your relationship has ended with your partner's death, you may not feel sexual for some time while you mourn the loss.

After he died I was celibate for a long while and then went through a long stretch of mourning and masturbation, always with a tremendous sense of grief. [a seventy-eight-year-old woman speaking of a time when she was in her fifties]

After a time of grieving most of us redefine ourselves as survivors with continuing needs for love, affection, and sexual expression. Then we may be ready to consider a new sexual partner.

When partners separate, some of us—particularly those who didn't initiate the breakup—may also lose interest for a while in expressing ourselves sexually as we grieve over the end of the relationship. Our self-esteem may be low and it may take us a while to regain sexual confidence. Or we may be ready to resume sexual activity right away. We may be surprised or even embarrassed by unexpected feelings of sexual desire.

Whereas married people sometimes take sex for granted, single people face continuing decisions about their sexuality, including the choice of being sexual with one person or with more than one.

I have been single for ten years and had many lovers. I like sex a lot; I went through what I call my sport fucking phase. I didn't have to love him—if I felt like having sex I had sex. Now I have two lovers. Sex is very nice with both these men. In fact it's better than it's been for a long time. [a fifty-five-year-old woman]

Many women want more emotional intimacy than can be found in a casual sexual encounter. Some of us have difficulty finding male partners who care about intimacy as much as we do.

It's hard to get emotional closeness and great sex to come together in one relationship. I had an affair and enjoyed it but we didn't have commitment, as I did with my husband. It's true what the books say: sexuality goes on all your life. But you can't split sexuality from emotion. To me sexuality means intimacy. [a seventy-year-old woman]

If we are dating again for the first time in many years, we may feel awkward and unsure of what to expect. How far will my date expect me to go? Can I get by with a goodnight kiss? Often, both men and women would be happy to have a friendly, nonsexual relationship, but feel pressured by certain expectations.

After I got divorced at forty-eight, I expected to have a man courting me like my husband did when I was a teenager in Venezuela. I was very naïve, so I had some surprises. I went out with a man and then he asked me to go up to his apartment to listen to music. So I said, "We just came from listening to music!" I was naïve, but I wasn't stupid! I wanted someone to hold my hand and say nice things, not to jump into bed with someone I didn't really know. [a fifty-nine-year-old woman]

Now I enjoy flirtations; when I don't worry about whether we'll have sex, it's totally fun. [a forty-eight-year-old divorced woman]

After about two years of brief and unsatisfactory relationships, I met a wonderful, warm, caring man, with a surprisingly developed feminist consciousness. How delightful to find that in bed he was exciting, passionate, and playful. [a forty-four-year-old divorced woman]

Among older women in 1990, 60 percent were unmarried, while nearly three quarters of older men were married.[7] When older men remarry they usually marry younger women. The man shortage, a hot topic among women of every age, can become critical in the second half of life.* What is often overlooked is that the majority of divorced women remarry. Among midlife women, 70 percent of women in their forties and 66 percent of women in their fifties are remarried within three years after a divorce.[8] Remarriage rates are dropping off as a growing number of midlife and older women savor their freedom and autonomy as unmarried women.[9] Yet the transition to an unmarried life can be difficult and painful.

Whenever I have been between relationships I have prided myself on being independent and not needing a man in my life. But now that I have no man in my life—now that I am not even casually dating, now that I have cut my ties with my long-distance lover—I realize that what I miss most is the physical contact. I am not even necessarily talking about sex, although that is very important to me. I miss the cuddling and holding and touching with affection. [a woman in her fifties]

Being single I miss that flow in marriage—when I was married if we didn't make love one day there was always tomorrow. [a divorced woman in her fifties]

What the hell. I'm really nicer than I used to be and now no one's looking. [a divorced woman in her sixties]

*When we are not in a primary relationship, our risk of HIV/AIDS may be higher. Women can also contract HIV/AIDS when they are monogamous but their partner is not monogamous or is an intravenous drug user. See pp. 96–97 for information on safer sex.

I wasn't only mourning my husband, I was mourning that there might never be someone else. [a seventy-eight-year-old widow]

Women who have lost a partner find many different solutions to the problem. Some marry again. Others choose a less formal although not necessarily less committed relationship, dating one male or female partner exclusively but maintaining separate living quarters, or living with a partner without marrying. Some women who are having trouble finding suitable sexual partners are learning to initiate both social and sexual interactions more often. Some of us, even some who never dreamed we would choose an unconventional life-style, are considering or trying out new kinds of relationships.

I keep wondering—is this the end of lovers? I can't really believe that. Yet in my experience few men my age are interesting and vital. Younger men? Sure, why not. But not too much younger or the experience gap becomes too much. I meet lots of interesting women and I am enlarging my circle of women friends. If I really connected with someone would I consider a lesbian relationship? Maybe. In the meantime, I am accepting myself in a new and different way. I am learning to treat and to nurture myself by doing the things I want to do and not doing what I don't want in a more honest way than ever before. [a woman in her fifties]

I feel such intense body hunger—for touching and stroking and for good old-fashioned sex. Sometimes I get together with an old friend. Neither of us wants it to be more than what it is now—good old friends with sex sometimes. [a forty-nine-year-old divorced woman]

I met a man fourteen years younger. We can laugh and talk and it feels so relaxed. He is very uninhibited sexually. We spend our time laughing and doing fun things. I relate so much better to younger men; they are less rigid about sex roles than older men. I like their values. [a forty-eight-year-old divorced woman]

I know a woman who is fifty-two who has a forty-year-old lover. She told me I have a hang-up about age, but I'm fifty-three, I'm afraid of getting hurt. Still, there's something to what she said: "If you're alive and beautiful inside, with all the experience and patience older women have, no twenty-two- or thirty-year-old can really compete. A fascinating older woman can be irresistible for certain types of younger men." I'm thinking about this and loosening up.

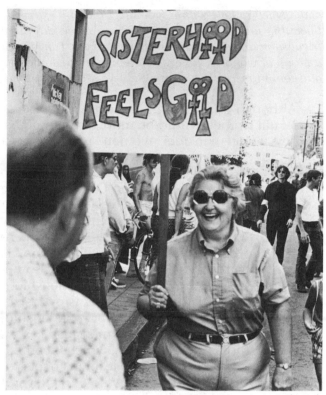

Cathy Cade

Sexuality between two women can be deeply satisfying. Some middle-aged or older women are, for the first time, considering or having sexual relationships with women.

I had an orgasm during a nonsexual massage which another woman was giving me. I thought, "What difference does it make what gender the hands are?" [a woman in her fifties]

My first sexual experience with a woman was at age forty. I found myself very suddenly and very intensely turned on to a good friend who was gay. No sexual involvement was possible since she was in a long-term relationship with another woman, but the feeling was clearly there. That summer I began to seek out women as sexual partners while on vacation. I was absolutely captivated by the sensations of holding and physically loving another woman. The combination of delicacy and strength was thrilling. And the softness . . . that double twofold softness of two women together. [a fifty-year-old woman]

I spent years trying to make it in the heterosexual world because my sexual identity was "wrong." When I finally allowed myself to love another woman fully, it was like coming home—home at last. [a woman in her sixties]

I grew up loving women—the way they walk, smell, feel; wanting to touch them, cherish them, love them passionately and overtly, but it was not until years later that I actually fell in love with a woman. I found it extremely liberating and also a wonderful way to develop deep friendships and associations in one's old age. I am part of a group of women who are developing mutual interests and commitments. [a seventy-eight-year-old woman]

Although it is sometimes suggested that heterosexual women would be more sexually active if they would consider women as partners, a recent survey of one hundred lesbians aged sixty to eighty-six found that 53 percent had had no sexual contact in the past year. One third of the 53 percent consider themselves celibate, but three quarters of that number are not celibate by choice.[10] It may be that the issue is not the gender of our partners, but our socialization as women, which conditions us to wait for someone else to initiate a sexual relationship.[11] Another study of twenty-five lesbians over sixty found that none, even those not in a relationship, had casual sex after sixty, but most had sex an average of three times a month, which is comparable to or more frequent than lesbian couples of all ages.[12] It is difficult to know how to interpret findings such as these because research on older lesbians is very limited.

Early in my life I knew that I never wanted to have children and I never wanted to marry. I had crushes on camp counselors and some girlfriends, but I also had boyfriends. At forty-five for the first time in my life I suddenly wanted to get married. My menopausal crisis! My lover was willing but then I realized that while it was a good relationship for a weekend in another city, I couldn't imagine being married to him. I decided marriage was not right for me and then I was celibate for twenty years. When I was sixty-five I fell in love with a woman who was twenty-three years younger than I was. Making love with a woman was not that much different from experiences I had had with men. But this was the most complete relationship of my life. It was romantic, passionate, sharing, intellectual. It was everything I had read about but never experienced—such fullness and balance. When the relationship ended I decided to go back to celibacy, the way I had lived happily for twenty years, but it was the hardest thing I ever did. Maybe I'm into twenty-year cycles and can look forward to another love when I'm eighty-five. That would be nice. [a seventy-two-year-old woman]

Many middle-aged and older women are celibate. Some lack the opportunity to meet partners, others prefer to be celibate.

In Colette's novel, Break of Day, *I discovered celibacy as a strategy for older women who too often see themselves as stripped of identity without a partner. Colette sees age fifty-five as the end of having lovers, but the beginning of an aloneness that is joyous and drenched in sensuality—particularly for the artist in all of us. It is a great gift to be one's self at last.* [Marilyn Zuckerman, a poet in her sixties]*

Sex and Aging: Physiological and Emotional Changes

As we age, we experience changes in our bodies that affect our sexuality. It's important to distinguish between the effects of the aging process itself, the effects of hormonal changes as we go through menopause, and the effects of illness, disability, and relationship difficulties. We don't need to resign ourselves to sexual problems as a natural, irreversible part of aging. As women, we have learned to come to terms with changes in our bodies; we can understand and accommodate ourselves to the changes of aging just as we did during menstruation and pregnancy. If you connect your sexual identity with the ability to have children, after menopause you may experience a sense of loss and a *temporary* drop in sexual desire. Some women report a need to mourn the ending of fertility, although such feelings are usually short-lived.

I know I wouldn't ever want to get pregnant again. Yet I'm aware that we derived great satisfaction from the thought that we could get pregnant if we wanted to. Sometimes we fantasize that we are making a baby, but it's not the same. [a fifty-one-year-old woman]

Many women in their fifties experience a reawakening of sexual interest once they no longer need to prevent pregnancy and once the pressures of child rearing are past.[13]

It's wonderfully freeing. I always hated the mess and the interruption of birth control. I was always anxious about getting pregnant and that put a damper on sex. [a forty-nine-year-old woman]

At times, hot flashes during menopause can interfere with sexual enjoyment.

My lover and I have had to be very creative to find suitable positions for lovemaking which take into account that one of us is bound to have a hot flash in the middle

*Her poems appear on pp. 12 and 428.

of it all. We discovered that lying next to each other, toes to head, gives us a good vantage point for genital play (toes are good for sucking too) without overwhelming each other with our wacky temperature controls. We'll be damned if such a thing can slow down our sexual pleasuring. [a lesbian in her fifties]

ORGASM

For many women, clitoral stimulation leads to orgasm. Yet until the mid 1960s, medical texts and marriage manuals followed Freud's famous dictum that the "mature" woman had orgasms only when her vagina, not her clitoris, was stimulated. Then sex researchers found that much of the sexual pleasure women experience occurs because of direct or indirect stimulation of the clitoris.[14] This information electrified the newly developing women's movement and contributed to a revolution in women's understanding of ourselves as sexually autonomous beings rather than sexual objects.[15] More recent research indicates that orgasm may occur as the result of clitoral stimulation, vaginal[16] and uterine stimulation, or a combination of both.

For many women, continuous clitoral stimulation is what most surely brings orgasm. Some women enjoy orgasms brought on by penetration of the vagina, which they describe as feeling "deep" or "uterine," and may find clitoral stimulation distracting if continued during vaginal penetration. In addition, increasing attention is being given to those women who report a loss of sexual feeling after hysterectomy;[17] they may miss the jiggling of the pelvic muscles and cervix that they had formerly felt during deep penetration. These new understandings lend further support to the idea that women's sexuality is complex and multifaceted. The main thing to remember is that you are the expert about yourself, and you can adjust your sexual pleasures to meet your changing needs.

Women who have uterine contractions during orgasm sometimes find that after menopause these are less intense, more spasmodic and irregular, and fewer in number. A few older women experience painful contractions, somewhat like menstrual cramps, during orgasm. This is more likely to occur if orgasm is infrequent. If this happens to you, try not to get into a cycle of worrying about it, because this condition is similar to the discomfort we experience when any seldom-used muscle is exercised and is less likely to continue if you have orgasms more frequently. If you have sex with a partner infrequently, or if the anxiety about the contractions interferes with your orgasm with a partner, you can help yourself by stimulating yourself to orgasm until you feel more relaxed and the contractions go away or become less painful.

SLOWER AROUSAL TIME

As a result of aging, both women and men become aroused more slowly.

You know you are middle-aged when a "quickie" takes forty-five minutes. [a fifty-one-year-old woman]

It's true that I need more time to be turned on, but everything balances out because I enjoy sex more once I do get aroused. [a forty-nine-year-old woman]

I've never been quick to have an orgasm and now it takes longer and I can't always count on it. I choose to make love because I want to be touched and stroked. [a fifty-five-year-old woman]

The slowing of sexual responses is similar to other ways in which our bodies slow down physically. If we believe social attitudes that "virility" or "sexual allure" means instant arousal, we may become alarmed as our bodies respond more slowly. This may lead to further anxiety and affect our confidence in ourselves. However, slower arousal time has its compensations.

When Jay used to lose his erection I would think that I had failed as a woman because I couldn't keep him aroused. But now I see that it can mean more time to play around and a chance to start over again so that lovemaking lasts longer. [a forty-nine-year-old woman]

VAGINAL CHANGES

As we age, the lips of the vagina, or the labia, become less firm, and less fatty tissue covers the mons, or pubic bone. This reduction in fatty tissue may decrease the pleasurable sense of fullness that was formerly part of your sexual response. The length of the vaginal canal may seem shorter, since the tissues are less elastic. The stretching of these delicate tissues may hurt on penetration or deep thrusting. In addition, thinner vaginal walls offer less protection to the bladder and urethra during intercourse and may result in bladder irritation or infection. Drinking a glass of water before sex and urinating after sex, as well as washing your genitals before and after sex, may help this condition. A hot bath feels good and helps relieve irritation after lovemaking.

The lower estrogen levels that accompany middle age may cause dryness or itching of the vagina, making intercourse less comfortable or even painful.* You may need more stimulation before you are lubricated enough for penetration. Dryness can also make it uncomfortable to have the vulva or clitoris caressed. Changing your lovemaking to allow more time to get aroused and expanding your repertoire to include more caresses—especially oral sex, which provides its own lubrication—before or instead of penetration may be all that is necessary.

A lot of hand play is wonderful because it does start the juices flowing. [a woman in her seventies]

I've always loved sex and I could make love for hours. Now, even though I'm excited, my vagina doesn't have enough juice. It's so frustrating—I want to, but it hurts. We have found that after penetration if he just waits and doesn't move for a while it stops hurting and then it's fine. [a fifty-one-year-old woman]

We can incorporate lubricants into our lovemaking now even if we never used them earlier in our lives. Try an over-the-counter product. Knowing that you are already lubricated may help you to relax and let your feelings of arousal build until your natural lubrication takes over. Artificial lubricants should not be expected to entirely replace natural lubrication, since without some of her own lubrication a woman is neither physically nor psychologically ready for intercourse.

If a woman feels pressured by her partner for rapid penetration, she may experience even less lubrication. Susanne Morgan notes that "lubrication is more than wetness: it is the first indication of arousal."[18]

There are several safe and effective lubricants on the market today, such as massage oils (with or without a variety of fragrances), vitamin E oil, apricot kernel oil, sesame oil, coconut oil, cocoa butter, and wheat germ oil. Some authorities, however, suggest using only water-based lubricants because oil-based lubricants don't flush out of the system as readily, and in older women they may cause vaginal infection.[19] Do not use petroleum products such as Vaseline for lubrication. Perfumes may be irritating to many women. Many sterile, water-based lubricants, such as Astroglide, K-Y Jelly, and Today, are available in drugstores. They vary in smell, taste, consistency, and how long they stay wet. Astroglide and Senselle are smooth, slippery, long-lasting lubricants that can be ordered through the mail (see Resources, page 461). You can order Trans-lube or Kama Sutra oils through ads in magazines. If surface lubricants used during lovemaking do not help, you may want to try a moisturizer, such as Replens. These products, made to plump up the vaginal tissues, are to be used regularly, perhaps three times a week. Application prior to sexual intercourse is not required. Aci-gel, for vaginal itching, is available with a prescription. When itching stops, go back to a nonmedicated lubricant.*

After my hysterectomy I started to experience discomfort with intercourse; my vagina was becoming very dry. There was no longer any pleasure in the activity; sex became something to avoid. Early on I started to use a personal lubricant with unsatisfactory results. Being a resourceful person, I dug deep into my past experience and remembered that the introduction of the spermicidal jelly with an applicator (which I used to use with my diaphragm) always produced the side advantage of easier intercourse. So I dug out my old plastic plunger-type applicator and filled it with the lubricant as in days gone by. The result was tremendous! My husband and I instantly noticed the improvement. The problem of getting the lubricant where I needed it the most was resolved. [a woman in her late thirties]

Some physicians prescribe estrogen for a dry vagina. This is a powerful drug that should not be taken without first considering all of its potential effects. (See chapter on Experiencing Our Change of Life: Menopause and pages 286–89.) An alternative to taking estrogen orally is the use of low-dose estrogen cream. It is important to note that estrogen is absorbed even more quickly when used vaginally than when taken orally. Because estrogen cream bypasses the liver, the risk of liver and gallbladder problems is reduced. However, the risk of other effects of estrogen is still present. If nothing else helps and you feel you must try estrogen cream, use as little as possible for as short a time period as is necessary to get the desired results. Apply the cream to the area that is most sore, usually the entrance to the

*Dryness may lead to small cuts and tears in the vaginal wall, which can increase susceptibility to HIV/AIDS infection (see pp. 96–97).

*For a fuller discussion of vaginal itching, see *The New Our Bodies, Ourselves,* 1992, pp. 604–6.

EXTERNAL GENITALIA

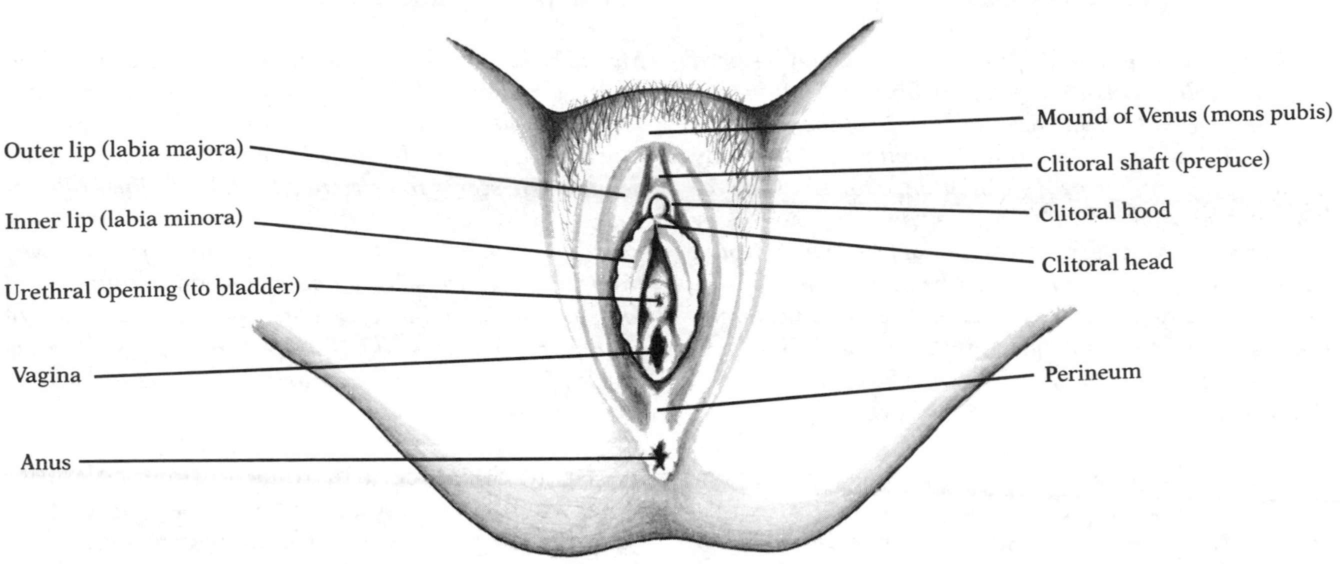

vagina. A week of such treatment will usually relieve soreness. English researchers found that only one eighth of the dosage usually recommended by American doctors is enough to plump up vaginal tissues.[20] The cream comes with an applicator with rings on the side that measure out 4 grams. You can measure a one-eighth dose if you use only enough cream to fill one of the small rings marked on the plastic applicator. If you can't use estrogen, androgen cream (which is made of 1 to 2 percent testosterone in a water-soluble cream) is another way to treat vaginal soreness and is used in the same fashion as estrogen cream (see pages 318 and 323 for the risks of using testosterone). These powerful substances are medications. They should never be used as lubricants at the time of lovemaking. Estrogen can be absorbed through the skin or tongue of your partner.

Clitoral Changes

The clitoris is always highly sensitive and grows even more so as we age. The hood of skin that covers the clitoris may pull back, so that the clitoris is fully exposed. If your clitoris becomes hypersensitive, you may not be able to tolerate having it directly touched or rubbed without lots of lubrication. Touching the mons, the clitoral hood, and the labia will stimulate the clitoris indirectly and provide pleasure.

Men Also Change

Men as well as women undergo changes in their sexuality as they age. Lower testosterone levels are sometimes a factor in loss of sexual interest for some men. Their sexual responses may slow down, and they may need a longer time of non-demanding genital stimulation before they attain a full erection. Once lost, the erection may take longer to regain.

A woman can help her partner to gain a full erection by putting pressure on the base of his penis, and massaging it away from his abdomen. This will press against the major blood vessels and hold the blood in the penis, creating an erection. It is important not to pull it up toward the abdomen, since this will drain the blood from the penis and diminish the erection. Another technique that some men like is to stuff a partially erect penis into the vagina and then the woman tightens her vaginal muscles rhythmically as a form of stimulation for both partners.[21]

Middle-aged and older men also experience changes in orgasm. They often don't need to ejaculate at the end of each sexual experience and may opt for orgasm every two or three episodes rather than every time they make love. Older men also need a longer time to renew their sexual energy after an orgasm before they can have another erection. But by delaying ejaculation and not pushing for orgasm after each lovemaking session, an older man can often rapidly become erect again. This means that both partners can enjoy frequent lovemaking and have orgasms when it feels right.[22]

My lover's divorce had left him feeling sexually rejected and vulnerable. When our relationship grew intimate, I made it clear that I didn't regard sex as a competition, but as a way for two people to express warmth and caring. My friend's "problem," delayed ejaculation, allowed us to prolong our lovemaking until both of us were ecstatically exhausted. Instead of the conventional problem of "would I come?" I worried at first when he didn't come, but he assured me that he didn't need to come every time. Sometimes we would resume our lovemaking in the morning and then he would have his orgasm, while I would sometimes have another. [a forty-seven-year-old woman]

Now there is longer playing around . . . and without fussing about whether it's going to be regular intercourse. We can bring each other to orgasm at any time. It's no longer goal oriented, so it's wonderful. [a woman in her late seventies]

Impotence is the inability to maintain an erection long enough to have intercourse. It is usually temporary. Sudden onset of impotence is usually the result of some unusual stress. Once the stress is removed, potency often returns.

I was getting angry because he seemed to be giving up sex. I was being solicitous—doing oral sex because I wanted it to work the first time after his operation. Then oh! It worked just like it used to! [a sixty-eight-year-old woman]

We enjoy each other. As far as sex is concerned, he is sensible. He understands he can't do what he used to do. Some men can't admit this and blame the woman, but not him. [a sixty-eight-year-old woman in a second marriage of thirty years]

He can't maintain an erection, so we mutually masturbate and it's very satisfying. [a sixty-five-year-old woman]

Although there is a sharp upward turn in male impotence after age fifty, a high percentage of men who become impotent after years of normal sexual activity can be helped by sex therapy. Worries about career and money or illness, fatigue, heavy meals, and too much to drink can all contribute to impotence. "This sensitivity to mental fatigue is the biggest difference between the aging population and younger men," say Masters and Johnson. "There is no way to overemphasize the importance that the 'fear of failure' plays in aging males' withdrawal from sexual performance."[23]

My husband was anxious about prostate trouble. He had been very ill and had a history of impotence. I want to say to him, "Relax, it's going to be okay," but I don't want to touch on the subject because I'm afraid he'll consider it a demand. He seems to be getting back his feelings of sexiness, but it's a slow process. When it's been so long [since we had sex] that I'm taking it personally or feel far away from him, I initiate it by doing something romantic. I dress up and do a dance, or I arrange a sexy situation of some sort—and it works. But he prefers to get it going himself because he's never sure if he's going to have an erection. [a sixty-five-year-old woman]

Up to 50 percent of male impotence (more than was previously suspected) may be caused by physical problems such as arteriosclerosis.[24] But when a partner has sexual problems or slows down sexually, whether because of physiological or psychological problems,* we may interpret it as rejection, or fear that it has something to do with our "diminished attractiveness."

Social stereotypes that men are "supposed" to have stronger sex drives than women and that women are "supposed" to be passive but alluring recipients of sex only aggravate the situation.

My husband became impotent. One of the grimmest things was the sense of helplessness and guilt. I wondered what I could do differently but was not able to speak about it openly because it was a big bad sad problem. We went months without sex and every time I would realize this I became enraged that he didn't want it. I thought maybe I should take the initiative, but he saw that as aggressive and as a demand, and he wouldn't even play around. I found that painful—we couldn't be physically intimate in any way without his seeing it as a threat. When we became preoccupied with his erections, I didn't have orgasm anymore. I was left hanging in the air. [a woman in her fifties]

SEXUAL AIDS

Many older women are enjoying sex aids that are available through mail-order catalogues or in department stores (see Resources, page 461). Although some people may find such toys objec-

*If the problem persists, your partner should consult a urologist to rule out physiological causes, or to get help for them.

tionable, others delight in playing with them. Generally, women find vibrators more effective stimulation than men do, and prefer electric vibrators that are not shaped like a phallus. These provide intense stimulation to the nerve endings around the vulva and clitoris.

I'd never be without one again! Sometimes I just want to be soothed and the sound and continuing vibration does that. Other times if I want to get really excited I know I can if I use my vibrator. For me it's a sure-fire way to have an orgasm. [a forty-nine-year-old woman]

Women who enjoy deep penetration sometimes prefer the phallic-shaped battery-operated vibrators. Yet many women find the weak vibration of these small, battery-powered vibrators does not provide sufficient stimulation to bring about orgasm.

Many women report that they like a sensation of fullness inside the vagina, and use dildos for this purpose. You can order dildos by mail or you can make your own from candles or vegetables (either raw or partially cooked). It is important never to use glass objects or anything that might hurt you or break. Always wash anything that has been in the anus before inserting it in the vagina.*

Some couples like to look at erotic films, magazines, or books, or to listen to sexy music or relaxing tapes or records of environmental sounds such as surf, forest sounds, or falling water. "White noise" such as the hum from a fan or air conditioner can block distracting noises and allow you to concentrate on your intimate environment.

ACCOMMODATIONS IN LOVEMAKING

Illness may bring about a temporary loss of sexual interest or ability to engage in sexual activity. Most illnesses do not mean the end of sexual activity but may require different ways of giving and receiving pleasure. With problems such as arthritis or back pain, fear of causing pain or being hurt can affect spontaneity. If a partner holds back in lovemaking or rarely initiates sex, her or his concern about illness may be misinterpreted as rejection. In fact, good sex can actually help relieve pain. It is distracting, and sexual stimulation releases neurotransmitters in the brain that block pain and produce pleasure.[25]

*Clean your sex toys often, especially between partners. See *Safer Sex Guidelines*, page 97.

People sometimes fear returning to sexual activity after an illness or surgery. Through self-pleasuring, you can rediscover your sexual self in private communication with your own body, trying out degrees of arousal that feel safe and comfortable. Once you feel reassured that your body is still capable of responding with pleasure, you may be ready to ask your partner to join you. Satisfying intimacy can hasten the healing process. Many women find they are more comfortable with a gradual resumption of lovemaking—touching, hand-holding, and caressing at first as a way to express closeness until they feel ready to resume full sexual relations.

If one person is unavailable sexually because of illness, it is always possible to lie together and hold each other and let feelings flow in a warm and close embrace. The most important thing to remember is that if you are open to trying new ways of making love you *will* be able to continue having sex. Even when you can't enjoy penetration or intercourse, you can still give and receive pleasure using a variety of techniques.

My husband had a series of operations last year—a penile implant—and he's still unable to enjoy sex. That doesn't matter so much to me. We still make love and hold and kiss. [a sixty-five-year-old woman, married forty years]

The following ideas may help when one of the partners is having physical problems.

Sex researchers encourage exercising sexual organs through Kegel exercises, masturbation, or lovemaking to help maintain muscle tone and lubrication. If you have not been sexual in a while, you may feel tight or dry at first, but you can overcome this with Kegel exercises (see pages 75–77) followed by gentle and slow resumption of sexual activity.

Let your partner know what feels good and what hurts during sex. You may want to do this by talking or by guiding your partner's hand away from tender areas, or toward places that feel especially good. Tell your partner what your present sensations feel like. Once you feel secure about being understood, you will be better able to relax and surrender to sexual pleasure without fear of pain.

Before making love, agree on a clear signal that you both know is a sign to stop if something hurts you. If a favorite position has become uncomfortable because of temporary or permanent aches and pains, experiment to find a position that feels better.

Ask for what you want in a positive way.

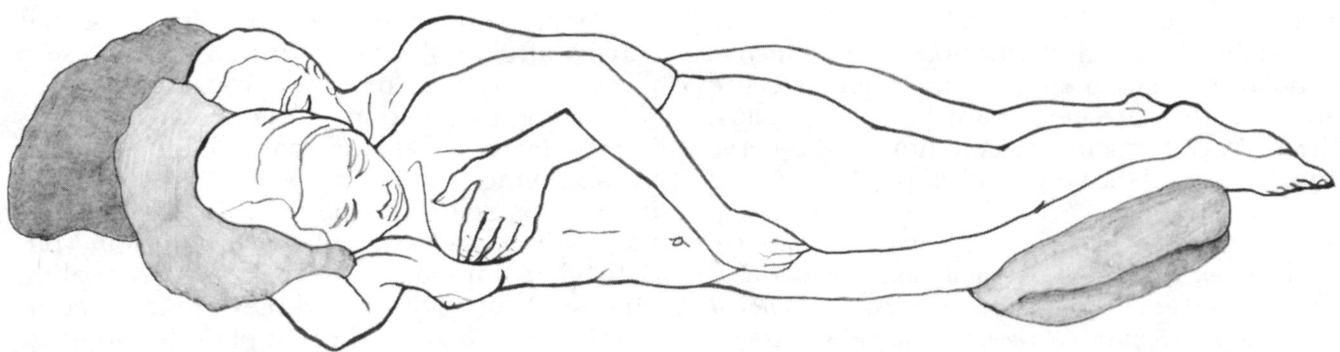

The "spoon position," where both partners lie on their sides and one has her back to the other, is excellent for cuddling and for lovemaking with or without intercourse. You can stimulate your own clitoris and breasts in this position or ask your partner to do so.

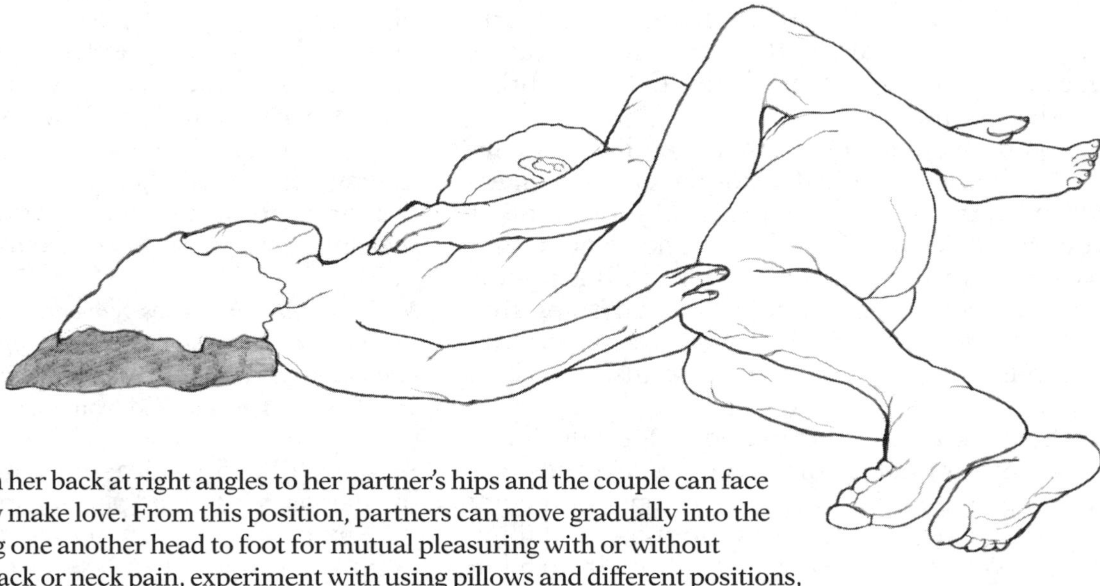

A woman can lie on her back at right angles to her partner's hips and the couple can face one another as they make love. From this position, partners can move gradually into the "69" position facing one another head to foot for mutual pleasuring with or without oral sex. To avoid back or neck pain, experiment with using pillows and different positions, or take turns pleasuring one another.

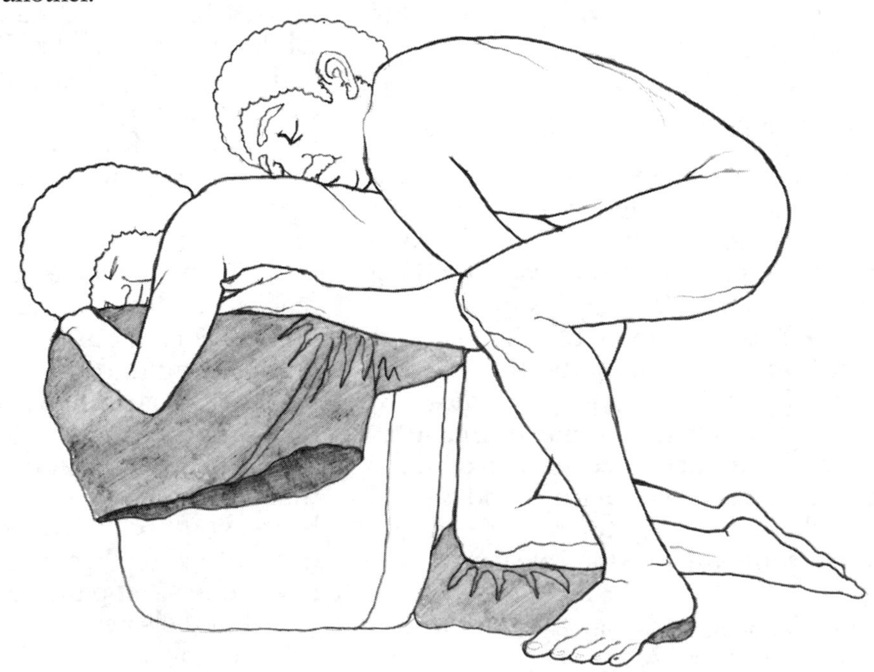

Use a low hassock or stool to lean on while kneeling, and your partner can hold you from behind; or stand and lean forward against a sturdy piece of furniture such as a bureau, and your partner can caress you.

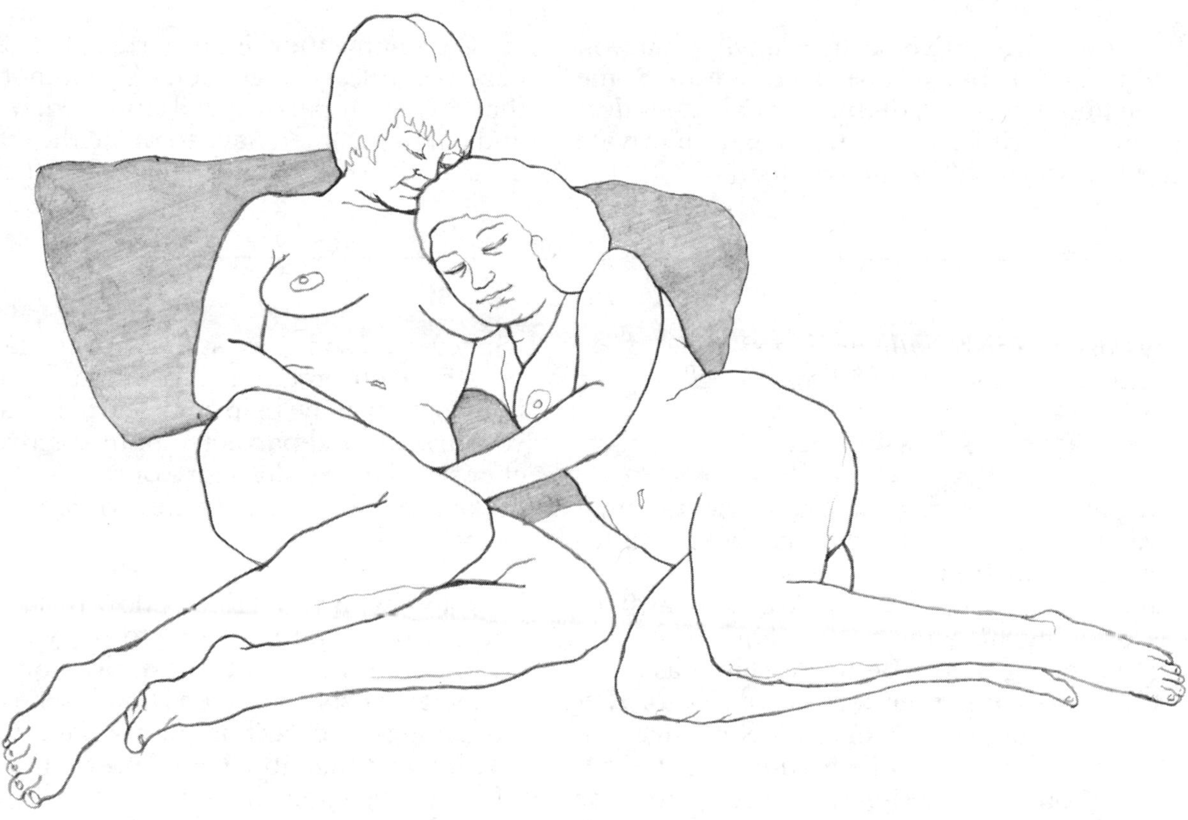

Having one partner on top of the other may be too stressful if either partner is having physical problems. Partners can caress one another or have intercourse in a sitting or reclining position. It can be comfortable to sit in an armless chair where one person sits in the chair and the second person sits on her partner's lap. Make sure the chair is sturdy. Sit so that both partners' feet touch the ground; this way neither person bears too much weight.

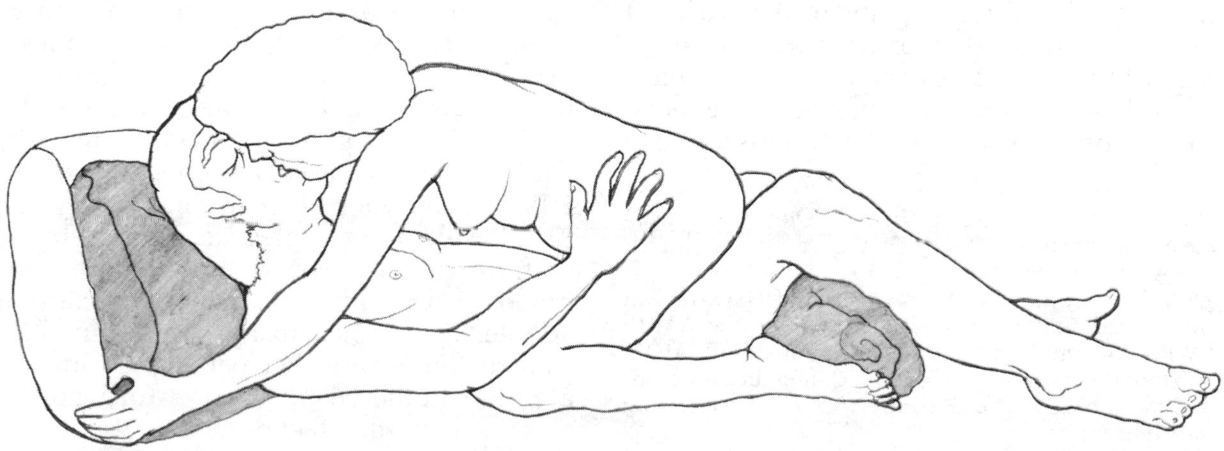

Change positions to allow for fatigue. The person who is ill or tired can lie on her or his back while the other partner kneels above. Several pillows can be used to advantage to support a back or be placed under the knees.

Offering an alternative sexual activity that you enjoy is easier on your partner's ego. Some women find it easier to discuss sexual issues during nonsexual times together. Look for a private time when you won't be interrupted.

Communication is important between partners regardless of gender. We cannot assume that a woman partner will know what we want and enjoy—women have to make the effort to be clear and explicit with each other. It's easy to

HIV AND SAFER SEX

by Christie Burke with thanks to Wendy Sanford, Liz Galst, and Allison Morrill

RESOURCES ON PAGES 461–62.

Regardless of our age or sexual orientation, if we are sexually active we may be at risk for sexually transmitted diseases, including HIV, the virus thought to cause AIDS. Today, HIV is growing at a faster rate among women than among men.* Being perceived as sexually inactive and therefore not at risk for HIV transmission, older women are less likely to be provided with information about safer sex. Women over forty, however, are one fourth of AIDS cases diagnosed among women.† In addition, older women who are infected with HIV may have difficulty obtaining a correct diagnosis and treatment.

Some older women experience an increased thinning and/or dryness of the vaginal tissues, which may result in small skin tears during sexual activity. These skin tears may allow HIV to enter the bloodstream, presenting an increased risk for transmission. (Vaginal lubricants like K-Y commonly used to reduce uncomfortable friction may reduce this kind of skin tearing.)

Negotiating safer sex may be difficult for many of us, especially those of us who have recently lost a long-term partner, have a history of physical or emotional abuse, or for whatever reason may suffer from a lack of power in our relationships. The following information may help you learn to talk to your friends and partners about safer sex, to choose to be sexually active or not, and if you are active, help you have fun while you protect yourself.

- Explore with your friends how to say "yes" to sex you want and "no" to sex you don't want. You may want to explore nonsexual ways to satisfy your needs for closeness and touching—such as hugs or massage.
- Think and talk about HIV prevention *long before* engaging in sexual activity. You could practice a safer sex "script" with a friend.
- Avoid drugs and alcohol and any situation that might impair your judgment and ability to practice safer sex.
- Be responsible and realistic. Keep your safer sex kit(s)—latex gloves, latex condoms, water-based lubricant, etc.—well stocked and close at hand by your bed and in your bag.

The most important aspect to staying safe is understanding the way you can get infected. HIV is a virus that is in all body fluids, but only in strong concentration in blood, semen, and vaginal secretions. Engaging in unsafe sexual activity (activity that allows fluid with a strong concentration of HIV to enter your bloodstream) puts you at risk. Besides unprotected sex, needle sharing with an IV drug user is the most common mode of transmission. Since precautions adopted in 1985, transmission from blood transfusion is rare. Yet persons so infected are more numerous in the over-forty population and can still infect others.

*See the 1992 edition of *The New Our Bodies, Ourselves* for a complete chapter with resources on HIV and AIDS in women.

†Judith B. Cohen, "Older Women and HIV/AIDS in the United States." Paper prepared for the AARP/CWPS Meeting on Older Women and HIV/AIDS, Washington, DC: Nov. 4–5, 1993. Conference proceedings available free. See Resources, p. 461, for ordering information.

hide our own embarrassment or reluctance to ask for what we want behind the assumption that "She must know, for, after all, she is a woman like I am." It's important to understand that every woman is different.

Choose a time of day when you are both feeling comfortable. Making love in the morning when you are rested can help if you tire easily. Men are more likely to have an erection in the morning. Time lovemaking to coincide with

SAFER SEX GUIDELINES

Higher-Risk Activities

(arranged by degree of risk from highest to lowest)

- **Anal Intercourse:** Rectal tissue tears easily allowing HIV to enter the body. Reduce tears by using a **water-based lubricant** (like K-Y). Ask your partner to wear **two latex condoms for extra protection.**
- **Fisting:** Putting a fist into the vagina or rectum is risky because it easily tears the skin tissues, and causes bleeding. **Latex gloves provide protection.**
- **Vaginal Intercourse:** Use a **latex condom** and if needed a **water-based lubricant** (like K-Y). Never use oil-based lubricants (Vaseline, vegetable oil) since they may cause condoms to break. Spermicide can be used inside the condom, in case it breaks. Consider using the new "female condom." See *The New Our Bodies, Ourselves* (1992), page 268, for information. **Nonoxynol-9, the active ingredient in spermicide, has been shown to kill HIV in the laboratory, and evidence of its effectiveness in people is growing.*** Some people have an allergic reaction to nonoxynol-9. In addition, some research indicates that repeated and frequent use of spermicide may cause skin irritation or ulceration and increase the risk of HIV transmission. If any of these effects occur, stop use immediately. You may want to try another brand.
- **Oral Sex on a Man:** Most risky if the man ejaculates in your mouth; also some HIV is in the fluid that comes out of the penis before ejaculation (precum). The safest activity is to use an **unlubricated latex condom** as soon as the man is erect enough for the condom to hold. Lipstick is oil based. Avoid using it with a condom. It is not risky to have mouth contact with intact skin on any part of the body, including the shaft of the penis, if there are no body fluids present.
- **Oral Sex on a Woman: Little evidence of transmission by this route.** Protection means using **large sheets of plastic wrap,** enough to **cover both the labia and anus.** Be more careful if the woman is menstruating or has a vaginal infection, as both could possibly transmit HIV.
- **Hand to Genital Contact/Finger Play:** Risk varies depending on the amount of activity, the amount and type of body fluid, and if you have cuts/sores on your hands. Protect yourself with **latex finger covers (finger cots) or latex gloves.**
- **Other Activities:** For rimming (mouth to anus) use plastic wrap. For water sports (sex partners urinate on each other) protect your eyes and avoid broken skin or cuts. **Clean your sex toys** (dildos, vibrators, etc.) by soaking them in hydrogen peroxide for fifteen minutes. You can use a condom on your sex toys. If no other latex barrier is available, cut up a condom or latex gloves.

Lower-Risk Activities

Use your imagination! You might try a hot bath with candlelight and flowers. Or perhaps some kind of fantasy play that can add spice to safer sex!

Low-risk activities include hugging, rubbing, "hand jobs" (hand stimulation with a minimum of body fluid present), mutual self-pleasuring (touching yourself while being held or watched), or massage. Kissing is also low risk except deep kissing where there are cuts, gum disease, or infections.

*Center for Women Policy Studies, *Woman-Controlled Microbicides for Prevention of HIV/STDs.* Fact sheet adapted from Christopher J. Elias and Lori Heise, *The Development of Microbicides: A New Method of HIV Prevention for Women.* New York: The Population Council, 1993.

maximum effectiveness of pain medications. Turn up the thermostat; a warm room helps you feel limber.

Creating a relaxed sexy mood with your partner can be a way to increase intimacy and release sexual energy. Changing the time and place for sex may keep it from seeming routine. The setting can make a big difference in whether you feel a surge of desire—an attractive, tidy bedroom free of reminders of illnesses can be an asset. Simply moving all the pill bottles into the bathroom may lift your spirits and put you in the mood for lovemaking.[26]

Mild exercise, yoga, massage, breathing and relaxation exercises, meditation, and prayer all reduce stress, counteract stiff muscles, and can be good preludes to making love. Taking a bath or shower together, listening to music, sharing a relaxing meal or quiet talk can help you and your partner feel close and connected.

Getting Help

Usually sexual difficulties can be resolved by talking things through in a spirit of mutual cooperation, but at times it may be necessary to consult a sex therapist or counselor specially trained to understand sexual problems.

Sex therapy usually takes less than six months. Clients are given sexual "homework assignments" that they carry out at home and then discuss with the therapist at the following meeting. Lists of qualified sex therapists are available through women's health or resource centers, SIECUS, or AASECT (see Resources for this chapter), or you can ask your physician for a referral.

Getting information from physicians can be a problem if either you or the doctor is reluctant to discuss sexual matters. Some doctors are comfortable with sexuality and are aware that older people have sex lives. Most, however, have little or no training in issues related to sexual functioning in general and many are ignorant or embarrassed about sex or have ageist attitudes. If you encounter a doctor who shifts the focus of your questions about sex into other areas or ignores or trivializes them, you may want to find another doctor.

The medical history your physician takes should include sexual problems in the past, changes in genital organs, and present sexual functioning. Your physician should also question you not only about the prescription drugs you take, but also about vitamin and mineral supplements and over-the-counter preparations.

Physicians rarely initiate a discussion about how an illness or medical procedure will affect sexuality, so you will have to introduce this topic yourself. Find out when you can resume sexual relations. Ask which activities you can resume and when. Be *very* specific in your questions and insist on explicit answers.

I accompanied my partner to the hospital where he was to have a prostate biopsy. The doctor gave a rapid-fire list of instructions on self-care for the days and weeks following surgery. When he mentioned sex, he said, "Sex, the same." I stopped him and asked, "Do you mean abstain from sex the same number of days as the previous instruction, or the same as usual, or what?" "Oh, two days" was the reply.

As instructed, we obediently abstained. When the two days were up we were eager to resume lovemaking. Proceeding in a gingerly fashion, we were gratified to find everything in good working order and had a lovely time. The following day, we began to feel turned on and started playing around. I was masturbating him with my hand, whereupon we were shocked to see a stream of bright red blood shoot forth from his penis. Since we had not yet heard the good news that the biopsy was negative, we were particularly frightened and upset. We called the HMO and spoke with a nurse on call who finally reached the doctor and relayed his new instructions to us. No sex for two weeks! Either he had misstated the original instruction, or he was changing it based on changed circumstances. When my partner returned for his follow-up visit, the young doctor was terribly embarrassed, as much out of surprise that we were "so active" at our age as for his error. [this woman and her partner are both in their late forties]

A nurse tells of a woman in her seventies who seemed inexplicably depressed after being told she could go home following a successful colostomy.* The staff had been impressed with the closeness between this woman and her husband and were surprised at her lack of anticipation about going home. Finally, she confided to the nurse, "I'm not the same as I was." She was concerned that the operation would make her unable to have sexual relations. Neither the doctor nor any of the nurses had reassured her or her husband that they could have sexual relations, assuming they were "too old" to care about sexuality.

Also ask your doctor how prescribed drugs

*See Cancer chapter for a description of colostomy (pages 361–62).

Resuming Sex after a Heart Attack

After a heart attack, fear of having another may cause people to delay sexual activity. Be sure your physician understands your interest in resuming sexual activity as soon as you safely can. People who have had a heart attack are usually able to have sex two to four weeks afterward, while bypass patients may reach this point in one to three weeks after they leave the hospital.[27] People who have been in the hospital for ten days, and have had a treadmill test, can have sex on the first day home, because a treadmill test is more strenuous than sex. If you can climb two flights of stairs without chest pain, palpitations, or shortness of breath, you can engage in lovemaking safely. If you suffer from angina, you may be able to take a nitroglycerin pill for the pain before lovemaking and then proceed.

Wait one to three hours after eating a full meal. Digesting your food takes an increased amount of blood. Your heart would have to work harder to provide blood during sex.

If you experience angina or pains in the jaw, neck, chest, or stomach, shortness of breath, and rapid or irregular heartbeats, tell your partner, rest, and take medicine if prescribed. When the symptoms disappear, you can resume sexual activity. If the symptoms do not stop, or if they start again, you need to get medical help.

will affect your sexuality. For example, antidepressant and antianxiety drugs may either increase or decrease your usual level of sexual desire. Some antihypertension medications interfere with blood entering the penis, causing problems with erection. Without exception, all drugs have a variety of effects in addition to the effect intended. Since pharmacists frequently know more than physicians about the effects of drugs, you may want to ask a pharmacist. See the chart in Helen Singer Kaplan's *The New Sex Therapy*, or check the *Physicians' Desk Reference* to discover the effects of drugs on sexual functioning.

Residents of nursing homes may have somewhat changed sexual needs due to illness or frailty, yet most still have sexual needs. Many nursing homes do not allow residents sexual privacy. All of us need privacy regardless of whether we are part of a couple, a single person, or whether we are heterosexual or lesbian. This human right is ours by law. Federal regulations state: "The patient may associate and communicate privately with persons of her choice . . . unless medically contraindicated (as documented by [her] physician in the medical records)."[28]

After Surgery

Our culture trains us to believe that "bodily perfection" is a prerequisite for good sex.* If a part of your body has been surgically removed, you need time to come to terms with the changes in order to feel ready to be sexual again. A partner's attitude is of prime importance in helping you to complete the healing process and regain sexual intimacy.

When I came home from the hospital after my mastectomy, my husband literally had to force me to remove my blouse before we made love. My scar did not turn him off, as I was afraid it would, and our lovemaking was good, and healing.

Many hospitals offer counseling to their patients after surgery; this has proved helpful to many people in the past,[29] especially to women who have had mastectomies or who must wear appliances as a result of ostomy surgery.

I "practiced" talking about my breast surgery with two of my best friends because I didn't see how I could tell a man I wasn't intimate with; yet how would I ever get that far if I didn't tell him? Saying the words helped me get familiar with the language I would be comfortable using. Then I did meet a man, and when I managed to tell him, he was very easy about it. I think I was more nervous than I needed to be, because afterwards it seemed to fall into place so easily. He likes me for me!

Conclusion

As middle-aged and older women, we have the experience and wisdom to manage changes, problems, and losses, and to find ways to continue to meet our needs for pleasure. We are in a

*See *The New Our Bodies, Ourselves* for a more extensive discussion and bibliography on sex and disability.

position to refine and enhance what we already know. We have learned to both give and receive, and to appreciate the fleeting moment and its pleasures. Our sexual selves become more integrated with our emotional and spiritual selves. We know how to value ourselves and our intimate loved ones and we can share our bodies as it best suits our desires. As long as we want it, sex can be a part of our lives.

NOTES

1. Bernard Starr and Marcella Weiner, *Starr-Weiner Report*. New York: Stein & Day, 1981, p. 35.

2. Cited in Timothy H. Brubaker, *Later Life Families*. Beverly Hills, CA: Sage Publications, Inc., 1985, pp. 36–45.

3. This idea appeared in *Feminine Forever* by Robert Wilson (New York: M. Evans & Co., Inc., 1966), and was common in many magazine articles decades ago. See the chapter, Experiencing Our Change of Life: Menopause.

4. Starr and Weiner, op. cit.; and Edward Brecher, *Love, Sex and Aging*. Boston: Little, Brown & Co., 1984.

5. Ewald Busse and Eric Pfeiffer, eds., *Behavior and Adaptation in Later Life*. Boston: Little, Brown & Co., 1968.

6. Reported in Jane Porcino, *Growing Older, Getting Better: A Handbook for Women in Later Life*. New York: Continuum, 1991, p.15.

7. Cynthia M. Taeuber and Jessie Allen, "Women in Our Aging Society: The Demographic Outlook," in Jessie Allen and Alan Pifer, eds., *Women on the Front Lines: Meeting the Challenge of an Aging America*. Washington, DC: The Urban Institute Press, 1993.

8. U.S. Bureau of the Census, Current Population Reports, P23-180. *Marriage, Divorce and Remarriage in the 1990's*. U.S. Government Printing Office, Washington, DC, 1992.

9. Jane Gross, "Divorced, Middle-Aged and Happy: Women, Especially, Adjust to the 90's," *The New York Times*, Dec. 7, 1992, p. A14.

10. Monica Kehoe, "Lesbians over Sixty: A Triply Invisible Minority," in Monica Kehoe, ed., *Historical, Literary and Erotic Aspects of Lesbianism*. New York: Haworth Publications, Inc., 1986.

11. Personal communication from Sarah F. Pearlman, a therapist specializing in counseling couples.

12. Marcy Adelman, as reported in JoAnn Loulan, *Lesbian Sex*. San Francisco: Spinsters', Ink, 1984, pp. 194–95.

13. William Masters and Virginia Johnson, "Human Sexual Response in the Aging Female," in Bernice Neugarten, ed., *Middle Age and Aging*. Chicago: University of Chicago Press, 1968, pp. 260–70.

14. William Masters and Virginia Johnson, *Human Sexual Response*. Boston: Little, Brown & Co., 1966.

15. Wendy Sanford, et al., "Sexuality," in Boston Women's Health Book Collective, *The New Our Bodies, Ourselves*. New York: Simon & Schuster, 1992, and earlier editions, as well as other feminist writing on sexuality. See Anne Koedt, "The Myth of the Vaginal Orgasm" in *Liberation Now: Writings from the Women's Liberation Movement*. New York: Dell, 1971, pp. 311–20.

16. Alice Ladas, Beverly Whipple, and John Perry, *The G Spot*. New York: Dell, 1982. The G spot is the name given to a part of the anterior wall of the vagina that may be especially sensitive to stimulation.

17. Lynn Payer, *How to Avoid a Hysterectomy* New York: Pantheon Books, 1987.

18. Susanne Morgan, *Coping with Hysterectomy*. New York: Dial Press, 1982, p. 163.

19. Personal communication, Myrna Lewis, coauthor of *Sex After Forty* (see Resources for this chapter).

20. G. I. Dyer, et al., "Dose-Related Changes in Vaginal Cytology After Topical Conjugated Equine Oestrogens." *British Medical Journal*, Vol. 284 (Mar. 13, 1982), p. 789.

21. Robert Butler and Myrna Lewis, *Sex After Sixty*. New York: Harper & Row, 1976, p. 156.

22. Masters and Johnson, *Human Sexual Inadequacy*. Boston: Little, Brown & Co., 1970, p. 323.

23. Masters and Johnson, "Human Sexual Response in the Aging Male," in Neugarten, ed., op. cit., pp. 277–78.

24. Thomas P. Hackett, *Sexual Activity in the Elderly*. Clinical Perspectives on Aging, No. 4. Philadelphia: Wyeth Laboratories, Dr. Irwin Goldstein of the N.E. Reproductive Center, University Hospital, Boston, quoted in *The Boston Globe*, Sept. 22, 1985, p. 34.

25. Barry Komisarik and Beverly Whipple, "Evidence that Vaginal Stimulation in Women Suppresses Experimentally Induced Finger Pain." Paper presented at June 1984 conference in Boston, Society for the Scientific Study of Sex.

26. Masters and Johnson, "Human Sexual Response in the Aging Male," in Neugarten, ed., op. cit., pp. 148–53.

27. "Sex and Heart Disease," 1990. Available from American Heart Association, National Center, 7320 Greenville Ave., Dallas, TX 75231.

28. Barbara Frank, *An Ombudsman's Guide to the Nursing Home Reform Amendments of OBRA '87*. National Citizen's Council for Nursing Home Reform, Revised, May 1993. Order from NCCNHR, 1224 M Street, NW, Suite 301, Washington, DC 20005-5183.

29. Mary Reid Gloeckner, "Partner Reaction Following Ostomy Surgery." *Journal of Sex and Marital Therapy*, Vol. 9, No. 3 (Fall 1983), pp. 182–90. See also Linda Dackman, *Up Front: Sex and the Post-Mastectomy Woman*. New York: Viking Penguin, 1990.

8

BIRTH CONTROL FOR WOMEN IN MIDLIFE

✦

BY PAULA B. DORESS-WORTERS, EDIE BUTLER, AND TRUDY COX

SPECIAL THANKS TO SUSAN BELL, JUDY NORSIGIAN, AND SUZANNE OLLIVIER

1994 UPDATE BY SUSAN BELL WITH SPECIAL THANKS TO JUDY NORSIGIAN

RESOURCES FOR THIS CHAPTER ON PAGES 462–63

Women continue to need up-to-date, reliable contraceptive information until they are sure they are well past their fertile years. This brief discussion of birth control is meant to highlight special contraception issues that affect women in midlife.

If you do not already have a basic familiarity with reproductive anatomy and birth control and would like to, we encourage you to turn to other resources, such as the Birth Control and Anatomy chapters in *The New Our Bodies, Ourselves,*[1] for more comprehensive information. A women-run health clinic or family-planning clinic is another good source of instruction and contraceptive services in many states. In general, nurse-practitioners and certified nurse-midwives who specialize in family planning are more thorough and knowledgeable than most gynecologists and will take much more time with each woman.

Women who are sexually active with men must continue to use birth control until they are past menopause. Middle-aged women often look forward to being free of the need for birth control, yet they may stop believing they are fertile when they still are. As early as our late thirties or early forties, our periods may become quite irregular, and those of us who are sexually active with a male partner may worry about whether a missed period means a pregnancy. Keeping track of the patterns in our menstrual cycles and paying attention to other body changes we experience can help us to distinguish them from signs

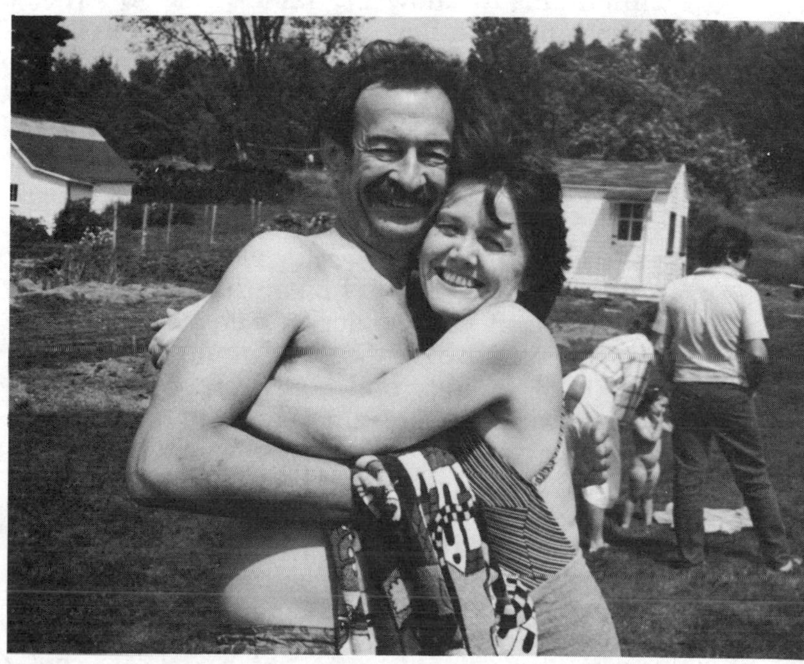

Judy Norsigian

of pregnancy. It can help us to talk with other women who are going through or have gone through menopause and to become familiar with the signs (see the chapter Experiencing Our Change of Life: Menopause). Continue contraception until one year after your last menstrual period. Women sometimes ovulate months or even over a year after menstruation appears to have stopped. If you are certain you do not want to become pregnant and consider abortion unacceptable, continue contraception until two years past the last menstrual period.

CHOOSING A BIRTH-CONTROL METHOD

Choosing a birth-control method is a very personal matter. We must weigh a lot of factors in making a decision. Each method's safety and effectiveness should be taken into consideration. Unfortunately, no contraceptive exists that is 100 percent effective and 100 percent safe. The risks of birth-control methods must be viewed in the context of the risks of carrying a pregnancy to term at an older age when a woman is more likely to have a chronic illness that would make pregnancy and childbirth risky. The most accepted measure of effectiveness is the failure rate—the number of pregnancies per 100 women using the contraceptive in the first year, as in the chart below. In evaluating a contraceptive's effectiveness for any group of women, it is important to know the failure rate for typical users and the failure rate when a method is used consistently and correctly (usually called the *lowest expected failure rate*).[2] Typical failure rates are strongly influenced by age, education, and socioeconomic status. Women under twenty-two are much more likely to experience contraceptive failure than women thirty and over. With barrier methods, very young women have failure rates 17 to 22 percent higher than women thirty and over.[3] Because older women are more likely to have the experience and maturity to use a method carefully and consistently, the lowest-expected failure rate may actually be closer to our own.

Recently, researchers have carefully reviewed studies of birth-control effectiveness and, as a result, they have revised their estimates of both lowest-expected and typical rates of failure (see chart below). The lowest-expected failure rate for a diaphragm's first year of use is 6 percent. That is, if one hundred women use a properly fitted diaphragm with spermicide consistently and correctly, six of them will conceive in the first year of using it. On the other hand, eighteen out of one hundred typical diaphragm users will conceive in the first year of use.[4]

FIRST-YEAR FAILURE RATES OF SELECTED BIRTH-CONTROL METHODS*

Method	Failure Rate in Typical Users[a]	Lowest-Expected Failure Rate[b]
Cervical Cap[c]		
Parous women[e]	36%	26%
Nulliparous women[f]	18%	9%
Male Condom[d]	12%	3%
Female Condom[d]	21%	5%
Diaphragm[c]	18%	6%
Foams, creams, gels, vaginal suppositories, and vaginal film	21%	6%
IUD		
Progestasert®	2.0%	1.5%
Copper T 380A	0.8%	0.6%
Norplant® (6 capsules)	0.09%	0.09%
Pill		
Progestin only	3%	0.5%
Combined Estrogen and Progestin	3%	0.1%
Sponge		
Parous women[e]	36%	20%
Nulliparous women[f]	18%	9%

[a]Among *typical* couples who initiate use of a method (not necessarily for the first time), the percentage who experience an accidental pregnancy during the first year if they do not stop use for any other reason.
[b]Among couples who initiate use of a method (not necessarily for the first time) and who use it consistently and correctly, the percentage who experience an accidental pregnancy during the first year if they do not stop use for any other reason.
[c]With spermicidal cream or jelly.
[d]Without spermicides.
[e]Women who have given birth.
[f]Women who have never given birth.

*Adapted from R. A. Hatcher, J. Trussell, F. Stewart, G. K. Stewart, D. Kowal, F. Guest, W. Cates, M. Policar. *Contraceptive Technology 1994–1996*. New York: Irvington Publishers, 1994 (in press). Reprinted with the permission of Contraceptive Technology Communications, Inc.

THE PILL, THE IUD, AND NORPLANT

By their middle years, many women have found a birth-control method that they consider convenient and effective. It may come as a nasty shock to many of them, then, to discover that the Pill, the IUD (intrauterine device), and Norplant pose special hazards to middle-aged women.

Oral contraceptives (or birth-control pills) contain one or a combination of artificial hormones that prevent pregnancy by suppressing ovulation. The Pill is the most frequently used and the most effective method of reversible birth control. Even so, Pill use declined in the late 1970s from a high of 10 million to 6 million users because of growing awareness among women of its hazards and risks. Many of the most serious negative effects are associated with high dosages of estrogen. Drug companies have reduced the estrogen content of the Pill, making it safer.

As a woman gets older, she is more likely to have a Pill-related heart attack or stroke. Women over forty with a second risk factor, such as diabetes or high blood pressure, and women over thirty-five who smoke are strongly advised *not* to use the Pill because of the increased risk of heart attacks and stroke. Although pills with lower dosages of estrogen seem to be safer than the pills produced in the 1960s, there are no data to support the claim that pills in current use have all the *positive effects* and none of the negative effects of higher-dose pills.[5]

Among women who *don't* smoke, taking the birth-control pill adds very little to their age-related risk, particularly for midlife women. *Smoking* while on the Pill is dangerous for women of any age. The risk of heart attack increases even for light smokers (one to twenty-four cigarettes/day), especially among older women, and Pill use further increases the risk. For heavy smokers (twenty-five or more cigarettes/day), Pill use compounds the risk of heart attack. By ages forty to forty-four, heavy smokers using the Pill will experience 421 more heart attacks (and 106 more deaths) per 100,000 women each year than heavy smokers not using the Pill.[6] For nonsmokers, Pill use adds little to the risk of stroke. **Smokers who use the Pill greatly increase their risk of stroke.** By ages forty to forty-four, heavy smokers using the Pill will experience 312 more strokes per 100,000 women per year than heavy smokers not using the Pill. A woman who smokes and uses the Pill can reduce her risk of cardiovascular disease if she stops smoking.[7]

Birth-control pills can cause a number of unintended effects and complications of varying degrees of severity. These effects may range from discomforts such as nausea, weight gain, depression, and increased susceptibility to yeast infections, to serious and potentially life-threatening complications[8] such as blood clots, heart attack and stroke, liver disease, and high blood pressure. It is dangerous for a woman at any age to use the Pill if she already has any of the above conditions, undiagnosed or abnormal genital bleeding, breast or reproductive-tract cancer, or a history of bile-flow blockage during pregnancy. Pill use is discouraged as well within four weeks of any surgical procedure and for women with mononucleosis or Gilbert's disease, liver tumor or history thereof, impaired liver function at the present time, or a past leg injury with phlebitis. Also, women with diabetes, gallbladder disease, or sickle-cell anemia are advised to avoid the Pill. There may be a relationship between the Pill and both skin cancer and cervical cancer, although researchers disagree and are currently studying this.[9]

Heart disease, stroke, and deep vein and pulmonary embolism are the main causes of Pill-related hospitalizations. Any woman who takes the Pill should see a health-care practitioner at least once a year for a complete well-woman gynecological exam, including a heart and blood-pressure examination. **Women approaching their forties should consider discontinuing use of the Pill.**

Some women who have intercourse very infrequently may be tempted to use the "morning-after pill" as birth control. This is not advisable because of the very high amount of hormones in this pill and the dangers associated with them, especially for women over forty (or smokers over thirty-five). Never use the "morning-after pill" without supervision from an experienced doctor or other health-care practitioner. It is not FDA approved as of mid-1993.

The IUD is a small device designed to be inserted through the vagina into the uterus. This procedure is done by a health-care provider. Some contain copper or synthetic progesterone; others are made of only white plastic. Currently, there are only two IUDs for sale in the United States, the Copper T 380 A (ParaGard) and the Progesterone T device (Progestasert).* IUDs may be more satisfactory than other methods of birth control for women who are at low risk of STDs (sexually transmitted diseases), who want effective long-term contraception, and who do not plan to have children in the future. For some women, IUDs may be a better alternative to sterilization.[10]

No one knows exactly how the IUD works. The most widely accepted theory is that the IUD causes an inflammation or chronic low-grade infection in the uterus. This causes the body to produce a higher number of white cells, which

*Most of the others have been recalled. Check with your health-care provider. The manufacturer may pay for removal.

may damage or destroy sperm or the egg and prevent them from joining; it may also hinder the buildup of the uterine lining, which must occur before implantation of a fertilized egg.[11] This does not preclude the possibility of conception, however, and does not protect against ectopic or "tubal" pregnancy (outside the uterus), a life-threatening condition.[12]

The Progestasert IUD contains synthetic progesterone and is sometimes prescribed to middle-aged women to control heavy menstrual bleeding occasionally caused by another IUD or by the menstrual irregularity of the perimenopausal years (see pages 324–25). The Progestasert IUD must be changed annually and is thought to cause a higher-than-usual rate of ectopic pregnancy.

One major risk of the IUD is infection. IUD-related infections can lead to damage to the fallopian tubes and/or uterus, sterility, and sometimes even death. Most doctors no longer recommend the IUD for younger women who may want to have children in the future. However, some middle-aged women may want to have a child, and no woman wants to risk a potentially life-threatening infection. There are other reasons that the IUD may not be an appropriate choice for women in midlife. Mid-cycle bleeding, common among IUD users, can also be a symptom of certain types of reproductive cancer such as cancer of the uterus and uterine lining. While these cancers are not common, they are found most often in women over forty. Such bleeding in IUD wearers may be either disregarded or misdiagnosed, thus delaying important treatment. IUDs are not recommended for women who have uterine fibroids, a condition also most common in women over forty. In addition, as women approach menopause, the uterus becomes smaller and the IUD can become deeply embedded and difficult to remove.[13]

The other most serious risk of the IUD is that it will perforate the uterus and travel partially or completely through the uterine wall. This is a serious emergency requiring immediate medical attention.

The IUD and pregnancy constitute a potentially dangerous combination. If you have an IUD in place and you become pregnant, have the IUD removed *whether or not* you intend to continue the pregnancy. If you remove the IUD, your chances of miscarriage are about 25 percent, while if you do not have it removed, the chance of miscarriage rises to 50 percent. If you do not remove it, you run the risk of an infected miscarriage, sometimes called a septic abortion. In extreme cases, this can cause the death of the woman as well as the fetus, and in most cases it is serious enough to require hospitalization. Women with IUDs should check out every missed period to be sure they are not pregnant or having a septic abortion. Of course, missing periods is fairly usual in the years prior to menopause, so this is yet another reason that the IUD is not a desirable method of contraception for women in midlife.

If the IUD has been your chosen mode of contraception and you plan to continue using it, it is critical to have regular examinations to check on the condition of the uterus around it, especially as you approach menopause, or if you experience increased bleeding. Any pelvic pain also needs to be evaluated immediately.

Norplant is a contraceptive implant containing a synthetic progesterone that lasts up to five years for women who weigh less than 154 pounds, and is extremely effective.[14] No one understands exactly how Norplant works, and its long-term safety has not yet been established. Women for whom birth control pills are dangerous should not use Norplant. The most common problem associated with Norplant is erratic, unpredictable bleeding for up to one year after insertion.[15] Mid-cycle bleeding can be a symptom of certain types of reproductive cancer, which, as mentioned, are most often found in women over forty. Thus, Norplant may not be an appropriate choice for women in midlife.

BARRIER METHODS

The diaphragm and other barrier methods are the birth-control practices most often recommended for women in midlife. See *The New Our Bodies, Ourselves* for detailed descriptions, pictures, and diagrams. In our thirties, forties, and fifties, many of us find that we use barrier methods more successfully than when we were younger because we have grown more knowledgeable and comfortable with our bodies over the years. For those of us who feel less comfortable with our bodies than we would like, using a vaginal barrier method is an opportunity to expand our self-knowledge and sexual confidence. Also, for women experiencing vaginal dryness, an increasingly common problem at midlife, contraceptive foam, cream, or jelly can provide additional lubrication. For women who have intercourse infrequently, barrier methods are advantageous because they do not have to be in place all the time. Barrier methods also provide some protection against sexually transmitted diseases.*

When the diaphragm is fitted properly and is used consistently and correctly, it has a failure rate of 6 percent. Most likely, the 6 percent failure rate exists because the diaphragm moves around a bit with frequent insertion of the penis, positions in which the woman is on top, and expansion of the upper vagina during intercourse. The typical failure rate is higher, about 18 percent.[16] Choose a health-care practitioner or clinic that allows enough time for you to practice inserting and removing the diaphragm several times. Too many practitioners omit this crucial step.

The diaphragm may be a risk factor for women who suffer from recurrent urinary tract infections.[17] Pelvic conditions such as a prolapsed uterus, a bladder that protrudes through the vaginal wall (called a cystocele), or any other openings in the vagina (called fistulas) are somewhat more common in midlife. If you have any of these conditions you may not be able to use the diaphragm, the cervical cap, or the contraceptive sponge. The "female" condom has been recently approved by the FDA. It will soon be available to women over the counter, without a prescription. Or your partner can use a condom, and you can add foam for additional protection. Some women find it convenient to purchase and keep a supply of condoms to offer to a partner who may not have one available. Used together, the condom and contraceptive foam offer almost 100 percent effectiveness against pregnancy with no dangerous side effects. They also help protect against STDs, including HIV.

Toxic Shock Syndrome (TSS)

As women in midlife, we are apparently less susceptible to TSS, but we are not entirely protected either. TSS is a rare but serious disease (see *The New Our Bodies, Ourselves* for more information), which primarily strikes menstruating women under thirty who are using tampons, especially high-absorbency tampons. However, a number of cases have been related to post-surgical complications or to use of barrier contraceptives, especially the contraceptive sponge, during menstruation, or to leaving a contraceptive in place for much longer than the recommended amount of time.

Every woman should be aware of the symptoms of TSS:

- A high fever, usually over 102 degrees
- Vomiting
- Diarrhea
- A sudden drop in blood pressure, which may lead to shock
- A sunburnlike rash

If you have these symptoms, remove the tampon or contraceptive at once and get medical attention immediately.

BIRTH CONTROL WITHOUT CONTRACEPTIVES

Abstinence is not the only alternative to the Pill, the IUD, or barrier methods. Sex without intercourse is an important birth-control option when we do not have access to safe and effective contraception, as well as an important variation in lovemaking. Fertility observation, or "natural birth control," involves learning from an experienced teacher to monitor and understand the hormonal changes in our bodies by observing the amount and quality of vaginal discharge, noting changes in the texture and position of the cervix, and keeping track of body temperature. In the years approaching menopause, however, menstrual cycles are apt to be erratic, making fertility observation a little more challenging. However, it can be a useful and interesting—even exciting—tool for monitoring premenopausal hormonal changes, and for women who are trying to get pregnant at midlife.

STERILIZATION

Sterilization, a *permanent and irreversible* method of birth control through surgery, is now widely available, and for married couples over thirty it is the most commonly used method of contraception.[18] Sterilization is a highly reliable method of birth control; the lowest-expected and typical failure rate for both tubal ligation (sterilization of the woman) and vasectomy (sterilization of the man) ranges from 0.1 to 0.4 percent.

A growing number of women and men in midlife choose sterilization because they are

*Condoms and spermicides containing nonoxynol-9 are among the contraceptives that offer some protection against sexually transmitted diseases (STDs) including HIV/AIDS. See box, pages 96–97. See also *The New Our Bodies, Ourselves*, 1992, chapters 14 and 15.

very sure they will not want to have more children. However, too many women still choose sterilization without adequate information and in desperation over the limited safety and effectiveness of other contraceptive methods. There is a deplorable history of sterilization abuse in the United States against middle-aged women,* poor women, women of color, and women who speak a language other than English. Primarily as a result of pressure from people of color and women's groups, regulations were enacted in March 1979 to protect women obtaining federally funded sterilizations. For example, the regulations require that a woman be provided information in her preferred language (orally and in writing) about the risks, negative effects, and irreversibility of sterilization, as well as alternative methods of reversible birth control. The regulations also prohibit overt or implicit threat of loss of welfare or Medicaid benefits if a woman doesn't consent to sterilization. The regulation especially relevant to middle-aged women is the one prohibiting a hysterectomy for the sole purpose of sterilization. **Hysterectomy—removal of the uterus—is major surgery, and should not be considered a method of birth control or sterilization.** (See the Hysterectomy and Oophorectomy chapter for more information.) Even now, after federal legislation has eliminated the worst abuses, too many women, especially non-English-speaking women, are not adequately informed of either the permanence of sterilization or its possible risks and side effects.[19]

Sterilization Procedures

Tubal ligation, popularly called "tying the tubes," blocks the woman's fallopian tubes so that eggs cannot pass through them into the uterus. It may be done either abdominally or vaginally, often through a laparoscope (see page 326). Serious complications are rare and the death rate is low (3 deaths per 100,000 procedures) compared with other surgery. The risk of death is greater when general anesthesia is used.[20] The skill of both the anesthesiologist and the surgeon is very important; be sure to inquire about the number of tubal ligations the surgeon has performed. Complications of laparoscopic sterilization may include puncturing of the intestine, bowel burns (with cauterization), perforation, hemorrhage, infection, and cardiac arrest. Some women experience a postlaparoscopic syndrome including heavy irregular bleeding and increased menstrual pain, which may create the need for repeated D and Cs* or, in some cases, lead to hysterectomies.[21]

Vasectomy, or male sterilization, is a much simpler and less expensive procedure with fewer possible complications than female sterilization. It can be done in a doctor's office in a half hour under local anesthesia. However, a vasectomy is not immediately effective, so use another means of birth control until the man has had twenty ejaculations. Tests should then be done on samples of semen.[22] The man is considered sterile after two negative sperm counts.

MISSED PERIODS AND PREGNANCY SCARES

If you miss a period, when you are not trying to get pregnant, consider whether it is a sign of pregnancy or a sign of menopause (see page 122). If you continue to be uncertain, it is important to have a pregnancy test early, so you can begin prenatal care if you decide to have a child, or make plans for an early abortion if you decide to terminate the pregnancy. If your periods have become irregular, you may want to wait until you have skipped two months before testing, but do not wait until a third month or you will not be able to have a less traumatic first-trimester abortion.

Many of the commonly used pregnancy tests cannot distinguish the hormonal changes of pregnancy from those of menopause; one test that can is a blood test called the Beta Subunit. In large cities it may be possible to have this test done at a drop-in clinic; however, in many localities you will be charged for an office visit each time you want the test done. (Medicaid and some insurance companies cover lab tests, including pregnancy testing.)

ABORTION

Middle-aged women who are routinely in good health have no special medical problems associ-

*Middle-aged women have been the chief victims of unnecessary and inappropriate hysterectomies. Too many doctors still regard a middle-aged or older woman's uterus as expendable.

**D and C* stands for *dilation and curettage*: the opening to the uterus is enlarged or stretched and the inner lining of the womb is scraped.

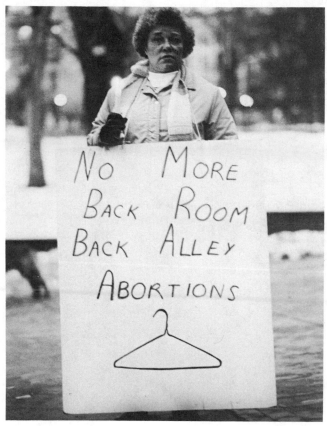

Ellen Shub

ated with abortion. A thorough medical history should be taken *before* an abortion and your physician should check for certain conditions. For example, fibroid tumors or a bladder that protrudes into the vagina may necessitate performing the abortion in a hospital.

Abortion is a vital option in controlling our fertility—and, therefore, our lives.* Whether or not abortion is any one woman's personal choice, safe, legal, and accessible abortion must continue to be available to all women who choose it. As the generation that fought for reproductive freedom, today's middle-aged women recognize the threat antichoice forces pose to the progress of women in every walk of life. Entering our postreproductive years does not weaken our resolve to defend the right to choice and to control over our bodies for ourselves, our daughters, and future generations of women.

*For more about abortion, see *The New Our Bodies, Ourselves,* chapter 17.

Notes

1. Boston Women's Health Book Collective, *The New Our Bodies, Ourselves.* New York: Simon & Schuster, 1992.

2. Robert A. Hatcher, et al., *Contraceptive Technology: 1990–1992, 15th Revised Edition.* New York: Irvington Publishers, 1990, pp. 133–36.

3. Howard W. Ory, *Making Choices: Evaluating the Health Risks and Benefits of Birth Control Methods,* 1983. The Alan Guttmacher Institute, 111 Fifth Avenue, New York, NY 10003.

4. James Trussell, et al., "Contraceptive Failure in the United States: An Update." *Studies in Family Planning,* Vol. 21, No. 1 (January/February 1990), pp. 51–54.

5. Boston Women's Health Book Collective, op. cit., p. 280.

6. Susan Harlap, Kathryn Kost, and Jacqueline Darroch Forrest, *Preventing Pregnancy, Protecting Health: A New Look at Birth Control Choices in the United States,* 1991. The Alan Guttmacher Institute, 111 Fifth Avenue, New York, NY 10003, pp. 75–76.

7. Harlap, et al., op cit., p. 78.

8. R. A. Hatcher, et al., op. cit., p. 247.

9. E. A. Holly. "Cutaneous Melanoma and Oral Contraceptives: A Review of Case-Control and Cohort Studies," *Recent Results in Cancer Research,* Vol. 102 (1986), pp. 108–17.

10. Boston Women's Health Book Collective, op. cit., p. 294.

11. K. Treiman and L. Liskin, "IUDs—A New Look," *Population Reports,* Series B, No. 5 (March 1988). Available from Population Information Programs, Johns Hopkins University, 624 North Broadway, Baltimore, MD 21205. Multiple copies are $2 each; free to developing countries.

12. Boston Women's Health Book Collective, op. cit., p. 295.

13. Bernard M. Kaye, et al., "Long-Term Safety and Use-Effectiveness of Intra-Uterine Devices." *Fertility and Sterility,* Vol. 28, No. 9 (September 1977), pp. 937–42.

14. Boston Women's Health Book Collective, op. cit., pp. 288–89, 292.

15. Ibid., pp. 290–91.

16. James Trussell et al., op. cit., pp. 51–54.

17. Betsy Foxman and Ralph R. Frerichs, "Epidemiology of Urinary Tract Infection: Diaphragm Use and Sexual Intercourse." *American Journal of Public Health,* Vol. 75, No. 11 (November 1985), pp. 1308–13; and Larianne Gillespie, "The Diaphragm: An Accomplice in Recurrent Urinary Infections." *Urology,* Vol. 24, No. 1 (July 1984), pp. 25–30, quoted in Kathleen O'Brien, "Lifestyle Factors and Urinary Tract Infections," *The Network News,* Vol. 12, No. 1 (January/February 1987).

18. Jacqueline Darroch Forrest and Richard R. Fordyce, "U.S. Women's Contraceptive Attitudes and Practice: How Have They Changed in the 1980s?" *Family Planning Perspectives,* Vol. 20, No. 3 (May/June 1988), p. 116.

19. See *The New Our Bodies, Ourselves,* pp. 300–302, for organizations working on this issue.

20. Hatcher, et al., op. cit., p. 391.

21. Boston Women's Health Book Collective, op. cit., p. 303.

22. Hatcher, et al., op. cit., p. 415.

9

CHILDBEARING IN MIDLIFE

✦

BY PAULA B. DORESS-WORTERS, TRUDY COX, AND EDIE BUTLER

SPECIAL THANKS TO JUDY NORSIGIAN, BARBARA KATZ-ROTHMAN, WITH THANKS TO PHYLLIS GREENLEAF AND JANE PINCUS

1994 UPDATE BY PAULA B. DORESS-WORTERS WITH SPECIAL THANKS TO JUDY NORSIGIAN AND JANE PINCUS

1994 UPDATE OF *PRENATAL GENETIC TESTING* BY ROBIN J. R. BLATT

1994 UPDATE OF *ALTERNATIVES TO MIDLIFE CHILDBEARING* BY ALLISON MORRILL

RESOURCES FOR THIS CHAPTER ON PAGES 463–66

More women today are choosing to have children in their middle years. Because we live longer and stay healthier longer, we can concentrate on other areas of our lives in our young adult years, and still choose parenthood well into our forties and even later if we are willing to use assisted reproductive technologies. Despite some of the added pressures of the middle years, such as more stressful and challenging jobs, new relationships, and aging parents, older women often have more experience at balancing life's demands.

I'm forty-three and becoming aware of the issues of old age, as I help my baby start his life. The advantage of having my children at thirty-five and forty-three is that I know myself; I knew I really wanted children. I know some things about what I need, what contributions I can make in addition to raising the children. I've made a commitment to photography and have a number of projects that I'm working on or looking forward to. Some of them are about lesbian family life.

At times I do feel a bit out of sync—with friends my age whose children are grown, with friends who have children the age of mine who are ten or fifteen years younger than I; or when I feel myself hitting my stride in photography and need to move at a slower pace partly because of the family commitments.

I've noticed that when I'm with friends in their fifties and sixties I envy their clean, quiet rooms. I tell myself, I've had this before and some day again this will be mine. I'm grateful to be intimately in touch with the stages and cycles of life. I asked the babies, "Is this too abstract?" They said, "Ba, Ba, Ba, Ba."

The best thing in my life is the joy of actually having a child. Eleven years ago when I was pregnant with my son, my marriage was in such terrible shape I almost had

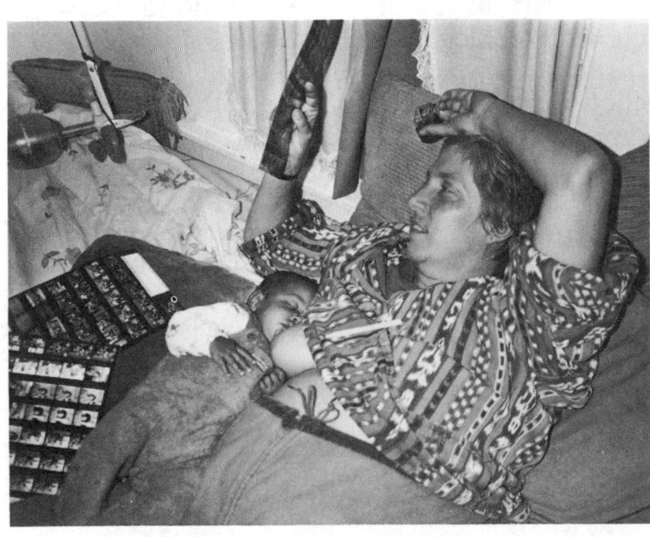

Lyn Stirewalt

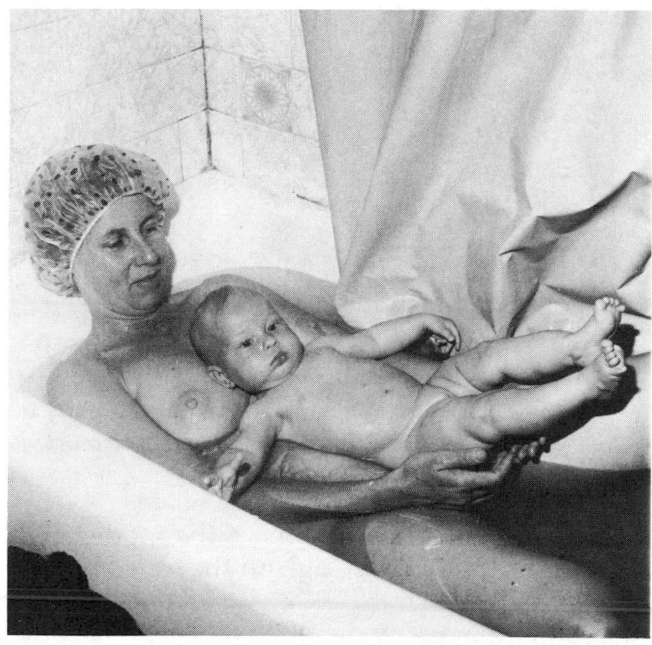

Lisa Roper

an abortion because I couldn't envision living my life with that much dissension. My husband wasn't supportive of me and so I figured he wouldn't be supportive of a child either. A sister had even made all the arrangements. Then the morning the abortion was scheduled, I decided not to have it, because I was thirty-four and I thought, I may not have the opportunity to become pregnant again. And with all the pressures and difficulties I have faced, some of my greatest joys have come from being a mother. The doctors referred to me as an "elderly primip," which made me laugh. I was healthy as a horse.

What saved my sanity when I was raising my youngster alone was that my mother lived next door to me. I never had to concern myself with finding a baby-sitter. My mother, like so many black grandmothers and aunts, provided care without my asking her and I could work whatever schedules I was asked to work. In fact, my son came home once and asked me what a baby-sitter was. [a forty-five-year-old woman]

For me, having children in my forties while raising two stepchildren seemed natural and appropriate. My age seemed irrelevant to me and to my husband, though sometimes it seemed to concern others when they found out. What is it like now to be fifty-eight and have a sixteen- and eighteen-year-old? Well, we do worry about getting it together for their college and our retirement, but other than that we don't feel very deviant and our kids don't seem to mind having "older parents." At least they don't seem to have much to say about it.

I was a forty-one-year-old first-time mother married to a fifty-three-year-old father of three children. In what some called an "advanced maturity" marriage, we needed time to be alone together as well as time to spend with our newborn, as well as time for his children from his former marriage and time for our dependent parents.

The difficulty of orchestrating all this with time alone for spiritual stretching and meditating seemed to increase with age. The demands on our energy and creativity were titanic. We felt we needed a minimum of one evening out per week and one weekend away alone together every six weeks because we would be sixty and seventy before there would be an "empty nest."

We might have managed this if we had forfeited privacy and hired live-in help, or had not moved when our newborn was a year old, leaving a network of friends built up during our adult years. Our marriage did not survive the stress. Paying attention to time alone and time together is a major challenge in combining midlife childbearing and midlife marriage.

CONCEPTION AND MIDLIFE FERTILITY

Women who want a baby in their thirties or forties may worry if they do not conceive right away. Some of us continue to produce eggs regularly up until menopause, while other women in their thirties gradually begin to produce fewer eggs, and thus have fewer opportunities for conception. The reduced fertility of women over thirty compared with younger women may be partly attributable to less frequent intercourse among longer-married couples.[1] So it is wise to be patient and allow enough time and opportunity for conception before assuming that there is a fertility problem.

Infertility is usually defined as the inability to conceive after a year or more of sexual intercourse without contraception.[2] Infertility increases only moderately with age.[3] Medical and lay media reports that exaggerate the degree to which fertility decreases with age have contributed to women's worries about their fertility.[4]

Infertility is becoming increasingly common at all ages due to environmental hazards and pelvic infections resulting from sexually transmitted diseases (STDs) and/or IUDs. If you have been trying to conceive for more than a year, you may want to read some of the feminist literature on infertility and new reproductive technologies (see Resources for this chapter) before going to see a health-care practitioner.

If you have taken a long time to conceive, you may be at risk for the "medicalization" of your pregnancy and birth. Doctors often intervene unnecessarily in midlife pregnancies with procedures such as Cesareans in order to "safeguard" the pregnancy of a woman who has taken a long time to conceive.[5] This is a concern because every medical intervention brings its own set of risks and complications. In considering the risks of midlife pregnancy, keep in mind that low fertility is a problem of conception, not of pregnancy. Once you are pregnant, you do not need to be treated a special way because you took a long time conceiving. However, a history of repeated miscarriages may require special care during pregnancy.

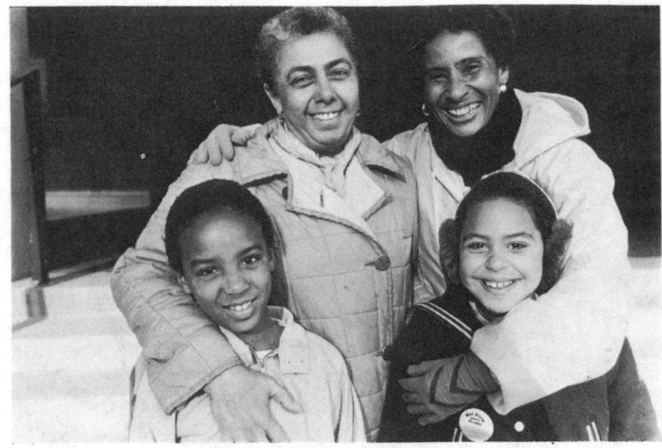

Marianne Gontarz

Childbearing for Women in Midlife

A major change over the past ten years has been the extension of women's "fertility deadline" from the early thirties to the early forties. What has brought about this change? Several factors stand out:

- Improved health and extended longevity of women
- Reliable birth control
- The women's movement, which has encouraged us to decide for ourselves whether and when we will have children
- More sophisticated prenatal testing and the availability of legal abortion
- New research that shows that some of the earlier assumptions and concerns about pregnancy and age have been incorrect or overstated.

Phyllis Kernoff Mansfield, a health educator, reviewed all the studies published in the United States that relate the age of the mother to seven pregnancy complications. She found that the vast majority of studies published before 1970 did not pass the simplest test for methodological soundness. The most glaring deficiency was the lack of a control group; that is, no comparison was made between older and younger women. The "problems" of older women were simply assumed to be related to their age, without accounting for other factors such as fertility history, general health, or number of previous pregnancies. When other factors were held constant, only Cesarean sections showed a definite increase in risk with age—and a C-section is not a complication but an intervention. Mansfield and her associates concluded that the general health and nutritional habits of the mother had far more influence than age on the outcome of a pregnancy.[6]

Contemporary women who first become pregnant in their thirties and forties have good results because they do not have a history of delayed childbearing due to pregnancy-related problems. These women have *chosen* to begin childbearing in their thirties and forties when they have found the right partner, when their job or career is going well—when they feel ready.

Other studies have also found that some of the risks formerly associated with childbearing in midlife have on more careful examination turned out to be associated with diseases or chronic conditions.[7] As we get older, we are at higher risk of developing such chronic diseases as diabetes, hypertension, and heart disease, as well as fibroid tumors, endometriosis, and scarring from operations and infections in the pelvic area, all of which can complicate conception and pregnancy. But these conditions affect only a relatively small number of women and do not warrant intervention in the majority of pregnancies in healthy older women. *Older women who do not have such conditions have no higher risk of a difficult pregnancy than younger women.*

The following is a list of factors that can complicate pregnancy and childbirth:

- Preeclampsia (toxemia), the presence of toxic substances in the blood, can lead to a much more serious condition called eclampsia, which in turn leads to convulsions and coma. Research has found the risk of this disease to be associated not with age, but with diabetes.[8] Diabetes is also linked to many other pregnancy and childbirth complications.
- Unnecessary Cesareans. A government study

found that a high national rate of 23.5 Cesareans per 100 births has brought no improvement in maternal or child health and in fact is associated with increased risk and complications. A national objective to reduce the rate of Cesareans to 12 to 15 per 100 births by the year 2000 is based on the assumption that one third to one half of Cesareans are unnecessary.[9] Doctors tend to intervene more readily in a prolonged labor when the mother is over thirty-five. They perform Cesarean sections more often and use painkillers and anesthetics sooner and in greater amounts. The use of anesthetics during childbirth has been associated with low blood pressure in the mother and respiratory problems in the newborn. And if a woman is apprehensive that she will have a difficult delivery because she is older, she may be more easily influenced to accept or to ask for drugs.[10]

My doctor was certain that my slow labor meant I had a "sluggish uterus," which he thought typical of older women. He was already preparing for a C-section when I went into transition. I later found out that my mother and sister had had similar labors. It was a family pattern. [a fifty-eight-year-old woman reporting on a first childbirth at forty]

- Women thirty-five and over are no more likely than women in their twenties to have premature babies, or babies who are small for their gestational age, according to a study of 3,917 pregnant women who were private-hospital patients.[11] The evidence suggests that the older mothers of today are more highly educated and more likely to be well informed about pregnancy, nutrition, and exercise. They are more highly motivated to take good care of themselves and to seek prenatal care; therefore they are more likely to have heavier, healthier babies.
- Race and socioeconomic status, not age of the mother, are the most significant factors predicting infant mortality in the U.S.* Women who have higher incomes have better access to a wide choice of good prenatal care and a wider choice of facilities. They can more easily purchase the additional food and vitamins they need during pregnancy. Recent funding cuts in health and nutrition programs and in prenatal-care services threaten to deepen the alarming disparity in infant mortality between white and black, the middle class and poor, and to slow the gradual decline in the national infant-mortality rate.[12]
- Maternal mortality is also shockingly linked to race and class-linked access to prenatal and other health care. Maternal mortality at all ages is three times higher for black women (18.6 deaths per 100,000 live births) compared with white women (5.4 per 100,000). By age thirty-five and over, the difference jumps to six times as high for black women with 57.5 deaths per 100,000 live births as compared with 9.7 deaths per 100,000 live births for white women.[13]
- Cardiovascular disease in the mother, not her age, is the factor that most increases the risk of infant mortality.[14] A study that eliminated those with hypertension from the study sample found that healthy black women over thirty-five had successful outcomes in pregnancy and birth.[15]
- Placental hemorrhage and other complications of the placenta have been linked to cardiovascular diseases such as hypertension.[16]
- Down syndrome is sometimes associated with the age of the mother; however, the father's age plays a role in one kind of Down syndrome.[17] Another type of Down syndrome is hereditary—the age of neither parent is a factor.

*See "Maternity Care in a Large Context" in *The New Our Bodies, Ourselves,* 1992, pp. 404–5.

NUTRITION

Everything in the Aging Well section deserves double emphasis if you are pregnant. Stay away from smoking, alcohol,[18] and drugs, and avoid caffeine. See *The New Our Bodies, Ourselves* for a more in-depth discussion of nutrition during pregnancy and of the effects of harmful substances on pregnancy. While age itself is not a risk, the chances of developing a chronic disease increase with age. Taking care of yourself often prevents disease, thus improving the outlook for a healthy pregnancy.

It is essential that you eat nutritiously while you are pregnant. Unfortunately, most obstetrician-gynecologists know little about nutrition and pregnancy, so you may want to talk to a nutritionist. Ask your health-care provider about her or his background in nutrition.

Eating well will ensure that you and your baby will be able to meet the demands of pregnancy, labor, and childbirth, and help ensure that your baby will have an adequate birth weight.[19] Low-birth-weight babies are more susceptible to complications at birth. Eating well also lowers the risk of complications such as anemia and toxemia, and reduces the risk of mental retardation in your baby. During pregnancy your body stores fats and fluids you will need if you breastfeed. Older women are a little more likely to have twins, creating an extra need for nourishment (an additional 100 grams of protein per day is recommended).[20]

In the past, doctors put a great deal of emphasis on gaining as little weight as possible during pregnancy. Pregnancy, however, *increases* your body's need for calories and protein; *it is not the time to diet.*[21] Monitor your weight to avoid a *sudden* increase in weight. This can be a sign of preeclampsia. It is best to eat as healthfully as you can and let your weight take care of itself. If you have a very low income, you may be eligible for the WIC (Women, Infants, and Children) program, a supplemental food program for pregnant and lactating women sponsored by the government. If you are on welfare, you may be eligible for a higher food allowance.[22]

Physical Activity and Exercise

Staying active is an important part of good prenatal care. You can swim, run, walk, dance, do yoga, whatever feels comfortable and does not tire you out too much. Physicians sometimes advise pregnant women not to "overdo it." They may be even more cautious with older pregnant women. Such advice can cause stress to women who are accustomed to exercise. It is important to keep up exercise at your accustomed level. If you have been sedentary, find ways to move more, beginning with walking and gentle exercise.

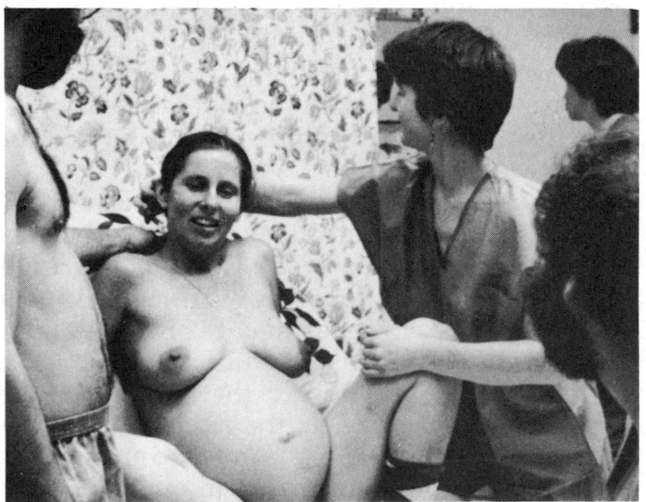

Ilene S. Hauck

I noticed that although I was one of the oldest women in my prenatal exercise class, I was in much better physical condition than the majority. Perhaps my regular swimming and dance made the difference. Clearly, one's emotional/physical condition rather than one's age is most important. [a forty-one-year-old woman]

The Kegel exercises (see pages 75–77 for description and instructions) can help during pregnancy to strengthen the muscles in the pelvic area, which can make the entire delivery process easier. See Resources for this chapter for books on exercise during pregnancy and childbirth-preparation exercises.

Getting Support

At any age, we want our pregnancy to include solid emotional support from our partners, friends, and families. That support can be especially important as we press through the maze of medical decisions and pressures that often accompany a midlife pregnancy. We may also be dealing with stressful situations, such as older children going through a turbulent adolescence or aging parents depending on us for support; we may have demanding jobs or careers; we may be worried about how pregnancy will change a relationship. Talking with other women often can be an important source of support.

When I first learned that I was pregnant, I was delighted, joyful, excited. And I assumed that people close to me would share my joy. Not so. My mother, my teenaged daughter, and my closest woman friend openly disapproved because I was unmarried. However, there were others—my sister, a close older woman friend and mentor, a male peer counselor, and other old friends who were happy for me. It was real important to my well-being to have warm support from people around me during my pregnancy. My prenatal exercise classes, besides readying my body for giving birth, also serve as an open forum for sharing concerns, thoughts, and resources with other pregnant women. It's always such a relief to suddenly step into a room where everyone is pregnant. The feelings of isolation immediately vanish. [a divorced woman in her forties]

An important source of support during pregnancy is a prenatal-care practitioner who will view you and your pregnancy as normal and healthy, while carefully monitoring any special medical conditions you may have. Although a late pregnancy can be as safe as an early one if a woman is healthy, older mothers run a high risk of having their pregnancies medicalized by health-care practitioners, causing worry and stress that can take a toll on your pregnancy. Thus, feeling optimistic and keeping stress at a minimum is an advantage medically as well as psychologically.[23]

In general, a midwife or a family-practice physician may be more likely to view midlife pregnancy as healthy and normal than an obstetrician. Obstetrical training is more intervention-oriented. The Pregnancy chapter in *The New Our Bodies, Ourselves* includes a detailed discussion of the kinds of care available and the issues involved.

A Massachusetts law requires hospitals to disclose their track record in perinatal (occurring during the period immediately preceding and following birth) care, so that a pregnant woman can find out the Cesarean rate as well as other birth practices at that hospital before signing up for childbirth care. Women are urged to find out as much as possible about prenatal-care providers and the facilities they practice in before making a choice. "We think the way change is going to occur is by parents' having more information and taking more responsibility for their own birth experiences," commented Beth Shearer of Cesarean Support, Education, and Concern, one of the fifteen consumer health groups that worked together to pass the Massachusetts bill.[24] Following this model, New York passed a more comprehensive bill in 1989, and advocates in other states have legislation pending.

PRENATAL GENETIC TESTING

Prenatal genetic tests for screening and diagnosis are either medical or surgical procedures performed with varying degrees of safety and accuracy on pregnant women, in order to provide information about the health of the developing fetus. The majority of pregnant women today are offered the maternal serum alphafetoprotein (MSAFP) test and ultrasound. Other tests such as amniocentesis and chorionic villus sampling may be offered.

Deciding about Prenatal Tests

Whether or not to undergo one or more of these tests is completely up to an individual woman. In making your decisions, you will want to consider factors such as your personal medical history and your views and values relative to pregnancy and child rearing.

Prior to testing, a woman may also want to consider genetic counseling to learn about her individual chances of having a baby with a genetic or disabling condition, and to discuss available pregnancy options. It is important for women to have information about each test, its risks and benefits to both the mother and baby, the disabilities being tested for, the safety and accuracy of the test, and whether the procedure is considered experimental or not.[25]

Prenatal genetic testing may provide information that will allow you to make an informed choice about your pregnancy. For example, knowing before birth whether your baby has a certain health condition could allow you to plan for specialized care at birth and thereafter, to relinquish your child for special needs adoption, or to terminate the pregnancy.

Prenatal testing requires a special set of skills in terms of assessment, test performance, and interpretation. The risk of complications is reduced when the physician performing the tests is experienced. Some women go to a specialist for these tests, but choose a less interventionist style of routine prenatal care.

Several writers on pregnancy have observed that the process of testing, waiting for test results to come back, and deciding on a course of action delays a woman's or a couple's emotional commitment to the pregnancy.[26] The very process of having a child involves unknowns and even with the testing that is available, many conditions cannot be discovered ahead of time. In our technological, medicalized culture, we may come to believe that the newly developed prenatal tests magically "prevent" disease and disability. We may be accused of not being responsible when we choose not to have them. Though tests may certainly be proper procedure in specific instances, it is not reasonable that they be done routinely—they may not always be safe for us or our babies, they further medicalize the experience of pregnancy, and they can cause unwarranted anxiety. Unfortunately, often the very existence of these tests pressures us into having them performed. Testing raises several difficult moral and ethical issues that each woman must consider carefully. For women, the right to reproductive choice is central to all other rights in life.

I felt I had to make the decision, before we knew the results, that if we got a diagnosis of Down's I would have an abortion. We talked to a genetics counselor before the test. She was very helpful—all the medical support staff were helpful; they made all the difference in my thinking of it as a positive thing we were doing. [a thirty-eight-year-old first-time mother]

I chose not to have an "amnio" because, after much soul-searching, I decided that I would be open to having a Down's child. My personal experience with adults who have Down's syndrome is that they are among the most loving people around. Though Down's children take more care, work, and commitment, they can develop into contributing creative adults. They play a very humanizing role in our society. [a forty-one-year-old woman with a long-delayed second pregnancy]

Because of my age, I was considered a high-risk pregnancy, but I did not consider myself one. I was healthy and ate well and had a strong family history. At this point in my life I wanted a child very much and felt prepared to accept whatever happened in terms of [the baby's] health. I also had had a miscarriage and felt the risk of another miscarriage, though slight, with amniocentesis, was great enough to warrant not *having any unnecessary intervention.* [a thirty-eight-year-old woman]

Though prenatal tests have their place, women are increasingly concerned about the way testing has become routine for women over thirty-five and increasingly pushed upon women as young as thirty. Prenatal genetic tests are being heavily marketed by commercial genetic laboratories. Many practitioners suggest testing to protect themselves against the possibility of a lawsuit in the event that a child is born with a condition that could have been detected by prenatal testing. It is important to remember that these tests cannot identify every possible condition, or guarantee a "perfect" baby. Those who administer the tests may not fully discuss the scenarios to expect following each test—the decisions and possibility of subsequent tests and procedures. Choose a practitioner who will communicate with you, who shares your views and will support your decisions.

ULTRASOUND

Ultrasound is an imaging technique using intermittent high-frequency sound waves to create a picture on a televisionlike screen. It can be used throughout pregnancy for many purposes, such as to confirm your pregnancy and estimate your due date, to examine the fetus and its organs, and to determine the position of the placenta. Ultrasound is used by itself or in conjunction with amniocentesis for one or more of the following: to help pinpoint the exact location and position of the fetus; to help determine the age and size of the fetus; and to check for structural abnormalities in the fetus. Ultrasound can be done either abdominally or vaginally. Vaginal ultrasound is a newer technique that some practitioners are beginning to use on the premise that it can be done earlier and will provide a clearer picture. Some women find it less uncomfortable than abdominal ultrasound, which requires a full bladder, but other women find it highly intrusive and uncomfortable. For some women it helps to insert the probe themselves.

Though ultrasound appears to be a safe test and can provide important information, its long-term effects are still unknown. You may want to consider using the test only when necessary. Ultrasound may be useful to provide information if bleeding occurs during pregnancy or to determine the presence of twins. Prior to the procedure, it is important to understand how the test results will be of use. Consider whether you really need to have this information early in your pregnancy. Ultrasound may be reassuring for a woman who has had prior problems with pregnancy, or has taken a long time conceiving. However, a randomized study of over 15,000 women demonstrated that screening of low-risk women does not improve perinatal outcomes.[27]

AMNIOCENTESIS

Amniocentesis can detect chromosomal as well as certain biochemical and metabolic disorders; it is most often used to test for Down syndrome. Amniocentesis does not detect every possible disorder and is not a guarantee of a healthy infant.

The test involves withdrawing a small amount of fluid from the amniotic sac by way of a large needle. It is usually performed between the sixteenth to eighteenth weeks of pregnancy, when there is enough amniotic fluid to give an adequate sample but the least risk of harming the fetus. Some researchers are experimenting with early amniocentesis performed between twelve and fourteen weeks. Amniocentesis results are usually available within two weeks after testing.

The risk of miscarriage associated with the test is estimated at 1 in 400 in large city hospitals specializing in such procedures; the risk is higher where the staff is not as well trained.[28]

Possible complications of amniocentesis include infection, leakage of fluid, vaginal bleeding, fetal injury, and a 0.5 percent risk of miscarriage.[29]

Amniocentesis is usually performed in a doctor's office. The fluid sample is often sent to a specialized lab for analysis. While many obstetricians will perform this test, it ought to be done by an experienced practitioner who does this test routinely, such as an obstetrician-geneticist. Costs can also be prohibitive, ranging from $600 to over $1,000. Many insurance companies, Medicare,* and Medicaid will pay for this test if a doctor states that it is necessary. Accessibility is still limited by geographic and financial barriers.

For women over forty, the chance of finding a health problem in the fetus is greater than the risk of miscarriage. Between ages thirty-five and forty, the odds are about even, and under age thirty-five, the risk of miscarriage is greater than the chance of finding a problem.[30]

Waiting for amniocentesis results can be very stressful. If a woman is having this test in order to decide whether to continue or terminate her pregnancy, it is important to realize that the results would not be available until the second trimester, possibly as late as twenty-four weeks, thus limiting her choice of abortion procedures.†

MATERNAL SERUM ALPHAFETOPROTEIN (MSAFP)

The maternal serum alphafetoprotein (MSAFP) screening test is used to identify women who may be at increased risk for fetal disabilities, including neural tube disorders (spina bifida and anencephaly), open ventral wall conditions, and Down syndrome. The MSAFP test is performed between fifteen and eighteen weeks of pregnancy. Produced by the fetal liver, AFP is passed into the amniotic fluid through the placenta into the mother's blood where it can be measured. Since the AFP level increases each week during pregnancy, the timing of the test is extremely important. Results are usually obtained within one week.

Because it is only a *screening* test, MSAFP cannot determine with certainty whether a condition exists. It can only be used to identify those women for whom further diagnostic tests may be helpful. There are situations where the tests will be incorrectly abnormal due to miscalculation of gestational age or the presence of twins. Accuracy is dependent upon the experience and awareness of the laboratory performing the test and the accuracy of accompanying clinical information.

An enhanced MSAFP screening test measures two biochemical markers, unconjugated estriol (uE3) and human chorionic gonadotrophin (hCG), in addition to AFP. Enhanced MSAFP screening can identify 60 to 65 percent of fetal Down syndrome as compared with approximately 40 percent using AFP alone.[31]

CHORIONIC VILLUS SAMPLING

Chorionic villus sampling (CVS) is a form of early prenatal diagnosis, used to detect chromosomal and other genetic abnormalities, performed between ten and twelve weeks. It is a highly invasive test and no longer performed at nine weeks because of complications that arose when performed that early. Timing is critical.

CVS is unable to detect neural tube conditions and disorders that can be detected with amniocentesis.[32] Because of this and its association with limb deficiencies and other fetal abnormalities, CVS is decreasing in popularity. The fetal loss rate associated with CVS is estimated at over 1 percent.[33]

OTHER PRENATAL TESTS

New genetic tests, such as embryoscopy,[34] preimplantation genetic diagnosis, fetal cell sorting, and others are on the horizon and must be approached cautiously.[35] Women should be fully informed before participating in any type of genetic test that is still experimental.

ALTERNATIVES TO MIDLIFE CHILDBEARING

As menopause approaches, some women speak of an urge to bear a child before it is "too late." One woman, divorced when her first child was young, and approaching her fortieth birthday, spoke of her wish to have another baby.

My son is sixteen and I suddenly have a strong urge to have a baby. I still want a family with children in it. I wonder if I'm really wanting a baby or if I just want to be part of a family, and it feels like a baby would give me that.

*For persons under sixty-five on Medicare, such as disabled women.

†For more information about abortion procedures, see *The New Our Bodies, Ourselves,* chapter 17.

If you decide that having a child biologically is not central to your wish for a family, you may want to explore alternatives such as communal living or foster parenthood. Another increasingly popular alternative is adoption. A forty-five-year-old single woman, determined to have her own child, decided on adoption because of her infertility.

I had a total hysterectomy, so that settled it as far as giving birth to my own child was concerned. At that point I was forty-two and realized that I couldn't fool around any more—I needed to go ahead—and I was very fortunate that a friend of mine worked for an international adoption-counseling center. One evening she told me there was a four-year-old girl available and asked, "Are you interested?" Something told me, "This is it, now or never." I was able to fly down and meet her first so I could get to know her and then decided to go ahead.

Be prepared for the possibility of bias against older women at state-run agencies. The unwritten rule is that a woman should not be more than forty years older than her adopted child. In addition, we deplore the discriminatory practices of state and private agencies that make it virtually impossible for an openly lesbian woman or couple to adopt children or to be foster parents.

While there is often a long waiting period (as much as seven years) to adopt a healthy white infant, social-service agencies have many older children and children with some medical or emotional problems who can be adopted immediately.

I didn't seem to have that need to have an infant. I felt I was older, so I wanted an older child! I felt it would work better for me economically, having to work and not earning enough to pay for day care. The adoption itself took all my savings. [a woman in her forties]

There are many adoptable children of color of all ages within the United States and from Third World countries. If you are considering adopting a child of a racial group different from your own, it is important to learn about the child's cultural background and heritage to help your child develop a sense of identity and to cope with racial prejudice.[36]

I took Spanish lessons for four months before she came. I was okay—I could get by. She was very kind—she didn't make fun of my Spanish, and that was all we spoke the first two or three months. [a woman in her forties]

At certain ages, the child may wish to conceal being adopted, or deny being of a different race or national origin than the majority of the community, in order to fit in. Even so, it is important to acknowledge and respect differences at all ages. As an adolescent or young adult, an adopted child often wants to explore her or his unique qualities including her or his ethnic background.

It helps to have friends of the same background as the child, who can be part of a racially diverse support system or extended family. Many support groups have formed in response to the multiple problems and challenges facing adoptive parents, especially those who adopt children from other countries (see Resources for this chapter). Such a group will put you in touch with other adults who are dealing with similar issues and will also provide playmates for your child.

Adopting a child can be both exhilarating and demanding.

Being a mother is wonderful. It's exhausting, challenging, fulfilling. I feel complete. There's no more of this nagging feeling that there's something missing in my life. I feel like I'm home. But she's a real challenge of a person to be with. Our cultures are different. We're very different people. Yet we've definitely made a bond. She wants very much to be close but at the same time she is testing a lot. She hits or bites or teases. She wants her way and has a hard time with no's. In the beginning she was more into pleasing but I think that she was raised in a strict environment and this is a much more permissive, loving environment. It's been hard for her to adjust to the change and it's been hard for me to get stronger in setting limits. But she's happy and I feel very lucky to have found such a lively and caring soul, too. Just a real good person. She's a challenge, she tests every area where I'm weak. It's good for me! We're both growing a lot in the process. [a woman in her forties who adopted a four-year-old child]

Notes

1. G. Mineau and J. Trussell, *Demography,* Vol. 19 (1982), p. 335. See also, J. J. Page, *Population Studies,* Vol. 31 (1977), p. 85.
2. Boston Women's Health Book Collective, *The New Our Bodies, Ourselves.* New York: Simon & Schuster, 1992, p. 500.
3. Jane Menken, James Trussell, Ulla Larsen, "Age and Infertility." *Science,* Vol. 233 (Sept. 26, 1986), pp. 1389–94.
4. Alan H. DeCherney and Gertrud S. Berkowitz,

"Female Fecundity and Age." An editorial in *The New England Journal of Medicine,* Vol. 306, No. 7 (1982), pp. 424–26.

5. Phyllis Kernoff Mansfield, *Pregnancy for Older Women: Assessing the Medical Risks.* New York: Praeger, 1986.

6. Ibid.; see also Donna Kirz, "Advanced Maternal Age: The Mature Gravida." *American Journal of Obstetrics and Gynecology,* Vol. 152 (1985), pp. 7–12. The author criticizes obstetricians' use of pejorative language to describe a middle-aged pregnant woman.

7. David A. Grimes and Gail K. Gross, "Pregnancy Outcomes in Black Women Age 35 and Older." *Obstetrics and Gynecology,* Vol. 58, No. 5 (November 1981), pp. 614–20.

8. Mansfield, op. cit.

9. "Health Objectives for the Nation: Rates of Cesarean Delivery—United States, 1991." *Morbidity and Mortality Weekly Report,* Vol. 42, No. 15 (Apr. 23, 1993), pp. 285–89.

10. Mansfield, op. cit.

11. Gertrud S. Berkowitz, et al., "Delayed Childbearing and the Outcome of Pregnancy." *The New England Journal of Medicine,* Vol. 322 (1990), pp. 659–64.

12. C. Arden Miller, "Infant Mortality in the U.S." *Scientific American,* Vol. 253, No. 1 (July 1985), pp. 31–37.

13. National Center for Health Statistics, *Health, United States, 1991,* Hyattsville, MD: Public Health Services, 1992.

14. K. R. Niswander and M. Gordon, *The Women and Their Pregnancies,* DHEW Publication (NIH) 73-379, Public Health Service, Washington, DC.

15. Grimes and Gross, op. cit.

16. P. Kajanoja and O. Widholm, "Pregnancy and Delivery of Women Aged 40 and Over." *Obstetrics and Gynecology,* Vol. 51 (1978), pp. 47–51; and Mansfield, op. cit.

17. L. S. Penrose, "Paternal Age in Mongolism." *Lancet,* Vol. 1 (1962), p. 1101.

18. Z. Stein and J. Kline, "Smoking, Alcohol and Reproduction." *American Journal of Public Health,* Vol. 73 (1983), pp. 1154–56.

19. See Boston Women's Health Book Collective, op. cit., p. 402, for a suggested daily diet for pregnancy.

20. J. A. Pritchard and P. C. MacDonald, *Williams Obstetrics,* 16th ed. New York: Appleton-Century Crofts, 1976, p. 531.

21. Boston Women's Health Book Collective, op. cit., pp. 401–2.

22. For more information, call your public health nurse at your local health department.

23. Phyllis Kernoff Mansfield and Margaret D. Conn, "Stress and Midlife Childbearing: Key Nursing Interventions." *Maternal-Child Nursing Journal,* Vol. 15, No. 3 (Fall 1986), pp. 139–51.

24. Richard A. Knox, "Law Signed Giving Parents Access to Cesarean Data." *The Boston Globe,* Jan. 1, 1986, p. 38.

25. Robin J. R. Blatt, *Prenatal Tests: What They Are, Their Benefits and Risks, and How to Decide Whether to Have Them or Not.* New York: Vintage/Random House, 1988. See also, Robin J. R. Blatt, *Prenatal Genetic Testing: A Consumer Guide for Women and Couples.* New York: Bergin & Garvey, in press, 1994.

26. Barbara Katz Rothman, *The Tentative Pregnancy: Prenatal Diagnosis and the Future of Motherhood.* New York: Viking, 1986.

27. Bernard G. Ewigman et al. and the RADIUS Study Group, "Effect of Prenatal Ultrasound Screening on Perinatal Outcome." *The New England Journal of Medicine,* Vol. 329, No. 12 (Sept. 15, 1993), pp. 822–27. See also editorial "Should Every Pregnant Woman Undergo Ultrasonography?" in the same issue.

28. Boston Women's Health Book Collective, op. cit., p. 430.

29. Daniel Siegel NICHD Study Group, "Midtrimester Amniocentesis for Prenatal Diagnosis Safety and Accuracy." *Journal of the American Medical Association,* Vol. 236 (1976), pp. 1471–76.

30. Rayna Rapp, "XYLO: A True Story," in Rita Arditti, Renate Duelli Klein, and Shelley Minden, eds., *Test Tube Women.* Boston: Pandora Press, Routledge and Kegan Paul, 1984.

31. Blatt, in press, 1994.

32. Miriam Schoenfeld DiMaio and Maurice J. Mahoney, "Chorionic Villus Sampling (CVS) Update." *The Genetic Resource,* Vol. 6, No. 1 (1991), pp. 15–16.

33. H. V. Firth, et al., "Severe limb abnormalities after chorion villus sampling at 56–66 days' gestation." *Lancet,* Vol. 337 (1991), 762–63. See also M. J. Mahoney, US NICHD Collaborative CVS Study Group, "Limb Abnormalities and Chorionic Villus Sampling." *Lancet,* Vol. 337 (1991), 1422–23.

34. Gina Kolata, "Miniature Scope Gives the Earliest Pictures of a Developing Embryo." *The New York Times,* July 6, 1993, p. C3.

35. Blatt, in press, 1994.

36. Joyce Ladner, *Mixed Families: Adopting Across Racial Boundaries.* Garden City, NY: Anchor Press, 1977. See also studies by Rita Simon and Howard Altstein, cited in "Black Children, White Parents," an editorial. *The New York Times,* Nov. 27, 1993, p. 18.

10

EXPERIENCING OUR CHANGE OF LIFE: MENOPAUSE

✦

BY PAULA B. DORESS-WORTERS AND DIANA LASKIN SIEGAL WITH HELP FROM NORMA MERAS SWENSON, FREDI KRONENBERG, AND LYNN ROSENBERG

IN THE PRIOR EDITION THIS CHAPTER WAS WRITTEN BY DIANA LASKIN SIEGAL, WITH JUDY COSTLOW, MARIA CRISTINA LOPEZ, AND MARA TAUB OF THE SANTA FE HEALTH EDUCATION PROJECT, AND FREDI KRONENBERG

RESOURCES FOR THIS CHAPTER ON PAGES 466–68

*Elizabeth Cady Stanton [the nineteenth-century women's rights leader] . . . described [menopause] as empowering. . . . Her "vital forces" formerly contained in her reproductive organs . . . were now "flowing" to her brain prompting her to leave her family for many months a year to pursue a career as a lecturer.**

Despite the fact that women live longer lives than ever before, providing us with wonderful role models of the potential of the postmenopausal years, women today are being exposed to a campaign of fear about menopause and aging. Menopause is increasingly painted as a time when we must be vigilant lest our bodies and minds begin to deteriorate and our bones to crumble, as if nature had made a mistake in the way our bodies are designed to function.

In the first edition of *Ourselves, Growing Older* we emphasized a self-help approach to menopause and we continue to do so. In recent years an escalating campaign promoting hormone use has changed the climate in which women experience menopause. Doctors sometimes urge women in their forties to begin hormone treatments before they even experience any of the signs of menopause. The many questions and comments we have received from women have persuaded us to address the issue of hormones in greater detail at the conclusion of the chapter. First we will discuss women's experiences of the change of life, and self-help approaches for managing its discomforts.

Women in the 1990s need tools to sort through a bewildering array of competing

*Lois Banner, *In Full Flower: Aging Women, Power and Sexuality,* New York: Vintage, 1993, p. 282.

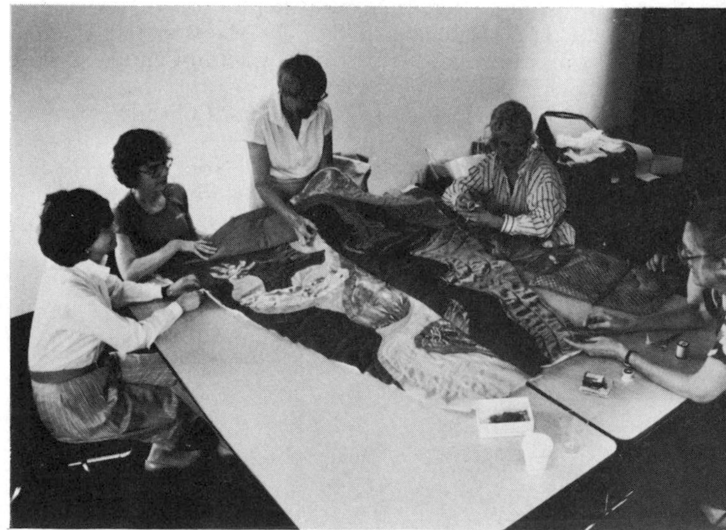

Seventy women worked on the Hot Flash Fan project.
Ron Schildnecht/Water Tower Art Association

claims and conflicting reports. In one study, when provided with clear information, women improved their knowledge scores about menopause and showed themselves capable of applying what they had learned to complex decision making. The overwhelming majority did not believe that the health-care provider should make all of the decisions.[1] Women need continued access to health and medical information in order to make informed choices.

We have compiled the most up-to-date information available upon going to press. Yet knowledge is continually evolving and new "spins" are put on old information. Thus, the tools and resources provided along with this chapter and in the Resources section for assessing and questioning information are as important as the specific research findings discussed.

We urge our readers to keep up with new research findings, but to be skeptical about exaggerated claims for the effects of hormone treatments. Knowing how to find and interpret information can be a key part of taking care of ourselves in the 1990s.

Consumer-health organizations such as the National Women's Health Network (see Resources, p. 482) and the Boston Women's Health Book Collective (p. 442) can provide you with information on new research that comes out between editions of books as well as keep you informed with articles offering critical perspectives. Periodicals such as *Hot Flash* (p. 446) and *A Friend Indeed* (p. 466) provide a forum for women to exchange ideas and experiences about menopause.

We hope this chapter will validate the broad range of experiences of women going through the change of life, and that the information provided here will offer each woman tools to live her menopausal transition with more zest, and to make choices based on her own values, preferences, and health status.

The Change of Life

The common folk expression *change of life* (often condensed to *the change*) describes well this transitional time in our lives. While it sounds less "scientific" than *menopause* or *climacteric,* the phrase *change of life* calls our attention to our capacity to change our lives and ourselves as we pass from our reproductive to our postreproductive years.

Menopause is a time when, if we have not already done so, we should learn to take as good care of ourselves as we do of others.[2] Many women become more self-confident and assertive and less interested in pleasing others.[3] Increasingly, women are writing about the change of life, or menopause, as a time of preparing for later life through emotional and spiritual transformation.[4]

[The menopause] is a rebirth of sorts, an incredible opportunity to rediscover who I am as a human being. The truth is that I have a very long life ahead, and now I can choose how I am going to experience it and what I'm going to do. It's exciting to be making a journey in response to myself rather than in response to the values placed upon me. [a forty-two-year-old woman]

The majority of women take the signs of menopause in stride and do not experience disruption of their daily lives. A community-based study of over 2500 midlife women found that the majority were "relieved" or neutral about menopause.[5] Nonetheless, many were troubled by discomforts they described as somewhat or very bothersome.[6] In the same study, 46.3 percent of women reported hot flashes during perimenopause (see below), and some evidence was found that women with a longer perimenopause were more likely to report hot flashes.[7]

Signs of Menopause

Menopause refers to the cessation of menstrual cycles or periods. We do not know that we have reached menopause until a year without periods has passed. **This chapter primarily describes natural menopause; surgical menopause can be quite different. See Hysterectomy and Oophorectomy chapter for additional information on surgical menopause.** *The climacteric* is a medical term that refers to the years when our periods start to become irregular (the perimenopause), until they finally stop (postmenopause). The average age of menopause is between fifty and fifty-two years of age, but an individual woman's menopause may occur any time from the forties to the late fifties. Cessation of periods before age forty is considered premature menopause. Smokers tend to go through menopause on average two years earlier,[8] thereby increasing their risk of bone loss[9] and other effects of an earlier reduction in estrogen level.

We speak of *signs* rather than symptoms of menopause. A symptom is a change due to dis-

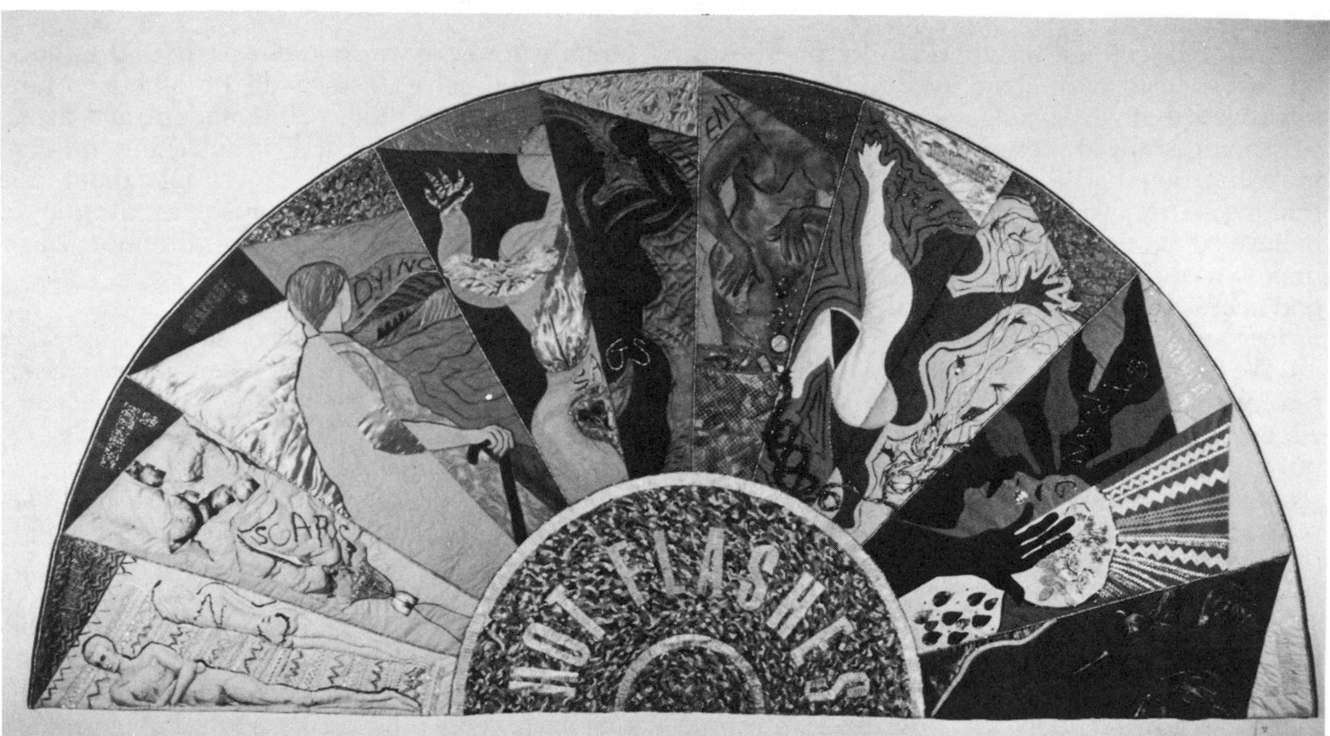

Hot Flash Fan completed. *Suzanne LaValley/Water Tower Art Association*

ease; menopause, on the other hand, is a natural event.

Three signs clearly associated with menopause are: cessation of periods, hot flashes, and vaginal changes. Cessation of periods is the only sign experienced by all women at menopause. Hot flashes are experienced by most Western women,* and vaginal changes by some women during or after menopause. Wrinkles and graying hair, which happen to both women and men as a function of the normal aging process, are not caused by menopause. Body weight and body composition changes may occur that may be related to the hormonal changes of menopause.[10] (See Weighty Issues chapter.)

Women at midlife may be subject to overtreatment when physicians view the normal changes of menopause as a deficiency disease requiring medication, or they may suffer from undertreatment and misdiagnosis of real symptoms of disease. Some physicians attribute to menopause almost anything reported by women at midlife, overlooking what might be symptoms of gallbladder disease, hypertension, and other serious conditions.[11] For example, profuse sweating, fatigue, and vaginal itching may be symptoms of diabetes,[12] and headaches and dizziness may be symptoms of other diseases.

*See *Menopause in Other Cultures,* pp. 127–28.

Changes in Menstrual Patterns

Our bodies may require years of changes, about four years on average,[13] before our well-established pattern of periods stops completely. Some women do not experience changes before their periods stop; but most experience some changes in the length, amount, and frequency of menstrual flow, often starting in their forties and sometimes their thirties.

During the premenopausal years, the hormones that control our menstrual cycles slowly begin to change their pattern.* During the perimenopausal years, the length of periods may change, menstrual cycles may become longer or shorter, or occasionally, a period is skipped, resulting in varying patterns of flow. Some periods may be ovulatory (producing an egg) and others may be anovulatory (no egg produced). If we have a cycle of reduced estrogen and reduced progesterone, the endometrial lining is thin and our flow may be lighter or last fewer days. During the perimenopause, menstrual cycles become more irregular and periods may be skipped for several months. Finally as our hormonal levels drop further, cycling stops and we

*For a detailed description of hormone patterns during the reproductive years, see *The New Our Bodies, Ourselves,* 1992 edition, Anatomy and Physiology chapter.

no longer have periods. This is the time when we are likely to experience hot flashes, though they may begin as we skip periods during the perimenopause.

Many women report occasional periods after their menstrual periods have finally stopped. At a workshop on menopause, two women reported having a period long after the cessation of their menses. Each started flowing when she took a sick parent to a hospital emergency room.

The *heavy period* (heavy bleeding or menorrhagia) is the most annoying and worrisome of perimenopausal patterns. Some women experience periods that are longer and heavier than normal and the flow may clot or gush. Or they may have a combination of patterns or fluctuating patterns. Sometimes the flow is so heavy that a tampon can be washed out of the vagina and even heavy pads cannot contain it. We may feel faint momentarily. We may fear or be embarrassed by so much blood.

At age forty-five I was dining in a foreign city when I felt the gush. I wiped myself as well as I could in the bathroom, made a pad out of paper towels, and managed to get back to my hotel. I reminded myself that menstrual blood is normal and that I did not have to worry or be embarrassed. I remembered that one of the first women to run officially in the Boston Marathon had her period the day of the race and had blood flowing down her leg. Everyone near me cheered her on and no one jeered at the blood. But still I felt better that I was in a city where no one was likely to recognize me. I had a few other episodes before my periods stopped last year. [a fifty-four-year-old woman]

Sometimes the periods become so extended and so close together that we seem to be having one continuous period. Heavy bleeding can result from one pattern of hormone changes in the perimenopause: prolonged estrogen with reduced progesterone, producing a thick or irregular endometrial lining that may not slough off completely or evenly.

Heavy bleeding is a pattern particularly common among black women, and frequently missed or inappropriately treated by health-care providers.[14] Black women undergo an exceptionally high rate of hysterectomies; it is not known how many are unnecessary. Women of color are underrepresented or not represented in the large major menopause studies; information about their patterns and medical needs is seriously limited, thus undercutting the ability of health-care practitioners to provide appropriate care.

Prolonged bleeding or more than a few brief

GLOSSARY OF SEX HORMONES

Estrogens are secreted by our ovaries. The primary form of estrogen secreted by the ovaries is called *estradiol.* Estrogen builds up the lining of the uterus.

Androstenedione is secreted by our adrenal glands and converted in our fat cells into *estrone,* the primary form of estrogen that continues to be produced after menopause.

Progesterone is secreted by the ovaries, adrenals, and placenta. It is responsible for the sloughing off of the lining of the uterus if fertilization has not taken place, for development of the maternal placenta after implantation, and for development of the breast glands. Progesterone is produced only in extremely small amounts after menopause. *Progestins* or *progestogens* are exogenous hormones,* made from natural or synthetic hormonal substances that produce effects similar to those produced by *progesterone.* The three words are often confused and used interchangeably.

Testosterone, sometimes called the libido hormone, is present in both women and men. In menstruating women it is produced in small amounts by both the adrenal glands and the ovaries, with the ovaries probably the most important source. After menopause or surgical removal of the ovaries, testosterone levels are lower.[15]

We refer to treatment with exogenous hormones as hormone therapy (HT) or estrogen therapy (ET), not hormone replacement therapy (HRT) or estrogen replacement therapy (ERT) as they are typically called. It is natural for hormone levels to drop after menopause, though our bodies continue to produce some nonovarian estrogens, primarily estrone.[16] **Therefore, we argue that exogenous hormones are not a replacement, they are added.**

*Note: All hormones described are endogenous (produced naturally by the body), unless they are specified as exogenous (produced outside the body). Numerous formulations and brands of exogenous estrogens and progestins are prescribed in the United States and abroad.[17]

episodes of bleeding after menopause may be a symptom of cancer, and should be checked by your health-care practitioner, who may recommend an endometrial biopsy or dilation and curettage (D and C), two methods of examining the lining or contents of the uterus. Beware of pressure to have surgery for bleeding unless tests show a malignant condition. Do not agree to a hysterectomy unless you have a confirmed diagnosis that warrants it, and a second opinion that verifies the first diagnosis. (See Hysterectomy and Oophorectomy chapter.)

There are many other helpful things to do to control the bleeding, such as eating a healthful diet, taking vitamin A (see discussion of dose on page 59), avoiding alcohol, and avoiding strenuous activity such as swimming or jogging when the period is beginning. Avoid aspirin and other drugs that slow down blood clotting. Ibuprofen (e.g., Advil, Motrin) may help for cramping or pain, and interferes less with blood clotting.[18] (See Hysterectomy and Oophorectomy chapter, especially pages 324–25, for more self-help approaches for menorrhagia.) Self-help techniques require months of learning about and observing our bodies' patterns and changes. This is part of the process of taking care of ourselves.

Though heavy bleeding is inconvenient, embarrassing, and scary, it can simply be one of several normal perimenopausal patterns. The only real health hazard (once a biopsy rules out malignancy) is iron deficiency (anemia). Have your hemoglobin checked and take iron, if recommended, but not unless you are actually anemic.

One medical approach to the problem of heavy bleeding is the use of synthetic progesterone (progestin) to compensate for the body's reduced production of progesterone or prolonged exposure to estrogen. When used at the very beginning of a period, progestins cause the lining of the uterus to slough off more completely than in previous cycles. The next period may then be lighter because the lining has not built up so thickly. Progestins may also be used to interrupt prolonged estrogen production, stimulate a period, and start a new cycle. Some women decide to try small doses of an oral progestin sporadically or for a very short time depending on the pattern of their periods. Beware of continuing the use of progestins for more than a few months, or injections that stay in the body for several months. Progestins do not alleviate all bleeding problems.

A more common and expected pattern is having lighter or fewer periods. The occasional "missed" period can be worrisome to women who are heterosexually active and fear they might be pregnant. In spite of scanty periods, you can still be fertile, so keep using contraceptives until you have gone for two years without a period. (See Birth Control for Women in Midlife chapter.)

Become familiar with your pattern by charting your periods and noting other body changes, and how they differ from pregnancy. For example, if when you miss your period, you are nauseous or have tender breasts, you may want to have a pregnancy test. If you are experiencing hot flashes, or possibly vaginal dryness, you are more likely to be menopausal. A follicle-stimulating hormone (FSH) test can be done to determine menopausal status, but it is rarely necessary or useful. An FSH level higher than 40 is menopausal, less than 20 is premenopausal. Thus, the test has a broad indeterminate range, and cannot tell you whether you will have another period or whether you can become pregnant. Better to let your body tell you.

Premenstrual Syndrome (PMS) and Menopause

Premenstrual discomforts such as swollen, tender breasts, water retention, and some tension or anxiety are not uncommon during the reproductive years. When severe enough these are considered premenstrual syndrome (PMS). Whether you have had such discomforts for years, or begin to have them in the premenopausal years, you can look forward to relief as your periods stop and your hormone cycles level out. This may take several years. Even women with only minor water retention and breast tenderness may still be aware of some cycling in their bodies after their periods cease.[19]

Medical researchers have no more idea why a minority of women suffer greater discomforts due to menopause than they know why some women are more distressed than others by menstrual cramps or PMS. Often they cover up their ignorance by "blaming the victim" for not taking care of herself, or for failing to accept her femininity or her aging. But even when we do all the "right things" and have all the "right attitudes" we may still need help with menopausal discomforts that become troublesome.

I searched for the truth about [PMS, mood swings, and] menopause but what I found didn't help me. I had to val-

idate my own experience. No one could explain why I had a hard time whenever my hormones shifted. I thought I was going mad at thirteen, I was depressed when I was pregnant, and I had unexplained depression and mood changes for the nine years between the ages of forty-five and fifty-four when my periods were changing. I was raising a daughter alone but I lived with people who were supportive and I tried everything: estrogen for two years, jogging, massage therapy, a woman's support group, homeopathic remedies. They helped a little but not enough. I even tried an antidepressant which did not help and caused me to gain twenty-five pounds. Once my periods stopped, I not only had an absence of depression but had a lightness and buoyancy, a state of being positively happy. I am fine now but I feel I lost a decade of my life. [a fifty-six-year-old woman]

Hot Flashes

It was a freezing December night when I lay in bed, dreading to get up and go down a long cold hall to an even colder bathroom. Then I had a hot flash and, all of a sudden, it was very easy to leave my warm bed! For the rest of the winter I used my nighttime hot flashes this way. My friends laughed when I told them that hot flashes are not all bad! [a fifty-nine-year-old woman]

In folk wisdom and humor, hot flashes are the sign most commonly associated with menopause. Surveys report that anywhere from 47 to 85 percent of women will experience hot flashes.[20] Many women never experience hot flashes at all.

For most women, a hot flash or flush can be nothing more than transient sensations of warmth. For others it is "perpetual summer." Some women report their hot flashes are pleasant and, as in the above example, useful. Some women experience waves of heat and drenching sweats, often followed by chills; some experience chills first. The flashes are often preceded by a brief aura, a sense of the coming flash. Feelings such as tension, anxiety, heart palpitations, and nausea may also accompany hot flashes or may precede and be relieved by the hot flash.

Hot flashes can begin when menstrual cycles are still regular or when they are becoming irregular. They typically continue for less than a year after the final menstrual period; however, for some women they persist for five, ten, or even more years.[21] In some instances, hot flashes first begin many years after menopause. Although they usually last a few minutes, the duration of some hot flashes may be shorter or longer. Their frequency also varies. Hot flashes may occur once a month, or once an hour, or several times an hour. They can occur any time day or night, though one study reports they are more frequent between 6 and 8 A.M. and again between 6 and 10 P.M.[22] Each woman has her own pattern.

At age fifty I skipped a period and had hot flashes at night for the first time during the month I was on jury duty for seven trials including two murder trials! I got my period the day after I finished jury duty and didn't have another hot flash for six more months. [a fifty-five-year-old woman]

We have few clues as to who is most likely to get hot flashes, how intense they might be, or how long the hot flashes might last. As ovarian estrogen declines, estrone (a postmenopausal form of estrogen) is produced in the fat cells. Women who are thin have lower levels of estrone than women who are heavier, and thus tend to have more hot flashes.[23] Generally, the body gradually adjusts to the lower level of estrogen and, for most women, the hot flashes stop or become infrequent.[24]

Many women report that their hot flashes are most disturbing at night when they are awakened. They may have to change their night clothes and sheets due to drenching sweats. The loss of sleep over many nights can cause fatigue, irritability, and a feeling of being unable to cope—much like depression. (See *Dealing with Insomnia*, pages 33–34.)

Women whose ovaries are removed before menopause, resulting in a sudden drop in estrogen levels, may experience intense hot flashes often beginning immediately after surgery, and vaginal dryness at an earlier age. Hot flashes occur more frequently and severely in these women (especially for about six months after surgery) than they do in women who go through natural menopause.[25] Most physicians prescribe estrogen treatment up to the age of a natural menopause. Even when the ovaries are removed after menopause, a woman may experience some hot flashes because small amounts of estrogen are still produced by the ovaries postmenopausally.

During a hot flash, the blood vessels most commonly expand (dilate) and blood flow to the skin increases. Though the skin temperature often rises 4 to 8 degrees during a hot flash and the sensation is one of heat or blushing, the internal body temperature actually falls.[26] This occurs because the body eliminates excess heat through increasing blood flow to the skin and through sweating. The rush of blood to the skin surface can cause reddening of the skin, lightheadedness, and a tingling sensation. There may also be a feeling of pressure in the chest, or anxiety. At the end of the hot flash, when the blood vessels narrow (constrict), some women experience chills, since body temperature has fallen below normal, and the temperature-control system is now trying to raise it back to normal.

Since my studio apartment had a patio door, I could easily step outside to cool off when I felt a hot flash coming. I felt shut in and constricted when that source of relief wasn't present in other settings. [a fifty-three-year-old woman]

At my first unexpected hot flashes I was afraid. I had in mind that hot flashes involved a loss of control, but when I paid close attention, I felt half in a dream state, flushed and physically lightheaded. Actually, it seemed like an altered state of consciousness, which wasn't that unfamiliar to me because I meditate. But I can see that for many women, it would be a new experience, one they'd fear and try to suppress. [a forty-two-year-old woman]

Only in the past fifteen years have researchers begun to study the causes of hot flashes. Their occurrence is related to a decline in estrogen levels. However, something else is also involved in triggering each hot-flash episode. Some researchers speculate that the hypothalamus (the part of the brain that regulates body temperature) is involved in a hot flash, perhaps through the release of some substance that triggers the hot flash. They are looking at the ways hormones interact with the temperature-regulating system.[27]

We hope that a better understanding of the mechanism of hot flashes will lead to self-help techniques rather than just to new drugs.

Self-Help for Hot Flashes

- *Keep track.* Chart your hot flashes in relationship to your menstrual periods and other events to see if you can find a pattern. The more you know about yourself, the better you'll be able to manage your hot flashes and the better you will feel.

From ages fifty-one to fifty-three I skipped many periods. Whenever I skipped periods I had hot flashes; the months I had periods I had no hot flashes. I began to see a pattern and could predict what to expect. [a fifty-five-year-old woman]

- *Keep healthy.* Some women have found that caffeine (coffee, tea, cola drinks, chocolate), alcohol, sugar, spicy foods, hot soups and hot drinks, and very large meals may trigger hot flashes. (See Eating Well chapter.)

Some women find that vitamin E minimizes or eliminates hot flashes and vaginal dryness. Vitamin E is found in vegetable oils (wheat germ, corn, and soybean), brown rice and millet, legumes, corn, and almonds. Egg yolks contain vitamin E but also contain very high levels of cholesterol. If you take a supplement, start with 50 IUs per day and find your effective level by increasing gradually up to 400 IUs per day. Avoid it if you are taking digitalis or are diabetic. Some find taking B complex to be helpful. Vitamin B_6 in particular (about 15 to 30 mg) is commonly used by Canadian women.

Many women report more hot flashes at times of stress. Try the methods described in *Disarming Stress,* pages 12–16, to relax.

- *Keep moving.* Activity relieves hot flashes, stress, and depression, and helps you sleep better. Exercise tones the body and improves digestive and cardiovascular health. (See Moving for Health chapter.)
- *Keep cool.* Dress in layers. Clothes made of natural fibers may be more comfortable than those made of synthetic material. When you feel a hot flash starting, take off some clothes. Go to a cooler spot, stand by an open window. Relax, take a few deep breaths. There is no reason to feel embarrassed. Fan yourself with whatever is at hand or collect fans to match your wardrobe as our great-grandmothers did.

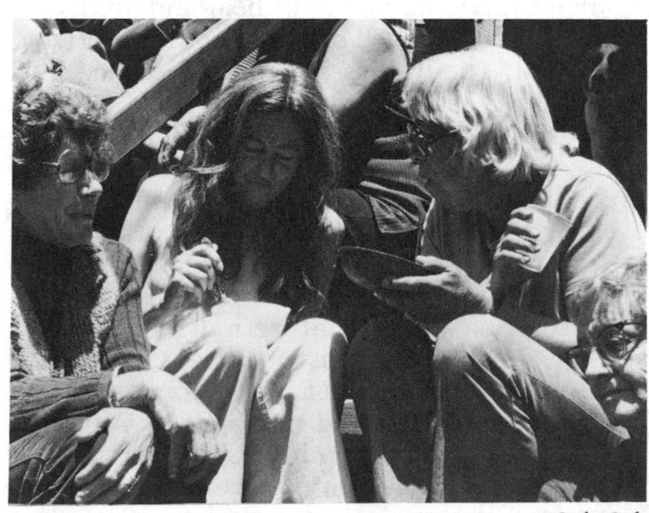

Cathy Cade

Drink something cool, place something cool where it feels best—on the wrists, temples, forehead. Shower. Visualize yourself in a cool place such as sitting by a lake with a cool breeze blowing. Lower the thermostat, or get a cooler, electric fan, or air conditioner. Before going to bed add a cup of table salt to a tub of warm water; lie in it until the water cools; rinse with cold water and go right to bed.[28] Sleeping in cooler rooms can significantly reduce the frequency and intensity of hot flashes, and reduce or eliminate the waking episodes due to hot flashes.[29]

- *Keep talking.* Break the taboos against menopause. Stay comfortable by letting people know when you are having a hot flash and reaffirm that it is nothing to be ashamed of. Use positive, not demeaning, humor. Tell household members or coworkers what is happening.

I never felt that I should suffer hot flashes in silence, so my husband and kids called me "Flash." When I told my husband it was the first anniversary of my last period he said, "Congratulations, Flash. You've done it." So we went out to dinner and celebrated that night. [a fifty-one-year-old woman]

Using Herbs*

by Judith Costlow
of the Santa Fe Health Education Project

Generations of women going through menopause have used herbal remedies. The interest in and about herbs is very strong and growing among women today. You can find herbs in health-food stores in every city across the country. They can be very helpful. Start by using them in the smallest amounts. Herbs are much slower acting than drugs, so a woman must be patient when starting to use them. Allow six weeks to try a particular herb or herbal combination before trying another, but stop taking any herb that gives you a bad reaction. You may want to test out several different herbs to find the one that is beneficial for you. Many health-food stores have their own special blend of herbs for menopausal signs. Some women prefer to try one herb at a time before trying a mixture of herbs. Some herbs, like ginseng and dong quai, have estrogenic activity and are often recommended for the discomforts of menopause. Estrogen from plant sources is slower acting and may not have some of the adverse effects of chemical formulations. Ginseng and dong quai are not advised for women with high blood pressure. Some herbs can be toxic if used in large amounts. It is best to follow the recommended dosages. If you have any chronic condition, be sure to tell the herbalist you consult and/or to pay attention to the contra-indications in the source book you use. An excellent source book on herbal remedies for midlife women is *Menopausal Years: The Wise Woman Way* by Susun Weed (see Resources).

If you have diabetes, tell the medical care provider who supervises your diabetes regimen about the herbs you are thinking of using. More research is needed about herbal remedies and medical conditions. You may want to consult an herbalist about which herbs to avoid, and how to prepare the herbs without using sweeteners or alcohol.

Get to know your herb store. The source of herbs can be important, since 80 percent of dried herbs sold in the U.S. come from other countries where pesticides that are banned here may be used. Read labels carefully and ask your supplier for information. You may be able to call companies that package herbs for sale in stores. Ask about their standards for quality and purity of their herbs, such as where and under what circumstances they are grown, and their process for verifying that such standards are followed.

Many herbs are sold both in dried form for making teas and in powdered form (capsules). Most herbs last longer in nonpowdered form, but there are a few exceptions like golden seal, ginger, and slippery elm. Dry herbs should be a color similar to their fresh color and their scent should be strong. Avoid brown, dull colors, and musty chemical odors when buying herbs.

*Information from *Menopause: A Self Care Manual,* by the Santa Fe Health Education Project. Order from P.O. Box 577, Santa Fe, NM 87504-0577.

Talking with others, sharing our experiences and feelings, acquiring knowledge about how our bodies are changing, and giving each other support eases our "change of life." A group of women coming together in a menopause support group or workshop to learn from one another, in a respectful, informative, and supportive setting, can effectively counteract fears and uncertainties with support and information. Much of the material in this section comes from women who have shared their experiences and their wisdom. By talking with other women we will continue to discover and exchange new self-help methods.

Vaginal Changes

As we age, the skin and mucous membranes in various parts of our bodies tend to become drier. The vaginal membranes become thinner, hold less moisture, lubricate more slowly, and become drier. To help alleviate this condition add moisture to the air in your house and drink eight cups of fluid each day.[30] Some women also suffer dry eyes and some a loss of saliva, which may be Sjögren's syndrome, a condition similar in many respects to arthritis. (See page 275.) For a very few women vaginal dryness is an early sign of menopause, others do not experience it until many years later, and many never do. In a community-based study of women ages fifty to sixty, only 20 percent of 1,109 women who were postmenopausal reported vaginal dryness, and only 15 percent of those to a degree that they regarded it as a "bothersome" symptom.[31]

Vaginal dryness can interfere with sexual spontaneity and pleasure, and be a challenge to deal with. Some women find taking vitamin E helpful. Do not use products that may cause or contribute to dryness, such as some prescription and over-the-counter drugs. Antihistamines, for example, dry other tissues as well as nasal tissues. Do not use douches, sprays, and colored or perfumed toilet paper and soaps that can irritate the tissues of the vulva. If itchiness develops, avoid scratching, which can irritate the delicate tissues and lead to infections and further problems. Aci-gel and other prescription ointments can help itchiness. Over-the-counter moisturizers such as Replens, if used regularly, can help dryness, and water-based lubricants, used at the time of lovemaking, can help as well. Try a variety of lubricants or moisturizers before considering use of a low-dose estrogen cream. (See Sexuality in the Second Half of Life chapter, pages 89–91, for more detailed suggestions.)

Women should continue after menopause to have pelvic exams and Pap smears—remind your older relatives and friends (see page 352). Exams can be uncomfortable when suffering from soreness or dryness, so tell your practitioner before the exam.

Changes in Mental Stability, Mood, and Memory

The myth that women go mad at menopause persists despite the lack of evidence for such a belief. The diagnosis of "climacteric insanity," based on Victorian ideas about women's lives, was not dropped from psychiatric diagnostic manuals until the 1960s.[32]

Some women report temporary mood swings, irritability, or a "cotton head" feeling[33] during the perimenopausal stage when hormone levels are fluctuating and readjusting. When this occurs, women need to know it will likely pass when cycling ends.

Sometime in my late twenties, I saw an article in a medical journal that showed a distraught-looking, middle-aged woman standing just behind a man who had a hand to his brow as though he had a bad headache. The caption promised that the medication being advertised was "for the menopausal symptoms that bother him *the most." The ad made me angry, but it scared me, too. Already, I had big mood swings as part of PMS. Would I become a monster in menopause? Twenty years later, I'm delighted to report that my periods have been gone for a year and my moods are steadier than they ever were.* [a forty-eight-year-old woman]

While the middle years have the potential for growth and enhancement, statistically many significant losses, such as an illness of our own or a loved one, job loss, widowhood, or death of others close to us, may cluster in the years between forty-five and fifty-nine. We are concerned that menopause is becoming a catchall for all the stresses and losses that women face at midlife. In one large study of midlife women, the cause of depression was more often multiple sources of worry due to caregiving roles and relationships than it was to menopause.[34] Depression may also result from fatigue due to interrupted sleep caused by night sweats and nocturnal hot flashes. (See above.) In mutual-help groups, women can find support not only for the discomforts of menopause, but for the multiplicity of losses, worries, and discrimination they may be experiencing as midlife women.

Despite the evidence of a growing number of older women in a variety of professions and creative activities, proponents of hormone treatments emphasize improvements in memory, cognition, and sexual functioning in an effort to convince women that in order to remain active sexually and competent in the workplace, they will require medical treatment. A recent study of eight hundred women from sixty-five to ninety-five years of age, half of whom had used estrogen treatment, and one third of whom were current users, found no effect of estrogen on cognitive function.[35]

THE MEDICALIZATION OF MENOPAUSE

Those of us now approaching menopause have had more choices and more information about our reproductive lives than our mothers and grandmothers ever had. Similarly, we expect to have access to current knowledge and to exert some control over our menopausal experience. Medical institutions and drug companies, however, flood us with information about the use of hormones to deal with menopause and related body changes, while neglecting basic research about the process of menopause itself. Paradoxically, this barrage of books, articles, sound bites, and advertisements from scientific, technological, and medical sources, and their popularizers, may actually reduce our control over our lives by medicalizing our change of life, thus cutting us off from traditional sources of information.[36]

When we rely entirely on medical experts and reject the experiences of older women in our lives, we are left feeling that we have no role models for dealing with life-stage transitions like menopause. We become more vulnerable to manipulative messages from the medical establishment and the media, whose chief objective may not be our health and well-being.

Contemporary women can re-create this traditional source of lore by meeting together in support groups where they learn that their experiences are common to their stage of life, and need not be frightening. Women learn to speak openly of their experiences, to sort out and assess a confusing array of information, and to share self-help approaches for managing minor discomforts associated with the signs of menopause.

The aging revolution means that as women we live nearly half our adult lives past menopause. It is a myth based on outdated views of women's roles that once our ovaries stop producing eggs, we are past our prime. Consider the irony of Sandra Day O'Connor referring to herself as "over the hill" to describe her postmenopausal status, when appointed as the first woman justice of the U.S. Supreme Court.

It is increasingly common for women to successfully take on new challenges in the years following menopause. Elizabeth Freeman started a business at the age of sixty-four:

I became aware of the energy and creativity of older women and I wanted to print the work of older, feminist women. The word crone, *generally derogatory in our society, originally meant "wise old woman." I conceived of a name for my publishing house by adding OWN (Older Women's Network), and Crones' OWN Press came into being. To me this period of my life has been most exciting and creative.*

Menopause in Other Cultures

Evidence is growing that cultural and social class differences influence the experience of menopause. A study comparing Mayan with rural Greek women revealed some interesting differences. Mayan women look forward to menopause, eat a diet high in carbohydrates and calcium, but no meat or dairy products, and do not report hot flashes. Greek women report more anxiety about menopause and growing older, and eat a diet more like ours. They report hot flashes but do not seek medical intervention.[37] Incidentally, Greek women smoke more than any in Europe.

In another study, Japanese women differed from North American women, reporting hot flashes at a much lower rate (indeed, no higher than people of other age groups, 10 percent of whom report hot flashes). The Japanese women tended to use herbal preparations rather than medications, and were less likely to use hormones at menopause.[38]

Looking at cultural differences shows us how ageism and medicalization can exacerbate the minor discomforts of this biological transition by making menopause a symbol of passing into the devalued status of an old woman. In cultures where women's roles and choices expand at midlife, anxiety about the menopausal transition is reduced.[39]

Through cross-cultural studies we can discover differences in diet and activity patterns that may influence how women feel at menopause. For example, a diet that includes rice (a source of vitamin E), soybeans, and herbs and vegetables (possibly high in naturally estrogenic properties) may explain why hot flashes are infrequently reported by Japanese women.

Medical Approaches to Menopause: Exogenous Hormones

The short-term benefits of estrogen for relief of menopausal discomforts, such as hot flashes and vaginal dryness, have been known since 1937.[40] In the 1960s and '70s, the idea of menopause as a "deficiency disease" was popularized,[41] and the use of estrogen was touted as having a wide range of youth-preserving, mood-elevating, and sexuality-enhancing effects, most of which were not true or remain unproven.

After reports in 1975 that women who used estrogen therapy were five to fifteen times more likely to develop endometrial cancer,[42] women became more skeptical of exogenous hormones, and hormone prescriptions declined. To protect against endometrial cancer, a form of hormone therapy combining estrogen with progestin (HT) was developed. In addition, the drug companies in the 1980s and '90s shifted their resources to discovery and promotion of other benefits of exogenous hormones, such as prevention of diseases associated with aging that can often be prevented in simpler and less risky ways.

Making Sense of the New Research on Hormones

Prior to the current emphasis on prevention of disease, a woman's decision to use hormones or not was based on a choice between short-term relief of menopausal discomforts and the possibility of certain risks. Women today are being urged to take hormones earlier, in some cases before experiencing any discomforts, or even signs of menopause, and to take them for longer durations and even indefinitely. Yet it is not clear whether women are buying this approach. The most popular reason for choosing hormone therapy is still short-term symptom relief.[43]

The growing body of research suggesting that estrogen treatment is protective against osteoporosis and heart disease contributes to the trend toward increased and longer-term prescribing of hormones.[44] Doctors may use these research findings to promote the idea that a woman is taking a risk by attempting to experience menopause and aging without benefit of exogenous hormones.

Many of the benefits found for estrogen may not apply to combined-hormone treatment, and the risks also appear to be different. There are insufficient long-term-study results for combined-hormone treatment to accurately assess its risks and benefits. It may be twenty-five years before researchers can provide us with this information.

The latest research reports, however, support the view that extended use of hormones increases the risks as well as the benefits. A meta-analysis* reviewing 265 studies published in English from 1970 to 1992 concluded that estrogen users are less likely to experience cardiovascular disease (CVD) and hip fracture; however, long-term estrogen use increases the risk of endometrial cancer, and there may be a "small" increased risk of breast cancer.[45] The "small" increase is reported in a companion article as 25 percent.[46]

Estrogen users do appear to have decreased rates of CVD, but hormone users may be healthier to begin with. The women in these studies who took estrogen postmenopausally were thinner, and more physically active, and had higher HDL (so-called "good cholesterol") levels, all of which lower their risk of CVD.[47] In addition, many of the studies excluded women with medical conditions from the hormone trials; thus the hormone users were at lower risk of CVD to begin with. These other aspects of hormone users' lives or health raise questions about the findings. Much of the research on hormones is done retrospectively in large ongoing studies; to resolve these questions requires randomized clinical trials. By assigning participants at random to hormones, placebos, or other treatment conditions their preexisting health would be equalized and thus the effects of the hormones or other treatments would be clearer.

If estrogen is shown to reduce heart disease, another important question is the mechanism by which this reduction occurs, and

*Some research reports employ a statistical technique called meta-analysis to provide a helpful overview of a body of research by "averaging over" the findings of multiple studies. Unfortunately the untrained consumer is not in a position to determine whether the meta-analysis was done well and with adequate attention to the quality or biases of the studies being reviewed.

PROS AND CONS OF HORMONES*

When Hormone Therapy[†] Is Appropriate

- Ovaries removed before age forty-five.
- High risk of fractures, especially if due to medical risk factors, such as ovariectomy or steroid use. If risk is due to life-style factors, consider changing them (as discussed in the Osteoporosis and Fracture Prevention and Aging Well chapters).
- Extreme menopausal discomforts, such as hot flashes and night sweats that are not manageable with other approaches. Vaginal dryness responds to estrogen cream and usually does not require pills.

When Hormone Therapy Is Inappropriate

Absolutely avoid the use of hormones, even if the above conditions apply, if you have any of the following:

- Past or present thromboembolic events (stroke, thrombophlebitis, pulmonary embolus, or heart attack)
- Breast cancer, endometrial cancer, or any other estrogen-stimulated cancer
- Severe liver disease or chronic impairment of liver function
- Unexplained vaginal bleeding
- Pregnancy or chance of pregnancy (hormone therapy could hurt the fetus)

Consider avoiding hormones if you have gallbladder disease; uterine fibroids; hypertension; migraine headaches; seizure disorders; heart disease; or kidney disease associated with fluid retention. Discuss risks and benefits with your health-care provider.

Risks and Other Drawbacks of Hormone Use

- Increases the risk of breast cancer after long-term use. Combined hormone therapy appears to be riskier than estrogen therapy alone.
- May double the risk of gallbladder surgery.
- Menopausal discomforts and bone loss may occur or recur when treatment is stopped.
- Nausea, weight gain, breast tenderness, uterine bleeding, fluid retention, and depression have been reported by some women.
- Return of monthly bleeding may occur with combined hormones. Estrogen alone increases the risk of endometrial cancer.
- Increased medical visits are required to monitor effects of treatment.

*Information adapted from *Taking Hormones and Women's Health: Choices, Risks and Benefits,* 1993. National Women's Health Network, 1325 G Street, NW, Washington, DC 20005.

†Women who use hormones should be aware that combination hormones protect women who have a uterus against endometrial cancer. Women who have had a hysterectomy and want to take hormones should take estrogen alone, because the progestins often diminish the beneficial effects of estrogen, may have other unpleasant effects, and may bring new risks.

whether this can be accomplished by other, less risky means. Evidence is growing that one way estrogen may reduce heart disease is by changing the lipid profile, i.e., by slightly decreasing LDL ("bad cholesterol") and increasing HDL ("good cholesterol").[48] It has also been suggested that estrogen treatment affects the contractibility of blood vessels. (See Hypertension, Heart Disease, and Stroke chapter for more information.)

We know alternative safe ways to reduce the risks of osteoporosis and fractures, such as by increasing calcium, exercising moderately, quitting smoking, reducing alcohol, and making our homes more accident-free. (See chapters 5, 6, and 19. A more detailed discussion of the pros and cons of hormone use to retard bone loss can be found in the Osteoporosis and Fracture Prevention chapter, especially pages 286–89.)

An important bioethical question is why use hormones at all to prevent heart disease or fractures in healthy women? Though much has been made of women's increased risk of heart disease after menopause compared with before menopause, women's rates of heart disease are lower than those of men at every age, and have been declining since the early 1960s. An epidemiologist who specializes in cardiovascular research testified as follows before a congressional committee:

> *There are alternative ways to reduce the risk of heart disease and fractures—for example, by participating in moderate physical activity and quitting smoking. However, we do not know how to reduce the risk of breast cancer. Despite these facts and despite the gaps in our knowledge about long-term effects of ERT and HRT, millions of American women are being urged to use these drugs. In my view they are being prescribed without adequate assessment of the risks, benefits and alternatives.*[49]

Hormones, like any medication, have risks as well as benefits. Some women may want to take hormones for a short time to relieve discomforts that disrupt our daily lives and sap our energies. In making this choice, we have to weigh the benefits of relief against the possibility that the discomforts will recur when we stop, that is, that we are merely postponing the transition, and that we are incurring risks that are as yet unclear. If we want to consider hormones for prevention of diseases, such as osteoporosis, we have to weigh a complex array of long-term risks and long-term benefits, as well as consider options for achieving the benefits by alternative means. A related policy issue is that it seems to be harder to get funds to study alternative means of managing menopausal discomforts than to study medical treatments, such as hormone.

The most serious risk of hormones, especially of long-term use, is the increased risk of cancer, especially of breast cancer. Results from two studies[50] have raised concerns that even relatively short durations of use may increase the risk of breast cancer. Some, but not all, studies suggest that use of estrogen alone for fifteen or more years may increase the risk of breast cancer by 30 percent.[51] The effect of combined hormone therapy has not been as well studied because this regimen has not been used for as long a period of time. However, the sketchy information available now indicates that combined therapy is at least as risky as estrogen alone, and possibly more risky.

The combined data from a review of twenty-four studies did *not* support the hypothesis that adding progesterone to estrogen treatment would reduce the risk of breast cancer, as it does for endometrial cancer. Women who take hormone therapy (HT) for more than ten or fifteen years increase their risks, including risks of breast cancer and other cancers, associated with their use.[52]

In summary, using hormones for prevention of diseases of the older years implies long-term use. However, a growing body of evidence demonstrates that the risk increases with longer-term use. If you choose to take hormones for an extended time, continue to reevaluate the risks and benefits by keeping up with new research and discussing it with your health-care provider. **If you have used hormones and decide to stop, taper your dose gradually.**

The indispensable 1993 report on the risks and benefits of hormone use by the National Women's Health Network makes a persuasive point regarding the weighing of risks and benefits:

> *Many women have an intuitive understanding of a little known statistic. The average woman who dies of heart disease loses eight years of life. Women who die of breast cancer lose, on average, nineteen years. Many women are uncomfortable taking a chance of increasing their risk of a disease which is always devastating and if fatal, often kills at a relatively young age.*[53]

Standards for using unproven treatments on healthy populations should be more stringent than those for treating persons who are ill and choose to risk something new as a possible cure. We question the ethics of attempting to flood a healthy population with an unneeded medication that may result in new risks. In any other situation we would call this an experiment.

Whether you take hormones or not, whether you take them for short-term relief of discomforts, or longer-term prevention of disease, is your decision. You will want to consider your own history, values, health status, and preferences as well as your understanding of the research studies.

Consider your choices carefully, but remember that the choice of hormone therapy or not is only one aspect of your change of life. Menopause is a normal part of a woman's life experience. We can learn from one another ways to manage the typical discomforts that occur. Our focus must be on our own growth and development as we contemplate the changes we want to make for ourselves during these and the following years. We must not be manipulated into regarding this important turning point in our lives as merely a choice point about medications.

At midlife we have the opportunity to expand

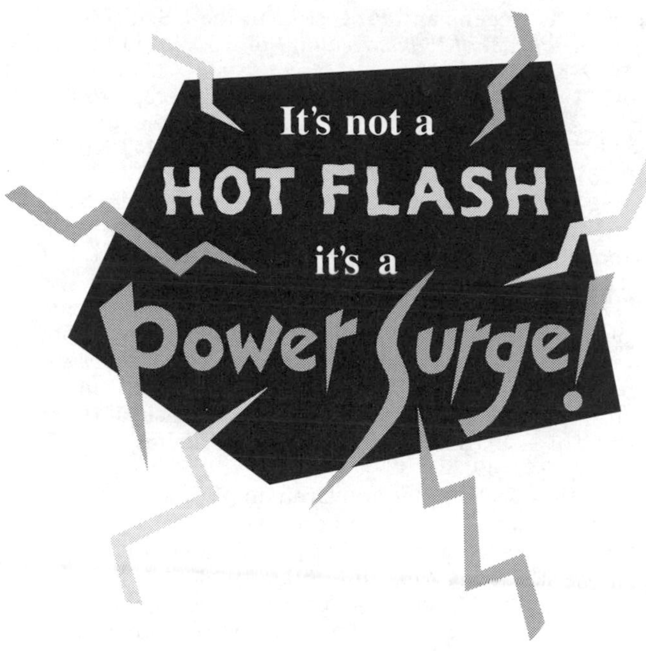

Logo reprinted with permission from Radiance: The Magazine for Large Women.*

our choices, to reach out for new, possibly long-delayed experiences, to create lives that reflect our values and desires. We need to be wary of the current trend to define us as an expanding market for drugs, cosmetics, and plastic surgery. Our considerable and growing numbers give us the potential of becoming a constituency with considerable clout. We can live our lives more fully and expressively. As Bernice Regan (lead singer of Sweet Honey in the Rock) says, "Menopause is a time to fly."

Notes

1. Marilyn Rothert, "Menopausal Women as Decision Makers in Health Care." Presentation at NIH Conference on Menopause, March 22–24, 1993. See also, Marilyn Rothert, et al., "Women's Use of Information Regarding Hormone Replacement Therapy." *Research in Nursing and Health,* Vol. 13 (1990), pp. 355–66.
2. Carol Gilligan, *In a Different Voice: Psychological Theory and Women's Development.* Cambridge, MA: Harvard University Press, 1982. Her thesis is that women develop morally through caring for others and later learn to care similarly for themselves.
3. Rosetta Reitz, *Menopause: A Positive Approach.* New York: Penguin, 1979.
4. See Resources for this chapter.
5. Nancy E. Avis and Sonja M. McKinlay, "A Longitudinal Analysis of Women's Attitudes Toward the Menopause: Results from the Massachusetts Women's Health Study." *Maturitas,* Vol. 13 (1991), pp. 65–79.
6. New England Research Institute, *Women and Their Health in Massachusetts,* Final Report, 1991. NERI, 9 Galen St., Watertown, MA 02172.
7. Sonja M. McKinlay, Donald J. Brambilla, and Jennifer G. Posner, "The Normal Menopause Transition." *American Journal of Human Biology,* Vol. 4 (1992), pp. 37–46.
8. Ibid.
9. John A. Baron, "Smoking and Estrogen-Related Disease." *American Journal of Epidemiology,* Vol. 119, No. 1 (1984), pp. 9–22.
10. Ann M. Voda, Nancy S. Christy, and Julene M. Morgan, "Body Composition Changes in Menopausal Women." *Women and Therapy,* Vol. 1, No. 2 (1991), pp. 71–96.
11. Catherine DeLorey, "Health Care and Midlife Women." In Grace Baruch and Jeanne Brooks-Gunn, eds., *Women in Midlife.* New York: Plenum Press, 1984, pp. 277–301.
12. Jane Porcino, *Growing Older, Getting Better.* New York: Crossroad Continuum, 1991.
13. McKinlay, Brambilla, and Posner, op. cit.
14. Toni P. Miles, "Menopause and African-American Women: Clinical and Research Issues." Presented at National Institutes of Health Workshop on Menopause, Current Knowledge and Recommendations for Research, March 22–24, 1993, Bethesda, MD.
15. Boston Women's Health Book Collective, *The New Our Bodies, Ourselves.* New York: Simon & Schuster, 1992, pp. 228–29.
16. U.S. Congress, Office of Technology Assessment, *The Menopause, Hormone Therapy, and Women's Health,* OTA-BP-BA-88, U.S. Government Printing Office, May 1992, p. 65. This invaluable document is available for $6 from the U.S. Government Printing Office, SSOP, Washington, DC 20402-9328. ISBN 0-16-037912-1, p. 18.
17. Ibid., p. 65.
18. "Heavy Bleeding," *A Friend Indeed,* Vol. 7, No. 2 (May 1990), pp. 1–3.
19. For more about PMS, see *The New Our Bodies, Ourselves.* New York: Simon & Schuster, 1992, p. 252. See also, Susan Lark, *Premenstrual Self-Help: A Woman's Guide to Feeling Good All Month.* Berkeley, CA: Celestial Arts Publishing, 1989.
20. Fredi Kronenberg, "Hot Flashes: Epidemiology and Physiology." *Annals of the New York Academy of Sciences,* Vol. 592 (1990), pp. 52–86.
21. Fredi Kronenberg, op. cit.
22. Ann M. Voda, *Menopause—Me and You.* Salt Lake City: University of Utah College of Nursing, 1984, pp. 7–8.
23. Yohanan Erlik, David R. Meldrum, and Howard L. Judd, "Estrogen Levels in Postmenopausal Women with Hot Flashes." *Obstetrics and Gynecology,* Vol. 59 (1982), pp. 403–7.
24. R. Don Gambrell, Jr., and Ann L. Hyatt, "Benefits and Risks of Estrogen Replacement Therapy in the Menopause." *Delaware Medical Journal,* Vol. 56, No. 4 (April 1984), p. 20.
25. S. Chakravarti, et al., "Endocrine Changes and Symptomatology After Oophorectomy in Premenopausal Women." *British Journal of Obstetrics & Gynaecology,* Vol. 84 (1977), pp. 769–75.
26. I. V. Tataryn, et al., "Post-menopausal Hot

*See Resources for Weighty Issues chapter.

Flushes: A Disorder of Thermoregulation." *Maturitas,* Vol. 2 (1980), pp. 101–7.

27. Fredi Kronenberg, et al., "Menopausal Hot Flashes: Thermoregulatory, Cardiovascular, and Circulating Catecholamine and LH Changes." *Maturitas,* Vol. 6 (1984), pp. 31–43.

28. Gregorita Rodriquez, curandera (folk-healer), Santa Fe, NM.

29. Fredi Kronenberg and R. M. Barnard, "Modulation of Menopausal Hot Flashes by Ambient Temperature." *Journal of Thermal Biology,* Vol. 17, No. 1 (1992), pp. 43–49.

30. Rosetta Reitz, op. cit.

31. New England Research Institute, op. cit., p. 9.

32. Lois Banner, *In Full Flower: Aging Women, Power and Sexuality.* New York: Vintage, 1993, p. 301.

33. Marian Van Eyk McCain, *Transformation Through Menopause.* New York: Bergin & Garvey, 1991. Chapter 3 contains a provocative exploration of alterations in mind-states experienced by some women in the perimenopausal years, and their meaning for our change-of-life transition.

34. John B. McKinlay, Sonja M. McKinlay, Donald Brambilla. "The Relative Contributions of Endocrine Changes and Social Circumstances to Depression in Middle-Aged Women." *Journal of Social Behavior*, Vol. 28, No. 4 (December 1987), pp. 345–63.

35. Elizabeth Barrett-O'Connor and Donna Dritz-Silverstein. "Estrogen Replacement Therapy and Cognitive Function in Older Women." *Journal of the American Medical Association,* Vol. 269, No. 20 (May 26, 1993), pp. 2637–41.

36. Barbara Ehrenreich and Deidre English, *For Her Own Good: 150 Years of the Experts' Advice to Women.* New York: Doubleday/Anchor, 1978.

37. Yewoubdar Beyene, "Cultural Significance and Physiological Manifestations of Menopause: A Biocultural Analysis." *Culture, Medicine and Psychiatry,* Vol. 10, No. 1 (March 1986), pp. 10–17.

38. Nancy E. Avis, Patricia A. Kaufert, Margaret Lock, Sonja M. McKinlay, Kerstin Vass, "The Evolution of Menopausal Symptoms." *Bailliere's Clinical Endocrinology and Metabolism,* Vol. 7, No. 1 (January 1993), pp. 17–32.

39. U.S. Congress, Office of Technology Assessment, *The Menopause, Hormone Therapy, and Women's Health,* op. cit., pp. 14–15.

40. Ibid., p. 4.

41. Robert A. Wilson, *Feminine Forever.* New York: M. Evans, 1966.

42. Kenneth J. Ryan, "Cancer Risks and Estrogen Use in the Menopause," an editorial in *The New England Journal of Medicine,* Vol. 293 (1975), p. 1200.

43. Rothert, op. cit.

44. Elina Hemminki, et al., "Prescribing of Noncontraceptive Estrogens and Progestins in the US, 1974–86." *American Journal of Public Health,* Vol. 78, No. 11 (1988), pp. 1479–81.

45. Deborah Grady, et al., "Hormone Therapy to Prevent Disease and Prolong Life in Postmenopausal Women." *Annals of Internal Medicine,* Vol. 117, No. 12 (Dec. 15, 1992), pp. 1016–37.

46. American College of Physicians, "Guidelines for Counseling Postmenopausal Women About Preventive Hormone Therapy." *Annals of Internal Medicine,* Vol. 117, No. 12 (Dec. 15, 1992), pp. 1038–41.

47. Lynn Rosenberg, Julie Palmer, and Samuel Shapiro, "A Case-Control Study of Myocardial Infarction in Relation to Use of Estrogen Supplements." *American Journal of Epidemiology,* Vol. 137, No. 1 (1993), pp. 54–63. See also, Grace M. Egeland, et al., "Premenopausal Determinants of Estrogen Use." *Preventive Medicine,* Vol. 20 (1991), pp. 343–49.

48. Meir J. Stampfer and Graham A. Colditz, "Estrogen Replacement Therapy and Coronary Heart Disease: A Quantitative Assessment of the Epidemiologic Evidence," *Preventive Medicine,* Vol. 20 (1991), pp. 47–63. See also Nabulsi, et al., "Association of Hormone-Replacement Therapy with Various Cardiovascular Risk Factors in Postmenopausal Women." *The New England Journal of Medicine,* Vol. 328, No. 15 (Apr. 15, 1993), pp. 1069–1116. See also Lynn Rosenberg, "Hormone Replacement Therapy: The Need for Reconsideration." *American Journal of Public Health,* Vol. 83, No. 12 (December 1993), pp. 1670–73.

49. Lynn Rosenberg, Professor of Epidemiology, B.U. School of Public Health. Testimony before Senate Committee on Labor and Human Resource, January 11, 1993.

50. L. Bergkvist, et al., "The Risk of Breast Cancer after Estrogen and Estrogen-Progestin Replacement Therapy." *The New England Journal of Medicine,* Vol. 321 (1989), pp. 293–97. Also, R. K. Ross, Studies of the University of Southern California. Presented at Hormone Replacement Therapy and Breast Cancer Risk: An Anglo-American Conference of the Royal Society of Medicine, London, September 1991.

51. K. K. Steinberg, et al., "A Meta-analysis of the Effect of Estrogen Replacement Therapy on the Risk of Breast Cancer." *Journal of the American Medical Association,* Vol. 265 (1991), pp. 1985–90.

52. Graham A. Colditz, Kathleen M. Egan, Meir J. Stampfer, "Hormone Replacement Therapy and Risk of Breast Cancer: Results from Epidemiologic Studies." *American Journal of Obstetrics and Gynecology*, Vol. 168 (1993), pp. 1473–80.

53. National Women's Health Network, *Taking Hormones and Women's Health: Choices, Risks and Benefits,* 1993. NWHN, 1325 G Street, NW, Washington, DC 20005.

11

RELATIONSHIPS IN MIDDLE AND LATER LIFE*

✦

BY DOROTHY FRAUENHOFER, LYNN SCOTT, PAULA B. DORESS-WORTERS, AND KRISTINE ROSENTHAL-KEESE

BECOMING A MOTHER-IN-LAW BY JANE PORCINO

1994 UPDATE BY DOROTHY FRAUENHOFER AND PAULA B. DORESS-WORTERS

RESOURCES FOR THIS CHAPTER ON PAGES 468–71

Women value relationships. For us middle-aged and older women especially, concern for interpersonal relationships has been a central theme of our lives. Most of us have worked hard to reach out to others, to express feelings of caring and attachment, and to be helpful when friends and family members are troubled. Throughout our lives our "people skills" have helped us get through some tough times.

As we move into the later decades of our lives, however, nearly all of us experience losses or changes in many of our most important relationships. When this happens, we fear the loneliness of being "unattached" and the emptiness of not being needed or valued. Many of us from traditional backgrounds were raised on homilies like "Blood is thicker than water," and were taught to avoid sharing confidences with "outsiders." Yet long-lived women frequently survive all of their close family members. Though we grieve for the loss of relationships we can never replace, we *can* overcome loneliness and isolation by reweaving and changing family relationships, nurturing old and new friendships, and especially by reaching out to other women to form new connections for support and intimate friendships. Our middle and later years can be a time of expanding choices and new opportunities.

EXTENDING OUR FAMILIES

This chapter speaks about extending, rather than extended, families, to emphasize our active role in expanding the conventional definition of family. Most women who have lived their younger adult years in a nuclear family with children extend their definition of family to include partners of children and, of course, grandchildren. Particularly in our middle and later years, we may also begin to think of our closest friends as a kind of extended family.

Family is important throughout our lives as a source of intimacy and connection. Whether we

*In this chapter we talk about many different life situations. We recognize and even celebrate our diversity as women. We have included in the chapter some material on relatively uncommon situations to extend to women the full range of alternatives that are available to all of us in our middle and later years. We hope this approach will raise consciousness and encourage women to unite across barriers of generation, race, class, and sexual preference that have divided us in the past.

choose a family similar to or different from the one we grew up in, most of us continue to value the love, acceptance, and intimacy of family life.

Being the center of a family network goes right on for us anyway, even though the children don't live at home any more. I am still embedded in family. Different people need me and us for different reasons. I've taken on my husband's family as well as my own, and he's taken on mine. I have two children by my first husband and my former mother-in-law is still living. My husband has three children and two of them have families of their own. Also my stepmother and stepfather, the second spouse of each of my parents, are still living and I, for various reasons, am their most responsible child. We have a stable happy marriage and my husband is a doctor, so we attract whoever is ailing. And we are both in the "support business," it's just how we are emotionally. [a fifty-seven-year-old woman]

I have two sisters who live upstairs. People are always surprised that we get along so well, living in the same house. My sisters never go out without coming by to ask me if they can get me anything. We weren't always like that. We were too busy with our own lives. Now we try hard to help each other. [a seventy-year-old woman, widowed]

Living with Loss

During our middle years, most of us first become aware of signs of advancing age in our parents, aunts, and uncles. We are shocked! These are not the elderly relatives of our grandparents' generation, but the stalwart adults who formed the strong, dependable landscape of our youth. Can it be possible that they are slowing down and needing help from *us?* This process can be a frightening reminder of our own mortality.

My father and all his family died in their late fifties. So, does that mean I have only four more years? I don't really feel morbid about it, but I live with a different perspective. [a fifty-five-year-old woman]

Most difficult is the not uncommon experience of a series of losses at midlife challenging our resilience and ability to cope.

Ten years ago, I lost both my sisters within three years. Then I lost Bob, the most wonderful man of my life. We married two years after we met. A year later, he was dead.

Now, my beautiful, intelligent, wonderful son has AIDS. His doctors call him a "long-term survivor." It's been really difficult to deal with his possible death. The family met to talk about his wishes around what he wants at the end. This is something we never expected to face with the younger generation.

How do I cope? I have always been a people person. I have many friends and organizational involvements. My marriage to Bob made me a more trusting person. Before Bob, I was bitter and didn't trust men. His love helped me accept Dan, whom I've known since I was thirteen. We became close after both our partners died, and spend a lot of time together. [a sixty-six-year-old woman]

Friends as Family[1]

For all of us, irrespective of marital status or sexual preference, women friends provide the support and continuity that enable us to enjoy new challenges and to cope with the changes and losses we face in the second half of life. With this awareness, growing numbers of us are learning to regard our friendships as lifelong relationships to be worked at and cared for "just like family." For those of us who grew up thinking of other women as our competitors, or as less interesting or less valuable than men, it has been rewarding to share our lives and our histories in women's groups and discover that women are, in fact, terrific.

My women friends hand-carried me through my divorce. When my marriage of sixteen years got difficult, my women's group helped me consider what to do. They recommended marriage counselors and therapists. A year later, when it was still clearly not working, my friends helped me find the resources I needed—books on the transition of divorce, referrals to lawyers, poems about women rediscovering themselves after painful losses. Getting hugs and occasionally back rubs from my friends kept me feeling cared for and connected. A friend who had been through a divorce came to the court hearing with me. When I couldn't afford new up-to-date clothes for going out to meet people, the same friend, now remarried and pregnant, suggested I borrow some of her nonpregnant outfits for the season. A single friend invited me to dinner to meet a divorced man she thought I would like. She and another friend loaned me some money so I could get holiday presents for my kids. [a woman in her forties]

Many of us are accustomed to forming primary emotional links with a man. But even when we live in a traditional way with a male partner, there is a high statistical likelihood that we will grow old in the company of other women. The divorce rate is rising and most married women outlive their partners.

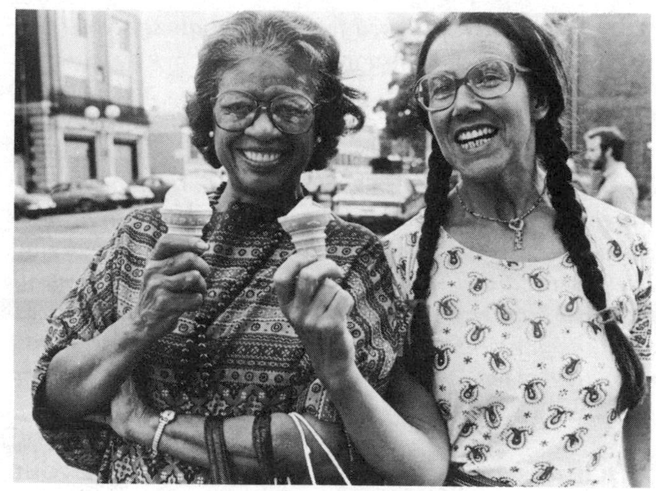

Marianne Gontarz

Because I was widowed young (in my early thirties), I had a series of short- and long-term relationships with men near my own age over the next twenty years that met my sexual needs pretty well. However, they did not always meet my emotional needs for closeness on a daily basis; they were not live-in arrangements, and in fact, more often than not, the man lived in another city or state. In my fifties, I became aware that even the sexual aspects of this type of relationship were not as satisfying as they had been, as my now middle-aged partner's sexual needs and problems often required that my attention be diverted from my own. At about the same time, a new friendship with another woman developed, with almost daily contact, and I recognized that the closeness and affection it was providing on a regular basis was meeting deeper emotional needs than the more sporadic sex offered by men my own age. [a fifty-four-year-old woman]

It's extremely important for women growing older to have a circle of women friends; there's no other way to guard against the inevitable loneliness. [a woman in her eighties]

If we have been raised to form our closest bonds with family members and others within an ethnically homogeneous community, we may be more comfortable having our most intimate friendships with those of similar background. However, it can be a pleasant surprise at times to find a kindred spirit in a more diverse setting.

I have often been shy about making new friends, but I am learning to reach out. I have just made a new friend. Though I am Jewish and she is Methodist, we share so many things in our life experiences that we could almost have been twins. Our ideas about the spirit, about religion, about life are so similar. We even share the experience of being estranged from our own children. We have helped one another and have found in one another sisters, extended family, friends for life. [a fifty-five-year-old woman]

Freda Rebelsky, an expert on adult development, observes, "So many good friendships start at times of our lives when we feel the most need for someone else to understand our pain.... From that we can develop the kinds of friendships that lead to lots of laughter, lots of joy, lots of sharing, and lots of growth."[2]

The greatest pleasure of growing old is remaining in contact with friends from church and in the community. I'm treasurer of the Older Women's League chapter here, and also the Black Caucus on Aging. I kept contact with my friends from childhood. I love people, all kinds of people. I don't give up a relationship easily. I only gave up one in seventy-two years, someone who really, really hurt me. I am friends with my ex-husband's second wife and went to see her on my vacation. She was so glad to see me. [a seventy-five-year-old woman]

I've just celebrated my seventieth year with a collective celebration of aging, together with friends of all generations, from two to eighty-two. What a warm and wonderful event, with food and drink and song and dance!

I am free and enjoying life. I concentrate on people and keeping up with relationships. I call or write perhaps ten to twelve of my friends every week. I keep a big stack of cards for every occasion, even those that say "just to say hello." When I travel, I rarely stay in hotels, because I have friends everywhere, male and female, and these are not sexual relationships. I've been courted recently, but I guess you might call me almost asexual. No, I never worry about being lonely or alone as I grow older, no more than those who have only their families. I've had friends come from halfway around the world to take care of me when I've been ill and I've done the same for them. [a sixty-two-year-old never-married woman]

Our Children Grow Up

For those of us who have raised families, being a mother was probably one of our most absorbing, time-consuming, and demanding relationships. We become parents in part because of our own needs to bond with others and to find fulfillment and meaning. Yet once our children are grown up and leave home, we must accept the fact that the daily caregiving part of mothering is done and must trust our children to take care of themselves, while we go on to take care of ourselves.

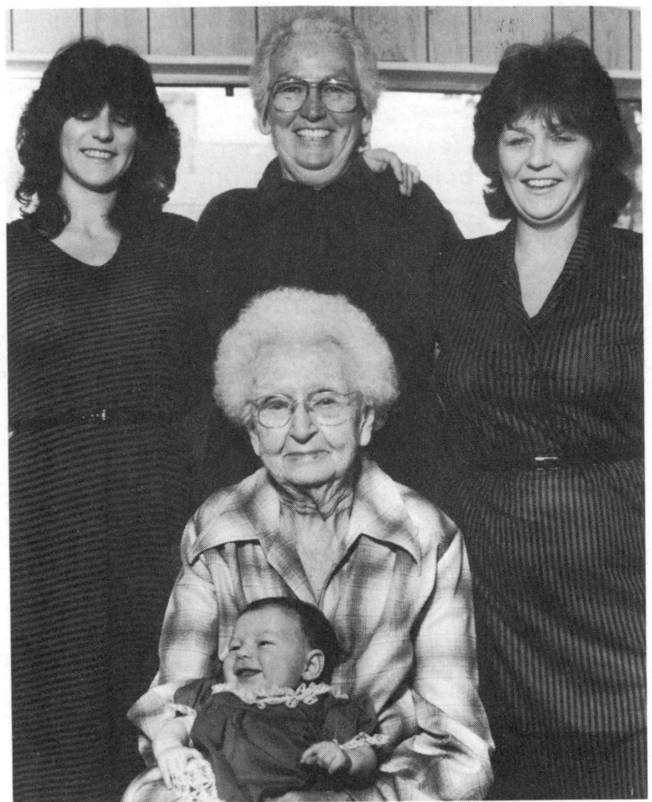

Teri Carsten

When we have meaningful work and other relationships outside the home—plans and goals to look forward to and other anchors for our identity and self-esteem—it becomes easier to let children go and to relish the freedom and opportunity of the next stage.[3] If we turn the concern and energy that we had directed toward our children toward meeting new possibilities, we can be happy and positive about the future, and as a bonus we give our children an optimistic view of growing older.

For some of us, the end of the caregiving years of mothering can present as much of a challenge and be as emotionally demanding as becoming a parent for the first time.[4] Some of us have to work at relinquishing control over our children's choices and giving up the dailiness of the relationship with them.

The way I get along with my kids is to realize that their lives are theirs and mine is mine. So I've learned to leave them alone to make their own decisions. When I was having trouble letting go of my youngest, my oldest daughter helped me. I now let them live their own lives. Actually, that's been my philosophy all along. I felt I had to prepare them to be on their own and make their own way. So I can't cry when they finally get to the point of doing what I had planned for them all along, can I? [a sixty-eight-year-old woman]

I really missed my children when they moved away but you have to "divorce" your children. One way I got over longing for my children was to think about the relationship I had with my mother when I was my children's age. I, too, had wanted freedom and control over my own life. Back then I didn't want to have to be with my mother all the time. I had my own friends. When I finally recognized this, the longing disappeared and I didn't worry any more. It's an act of love to want your children to live their own lives. [a sixty-five-year-old woman]

Others of us look forward to the time our parenting obligations will be fulfilled.

I have had this job for twenty-five years and I am looking forward to being "Parent Emeritus." I have never lived alone, never, ever. So it's going to be a whole new experience when the last one leaves. I've been happy when each one left, even my oldest daughter, who was really easy to raise. When I think of sitting across the breakfast table from my ex-husband and trying to find something to talk about, I feel lucky not to be in that situation. Sometimes I think, "Does this mean I'm going to grow old alone?" I don't really look forward to that. On the other hand, I don't want to do a lot of things like accounting for my time, preparing meals, having someone sick. So, I think it's a new challenge! I may end up finding out that I simply hate living alone, and then I'll do something about it. But I hope I'll like it because I want to have the extra space when my four kids come back to visit. [a fifty-year-old woman]

Having children return home or make new demands for support and nurturing after they have left home and been on their own is a prevalent concern of middle-aged women today. Though we may now feel ready to begin a new life of our own, there is always the possibility that we may be called upon to share our resources once more.

My twenty-eight-year-old son moved back into our apartment when he was discharged from the Air Force. It was supposed to be temporary until he could find an apartment, but after a year he's still here. He says he can't afford to pay $400 a month until he finds a steady job. Then my daughter moved back when she and her friends were evicted. I was looking forward to peace and quiet, but here I am. [a sixty-year-old woman]

Some parents find it possible to live with adult children, and sometimes grandchildren, but the transition from the mother/child relationship to one of independent and mutually respectful adults is a very difficult one, and may not be possible for everyone. It requires willingness to compromise, clarity about individual as well as family goals and values, and the weathering of crises.

At the other extreme, some adolescent and adult children may want to put the maximum possible distance between themselves and their parent(s). It is natural to grieve if your child does not wish to see you or be close. Don't add to your feelings of rejection and loss by perceiving this situation as a personal failure, however. Try to remain warm, understanding, and open to communication while keeping busy with your own life. Chances are that once your child feels more secure in her or his independence, she or he will once again want to be in touch with you. There is little you can do but accept the fact that your child, for whatever reasons, does not want to be close for the time being. Sometimes the closer we have been to a child, the more extreme is the need for separation.

I decided that if my daughter did not want to communicate with me, I would respect her wishes; that in doing so, she would learn that I am indeed a separate person and might become curious about this person who is separate, who respects her, and who is no longer "available mother." And that this separation would help me grow as well as help her grow. [a fifty-three-year-old woman]

I wasn't prepared for the intensity of the changes in my teenage daughter. As I look back on it, I think we were each experiencing hormonal changes at opposite ends of the continuum. She was so changeable—one minute happy, another minute depressed. One moment she needed me and acted like a sweet child again, and another time she's telling me she knows more about everything than I do. Those were stressful years. Now that she's working and has her own apartment, we're great friends and everything seems to be in balance again. [a forty-nine-year-old woman]

Barring serious financial, emotional, or health problems, the parent-child relationship, which was based on dependency, should now be based on mutuality: mutual recognition of each other as separate personalities, mutual respect, and mutual helping.

There may be times when a mother finds herself in need of help from her children. Many women are particularly reluctant to accept help from children even when freely offered.

My son is a doctor but it took me a long time to recognize his skills. I continued to think of him as my little Johnny—messy, awkward, and uncertain. Then some of my friends became his patients and were constantly praising him. I began to see him in a different way, began to ask him questions about my health and to seek his advice. Now I go to one of the doctors in his clinic and my son takes care of me by consulting with my doctor. [a sixty-eight-year-old woman]

My daughter is always buying me something, even if I need it like a hole in the head. She wants me to look good. She always notices if I don't wear it. My daughter wants to give me something. She wants to take care of me. I think she would like it better if I were more dependent. [a sixty-eight-year-old woman]

Though it is hard for us to give up our role as the helping or caring person within the family, it may help to think of receiving help as part of the mutual exchange of family caring.

I really don't like being dependent on my children, but what can I do? I have to face reality. I'm sure they know that for many years they were dependent on me. I really tried hard to help them, protect them, give them a good education. I suppose it's my time to receive help from them. [a woman in her seventies]

When I was between jobs, my son emptied out his bank account and sent it to me for my birthday. He wrote, "This is for you to use as an interest-free loan. You'll pay me back when you are able to." I hadn't asked for help, but somehow he got the idea. It made me feel that all that nurturing and caring had made an impression. [a fifty-nine-year-old woman]

I never quite had the relationship with my own mother that I now enjoy with my daughters. We travel together, go to movies, plays, and often do our shopping together. I can't explain how it came about, especially when I consider the tumultuous times we went through during all their adolescent years. I was patient and sort of waited for them to grow up—you know, sort of let them scream and yell their way through it. Now, they are well adjusted and successful and great fun to be with. [a sixty-one-year-old woman]

Becoming a Mother-in-Law

Mothers-in-law have been the source of every type of commentary from humor to outright derision. These woman-hating barbs reflect the low regard in which older women are held in our society. The conventional rivalry between a woman and her daughter-in-law, supposedly competitors for the attention of the man, epitomizes the very essence of the intergenerational barrier between women that this book seeks to change.

It is eye-opening to look at the two roles of grandmother and mother-in-law together. It is evident how little the stereotypes conform to the reality of our lives. After all, the sweet, loving, gentle soul that a grandmother is supposed to be and the critical, interfering busybody that is the caricature of a mother-in-law are often the same woman.

Mothers-in-law have traditionally been advised to "mind their own business." This can be in practice a very difficult prescription, because for so many years, your child *was* your business. Yet once your child is grown up, and certainly once she or he is in a serious relationship, you are not expected to offer help unless it is requested, or advice unless it is sought. The in-law relationship is one in which we have no choice at all. Perhaps that is part of its difficulty. Whether we like our son- or daughter-in-law, his or her parents, and the other in-law relatives is almost a matter of chance. We must suspend judgment and simply accept the mate that our child has chosen. This is a way to show love and respect for your child.

It is difficult to see your child make a choice that you disapprove of or consider harmful. It is particularly hard if the choice means that your child will live far away from you, either geographically or emotionally, by choosing a lifestyle that is very different from yours.

The best part of our trip to Australia was getting to know our son-in-law. He and I took long walks on the beach, had breakfast together, and visited with his mother, who told me all about him as a young boy. When he took us sailing for a week, his skills and interest were apparent.

There had been problems between us before, but I approached this trip with a positive attitude. I traveled 6,000 miles to discover that my son-in-law was very lovable. I should have known, since my daughter had been telling me so for years. [a woman in her sixties]

You have had some twenty or more years to transmit your values to your child. The entire family relationship will be strengthened if you can trust that your child has absorbed those values. It would probably help both of you to let your child know that you still love her or him and want to maintain a caring relationship, whether you approve of the chosen partner or not. Resist the temptation to say "I told you so" if their relationship does not work out. Your child and maybe even the former partner may need your continued support. They will feel freer to turn to you if they have not been made to feel defensive.

As if being a mother-in-law were not difficult enough in itself, many of us now have the additional confusion of being a "something-or-other" to our child's live-in lover. Perhaps a new title would change the whole view of this difficult relationship. Perhaps, just as we talk of love relationships and love children, we should also speak of mothers-in-love.

In traditional cultures, the roles and obligations of the parents of an engaged or married couple are formally defined. Today, however, it may take time to recognize a relationship as serious and lasting. Without guidelines to tell us what our role is during the courtship's progression, we may feel at a loss in determining where we fit in the couple's life.

My daughter has been living with her friend for four years and I'm just beginning to treat him more like a permanent presence. I've begun addressing letters to both of them. He's becoming less like just a boyfriend and more like a son-in-law. [a sixty-one-year-old woman]

My son and Deborah dated in college and since that time have shared an apartment. I like her and she and I have a good relationship, but I don't know the rules. What expectations should I have for holidays and when should I invite them? Last year was the first time I gave Deborah a birthday present. I felt good about acknowledging her relationship with my son. [a fifty-four-year-old woman]

Some of us who considered ourselves open-minded and "modern" have surprised our children and even ourselves by being upset over the nontraditional and unexpected choices our grown children may make. We may discover that we unconsciously harbored a fantasy of a partner from a similar religious or cultural background, reflecting a wish to have our children carry on our family traditions into the future. If this happens, or if our children choose not to marry and have children at all, or simply delay these choices,[5] we may find ourselves feeling anxious, guilty, and wondering what we have done wrong.

The issue of children who delay having children or choose not to have them may be a major part of the dilemma for parents of those who choose a partner of the same sex. This can be a problem even for parents who *can* accept their child's sexual preference. There are also many other issues that come up for parents of a gay or lesbian child. Support groups have been formed so that the parents can talk about their feelings and come to understand their children's choices (see Resources for this chapter).

Our favorite in-law is our daughter's woman friend. They have lived together happily for over four years, and are an important part of all family gatherings. I have found this new member of our family particularly sensitive to both the joys and sorrows in my life. I feel most comfortable to just drop in on them and to share the experiences of their life—but also, to know they want to share my feelings, too. [a sixty-two-year-old woman]

BECOMING A GRANDMOTHER

One cannot deny the pleasurable feeling of self-renewal that is experienced by grandparents. To see a new generation coming, perhaps carrying on our features, talents, or idiosyncrasies, is most fascinating.

Being a grandmother is one of the great experiences of life, especially today, when we don't take the miracle for granted. There is no question that having a grandchild come to visit is demanding physically, mentally, and emotionally, especially when the grandmother is also working. Our three-year-old granddaughter has just left after a four-week visit. As the wildflowers in the juice glass fade, I try to decide which of the twenty-one crayon and watercolor pictures to keep taped to the banister. I rescue a 1950 miniature trailer truck her father used to play with from under the bed and hear her say proudly, "I'm bigging!" I see the world anew through her eyes and hope I'm still bigging too. [a woman in her seventies]

Some women look forward to having a less stressful relationship with their grandchildren than they did with their children, especially if they were too busy or too unsure of themselves to have fully enjoyed the early years of their children. Women whose economic conditions have improved over the years may take special pleasure in indulging their grandchildren in ways that they were not able to with their own children. Unfortunately, this can become a source of friction, so be sure to discuss treats and presents with your own child in advance.

A new stage in the mother-in-law relationship often follows the birth or adoption of our first grandchild. At that time we become more like colleagues or peers to our daughters or daughters-in-law, and can relate to each other as one mother to another. While we may be able to be closer to them than we were in the earlier honeymoon-couple/in-law phase, it is important to continue to respect the autonomy of our adult children, as well as their authority as parents.

In our culture, which is still too much in the grips of the adoration of youth, becoming a grandmother often bears a stigma for a still-youthful woman.

When my daughter called me from Florida to tell me I was now a grandmother, I was not in the least elated. I had recently remarried and was seeing myself as a young, passionate lover. I didn't want to think of myself as a

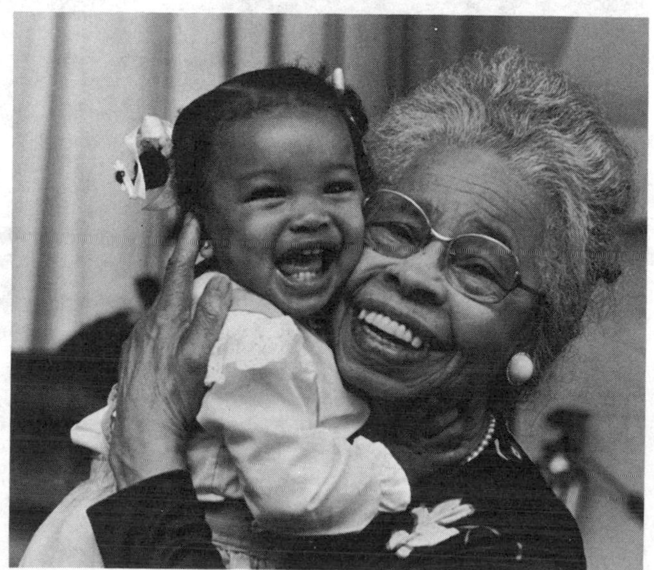

Cathy Cade

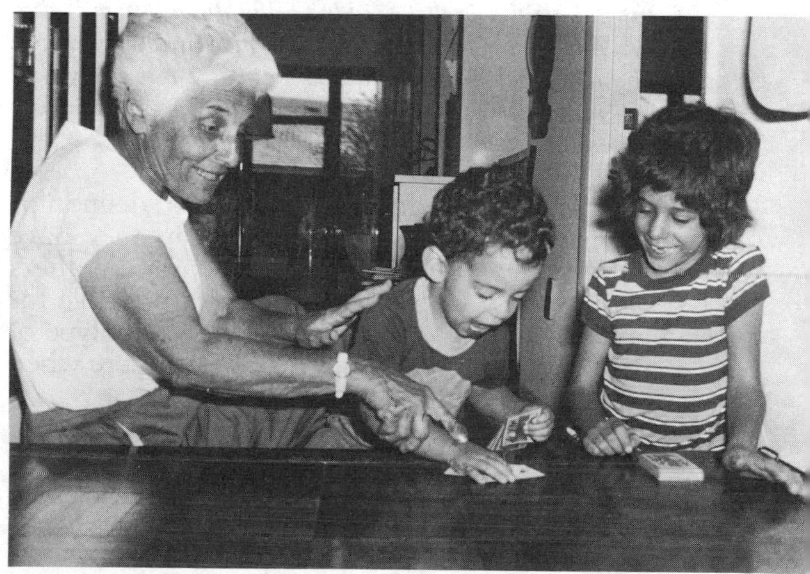

Ellen Shub

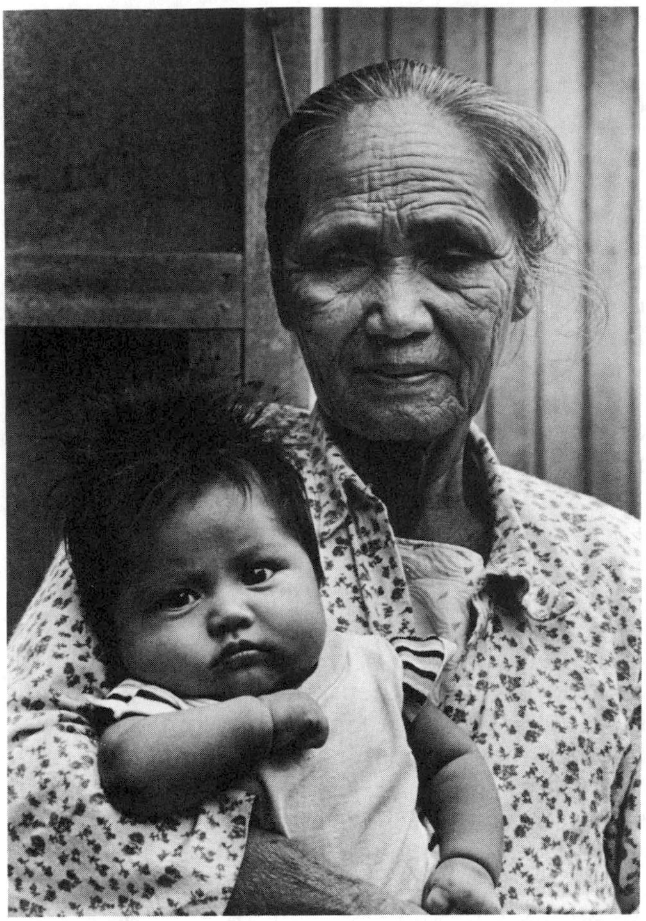

Jerry Howard/Positive Images

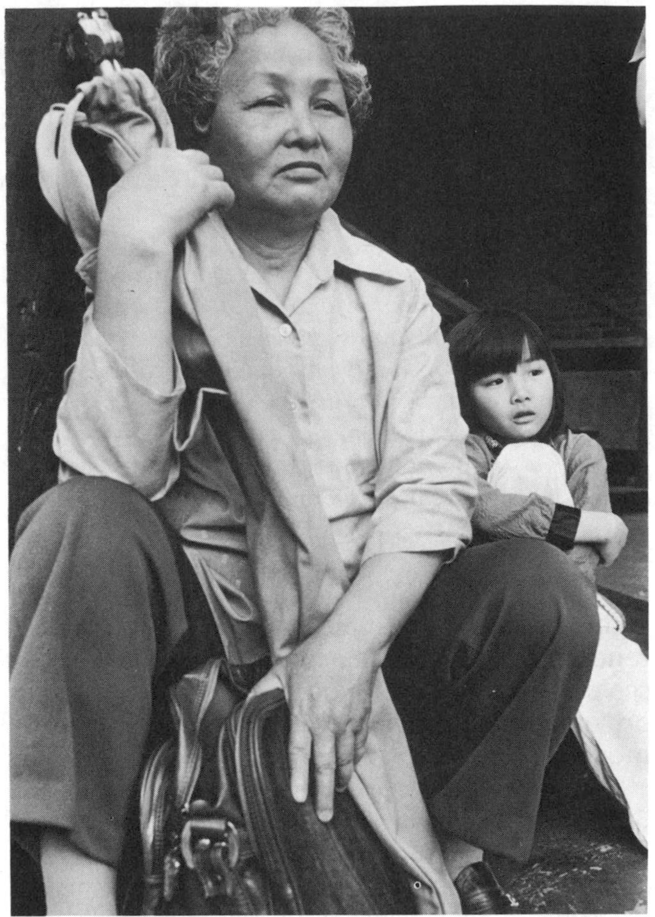

Marianne Gontarz

grandmother. That was because of the picture I had of my own grandmother—a fussy, domineering, and strict woman who took care of us when my mother worked. I think when my daughter first informed me of the birth of my grandchild I felt I couldn't fulfill the role expected of me. And I didn't want to. I finally made my own decision about our relationship but sometimes I feel guilty that I'm not a good enough grandmother. [a woman in her fifties]

Today's grandmothers want to define for themselves the specific relationship they have with their grandchildren. Few grandmothers want to baby-sit regularly or be responsible for child care. Most women resist the stereotype of the "doormat" grandmother, always there when anyone needs her.

I have an unwritten understanding with my children: I do not baby-sit my grandchildren. I entertain them. I invite them—but I'm not called in as a baby-sitter. I think baby-sitting damages the relationship. They know when I'm with them I'm there because I want to be and because

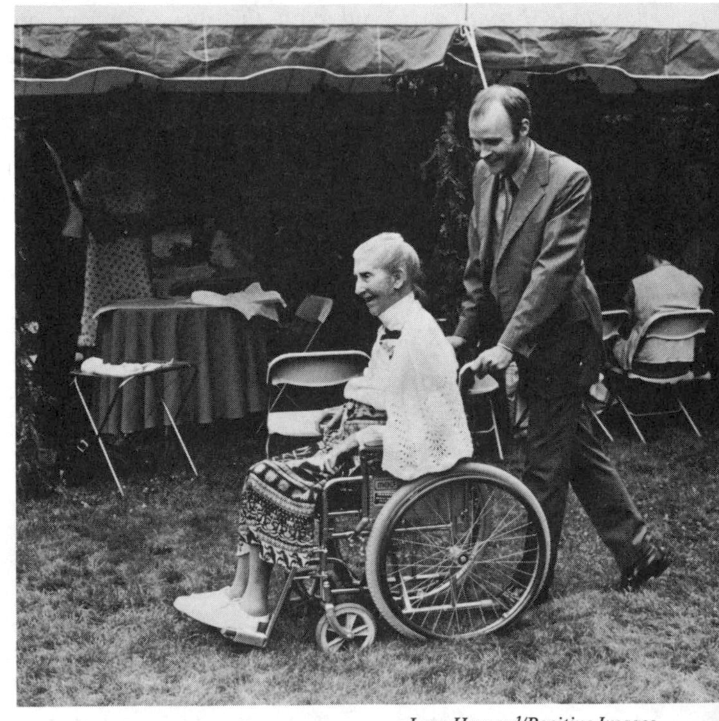

Jerry Howard/Positive Images

I enjoy their company. And I invite them on that basis too. I don't want to be considered a baby-sitter because that's not the relationship I want to establish with my grandchildren. [a seventy-four-year-old woman]

Some women, however, enjoy taking care of grandchildren.

I'm going to do my first stint of grandchild care for my nine-month-old grandchild this summer. My daughter is signed up for a four-day course. I really love children and I think it will be fun. I'm looking forward to it. I'm a little ticked off that her husband isn't doing it, but I'm really staying out of that. And it's nice to do something concrete for my oldest daughter. She's just consistently very giving and thoughtful. [a fifty-year-old woman]

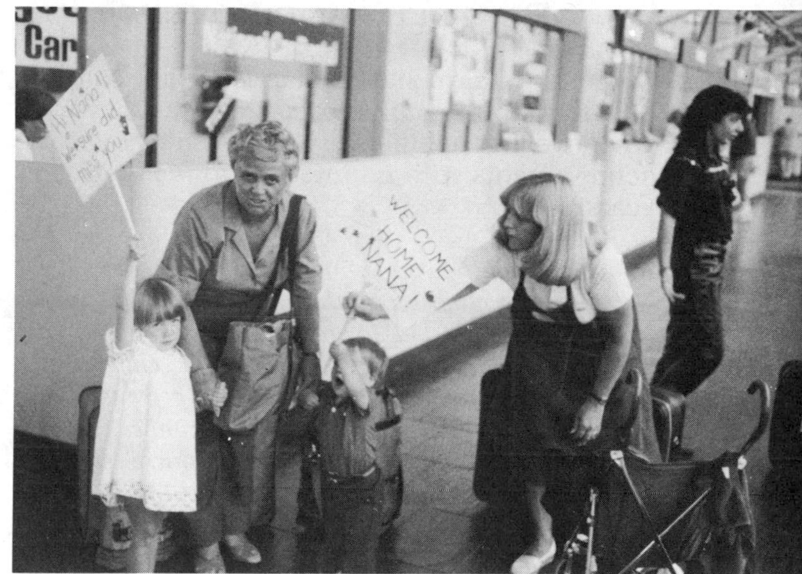

Peter Lantos

Some women care for grandchildren because of the illness, incapacity, or death of the child's parents. Often when we do this we are deeply anguished ourselves and need support.[6] Other grandparents experience pain at losing contact with their grandchildren after the parents have been divorced or separated. It is important to realize that such things happen and to build good relationships with our children's partners. If you cannot work things out with your child's former partner, it can help to have the advice and support of an organization involved with grandparents' issues (see Resources for this chapter).

Some women find it easier to ask their older grandchildren for help or companionship than they do their own children. Conversely, a grandparent may offer help in a way that complements what parents can do, or that fits better with what a young person wants.

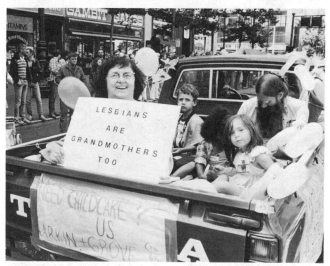

Cathy Cade

When one of my grandsons got himself into a jam with jobs during his senior year in high school and couldn't make it home to dinner, I invited him to come have dinner with me. I would set my dinner hour to accommodate the time when he could make it because I thought it was unhealthful for him to be skipping meals.

I don't feel hesitant about asking them to do things that I don't have the strength to do. My sixteen-year-old grandson is very strong and if I have a piece of shrubbery I can't uproot, I call him up and ask him, and he does it. Sometimes I pay them, especially if it is a special skill that they should be paid for. My other grandson services my car and I pay him for it, but when I need someone to pick me up at the airport, he comes and meets me and picks me up and, of course, I don't pay him for that.

I have a very easy relationship with my grandchildren now. I hope that they consider me as a friend and not as an authority figure. That's what I aim for. I'm not the kind of grandmother you put a lap robe over. [a seventy-four-year-old woman]

I want to do something with the money I have left so my children and grandchildren will have memories of me—not just leave it to them and have them buy a car or some material thing, and that's the end of it.

I have two grandchildren here and two in New York. When they were all about eight or nine I started taking them on trips. I usually take one of the Massachusetts grandchildren and one of the New York grandchildren on each trip, because I want them to know each other, too. So, now they have been to lots of places that they will always remember. And we have wonderful pictures, too. [a woman in her seventies]

PARTNERS AND LOVERS

Some of us have stayed married for decades to partners who remain as dear to us as they were when we first fell in love. We can enjoy our joint achievements with no interruptions in our later years.

I am sixty-eight years old and have been married to the same man for almost forty-three years. In earlier periods we had more ups and downs, preoccupied as we were with the ambitions and pressures of work, child raising, and developing our identities as separate persons. We are more capable now of appreciating one another and have a more relaxed and confident view of ourselves and a greater sense of gratitude and contentment that we have each other. I think we have come to have a kind of pride in each other, in the kind of person we each have become.

From the beginning of our much-valued marriage, we agreed that we would each gather gifts of knowledge, skills, and a wide variety of disciplines to bring to our relationship so that it would prosper and serve as a measure of our own growth.

After forty-six years we have learned that we cannot change each other and that it is not weakness but rather strength to be willing to adapt. We have also learned that it is a myth that one member of a long-term relationship is always dominant while the other is a follower. Over the long years, we have taken turns at being leader, in both good times and bad.

Today, as we near our seventies, our daily lives are rich in shared experience and in appreciation of the many aspects of human love. We are both lucky and skillful in maintaining our sexuality as a happy resource in friendship and communication.

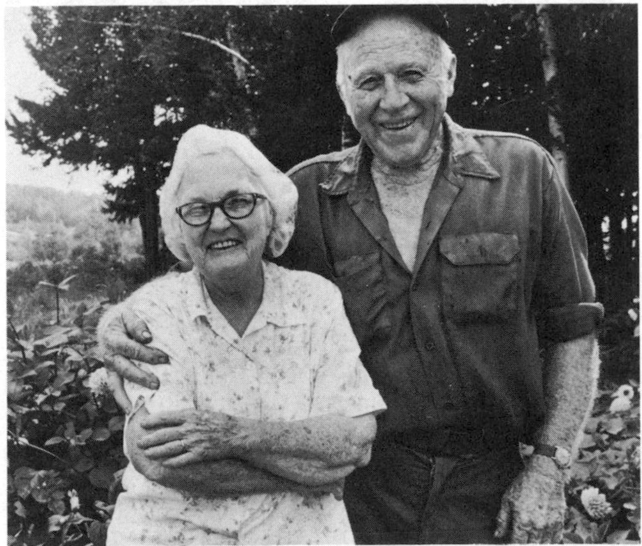

Marianne Gontarz

For many women, the demands of raising a family have meant delaying or holding back our individual aspirations. After the children have grown, however, the husband's life outside the family often continues as before, while the wife may face a total redefinition of all her roles, even if she has been employed continuously outside the home—but especially if she has not. Most households are arranged around the personality or the employment needs of the husband and the developmental needs of the children. The changes we women go through inevitably make waves in our relationships and challenge us to rework our ways of living with our partners. Some men are flexible, secure, and caring enough to understand and accept the required adjustments, but in many relationships a period of renegotiation may be needed.

My husband didn't like it when I got a studio away from the house to do my artwork, but I did it. I don't ask permission any more. When I want to go somewhere, I say, "I'm going," not "Is it all right if I go?" I'm going to travel for a month by myself. That would have been inconceivable ten years ago. So this has been a long slow process of changing myself and my marriage. At first, we had a lot of fights and arguments and we started to say, "Let's call it quits." But somehow the love kept it going and we decided to go to a therapist. After a while, my husband began to appreciate some of my changes. One of the nice things about aging is that after so many years of coping you begin to see that problems aren't insurmountable. You know you've solved them before and so you can see the light at the end of the tunnel. We have finally learned to accept each other as we are. If the positives outweigh the negatives in a relationship, then it is worth saving. No relationship is a bed of roses. [a fifty-seven-year-old woman]

My husband worked in an automotive factory on the line for more than forty years. Sometimes he worked double and triple shifts during the good times. He provided well for me and our six children and all the kids finished college. We had money in the bank and looked forward to the time when he could come home and relax. We never dreamed this would cause any problems, but it did. For about a year after he retired we fussed and fought. Then, even though I hadn't worked since my youngest was in kindergarten, I went out and got a job as a saleswoman in a department store in town. He resented that—wanted to know who would cook and keep the house. I said, "You can." The biggest surprise was that he learned to cook. Every day when I come home he has dinner on the table. We have learned to enjoy each other's company and we are both happy with our new life. [a sixty-eight-year-old woman]

When partners carry out the tasks of marriage and family building as "shoulds," putting aside their own needs for growth and development, unmet needs and resentments fill the void left by the children's departure. These may have begun to surface during the children's adolescence. Partners in long-standing marriages need to have individual and shared goals to keep themselves and the relationship vital. A challenge of midlife marriage is to develop new goals once the family-building stage is completed.

There are so many aspects to a marriage: love, children in common, mutual friends, common interests—each a thread that keeps a marriage together. Sometimes only one or two of these threads have remained unbroken, yet the partners are reluctant to separate. Often the transition of grown children starting a life of their own, or the sudden understanding that an unsatisfactory marriage will forever prevent us from achieving our life goals, becomes the needed push toward the dissolution of a long-standing partnership.

After twenty years of marriage my husband and I decided to divorce. We had gotten along badly for many years and whatever was left of our relationship was finished long before we made this decision. The one thing that was hard to give up was our group of friends. We engaged in a very active social life and actually had fun going out often in social groups. Our friends were astounded—many people called us the "golden" couple, always happy and having fun. They never dreamed my husband was an alcoholic—though still successful in his work—and his drinking and affairs with other women corroded our family life. [a forty-five-year-old woman]

Women who initiate a divorce themselves may feel the exhilaration of a new beginning, or at least the energy of acting on long-repressed feelings. That energy can give us the courage to face the changes of marital separation.

I was trained to be a lifetime servant and didn't believe that life could be fun. Through counseling and group therapy at our battered women's outreach, I have discovered my inner strength, and that I deserve the best life has to offer. I am now divorced from my battering husband. I wrote many poems tracing my experiences from darkness to light, from bondage to freedom. I think this journey of self-discovery is what every woman tries to take. [a thirty-nine-year-old woman]

Leaving my marriage to an abusive husband was a real liberation for me. No more waiting up at night until the wee hours, listening for his footsteps, trying to determine how drunk he would be. No more fighting off his sexual advances when he was too drunk and impotent to do much about that anyway. No more having to take the children's side constantly because I felt I had to make up for his emotional abuse of them. The night I packed everything in the car to leave, he padlocked the gate and slashed the tires. I called a locksmith and AAA and before dawn we were on our way. I was forty-four years old and starting over after twenty years of marriage.

Breaking up a marriage is rarely an impulsive decision for women, and often it is preceded by years of gradual preparation. Preparation for financial self-sufficiency can be a significant step toward emotional readiness to withstand the pain of separation and the challenge of being on your own.

I had tried numerous times to get my husband to move out of the house so I would feel safe, but I did not succeed until I started an internship at a hospital. I guess he finally realized that I meant it when I said I wanted him to get out when he saw that I was preparing to support myself. In addition, I stopped covering up for him: I stopped cleaning up the messes he made smashing things; I stopped the crisis interventions; I stopped trying to act as his therapist. Instead, I went to a divorce and mediation center. Mediation turned out to be impossible since my husband refused to talk. The mediator told me to get a divorce attorney, which I did. [a fifty-two-year-old woman]

When it is our partner who initiates the breakup of a marriage or a long-term relationship, the feelings of pain and rejection can be devastating, especially if he or she has left us for a younger lover.

I'm so bitter—I sometimes feel like totally destroying him. I gave twenty-five years to this marriage—making sacrifices, taking care of the children, taking his shit. Now he's with this girl young enough to be his daughter. I have been in therapy for a year trying to cope with it. It's helped me handle my anger. Yet I feel exploited. He took my youth, my beauty—he destroyed that. My innocence, too. I long for that sometimes. [a fifty-year-old woman]

Divorce

Divorce is having
all your teeth out one by one.
First the incisors wear down dull
as your grandfather's carving knife,
then the eye teeth go blind
lose their dogged bite.
The molars cease to grind out love
and then the judge excises
the impacted wisdom of the wedding
and you bleed and bleed.

Jane Strete

I had never allowed myself to face the possibility of divorce. I was so fearful at the thought of being on my own. I was in shock, briefly, and then I was sad, frightened, and lonely. For six months I believed I could get my husband to come back. Finally I began to accept what had happened and to look ahead to my own future.

I got my former husband to share in the care of our youngest son so I could go back to school. Then I lived with a group of older people; that created a new home for me and helped me to feel less lonely.

Today I am living on my own as a single person, going to graduate school in a city 800 miles from my former home and building a new life. I see myself as a dependent person acting independently. I'm a risk-taker, that's what's helped me make the changes I've made. [a sixty-year-old woman]

The breakup of a marriage, however devastating it may seem, carries with it the potential for a new life. With age, we grow in maturity, experience, and confidence, qualities that have a beauty and power to attract in their own right. Best of all, these are qualities that reflect how we feel about ourselves and do not depend on the perception of others.

Widowhood or Loss of a Partner

Since women usually live longer than men and are often younger than their mates, widowhood is the experience of the majority of married women. The average age of widowhood in the United States is fifty-six, and the average widow lives for eighteen years after her husband's death.[7]

My youngest son had just decided not to stay in college. I remember driving along thinking that now my husband and I could plan for our old age. When I got home I got a call about my husband. He died suddenly just as I was about to turn fifty-eight. [a seventy-eight-year-old woman]

The experience of widowhood varies according to the time of life in which it occurs. If you have lived with a partner happily for four or five decades, and perhaps raised a family together, your grief may be tempered by an awareness of the good fortune you shared together. Yet if you are in your seventies or eighties and in failing health yourself, you may have less emotional and physical energy to rebuild your life as a single woman. Women who are widowed young often are devastated by the shock and overwhelmed with the responsibility of raising and educating children on their own, yet the younger you are the more likely you are to eventually recover from your grief.

Many recently widowed women report that they imagine their partner is still there and catch themselves starting to talk to him or her. They worry that they are losing their minds. However, this is not unusual behavior in the early months of widowhood. It may seem inconceivable to many a recently widowed woman that she can ever find happiness again, or comfort, or even peace of mind by herself or with a new love. Gone is the companionship, the sexuality, the economic partnership, the intimacy of many years. Some of these pieces of the lost relationship will never be replaced; for others perhaps only a pale substitute can be found.

I think I'm still depressed. I don't think I've gotten over it—after twenty years I still feel his presence. When I lost my husband I cried and cried even though I had a lot of support. People would talk to me, try to reason with me—still I just wanted to die. But then always my mind would come back to "I have three sons who still need me. I can't just die." [a sixty-five-year-old woman]

In the last four years I have come from the depths of despair to feeling that life is good and that there still is a reason and a need for me to be in this world. At the beginning I continued to live because I felt my children had been through enough and they didn't need any more grief. It took a long time before I started to live for myself. I functioned extremely well most of the time (everyone always said how well I coped) but felt like I was just going through the motions, waiting for my husband to come home. [a woman in her fifties]

Particularly stressful is loss of a partner in a relationship that was not publicly acknowledged. If you have lost a lover and few of your friends and acquaintances knew of the relationship, you may feel quite alone with your grief, and have to carry on without the usual social supports that are mobilized for the widow. Even if you have been open about your relationship, friends may not fully appreciate the depth of your loss.

Recently I vacationed with friends who had been friends also with my deceased partner-in-life. A guest arrived with slides of earlier vacations, including pictures of my lover.

*I objected that if I had been a man who had been recently widowed, they surely would have asked if I would object to showing the pictures. One friend responded that she wanted very much to see them. She blanched when I suggested that she might feel differently after the death of her husband. Clearly, she thought that my relationship to Karen differed from her marriage; she evidently also thought my love differed from her friendship with Karen only by degree. Heterosexuals really do not understand what lesbians feel for their partners, even when they know us well. All of these friends had known Karen and me as lovers and had sent me bereavement condolences when Karen died.**

For a few women, the death of a spouse is a relief from a relationship that they may have wanted to leave earlier but for one reason or another were not able to. This situation can also be painful, as we grieve for the kind of relationship we might have hoped for when we first married.

For years I stayed in a marriage with an abusive husband because I was always afraid to divorce for economic reasons. After all, where was I to go and how would I be able to support myself? I did miss him for the year following his death. I never minded taking care of him while he was ill. After all, he was family. But I did resent all of the earlier years when he was so dominating and critical. Being a widow is my first freedom. I have a good relationship with my children and with my brothers and sisters. I have friends of long standing. I don't mind being alone at all. No one yells at me . . . I do what I want. [a seventy-eight-year-old woman]

It is not uncommon for recently widowed women to continue to receive guidance from their husbands, in dreams, in daydreams, in convictions that "this is just what he would want me to do." Women who were accustomed to relying on a husband, who have not had a lot of experience making their own decisions, may need time to accept that the ideas they are willing to trust, the advice they consider wise, come from themselves.

I still have dreams—not as often as I did when Bill first died—that he is giving me advice on how to do things. And it is always good advice; I listen to it. If I am ever undecided about something, he seems to come in my dreams and tell me what to do. [a sixty-seven-year-old woman, five years after the death of her husband]

Once a woman experiences some of the satisfactions of doing things for herself, she may begin to realize that she has many of the competencies she formerly ascribed to her husband.

Getting more education or a better-paying job is part and parcel of this process for many widows. Yet some women are reluctant to assume their independence and to feel the possibility of being active and powerful, as if managing for themselves would be disloyal or would diminish the importance of their past relationship.

Eventually, widows must restructure their lives as single women. We appreciate old friends who continue to call, to invite us and include us in their lives, but we may be disappointed in some who maintain the Noah's Ark system of social life: couples only. These friends may simply be afraid to confront the widow's grief. By avoiding her they can deny the possibility that death could disrupt their own relationship.[8]

While well-meaning friends and family may tell a widow to make new friends, find new interests, and create a new life for herself, many recently widowed women may need at first to reminisce about the past relationship, relive its good moments, hold on to the sense of the continuing presence of the lost spouse. If the relationship was a deep and involving one, then a widow's new life must be made out of parts of the old, and some of these parts must now be retrieved from the ended relationship. This is a way that many widows preserve the continuity of their lives.

My children, family, and many friends have been extremely supportive. Contrary to the experiences of many widows, the friends who are couples and who were friends of my husband and myself have continued to include me in their social lives. For the first two years or so it was usually too painful and I preferred not to spend too much time with them, but they were persistent and continued to invite me. In the last several months I have

*Excerpted from an unpublished manuscript by Carolyn Ruth Swift.

felt more comfortable and it is easier and even pleasant to join them sometimes. Most of my other social life is with women friends and family. I haven't "dated" at all but feel that if the opportunity arises I am ready to consider a new relationship. [a fifty-two-year-old woman]

Married friends, adult children, and relatives usually find themselves inadequate to the task of comforting a recent widow. Once the apparent emergency and the immediate needs are past, the widow is expected to pick up her own life and take care of herself. This is the time when the grieving person tends to feel most abandoned and helpless. But our lifetime habit of forming friendships and creating extended emotional "networks" contributes, according to researchers, to women's greater ability to survive after widowhood.[9]

Only someone who has actually been through the same experience can fully appreciate and meet the continuing needs of a grieving widow. This is why various kinds of widow-to-widow networks—both the ones that deal with practical matters such as balancing a checkbook and the ones that focus more on emotional issues—have been growing.[10] Being part of a group of women dealing with loss helps us understand that grief is appropriate and normal. In such groups we can feel freer than we do among family and friends to expose the depth of our pain and loss, knowing that we will be understood.

BEING SINGLE

Contrary to the prevailing stereotypes, a study of fifty single women aged from sixty-five through the mid-nineties found that those women who had never married were as embedded in relationships and social networks as women who were presently, or had been, married. For many women, the world of work was an important source of friends, but in retirement many went on to initiate new friendships with neighbors or members of organizations to which they belonged. Families were also a significant source of important relationships, especially siblings.[11]

These women understand the importance of friendship; they have had the lifelong habit of reaching out to other women and the freedom to do so. Women who have been single all their lives are probably less likely than married women to go through midlife upheavals.

Older single women we spoke with expressed satisfaction with their lives and their choices.

Single? I feel great about what I've seen and what I've passed up. I haven't missed a thing. I have a good many friends. Most of my closest friends have been married, a few single. I made matches but not for myself, even though I did have three different engagement rings which they never would take back. I eluded all attempts to marry. If I had my life to live over again I think I would marry—it's nice to have children. But being single has given me a lot of freedom to do what I want when I want. I help others solve problems, rather than have my own. My relationships have grown richer. My friends and I appreciate each other more. Many of us are still around and we've gone through a lot together. Today, we have a little more in material comfort than we started out with and we have friendships that have lasted a lifetime. [a seventy-two-year-old woman]

In generations past, marriage was the norm for women, and the main concern of their families. Not to marry was to be an outsider. Singleness was a stigma.

I was a pediatrician for forty-odd years, of which I am proud. But do you know what? At family gatherings and in the old neighborhood they still see me as the one who didn't marry. Not as the first in the family to go to college. Not as one of the first Catholics admitted into the fancy medical school I attended. Not as a well-known physician in Philadelphia. No, just as Sally, "the one who never got married."[12]

Often it is only in the middle years, when the supply of potential mates is dwindling and

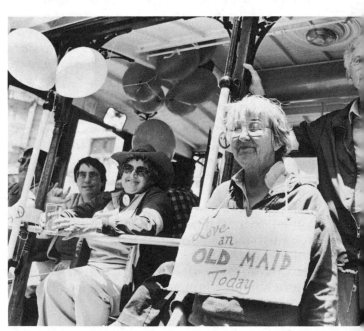

Cathy Cade

it becomes clear that one's life-style is firmly established, that women admit to themselves that they have made a choice and that they are happy with it.[13] Some women for whom sexuality has not been a priority may have truly preferred to be celibate. Others have guarded their personal freedom by making their sexual lives, with men or with women, a small and perhaps temporary part of their lives. Whatever the reason, once the choice is recognized and accepted, it opens up new possibilities for security and comfort. Buying a house, deciding on a new geographical location, joining resources with other women in business or leisure, and providing for old age all complete the life of the single woman.

In later years, loneliness and isolation can be a serious problem for older women who have outlived their friends, spouses, or partners. If you are feeling isolated, if your neighborhood has changed and you find you no longer know many people, senior citizens' centers can be good places to find new activities and to meet people.

I say to them, why don't you just get out and come on up to the center? Everyone misses you there. We're really getting that garden we started in shape. It's beautiful! But we need your help. I know how hard it can be sometimes to get out with all the aches and pains, but we have to keep going. [a sixty-eight-year-old woman]

You can't just sit and wait for someone to come to you. They won't. Let's face it, old people are easy to forget, not through any fault of their own but because everyone is so busy these days. Young people don't have the time to sit around and talk. So we have to make more of an effort ourselves. I call my folks even if they don't call me. I know some people who just sit around all alone and then get mad if nobody calls them. They've got the telephone right there and probably have more time than a lot of people to make the calls and keep in touch. [a woman in her seventies]

For women who've been divorced or widowed after a long marriage, it is not easy to begin again. Perhaps you have spent most of your adult life within a family where you had to expend little energy to maintain comfortable contact with close friends. Close association with your family and your husband's family and with friends who also socialize in couples may have met all your social needs. Now you have to become more assertive in reaching out to others.

EMPOWERMENT STRATEGIES IN RELATIONSHIPS

by Dorothy Frauenhofer

- Make a list of all the good things you do for others. Make a list of all the good things you do for yourself. Are you shortchanging yourself?
- Keep a continuing list of your strengths. Try to reach a list of one hundred. Join groups whose endeavors inspire you to develop your strengths.
- Rid yourself of negative thoughts about yourself. Replace them with thoughts from your strengths list.
- Do your negative thoughts come from others in your life? Consider ways to spend less time with those who reinforce your negative view of yourself. Reach out to others who appreciate your strengths and support you.
- Are you close to someone who is abusive? Consider ending that relationship, or at least making it less central in your life.
- Visualize yourself using your strengths to create healthier relationships, a new environment, a new job. Be creative and open-minded. Visualize being the strong, healthy, powerful person you wish to be.

I needed a new social life. With older couples, you begin to feel you don't belong with them any more. I looked for single people to be with because they understood my problems. After my divorce I wanted to talk about the hurt and disappointment, but my married friends didn't want to hear about it. Perhaps they didn't want to acknowledge that it could happen to them too. So we grew apart.

I had a girlfriend who was a widow. She said, "You can't sit home." We Latin people love to dance and go to parties, so she took me to a party at her church for widowed people. When I protested that I was not a widow, she said, "Who cares?" At first, it was a mixed group of mostly widowed people. Recently, more divorced people have joined the group. [a sixty-year-old woman]

NEW PARTNERS

Many women are eager to find a new partner, if not immediately after their marriages end, certainly at some point thereafter. This is when the insecurities of aging, of changing values, and of confused expectations come into play. It is perhaps useful to consider that we are not starting over from the beginning, but from where we are right now. The search for love, companionship, and new friendships may take us down some roads we never thought we'd take. Many women try new activities such as community theater, adult education, or political-action groups that suit their talents, interests, and time schedules. Although it's a bit like entering a sweepstakes (the odds for finding true love may not be so good), the fun of new activities and sometimes curiosity about who is "out there" can be very energizing. Consider reaching out beyond your usual circle. You may find new friends who are appropriate to the new person you are in process of becoming.

I want someone like myself, with some education, but not so smart that I would bore him, someone I could get along with. I almost married again. I met someone who took the time to get to know me. I was unhappy and he lifted me out of my unhappiness. He made me feel that I deserved love and respect when I had been feeling that I was "finished" in my forties, an old bag. I was afraid that I would end up living in a rooming house or having to move in with one of my kids, so I was going to marry him. But he was old-fashioned. He wanted to do things a way that I used to like, but that I don't want any more. He didn't want me to work after we were married or to own my own house. We couldn't seem to agree on anything so the relationship fizzled out. But he did me the big favor of making me feel valuable, that I was a mature, beautiful woman, even though I was no longer young. [a fifty-nine-year-old woman]

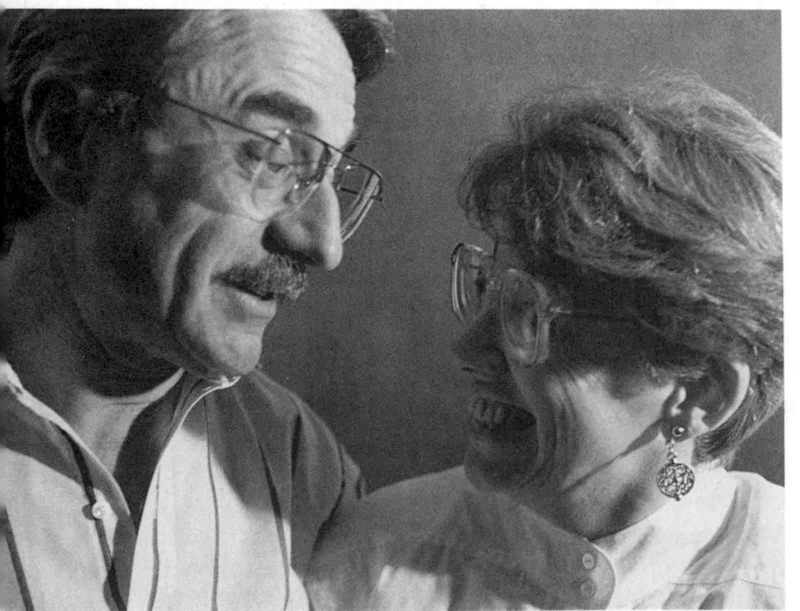

Ben Doress

Some women find someone they care about enough to risk a second marriage. Remarriage can be challenging, yet experience and maturity can make it an easier adjustment than it was the first time around.

My present husband is more supportive and less critical than my first husband. We're very different and that makes this marriage astonishing and full of surprises. If we'd married young the differences between us would have overwhelmed us. In middle age the differences are sort of a lark—they're intriguing. Here's this person who has to watch baseball. In my twenties I would have felt quite critical because I would have thought it reflected on me and my taste in men, but when you're fully formed in your middle years it doesn't bother you. Instead the differences between you keep the relationship surprising and fresh. [a fifty-seven-year-old woman]

Lesbian Partnerships

Over the years, some women who were thought to be single have in fact been in discreet lifelong relationships with other women, which for reasons of public opinion had to be kept secret. Though the social strictures are less severe than formerly, many women are still understandably reluctant to make their sexual preference known. For other women, however, the relaxation of social attitudes has provided a liberating atmosphere in which to exercise new options. Some women, after years as wives and mothers, turn to a lesbian relationship and become part of a community of women. Whether our friendships with women will also include sexuality is a matter of very personal preference, but knowing that there is such a possibility can be very liberating.

I feel so lucky to have the choice in this period of women's liberation to leave behind society's negative attitude about women and instead be a woman-identified woman. How rich we are in wisdom, experience, talents, and skills! I believe we have within us the necessary balance to turn the society around and I am a part of that movement! [a woman in her fifties]

Around the age of forty, I began realizing that I was sexually attracted to women, but I continued to date men until I fell in love with a woman at age forty-five and began a long-term relationship. I was married for sixteen years and have two adult children. I am now in a rela-

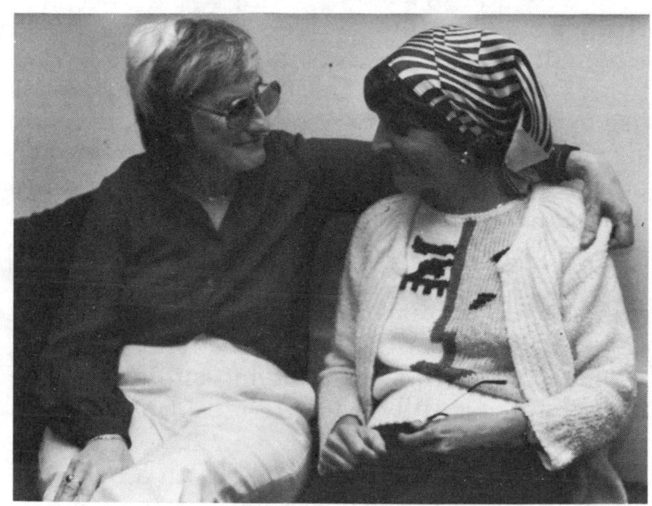

Elizabeth Furdon

tionship with a West Indian woman which has presented me, as a Jewish woman, with numerous challenges in terms of cultural and racial differences.

I feel that my life would be far more limiting if I were still heterosexual and erotically dependent on men. I find traditional men of my age sexist, controlling, patronizing, and unable to express emotion . . . qualities which are unattractive and boring.

Although the stigma and restrictions of homosexuality certainly affect me, I love being a lesbian. I love the companionship of women and a life-style where my relationships are primarily with women. [a woman in her fifties]

The advantage of such a "coming out" is the existence of a ready-made supportive community that the new lesbian can enter. Yet as the following experience shows, acceptance may take a while.

After twenty-five years as wife and mother, the label I heard when I first mingled with lesbians was that I was not a real lesbian. I didn't understand—after all, wasn't I in love with another woman? I was confused and intrigued at the same time that lesbians expected me to be strong, self-supporting, with a place out there in the world. No one was interested in the passive, unopinionated woman I had been who knew how to use her body seductively for attraction and approval. I had to learn how to be with lesbians—to develop my knowledge and creativity at a deeper level than I had ever before been challenged to do.

Now I realize that I was still acting like a privileged heterosexual princess. Even though lesbians depend emotionally on others, they are usually self-supporting. I had never been trained to be that and I still expected, on some level, that someone would take care of me. I am grateful for the lesbian community's higher expectations. I have discovered a lot of inner strength and know now that I can be financially, emotionally, and mentally self-supporting, and that is freedom! [a fifty-four-year-old woman]

There are, of course, risks in changing sexual orientation. Those who are close and dear to us may find the change too drastic and withdraw, or refuse to accept our newfound selves, friends, or lovers.

I was involved with a woman and my daughter said, "Are you planning to come to Thanksgiving dinner?" and I said, "Oh sure I am, and I'd like to bring Elaine with me too." She said, "I don't think that's a very good idea. The families have talked about it and we thought it would be better if you just come alone." Then she added, "Why don't you come and just try to act like a real grandmother?" That taught me a great deal because I did not want to come to Thanksgiving dinner and act like a real grandmother because I don't know what that is. "What the hell is that? A real grandmother!" I said. "There isn't a model." [a sixty-three-year-old woman]

I remember the morning I greeted my friend of twenty years with the usual hug and kiss, then sat her down to tell her I had become a lesbian. She listened as we talked for hours, and told me she didn't understand at all, but would remain my friend. When she got up to go, and I approached her for a goodbye hug, she put out her hand at arm's length and said, "I cannot hug you anymore." That really hurt. [a fifty-four-year-old woman]

If we come from a social world where women and men mingle, we may long for the comfort and security of social acceptance. We may be fortunate in carrying some friends over from former days, but they, too, now lack our experience. Realizing that we may lose old friends both compels and enables us to embrace a concept of "family" that includes a larger community. Maintaining relationships is an important value of the lesbian community and women who formerly were lovers often remain close and supportive friends.

The lesbian community that we see at women's dances, at concerts, in bars, often seems to have found the key to eternal youth. Already disoriented in many ways, an older woman new to lesbian life may miss the companionship of women her own age. In some large cities, organizations specifically for older lesbians (and gay men) can help you meet other women your age. It is important to find a balance between former friends and new friends who are lesbians, even if you find yourself among women your daughter's age. Changing your sexual preference can make you feel insecure for a while, and you will need other lesbians for support. It is a rare old friend who can talk with you about your new self-discovery without questioning your choice or feeling threatened by it.

As lesbians, we have sharpened our wits and shaped our viewpoints on discrimination and the struggle for survival. We are drawn, as are many women, to the fight for women's rights over our bodies, for our rights not to be abused sexually, emotionally, or physically, for the restoration of health to the earth, for peace and a decent standard of living all over the world, and for the rights of those of our loved ones most vulnerable: children and frail elders. For some of us the work is never done as long as we feel the pinch of discrimination in our own lives. [a fifty-six-year-old woman]

LIVING IN COMMUNITY

It is important for women at any age to overcome the notion that we are somehow incomplete if we are not married or involved in a long-standing sexual relationship. The middle and later years can be a time to achieve a balance between companionship and solitude. It can help to stop thinking of our unpartnered state as aloneness, and to think of ourselves instead as moving toward living in community. We have many choices to make in this new way of life.

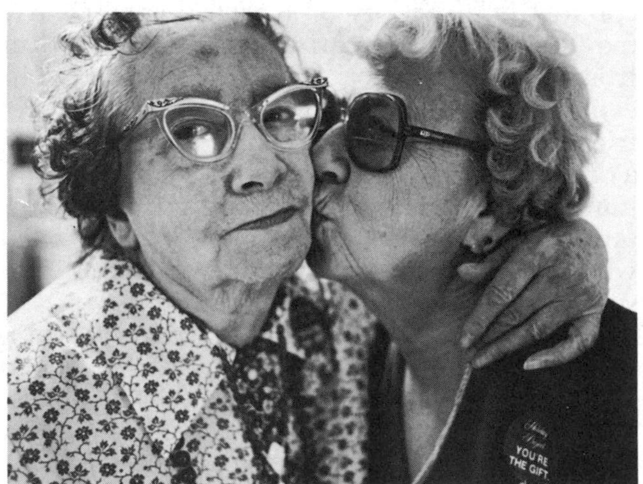

Marianne Gontarz

How big a community feels comfortable, and whom do you want to include in it? Do you want to see friends more often? Think about what you like to do and which of your friends would enjoy sharing that activity with you. Reaching out to other women in similar circumstances to yours can be a good source of new friendships. Women's and senior organizations, community activist groups, adult-education classes, and exercise and recreational activities are just a few of the many ways to meet new friends. Do you want to consider a group-living situation? The next chapter is full of helpful ideas and ways to begin exploring.

If you find yourself excited about a new creative pursuit or political agenda, you may find as you join groups or classes that you meet new people who share your passion, a wonderful basis for new friendships. We are never too old to begin new friendships.

NOTES

1. Heading borrowed from a book of the same title by Karen Lindsey. Boston: Beacon Press, 1981.

2. Freda Rebelsky, "Friends: Who Needs Them? Part II," a lecture reprinted in *The Community Church News,* November 1986, 565 Boylston St., Boston, MA 02116.

3. Lillian B. Rubin, *Women of a Certain Age: The Midlife Search for Self.* New York: Harper & Row, 1979.

4. Zenith Henkin Gross, *And You Thought It Was Over: Mothers and Their Adult Children.* New York: St. Martin's Press, 1985.

5. Susan Christian, "Grandparent Anxiety." *Modern Maturity,* December 1983–January 1984, pp. 32–35.

6. Meredith Minkler and Kathleen M. Roe, *Grandmothers as Caregivers: Raising Children of the Crack Cocaine Epidemic.* Newbury Park, CA: Sage Publications, 1993.

7. Phyllis R. Silverman, *Helping Women Cope with Grief.* Newbury Park, CA: Sage Publications, 1981.

8. Ibid.

9. Knud Helsing, Moyses Szklo, and George W. Comstock, "Factors Associated with Mortality After Widowhood." *American Journal of Public Health,* Vol. 71 (1981), pp. 802–9.

10. Phyllis R. Silverman, *Widow to Widow.* New York: Springer, 1985; and Silverman, op. cit.

11. Barbara Levy Simon, *Never Married Women.* Philadelphia: Temple University Press, 1987.

12. Barbara Levy Simon, "C'est la Vie: Never Married Old Women and Disability: A Majority Experience." In Michelle Fine and Adrienne Asch, eds., *Voices from the Margins: Lives of Disabled Girls and Women.* Philadelphia: Temple University Press, 1987.

13. Nancy L. Peterson, *The Ever-Single Woman: Life Without Marriage.* New York: Morrow, 1982.

12

HOUSING ALTERNATIVES AND LIVING ARRANGEMENTS

✦

BY MICKEY TROUB FRIEDMAN

SHELTER POVERTY AND DISPLACEMENT BY CAROLINE T. CHAUNCEY

SPECIAL THANKS TO ELAINE OSTROFF FOR HELP WITH SECTION ON ADAPTIVE ENVIRONMENTS

1994 UPDATE BY MICKEY TROUB FRIEDMAN

RESOURCES FOR THIS CHAPTER ON PAGES 472–74

WINDOW LOCKS

Today I'm installing my condominium window
locks. Measure with the eye, then with scout
knife awl begin the screwhole. Drill. The bit
sticks. Turn the drill backward. It slips
off the bit. Work out the bit, replace it
in the drill. Measure screw against
finger at depth of hole on bit.

I could pay to have this done; but I save
money, enjoy the doing, keep out the cold
and some rampaging man on a ladder.
Til now all my locks were screwed in
by father, carpenter, husband. I searched
out this do-it-myselfing, raced after,
hounded, tackled, captured it
roll ecstatic with it now in my arms.

Try installing your own window locks.
You'll know why carpenters are proud,
insist on cash-in-the-palm. I am my own
journeywoman, nurtured by past lives, taught
by my father in his hobby shop, by handling
my mother's carpenter-father's tools.
I know these locks as I knew my babies'
bodies. The heat of my arms turns the drill.
I can install my own life.

Jane Strete

Housing is an important issue for everyone, and can be a critical one for middle-aged and older women. Beyond the need for a safe, comfortable, affordable place to live, having a sense of "home" is a vital part of identity, security, and community. Home is the center of life and, for many women, of work as well. Home, with its treasured mementoes and familiar furnishings, provides a link to the past and a feeling of rootedness.

As younger family members leave to live on their own, we may find ourselves rattling around a once-crowded house or apartment. We may move, alone or with a partner, to a quieter setting or a warmer climate upon retirement. As widowed or divorced women, we may find a formerly congenial suburb no longer hospitable and seek the companionship of other single women and men in an urban environment. We may revel in a room of our own, perhaps for the first time.

Whatever our circumstances, as we grow older most of us will experience a multiplicity of changes in health, income, family structure, and way of life, which in turn will influence both our housing preferences and the kind of housing available to us. Where we live and how we live is such an intrinsic part of our daily existence that even thinking about making a change can be

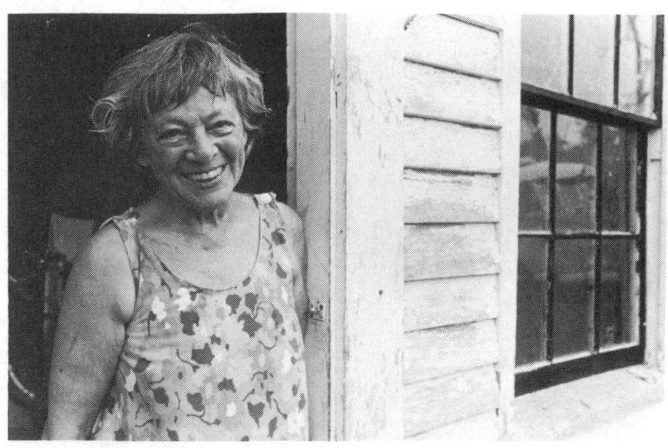

Marianne Gontarz

unsettling. But once you get started, simply by reaching out for information you begin to make connections with others engaged in the same search. The process itself contributes to creating a support network for the present as well as contacts you can draw upon in the future.

Shelter Poverty and Displacement

Maintaining an affordable home that meets our needs is one of the key challenges of our middle and later years. "Shelter poverty" is defined as spending so much money on housing and fuel that not enough is left over to meet other basic needs. Experts estimate that, ideally, no more than 30 percent of one's income should be spent on shelter. But 30 percent of a low income is simply not enough for decent housing, so many people who are technically above the poverty level are in reality "shelter poor." Nearly one third of the population spends more than 30 percent of its income on housing, and in more than 2 million households, total shelter costs take up a whopping 85 percent of the budget. Many older women live alone, and consequently their per-person housing cost is higher than for those who share housing with others.

With incomes either fixed or diminishing and the costs of both owning and renting a home steadily rising, shelter poverty thus becomes a major concern for older women. Housing problems associated with aging are even more difficult for black and Hispanic women, who are almost twice as likely to live in rental housing as are all other elderly. The National Urban League calls this "double jeopardy." Having more housing options available can help solve many of the problems women face in the second half of life.

The Housing Shortage and Homelessness

To keep up with the escalating demand for new housing, the federal government estimates that the construction industry would have to provide 2 million new housing units per year. But the gap in reaching that goal continues to widen. The tight housing supply is reflected in the low vacancy rates found in many major cities—often less than 5 percent.

Joining the ever-increasing number of homeless are younger individuals and families. Estimates range from a half million to over 2 million Americans becoming homeless in a year,[1] depending on who is describing the problem. The 1990 census found it impossible to determine an accurate count.

Adding to the problem of homelessness is the disappearance of single-room-occupancy (SRO) hotels in urban areas. Though these hotels are often dirty and dangerous, they are sometimes the only housing option available for many older people. In recent years, such hotels have been remodeled or torn down to make way for urban-development projects, with little thought given to finding new housing for the displaced former tenants. In some large cities more than 80 percent of the SRO units have been lost to condominium conversion and other redevelopment projects. Changes in the housing market have also resulted in the loss of lodging houses, which formerly provided a convenient or affordable housing alternative for some older people in many communities.

In New York City, the housing shortage has become so severe that special shelters for the elder homeless have been created. Contrary to prevailing stereotypes, these shelters serve many elders who are well educated and some who had owned their own homes in the past. Some had been evicted for nonpayment of rent and others lost an apartment when the building they lived in became a cooperative or condominium or was torn down. Some have incomes too low to qualify for market-level housing, but too high to qualify for subsidized housing.[2]

A number of activist and advocacy groups are working to end homelessness. The Community for Creative Non-Violence, based in Washington, D.C., studied thirty cities exhaustively and published the results in an excellent book, *Homelessness in America.*[3] Rosie's Place, a drop-in center, emergency shelter, and lodging houses in Boston, offers a place for women not only to sleep but also to eat and socialize, and get off the streets permanently. It serves 200 women daily with 25 staff and 300 volunteers. It has been offering its unique support for seventeen years, working with many civic and church groups, and is opening a residence for ten women with HIV/AIDS.

Also in Boston, The Committee to End Elder Homelessness, started by a group of women ages forty-seven to eighty-two, developed a congregate house for nine elderly homeless women. It sponsored a one-day survey of shelters that found 98 women among the 460 homeless persons over age fifty, more women than in previous estimates, and a higher percentage than among the younger homeless. Five of the homeless women were over seventy-five years old!* The committee has an outreach program for finding housing for homeless elders and is now developing a forty-six-unit building for women and men.

Construction of new housing is very slow. Low- or moderate-income housing is only marginally profitable, so the trend is toward building luxury apartments, condominiums, and expensive single-family homes. As the upwardly mobile move into newer and better housing, their former homes become available to lower-income households, but when this filtering process slows down, due to a shortage of new housing at all income levels, the overall quality of affordable housing declines. This presents particular problems for older women. If you are fortunate enough not to have to deal with these issues in your own life, you may want to add your voice and/or contribute money or resources to help address this problem.

**Old, Alone and Homeless: A Survey of Boston's Homeless Elders* is available for $4 from the Committee to End Elder Homelessness, Inc., 30 Wallingford Road, Boston, MA 02135.

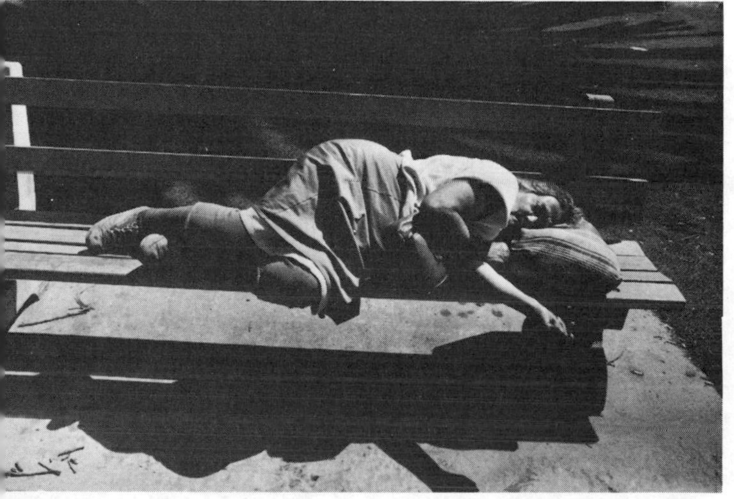

Norma Holt

WHEN NEIGHBORHOODS CHANGE

The evolution of a neighborhood is usually inevitable, but for elders, both improvement and deterioration can create problems. Gentrification can occur when developers or private investors buy inexpensive homes or buildings in moderate-income neighborhoods and renovate them, often for resale to more affluent buyers. With gentrification, property values rise—and with them, property taxes, building-code requirements, and rents. Along with the pressure of these added expenses, we may feel abandoned when friends move away or we may face a significant loss as the corner grocery is replaced by an espresso café. Even though gentrification increases the sale price of our homes, that money may not go far enough toward finding us an appropriate or comfortable replacement and it may be difficult for a woman on her own to obtain a mortgage or home-building loan.

Neighborhood deterioration can also make us feel uneasy or isolated. Programs to increase safety may not be reassuring when we feel threatened by street crime and an inadequate police presence. Banks' illegal practice of refusing to invest in low-income or minority neighborhoods, called redlining, may hasten the deterioration process. Loans are denied to people of color at twice the number that they are denied to whites, even when incomes are the same. Government agencies refuse to "test" real estate agents or landlords, and laws are often not enforced. However, there *are* legal ways for residents to preserve services and to press for reform.

IF YOU ARE A RENTER

There is no need to talk here about the many landlords who enjoy good relationships with their tenants. Our concern is with dishonest landlords who use such illegal tactics as verbal harassment, neglect of necessary repairs and safety precautions, reduction in utility service, or even deliberate damage to their own buildings to force out unwanted tenants. Such practices have shortened the lives of many elderly poor, including many women who may find it extremely difficult to defend themselves because of language

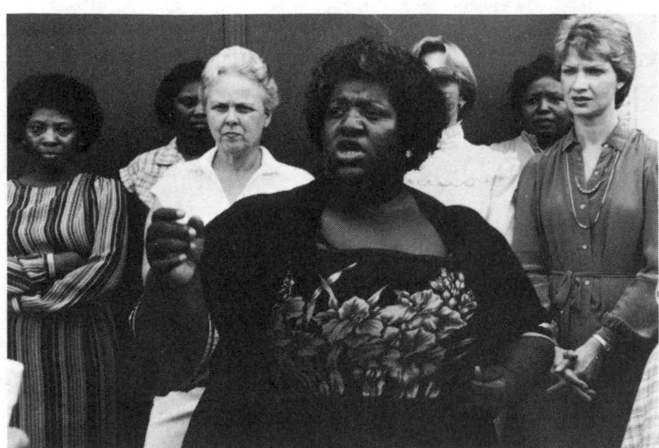

Elana Freedom

Tenants' Rights*

Regulations and ordinances to protect tenants can be complex, and vary so much from state to state that it would be impossible to summarize them here, but legal services for low-income elderly exist in every state and provide free assistance. This kind of help is provided in both urban and rural areas.

These five general principles of landlord-tenant law have nationwide applicability:

1. In most states, there is an implied "warranty of habitability," which means the landlord is required to provide decent housing in exchange for the payment of rent.
2. Most states have protection against evicting tenants in retaliation for their complaints about housing conditions.
3. In almost all states a landlord must use judicial procedures to evict tenants. A landlord cannot physically eject a tenant without a court order.
4. The Federal Fair Housing Act prevents discrimination against tenants on the basis of race, color, religion, national origin, physical or mental handicap, age, and sex. Discrimination on the basis of sex has been interpreted to also prohibit sexual harassment.
5. Most states have strict protections for tenant security deposits.

*Personal communication from Catherine M. Bishop of the National Housing Law Project, Berkeley, California.

barriers, lack of education, frailty, fear of retaliation, or because they don't feel comfortable "making a fuss." Don't allow yourself to be coerced. Find out what your rights are. Most tenants are unaware of their rights, as are many social-service professionals who work with them. Laura Monroe, an attorney with Greater Boston Legal Services, stresses that "it is very important to make good use of your day in court. There is nothing trouble-making about exercising your rights. Rights that are unused are like no rights at all."[4]

For those who want to get involved in advocacy, there are several good books available and opportunities at all levels to make an impact on housing policy. Federal cutbacks tightening income requirements and directing less money to large subsidized-housing complexes, coupled with escalating need, make this a time when advocacy is especially crucial. Get on political-action mailing lists, find out when hearings on housing will be held by your state legislature and by local agencies and organizations that share your concerns. It's an important time to add your voice to these issues! (See Resources for this chapter for a list of ways and places to add your voice.)

Getting Help from the Government—for Tenants and Prospective Owners

Federal subsidies for housing come in three major forms: vouchers, which enable renters to live in private housing; public housing projects, in which construction and operating costs are subsidized; and private or nonprofit subsidized housing. Commonly called "Section 8 subsidies," vouchers or certificates are administered by the U.S. Department of Housing and Urban Development (HUD). Only one fourth of households eligible for subsidies obtain them, however, and there can be a three- to five-year wait. Nevertheless, they are still worth applying for. If you do get one you can continue to live in your present apartment, paying no more than 30 percent of your income for rent—HUD pays the rest. Landlords *must* agree to accept government reimbursement and to comply with federal building codes for health and safety. The programs are complex; some offer the subsidy directly to income-eligible tenants and others offer it to owners or developers. To find out if you are eligible, how to apply, and how long the waiting lists are in your community, contact your local housing authority or state office on aging. Ask them about other programs in your area that may be more feasible for you.

Federal subsidies are also available to help defray fuel costs for both renters and homeowners. On the average, persons over sixty-five spend 30 percent of their income on energy.[5] The Federal Low Income Energy Assistance Program provides subsidies for households that meet certain income requirements. The program is badly underfunded (serving only one third of the eligible households), but priority is given to the elderly. An average subsidy is enough to cover between 20 and 30 percent of energy expenses. In addition, many states and some private agencies and utility companies offer consumers free energy audits and low-cost weatherproofing assistance.

If your apartment house is being converted to condominiums or going co-op, it may be worthwhile to buy your apartment if you can afford to. It may prove cheaper and more appropriate for your needs. Although the purchasing and operating costs for an apartment are usually lower than for a house, the tax advantages are the same. Federally insured mortgage and loan programs with lower-than-market interest rates offer additional assistance. HUD offers low-interest loans for condos, co-op housing, mobile homes, and rehabilitation of existing homes. Section 202 loans, available to nonprofit sponsors for new construction, are the only loans targeted specifically for elders and the disabled. The Farmers Home Administration offers several programs for those in rural areas: grants, loans at very low interest rates, and a rental assistance program [FmHA 515] similar to HUD's.

If You Own Your Own Home

Home-Equity Conversion

Home-equity conversion is a method that allows homeowners to convert some of what their house is worth into cash by selling it in advance, while continuing to live there for a number of years or for the rest of their lives. The term *home-equity conversion* covers a number of variations on this arrangement; information about them is continually updated (see Resources for this chapter). In one type of home-equity conversion, the "reverse mortgage," the homeowner receives monthly payments from a lender (usually a bank) that must be repaid at the end of the term. A reverse mortgage is useful only for a person who wants to stay in her home for about five to eight more years before moving to another situation. A "lifetime reverse mortgage" is more useful in most situations because it allows the homeowner to stay in her home, keep the title, and receive monthly payments plus a subsidy for maintenance. At the homeowner's death, the house becomes the property of the lender. It is preferable to make this arrangement with a prospective heir rather than with a financial institution. If you borrow from a relative or friend, you must still protect your legal right to stay in your home. Make sure all parties understand the agreement. In a "sale-leaseback," a public or private investor buys the house and agrees to lease it back to the original owner for that person's lifetime. If you enter into such an agreement, be sure that it provides for your right to stay in the house even in the event of a subsequent resale by the new owner. Some plans allow

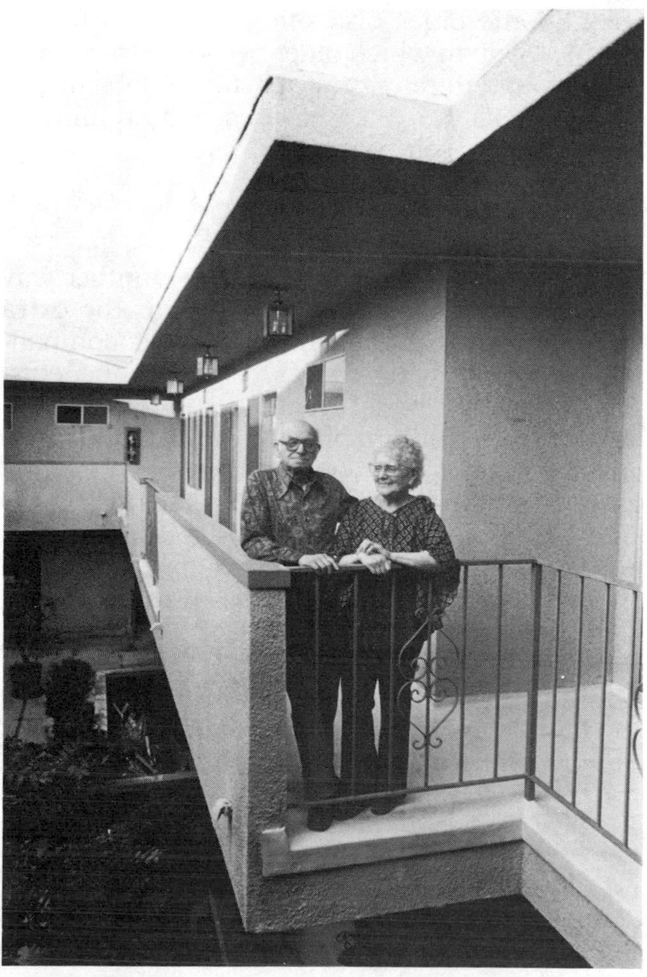

Jerry Howard/Positive Images

the original homeowner to retain occupancy for a specified time only, or to defer property taxes and the cost of basic repairs until the property is sold, either after the original owner's death or if she decides to move.

Homeowners interested in converting home equity into cash should seek professional advice regarding the tax and estate-planning issues involved in these complex transactions before proceeding. Such plans may also have an impact on eligibility for Medicaid, SSI, or other government benefits, since the regulations often allow for home ownership but limit the amount of cash or other assets a recipient may have (see Money Matters and Women's Health and Reforming the Medical Care System chapters).

TAX RELIEF

In many cities and towns homeowners over a certain age can obtain tax abatements, tax reductions, or tax deferrals, through which they postpone paying property taxes until the house is sold. Deferrals can also be obtained for repair costs. Some cities also offer tax work-off programs, through which older people work at minimum wage in temporary part-time jobs in city government until they have earned an amount equivalent to their property taxes.

TAKING IN RENTERS

Sharing the space in your home is another way to reduce housing costs. Along with the extra income, such an arrangement can offer companionship, help with chores, or other benefits. There are a number of creative ways to be a landlady with a minimum of aggravation. Tailor your arrangement to suit your needs for privacy and draw up a written agreement that includes a specific provision for evaluating and renegotiating it in the future. For example, a woman with three children still at home decided to rent rooms but keep the kitchen for her family's use.

There are always the mistakes (and the learning by them). It's important to have a contract so that everyone's expectations are understood. I've had numerous successful, delightful, and profitable experiences with tenants in the past eight years, and will continue to share the house as long as the arrangement works and the space is there. As a side benefit, I have made some good friends with whom I keep in touch. I feel that the rhythm established in this house is to allow a leisurely and pleasant "passing through" for a number of people, giving them time to think of the next step in their lives without the threat of having to leave. Keeping a business relationship and a comfortable psychological and physical distance helps each of us maintain our own private space.

A seventy-six-year-old woman who retired and worried about how to maintain her 130-year-old house with Social Security as her only source of income began renting rooms on a short-term basis to families of hospitalized people.

The first year I did this, I used to get so upset. It's hard not to feel bad for them. I'd think, what if I was far away from home? I'd want someone to talk to. If they have a motel room they go back and it's cold and lonely. Here they can come in and talk awhile. Somebody asked me if I was afraid to have strangers in the house. I told them that once someone comes in the front door, they're not a stranger.[6]

The bed-and-breakfast concept is growing in popularity, with benefits for both traveler and host.

I had moved into this seacoast community because I wanted to return to my roots. I decided to capitalize on my location and take people in overnight on a limited basis. This would not only supplement my income but add some spice to my life. And of course, one of the good things about bed and breakfast is that you can say no if you don't feel like having guests. [a seventy-nine-year-old woman]

LIVING ALONE VERSUS LIVING WITH OTHERS

One important decision to make is whether you want to live alone or with others. For some of us, the thought of having to accommodate the timetables, moods, habits, and needs of others may be a deterrent to shared housing. This may be especially true if we have often done that in the past—for parents, partners, roommates, spouses, and children.

I like living alone. It's peaceful. There's nobody to boss me around. The hardest time for me was when my husband first went to the hospital. We were married thirty-three years and did everything together. Work, too. He was a fine carpenter and we had an antiques business. His doctor told me I couldn't live alone "out there in the woods," but I told him since I was a little girl someone has always told me what to do. Then, after my husband died, I was almost crazy, but I got hold of myself, and I fixed a rocking chair that was in such bad condition that he had said *he'd never fix it. Well, I did—and I sold it for $35.00! So I found out I could get along alone. And that was twenty years ago and I'm still at it. At seventy-six, I work as much as I want to, and I do get out and see people—but only when I feel like it. I even helped fix my own roof last summer! People are always asking me why I don't have a telephone. Well, I don't need one! I have so many friends here, and I can always walk down the road and use my neighbor's phone if I have to. And besides—I still ride my bicycle whenever I want. One of my friends and I cook dinner together almost every night, either at her house or mine. And sometimes we go out to eat. We pick apples, strawberries, go fishing, arthritis or not. I'm a very lucky person!* [a seventy-six-year-old woman]

I like quiet—I don't *like silence, there is a difference—and depending on how I am feeling, I may have the radio or TV on even if I am not paying attention, because it is too silent otherwise. In talking with others, I gather that this is not at all unusual. I do miss sharing a home with someone and yet I must say that I also really like the fact that I have a wonderful home which I have put together by myself. I like being able to do what I want when I want.* [a woman in her fifties]

Still, many of us find that no matter how active we are, how full our social or professional lives, living alone can be painful.

In spite of supportive children and a large circle of friends, I really don't like the idea that I may be living alone for the rest of my life. I even tried having a dog but the disadvantages and limits to my freedom outweighed the joy of having her there to greet me as I opened my door. She is now romping happily on a farm, while I am often lonely and wondering what's next for me. [a woman in her fifties]

One of the reasons I opt for shared living in some form is that it can provide a balance which most of us need: privacy along with an opportunity for informal companionship. I even like the adjustments I have to make when my pattern comes in conflict with others. There is great satisfaction in learning to agree and work together in running our joint enterprise. I've found that a sense of being at home is a realizable goal. It may be greatly different from the home we grew up in or that we had when we were on our own, but it can have as much validity as those other homes. [a woman in her seventies]

SELECTING A HOUSEMATE

How we go about finding someone to live with can vary with our individual circumstances. Some of us are lucky enough to have a close friend with whom we can share a house. Or we

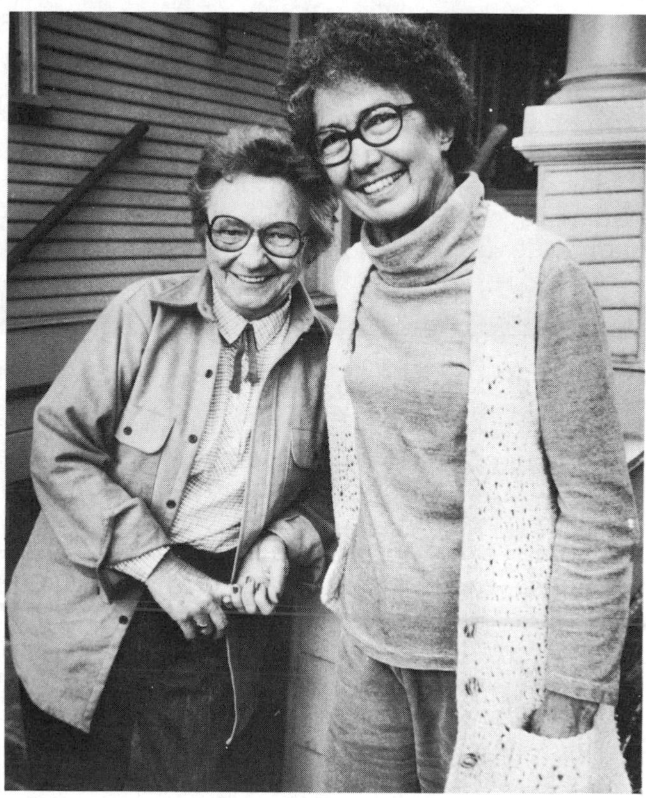

Nick Lammers

may start out with a temporary arrangement and find it so successful that it becomes permanent.

I met a teacher at the institution where I did volunteer work who was urgently looking for an apartment. She moved in temporarily with my father and me. She was helpful in doing things for my father that I didn't have time for, such as watching the ball game with him or taking him for a ride. I in turn would get the meals. After my father died, we just kept living together. For twenty years my roommate and I have had very separate but compatible lives. Financially she is better off than I am. It would be difficult for me to live alone on my shrinking pension. We still split everything right down the middle, except that she always had a car and I had household furnishings. I eat at home and entertain more than she and we often don't have lunch or dinner together, but we split everything. I became a "member" of her family, an adopted sister. When I have been hesitant to spend my more limited money, she will say "I think you should do it" and will provide the funds. Whatever happens, happens, but after twenty years of being roommates, I would expect us to stay together. In my will I leave everything to her. [a seventy-two-year-old woman]

If there is no one in your circle who is interested in shared living and if you have never advertised for a housemate before, you may want to get some help. In addition to informal or private arrangements, specific home-sharing programs may exist in your area. Check with women's centers, social-service agencies, senior centers, Area Agencies on Aging, or your state department of elder affairs. Check also with your church, synagogue, YMCA, or other community agency. If you want help choosing, checking references, or saying no to someone, a social worker or other neutral third party can serve as a mediator and can provide support.

If you can afford to own your own home, you may want to explore cohousing. Residents build and own their own homes on cooperatively owned land with the purpose of creating an intentional community. (See Resources, page

TIPS FOR SUCCESSFUL HOME SHARING

by Fran Roberts

1. Spend some concentrated time together before you make a decision to share a home. Take a trip together, share a vacation house, spend a long weekend in each other's present homes.

2. Try to be clear, not only with a potential housemate but also with yourself, about your real plans and hopes for the future. If they include the possibility of marriage, remarriage, or a continuing relationship that may be uncomfortable for your housemate(s), or if for some other reason you have doubts about how permanently you'll stay in the house-sharing situation, discuss the matter honestly. If you're not sure about the permanence of your plan, it might be better to share a rental arrangement.

3. Discuss every aspect of your arrangement in advance, especially what provisions you want to make in the event that one person dies or chooses to withdraw. For example, does the remaining partner have lifetime use of the home and its furnishings? Can the remaining partner buy out the other's share? What provisions do you want to make for heirs? After you have mutually determined what you want to accomplish, work with a lawyer to develop the documents necessary to achieve your goals. These might include a written contract, a trust agreement, and new wills. Tell your family what's been decided.

4. If you're planning to share a house by owning it jointly, it often works out better not to share a house that one partner already owns. It's easier to establish new ground rules and break old patterns in an environment that is new to everybody. This can be especially important if either woman has children living at home. If you must consolidate into one partner's house, bring some of the other partner's things in and buy some new things together as soon as your budget allows.

5. You will need to clarify which decisions you will make individually and which jointly. It usually works best when both partners have a reasonably equal amount of spendable income, because without financial equality, joint decision making—the core of a successful relationship—is much more difficult. However, where there is a strong desire to live together and where all parties believe in the principle, it can also work for each to contribute according to her means, recognizing the value of nonmonetary contributions to a household.

6. Set up a joint bank account for household expenses in addition to your personal accounts. Discuss recurring expenses such as utilities, fuel, and mortgage payments, and how they will be handled, as well as major obligations such as property taxes, insurance premiums, housing maintenance, and improvements.

7. Set up a "kitty," or petty-cash fund, for day-to-day expenses such as groceries, and contribute equal amounts, preferably at the same time, to avoid confusion.

8. Be prepared for a few raised eyebrows from people who are curious about whether there is a sexual basis to your relationship, and decide together how to deal with this. Don't be surprised or dismayed if some jealousy erupts from a child, sibling, or close friend who feels threatened by her or his displacement in your life. Consideration of the needs of family and friends—and time—will work wonders in reducing tensions caused by the novelty of your living arrangements.

473, for information on the subject of cohousing.)

What Makes Shared Living Work

The most important factor in the success of shared living arrangements is the willingness of all parties to change and compromise.

Living involves changes. Shared living is no exception. I have seen many changes both in situations and in the people who have shared them. I like it that way. Static living can be a bore. [a seventy-eight-year-old woman]

Another factor is respect and consideration of the desires, responsibilities, and needs of each person involved. Does one housemate have a child who is away at school but still living at home during part of the year? Or does one invite grandchildren for school vacations? Do any of you have frail or elderly relatives who may need temporary care? How will your prospective housemate(s) react to a short visit from a friend or lover (old or new), or an extended visit by an adult daughter or son who returns to the nest after a broken relationship or a lost job? Though no one can foresee the future, such issues should be clarified as much as possible before, not after, people decide to share a home.

Once housemates are living together, periodic house meetings or discussions are useful for evaluating how things are working out, airing differences, and negotiating changes.

Two women in their fifties, each having raised two children, decided to combine their resources and share their lives. One is divorced, the other widowed. On the opposite page the latter offers some suggestions that have worked well for them.

Communal or Group Living

This is an alternative that is usually associated with younger people but can work well with any age group or with persons representing a range of ages. It is usually an informal arrangement planned and carried out by the residents themselves without the help of agencies or professionals.

At midlife and newly divorced, Betty Dexter moved to Maine, where she took a course in house building and with her children built a fine house in the woods. As her children began leaving home, she realized that limited job and social opportunities began to outweigh the value of the rural tranquility she had earlier sought. Ever a woman of action, she investigated housing opportunities in a nearby large city, and was courageous enough to risk another new beginning. Her story is on the next page.

Intergenerational Living

While many older people enjoy the company of their own generation, others have a strong preference for mixed-age housing. Young adults with no family members nearby can turn to older housemates for counsel, inspiration, and wisdom, while older women who either have never had children, live far away from their children and grandchildren, or have outlived all their family members can enjoy the companionship of younger housemates. The energy of the young can be channeled toward repairs and maintenance, snow shoveling, spring cleaning, heavy shopping, while elder housemates contribute time and skills to less physically demanding jobs.

Many old people prefer not to uproot them-

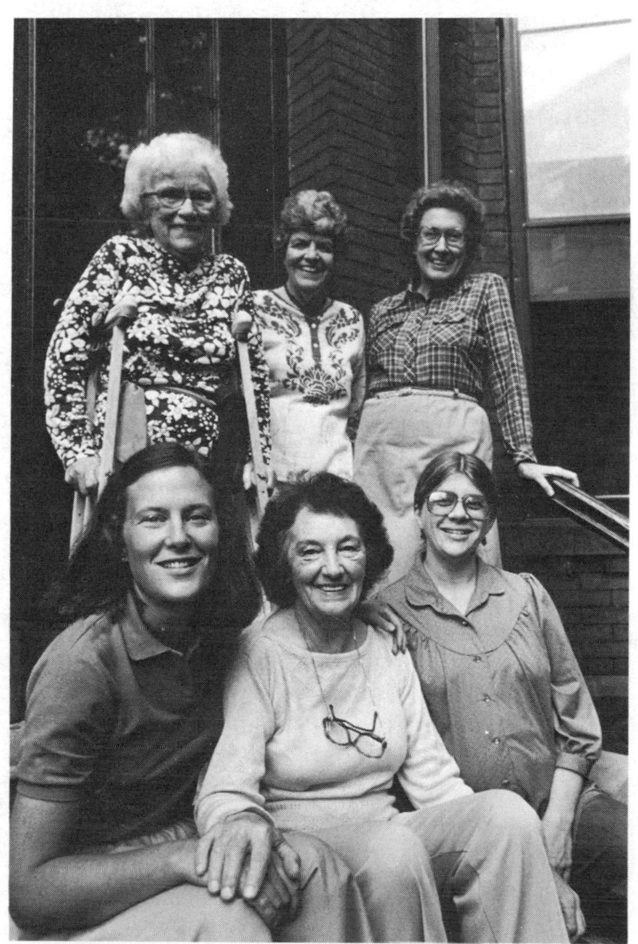

Sarah Putnam

selves from long-established ties to friends, neighborhoods, churches or synagogues, clubs, health-care practitioners, or the comfort of familiar places. Having learned to cope with public transportation, social-service systems, medical resources, and other benefits or aggravations of a particular environment, they'd rather accommodate having new housemates than move to a new community.

The most familiar form of intergenerational living is the tradition of members of the same family sharing a house: either younger persons

Cheaper by the Dozen

by Betty Dexter

When people hear that I live with eleven other people, they raise their eyebrows and ask, "You're fifty-eight, why do you want to live like a hippie?" "How do you stand the noise?" "Don't you want privacy?" "Do you have a lock on your bedroom door?"

I really don't know where to begin—the image of group living, in so many minds, is one of chaos, dirt, nightly orgies, and deafening stereos. Our house has none of these. We are a multigenerational group of adults who want to save money and who believe that community is healthier than aloneness. Otherwise, we are the same as the rest of the world: we like our home clean; we want love, not one-night stands; and we enjoy solitude as well as festivity.

Where my life greatly differs from that of most single women my age is in the area of responsibility. I do not want to pay for, insure, repair, polish, paint, tend, display, or worry about a house and its furnishings. But I want to live well. To me that means not only comfort and good food but stimulation and fun. Group living provides all of these and much more. I'm not living barricaded behind multiple locks because I fear unfamiliar steps outside my door. My social life is based on a bunch of people doing things together. In our house there are joggers, music and art lovers, and sports fans. Some people love board games while others retire to their rooms with a new book. I and two others are theater buffs. But most important, all of these pursuits are guilt-free because the time for them is not stolen from our duties.

How do we run a sixteen-room house and still have lots of leisure? Organization. It's not a perfect world and sometimes people slack off, but on the whole this is the grand plan:

Decision making:	Everybody attends house meetings twice a month.
Food shopping:	Rotation (two persons responsible for each six-week period).
Cooking:	Everyone makes her or his own breakfast and lunch. Twice a month each member cooks dinner for the group and cleans up afterward.
Kitchen cleaning:	Rotation (one person every twelve weeks; the job takes three hours).
Painting:	Everyone paints her or his own room. We have a once-a-year painting party at which everybody paints the common areas.

Other jobs, such as figuring and paying bills, cleaning bathrooms and living/dining/-guest rooms, and performing minor repairs, are done by those who choose them. If a person gets sick of some job, he or she asks for a change and somebody swaps. When people leave, jobs are rearranged so nobody ends up, as the average housewife does, doing the same old jobs for a lifetime. If you have a bad back, you never have to lift a storm window. If you're hopeless at math, forget it, the bill payer will struggle with the bank statements.

At present my jobs are cleaning the living and dining rooms and washing the house linens. I usually devote Saturday morning to these chores. Besides that, I cook two big dinners monthly and in exchange I get twenty-two free evenings in which I come moving in with parents or older relatives, or an older parent coming to live with adult offspring and their children.

I am so fortunate that I still live in the house and in the town where I grew up and had my [medical] practice. Although I never married, I felt as close to my sisters' children as if they were my own, and now it's their children who live with me and help keep this place going. I do all the cooking and some of the cleaning, and it works out just fine for all of us. [a woman in her eighties]

Though it is common today to look back with nostalgia at extended-family living arrangements, not all of these were idyllic. Many families lived together under the pressures of tradition or economic necessity, while chafing at the limitations on their freedom. Today, families who share a house are more likely to *want* to live together and to have compatible values and lifestyles.

I've often wondered what my son and his family get out of living with me. My son and daughter-in-law both work and make good money, but they've never said anything about wanting to buy a house. I think I give my grandchildren a certain amount of security, especially because their parents aren't always there. If they want anything or need anything they come and ask me.

What do I get out of it? Respect and being comfortable in my own home. I feel safe and I enjoy the contact. They clean the house. My grandsons take care of the yard, though I wish I didn't always have to tell them to. But when I do they are very polite and say, "Yes, Grandma," and it's done. [an eighty-five-year-old woman]

If you are thinking of sharing a home with your parents or adult children, you should ask yourself some hard questions. Can you coexist as adults, or are there still unresolved power struggles between you? Are you—or they—flexible enough to adapt to new dynamics, new roles?[7] As with any other group-living situation, mutually agreed upon ground rules and periodic reevaluation will help establish an equitable distribution of responsibilities and resources.

After my mother died, my dad took early retirement and came to live with us in the country. I don't even know who asked who. It just sort of happened. Things worked out really well for a while and then he began to seem depressed. He was still "young" in many ways—had kept up with old friends in the city and talked a lot about working again. In the beginning he enjoyed baby-sitting for our boys, but as they grew older, my husband and I realized his attitude about discipline was different from ours and we often felt we wanted more control over our kids' lives. It began to be tense all the time—the boys felt torn in their loyalties and my dad felt unappreciated. It was really hard to begin, but we finally talked it out. We did this at the urging of a friend who had correctly

---

home, put my feet up, and wait for the dinner gong. I make two trips to the grocery store every sixth week with my "shopping buddy." About four times a year I do kitchen cleanup.

There! The drudgery's finished; now let's talk about other aspects of group living.

1. *One's mindset:* If you're a woman who is upset if the house does not reflect *your* taste, then you'll have to decide whether that's important in the great scheme of things. If it is, then don't move into a group house where the common rooms belong to everybody and are dioramas of diversity. This was a stumbling block for me. I now confine my decorating efforts to my own bedroom. If you haven't missed an issue of *Better Homes and Gardens* in years, think about this, because you don't want to be apologizing for your home.

2. *One's role:* In my first group experiment, I took in to live with me two young men who had been orphaned early in life. (I had lost custody of my own ten-year-old son just three months earlier.) Of course at the time I didn't see any connection, but shortly thereafter I found I couldn't say the things that needed to be said to make the house run well. I was too sorry for motherless boys during that period.

3. *One's openness to change:* I think you have to let go. Admit there is more than one way to wash lettuce; try exotic dishes you'd never make for yourself; go along with the gang to a "far-out" film. (I'll bet next year you won't even call it far-out.)

But finally, best of all, if a middle-aged woman stays alert and tuned in, she can become a star in *Group Living,* the only soap opera I know that runs seven days a week all year round without reruns or commercial interruption!

guessed that Dad wanted "out." He just didn't know how to tell us. We all had to acknowledge that the arrangement wasn't working any more. He's now on his own, happily back in the city, working part-time. He spends holidays with us and we're friends again. [a woman in her forties]

A new variation on the familial pattern of intergenerational living is that of unrelated persons of different generations sharing a home. A university program that was among the first to match people who had extra space with those who needed housing found that some of its most successful matches were between young adults and elders.

Mrs. D. is a woman in her early sixties who was widowed two years ago. She owns her own three-bedroom home in a suburb of Boston where she works daily as an accountant. She has a large circle of friends, mostly other widows. Because she is used to caring for someone and having someone there in the evenings, Mrs. D. requested a housemate from a local home-sharing program. Her first match was a young woman in the area for a six-month education program. That worked out so well that Mrs. D. has applied for her second match.[8]

After years of taking students into her home, one woman was cared for through a long and lingering illness by these same young people. Although they no longer lived with her, they took turns coming in and seeing to her needs. A lovely circle of caring![9]

Accessory Apartments and ECHO (Elder Cottage Housing Opportunity) Housing

One variation on intergenerational living is for an older person to live in a separate apartment, perhaps created specially for that purpose, in a single-family house occupied by her children or grandchildren (or other younger relatives or friends). This concept, called accessory apartments, is becoming increasingly popular in suburban communities across the country. It has a number of advantages, providing independent living for both generations with the opportunity for easier visiting and the reassurance of help and support when needed.

After I became a widow, I lived alone for twenty years and traveled all over the world until I was ninety-one, when I broke my hip. While I was recuperating, my only daughter and her husband fixed up an apartment for me within their house. I ate most of my meals with them, and we got along splendidly.

In ECHO housing, an older person lives in a small, separate unit built on the same lot as the home of a relative. With this arrangement, maximum independence can be maintained while assistance is close by if needed. This arrangement is more common in other countries. In the United States zoning regulations often forbid a second building on a single lot, or a second dwelling unit in a "single family" home. However, such regulations can sometimes be modified or changed. Or you can apply for an exception, variance, or special-use permit; since these apply to only one dwelling, neighbors are less likely to object, particularly if the new unit houses a family member.

Manufactured and Mobile Homes

The Office of Technology Assessment, a congressional agency, reported recently that the United States is lagging behind other nations, particularly Sweden and Japan, in developing high-tech, factory-produced housing components that could make home building significantly less expensive. Antiquated housing-industry regulations and local zoning ordinances continue to retard progress in this promising approach to providing well-designed housing at lower cost.[10]

Some women have found "mobile" homes[11] a low-cost energy-efficient alternative to conventional housing, either on their own land or in a trailer park. Zoning may be a problem, but recent technological and esthetic improvements in prefabricated houses or components (i.e., preassembled walls, windows) have inspired a new look at such restrictions. Recognizing the necessity for moderately priced housing, a growing number of communities have mandated that some land be set aside for such homes.

After my husband died my house was just too big, but I knew I could take care of a mobile home. So when I sold the house, I kept an acre to put this on. I added a base and two porches, so I could sit out in the summer, and I can walk to my job at the library—I've never driven, you know. I've lived in this village since I was thirteen. I know a lot about the history and I want to be a part of it. Lonesome? I'm seventy-six and I can't stop long enough to be lonesome! Besides, I have an extra bedroom and my divan opens up, so I have plenty of room whenever my grandchildren visit. I like being independent. It's been the perfect solution.

We have heard reports of women's communities developing in trailer parks, as women who moved there with their husbands upon retirement elect to stay after widowhood. The women establish firm friendships and help one another with routine and emergency situations.

When We Begin to Need Help

As the average life expectancy lengthens, and as more of us grow older, the connection between housing and health becomes increasingly crucial. It is particularly critical to have available a range of supportive services to be used as needed: community-based health and therapeutic-care programs; household services; home-delivered meals; respite care; friendly visitors; and a variety of emergency-response systems, from a telephone reassurance program to devices worn around the neck at all times. One or more of these can enable us to age "in place" and maintain a greater degree of independence than is possible in a supported residence or a nursing home.

Adapted Housing

Before we make a hasty move because of a sudden or gradually worsening disability or illness, an important alternative to consider is adapting the housing we already live in. Western culture is oriented to the individual and teaches us to look within ourselves for the causes and solutions to problems, but sometimes the problem is in our environment. We may panic and assume that because of changes in our physical condition we can no longer live on our own, or in a familiar and loved home. Yet it may take only minor and inexpensive changes, such as grab bars, railings, or ramps, to make a place safer and more livable. Changing the environment to meet our changing needs can be a liberating and expressive act that can give us a great feeling of personal power.

A new federal incentive for home adaptation, the Fair Housing Amendments Act, establishes the right of tenants, effective in 1991, to adapt their homes when changes are needed "in order to have full use and enjoyment of their premises." The tenant must bear the expense of the changes, must assure the landlord that they are done in a competent manner, and in some cases, must restore the premises to the original condition upon moving. Widening doors, installing ramps, and removing thresholds are some examples of changes that may be allowed in common as well as in individual space. The law also requires landlords to accommodate a tenant's needs for changes such as a closer parking space or changes in trash collection practices.[12]

Financing of home adaptations can be problematic and require a bit of research.[13] Check your city planning office for state or federal loans. Grants may be available from Centers for Independent Living (see Resources) or state rehabilitation agencies. In some states, Medicaid will pay for certain home adaptations on the criterion that making this investment is cheaper than incurring nursing-home costs.

Adaptations to consider are: clamp-on levers, handrails, bathroom grab bars (toilet and tub), electronic-appliance control units, lever door-handle set, single-lever faucet, widening of interior doorway, interior stair lift, and exterior wheel chair lift. If any of these are needed, get several estimates and compare prices, as there is a huge range.

Small accommodations for comfort or safety can sometimes be made at little or no cost—for example, a simple change in placement of furnishings. A first-floor bedroom can be set up when you need to limit stair climbing by moving a day bed or lounge into an infrequently used downstairs room. Moving chairs and getting rid of scatter rugs can help prevent falls. The willingness to make minor changes may make a big difference—or forestall a larger change.

Home Care and Social Services for Independent Living

Home-care services are a central part of independent living. Though such programs are cost-effective, misguided penny-wise budget cutters have reduced or eliminated them in many areas, prematurely forcing formerly independent people into institutional living. Housing activists must be aware of the importance of home-care services and work toward strengthening, expanding, and coordinating them with other community resources. Such services should be available to all who need them on a sliding-fee-scale basis, thus expanding the availability of beds for those who really need to be in a health-care facility. (See *Home Care and Community Services* section, pages 216–17, for a description of types of services available in many communities.)

Senior Apartments or Senior Housing

Senior housing usually refers to low-cost apartments built for elders and subsidized by federal, state, or local agencies, or by private nonprofit sponsors. For those who find comfort and security by living primarily with others whose values, history, and culture are similar to theirs, religious, cultural, professional, and labor organizations often sponsor low- or moderately priced housing. When such housing is subsidized by federal funds from HUD, it is more likely to be mixed-income housing, as applicants with housing subsidies must be accepted. A specified package of health and support services may be included.

For many older women, having a subsidized apartment means being able to live within their means in adequate rather than substandard housing.

I live alone in the elderly apartments. They're ideal. After all, when you're getting along on Social Security, you can't do any better, because you've only got to pay the rent and the telephone. And they shovel out the snow! [a seventy-five-year-old woman]

Many single and widowed women enjoy having so many potential friends and companions right in the building.

I live alone, but I'm never alone. I'm bouncing out all the time and knocking on the door here and there. We're all back and forth all the time. And at Christmastime, I do the tree trimming in the lounge. We have a big Christmas tree in the upper hall and it's real dressed up and nice. [a woman in her sixties]

For women who want to keep busy and active despite limitations on their mobility, having a variety of activities available where they live may be the ideal solution.

At the time of my involuntary retirement I was eligible to apply for senior housing, which I did. This opened up a new way of life. I am living among my peers, with whom I have much in common. This is a wonderful housing complex with so much to do. I have joined the art group and the choral group, a discussion group, a nutrition group, and the tenants' group. I am also board secretary of a Jewish women's organization and do volunteer work sending out cards. People tell me I'm hard to reach at home. Gee, I wonder why?

I can just about navigate around the building, but I am very limited with walking any distance. I've had two unsuccessful knee replacements. I wonder what I'd do if I had a good pair of legs. [a woman in her seventies]

Many communities have adopted innovative solutions to the shortage of housing for elders. In Hallowell, Maine, an industrial building overlooking the river has been remodeled into apartments. It's within walking distance of town activities. In Virginia, a large building, rehabilitated and funded by church groups, now contains efficiency apartments and serves communal meals. If a resident has exhausted her funds, contributions from the church are used. A ninety-nine-unit cooperative built in 1984 in Chicago, sponsored by the Illinois Association of the Deaf, is specifically designed for older hearing-impaired people. In New York City, a seventy-one-year-old blind newsdealer and activist designed a two-hundred-unit apartment building for other blind adults.

Scattered-Site Housing

Another concept is to have a network of social services available to elders who live in separate apartments dispersed over a designated geographical area. For example, the Jewish Council for the Aging in Washington, D.C., started a Group Homes program in 1973 for those who are mobile and able to do most things for themselves. For a basic fee, in addition to their housing, residents receive food, a daily newspaper, local phone service, and the services of a homemaker and a social worker. The residents enjoy the warmth and companionship of this type of housing and the knowledge that their basic needs will be met.

A similar model developed in Philadelphia by the Quaker community encourages residents to live in twos and threes in apartments where health and social services can be delivered to them with efficiency and economy.

Congregate Housing

Congregate housing is specially planned, designed, and managed multiunit senior housing. Each self-contained unit typically includes a bedroom and bath, possibly other rooms, and in some instances a small kitchen. Common space for shared cooking, dining, and group activities is centrally located, to be shared by several residents. Supportive services such as housekeeping, transportation, social and recreational activities and sometimes meals are provided if desired, usually for a fee. The staff is trained to respond to health changes or other needs. Home care, such as help with bathing, or physical therapy, can also be delivered here, if needed.

Congregate housing is an excellent concept but little is being built because there is so little funding available for the social services that were to be an integral part of the package. And the renovation of older buildings (large homes, phased-out schools, etc.) is often thwarted by obsolete regulations or building codes.

Sometimes congregate housing is described as independent living. I feel this is unfortunate. With this understanding, a new resident might come in feeling no need to change her way of living in the common spaces of the apartment. If she always cooks for a whole hour at 6 P.M., or doesn't like to work with other people, there will be trouble if another resident has the same feeling. The way I feel congregate living should be described is interdependent living. This conjures up a give-and-take, an accent on cooperation with others rather than insistence on one's own way. It puts the emphasis on mutual support. And it provides the opportunity for little successes. We can learn to live together by trying out procedures, discarding some, and working out more effective measures. [a seventy-eight-year-old woman]

SUPPORTED GROUP LIVING

Rest homes and board-and-care homes are subject to less regulation than nursing homes, although most states have tightened their restrictions in the last few years. These homes provide shelter, food, and a twenty-four-hour resident staff person. Such residences should be located near sources for in-home services. If a nurse or personal-care attendant is needed, the care is usually only part-time and for an additional fee. The greater independence of such residences as compared with nursing homes may be attractive to those who do not require daily health and social services; however, some elders who live in such settings may need more skilled care over time. Periodic evaluations remain important.

The line between independent group living for the elderly and assisted group living is easily blurred, and different states have different laws regulating various aspects of group residences. It is important to have enough regulation to weed out those homes that are unsafe, poorly run, or exploitive, while not discouraging innovation by and for those who are able to manage well by themselves.

A big old place which was vacant for ten years has come back to life down in the village. It's now a residence for nine people, and you can rent a room (which includes three meals and laundry) either on a monthly, seasonal, or yearly basis—even weekly for recuperation, respite, or just to try it out. The first person who signed up went back to her own house and garden in the summer, and returned there in the fall. It's privately run and open to all ages, but has attracted mostly older people from right around here. Because it was an inn at one time, each room has its own bath—that would be important to me even if I had to give up other areas of privacy. The location is ideal—within sight of the church, town library, community center, firehouse, and—even more important—it's next to the post office, which is the social center of town. There's a boarding school right up the road,

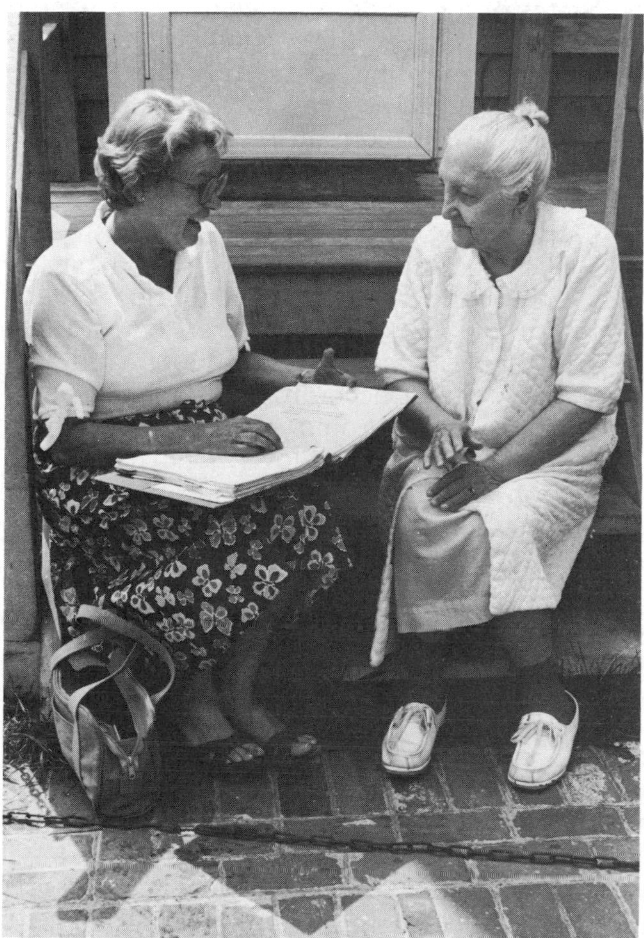

Norma Holt

which provides some cultural activities as well as a chance for some interaction with teenagers far from home. People from the community come for lunch or craft workshops. My friends and I feel comfortable knowing the house will be there for our parents or for us if we can't be as independent as we are now, or don't want to be. [a woman in her fifties]

I went shopping for a place to live near my daughter and her husband and I found an ideal place. It's a small group residence and there's another woman there in her nineties too. I moved in for a trial month and then permanently. I have a first-floor room and can use my walker when I need to. An old beau of mine lives nearby so I called him and now he takes me for a weekly drive and dinner out. My daughter and granddaughter come over often, too. [a ninety-three-year-old woman]

Retirement Communities

These communities range in size from a single building to whole "villages" or towns, and offer a variety of services and recreation. They may be built, sponsored, and managed by nonprofit organizations, profit-making companies, or a combination of both.

The Clovers Retirement Community

*by Kathleen McGuire**

The Clovers are a group of seven women who met between 1976 and 1978 through a self-help, peer-counseling group called Changes. By 1978, individual members of the group began to move all over the United States and Canada. We decided that we did not want to lose these good friendships to distance and time, so even though we were only in our early thirties then, we had a great idea: Why not commit ourselves to be lifelong friends and to care for each other when we became elderly? The Clovers Retirement Community was born.

We committed ourselves to a yearly reunion and a yearly contribution of one hundred dollars each to the retirement fund. By 1986, we had six reunions and our money-market account. We had Clovers T-shirts, a round-robin newsletter, a photo album, an archive, a Clovers Chorus and collection of affirming songs, and a phone chain and support network that was activated whenever a Clover was in need.

The dream was for a piece of land on which we could all retire together. Basic to the group are skills of empathetic listening and experiential focusing, which we learned in the Changes self-help community. Even our commitment to listening skills, however, was not enough to avoid the conflicts of personality and goals that affect almost all groups. Ours: those who wanted deep personal growth and interpersonal conflict resolution at reunions versus those who wanted a lighter, more vacation-like time—personified as a conflict netween two strong leaders.

At the 1986 reunion, we had a major blowup, and since then have not met as a group, although there have been mini-reunions of two to four people. In 1989, the treasurer dispensed an equal share of the retirement fund to each person.

The net of relationships remains. One member has continued to circulate among all the members, tying them together indirectly. Deaths of parents, divorces, and brushes with cancer have softened angry feelings and drawn us closer. There's talk of a reunion in the summer of 1994, and everyone is talking to everyone else through Christmas letters and emergency phone calls when someone needs help.

Many of us have gone on to become landowners, so there are a number of potential sites for retirement. Members still talk of our long-term dream. I expect it to happen. We're in our early fifties now and have twenty years to continue building relationship. What other great options are there for that time when family, career, and partners no longer demand us and illness reins us in? I think the clovers will take care of one another.

*See Resources, page 449, for Kathleen McGuire's book on starting and maintaining a supportive group or community.

Life-Care or Continuing-Care Communities

These offer independent apartment living for people who are in relatively good health, with medical and support services nearby. Many include a nursing home on the premises. A resident may move from a residential part of the community to another building or section that offers intermediate or skilled nursing care. In return for a sizable entrance fee, as well as monthly maintenance charges, residents are guaranteed a permanent place to live and a specified package of medical and nursing benefits, which can be increased or decreased according to the resident's changing needs.

The type and level of available care should be specified in a written agreement. The agreement should also clearly state your right to terminate the contract and receive a refund should the arrangement become unsatisfactory for any reason. It should state the conditions under which you might be involuntarily discharged or moved and what alternative care provisions will be made in such a case. Another question that must be answered is what happens to your assets if you die shortly after entering. Can your investment be returned to your estate, or does it remain the exclusive property of the retirement community? In some situations, you can buy your unit under various conditions and limitations, and the equity in it passes to your heirs when you die. One small liberal arts college in Connecticut, which built a nonprofit life-care community on its campus, guarantees a refund of two thirds of the entrance fee should you leave the community at any time.

Various financial and management problems, however, have closed some life-care communities in recent years. Whether nonprofit or for profit, such communities need regulation. Be a prudent, knowledgeable consumer: obtain information in writing, and have the community's financial statement reviewed by your accountant, estate planner, or lawyer.

THE TRANSITION

When we begin to consider a possible move for any reason, it's a good idea to look as far ahead as possible—to visualize future needs, not just those of the moment. Become informed about what's available *before* you need it. Try to arrange a short-term stay. Once your house is sold and furniture dispersed, it can be hard to go back to your former life-style.

When my husband died, I felt very much alone in a large house which had been built for us over fifty years ago. The chance to move into an apartment building (where over a dozen of my friends live) came along five months later, but I wasn't sure I would really feel "at home" there. Fortunately, my grandson and his wife were house hunting in a nearby community, and I asked them to live in the house for a year, to give myself a "fallback." Within a few months I was sure I did not want to go back to that big, empty house. Meanwhile, they had grown to love it there and decided to stay. I now enjoy being their guest for Thanksgiving and other family gatherings, without having the hassle or the work of feeding an ever-expanding clan. [an eighty-year-old woman]

A small group of pioneering feminists in the Appalachian area of Ohio purchased a 150-acre hill farm and are developing a collectively owned land trust with individual homes, meeting spaces, and a guest house. They call themselves the Susan B. Anthony Memorial UnRest Home.

The Susan B. Anthony Memorial UnRest Home (SBAMUH) is a rural women's community of four residents and several nonresident members, ages 40 through 68, who are ardently feminist, ecologically attuned, and politically active. Major decisions are made by the Board of Directors and resident members using consensus, with input from nonresident members. We seek a balance between individual freedom and the welfare of the community as a whole. Above all we desire safe, congenial, inexpensive living space for feminists.

Our community is intentionally intergenerational, with class and religious differences. We are eager to include more women and lesbians. We welcome old women and look forward to ethnic diversity.

SBAMUH is located 10 miles from Athens, Ohio, home of Ohio University, a campus of 18,000 students, and 15 miles from Hocking College, with 4,500 students. We are part of a growing women's community in southeast Ohio, with monthly gatherings, a coffeehouse, a newsletter, a women's center, a N.O.W. chapter, and a women's chorus. Residents are involved in feminist and lesbian activism, antiracism and justice issues, conservation, and recreation. We operate a campground available to individuals and groups of women (by advance reservation only).

Our 151 acres are very scenic, with narrow valleys, steep ridges, waterfalls, rolling fields, and a swimming pond. It is serviced by a little-traveled but good gravel road, electric lines, and telephone lines. New residents can build a dwelling, bring in a mobile home, or temporarily share the farmhouse.

Pioneering a feminist community could be the most challenging and rewarding experience of a lifetime. Feminists who are seeking residential community are invited to contact us (see Resources, p. 473) via letters or tape cassettes. Getting to know one another well is essential for sound community building.

The great American dream of home ownership, or at least of having a private apartment, has for some been transformed into a bad dream of isolation, escalating rents, taxes, and maintenance costs. Yet these forces have pushed a growing number of women to think creatively of change, and to formulate a redefinition of family and community. What these stories have in common is a spirit of innovation, commitment, and mutual support grounded in long-range planning. We hope more and more women will be inspired by these examples to explore new ways of living that will enhance their later years.

NOTES

1. "Study Finds Vast Undercount of New York City Homeless." *The New York Times*, Nov. 16, 1993, pp. A1, B4.
2. "New York Shelters Meet Special Needs of Elderly." *The New York Times*, Mar. 29, 1987, p. 38.
3. Mary Ellen Hombs and Mitch Snyder with foreword by Daniel Berrigan, *Homelessness in America*. Washington, DC: Community for Creative Non-Violence, December 1982.
4. Anthony Barnes, "Unfamiliarity with the Law Heightens Tenant Problems." *Boston Seniority*, January 1985, pp. 1–2.
5. Coalition on Women and the Budget, *Inequality of Sacrifice: Women and the Reagan Budget*, section on public housing. National Women's Law Project, Washington, DC, March 1984.
6. John Ferland, "She Makes MMC Visitors at Home." Portland, Maine, *Press Herald*, Oct. 2, 1984.
7. Barbara Silverstone and Helen Kardel Hyman, *You and Your Aging Parent*. New York: Pantheon, 1982, pp. 148–50.
8. Personal communication from a woman on the staff of a town-sponsored home-sharing agency.
9. "MG's Friends." *Boston College Magazine*, Fall 1984, pp. 26, 27.
10. Washington (AP), "Report Finds U.S. Housing Held Back by Poor Research." Portland, Maine, *Press Herald*, Sept. 16, 1986.
11. Formaldehyde, used in the construction of mobile and some conventional homes, may cause cancer. If you are concerned, check current standards with HUD and the Environmental Protection Agency. Ann Mariano, "Cancer Risk Seen in Mobile Homes." *The Washington Post*, Apr. 26, 1987.
12. Center for Accessible Housing. Fact Sheet 1. The Fair Housing Amendments Act of 1988. Fact Sheet 2. Reasonable Modification of Existing Premises (See Resources, page 472).
13. Consumers Guide to Home Adaptations, 1990. See chapter 20, "Funding for Home Modifications," Adaptive Environments Center (See Resources, page 472).

13

WORK AND RETIREMENT

✦

BY EDITH STEIN, PAULA B. DORESS-WORTERS, AND MARY D. FILLMORE

SPECIAL THANKS TO TISH SOMMERS

1994 UPDATE BY MELISSA KESLER GILBERT WITH SPECIAL THANKS TO RUTH HARRIET JACOBS

COMPARABLE WORTH, OR PAY EQUITY BY ROSLYN FELDBERG

RESOURCES FOR THIS CHAPTER ON PAGES 474–77

All human beings need the sense of achievement and accomplishment that comes from satisfying and socially valued work. For middle-aged and older women, work outside the home provides a sense of mastery and increased self-esteem. Social scientists used to believe that jobs for women conflicted with the homemaking role, but contemporary research shows instead that multiple roles for women are more likely to bring multiple satisfactions rather than stress and conflict, especially when the jobs are good, pay well, and provide opportunities for achievement. Having an external source of rewards and respect, earning our own money, and meeting new coworkers and friends bring us greater independence from our families and provide a hedge against the isolation and feelings of obsolescence that can plague older women.

Dramatic demographic changes have taken place in the past twenty years; more jobs for women have opened up and more women are in the work force. Today almost 60 percent of all women are employed for pay and women aged fifty-five and over constitute a growing segment of the American labor force.[1] Women continue to enter many fields traditionally closed to them, and have almost doubled their numbers in executive, administrative, and managerial occupations over the past decade.[2] Despite these gains, the recession of the early 1990s has slowed down the flow of women into the labor force and has generally worsened the employment picture for many of us.[3] These developments present not only special challenges and pitfalls for older women, but special opportunities as well.

Women often find new directions in work and education at a time in life when men worry about their time "running out." Perhaps women's less conventional career paths can provide a model of what is possible for all workers in the second half of life. Yet it is also true that many women find themselves in dead-end or entry-level jobs, or frozen out of the work force altogether, at an age when men are at the peak of their earning power. By their fifties and sixties, choices narrow considerably and making a change becomes increasingly difficult. Many communities have agencies that provide help to women and men over fifty-five who are seeking employment. The road to the rewards and satisfactions we seek can be a rocky one.

DISCRIMINATION

As women, we face sex discrimination throughout our work lives, and some of us face other forms of discrimination as well. Well-docu-

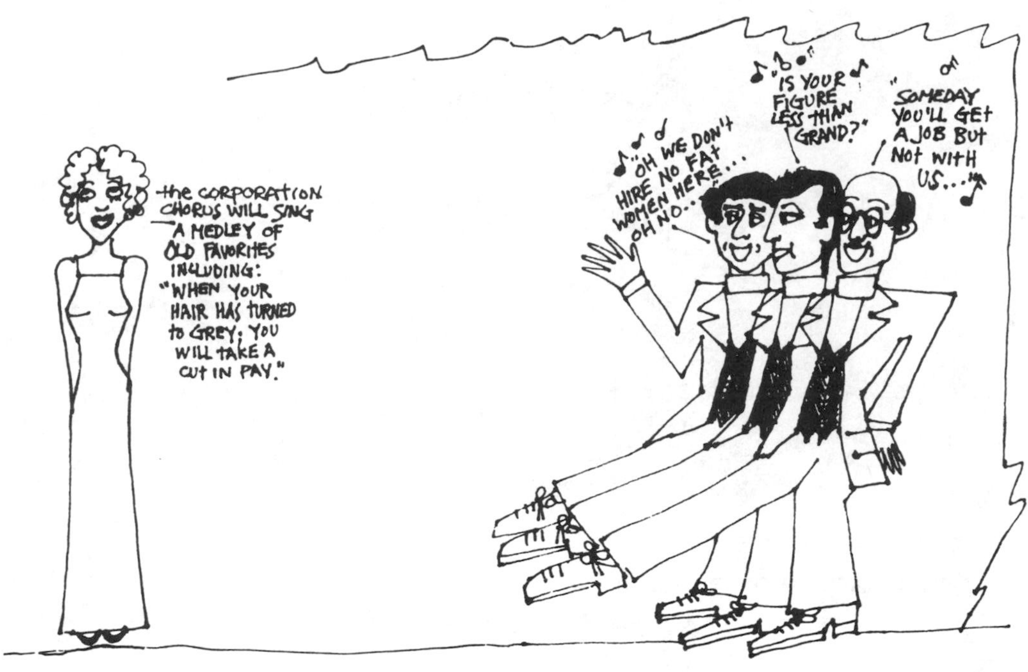
THE CORPORATION CHORUS WILL SING A MEDLEY OF OLD FAVORITES INCLUDING: "WHEN YOUR HAIR HAS TURNED TO GREY; YOU WILL TAKE A CUT IN PAY."
"OH WE DON'T HIRE NO FAT WOMEN HERE... OH NO..."
"IS YOUR FIGURE LESS THAN GRAND?"
"SOMEDAY YOU'LL GET A JOB BUT NOT WITH US..."

Nicole Hollander, from her book I'm in Training to Be Tall and Blonde *(New York: St. Martin's Press, 1979)*

mented government publications report these shocking facts:

- Women earn only 70 percent of what men earn, though women and men are, on average, equal in years of education completed.[4]
- Women are two thirds of our country's contingency work force—part-time or "temporary" employees with low wages, few or no benefits, no health insurance, no worker protection, few opportunities for skill training, and little chance of qualifying for pensions or significant Social Security benefits.[5]
- Women college graduates earn, on average, less than male high school graduates.
- Sixty percent of all women workers are concentrated in low-paying, traditionally female occupations in the sales, service, and clerical sectors with few opportunities for advancement.[6]

In addition to sex discrimination in employment, many women also face discrimination because of race, class, sexual orientation, or disability. Though black women work more continuously than white women, they earn only 82 percent of white women's income.[7] Older black women are three times more likely than white women to work in service occupations; one third of those over sixty-five who are employed work as private household workers.[8] Over the past decade, Hispanic women have increased their employment by 94 percent; married Hispanic women contribute a substantial 32 percent of their family's income.[9]

The Compounding of Age and Sex Discrimination

When we reach our middle years, the discrimination we have faced throughout our lives is compounded by age discrimination, which continues to be common despite laws against it. Contrary to widespread employer prejudice, older women are reliable workers with low attrition and low absenteeism.[10] In fact, the official unemployment rate for older women is low because they seldom change jobs. However, the recession has brought increased job loss for older workers, many of whom are concentrated in declining industries.[11] Displaced women workers are less likely than men to find a new job, and are more likely to be paid less upon reemployment. Older women are unemployed for a longer duration (fourteen weeks) than younger women (eight weeks).[12] The official unemployment rate is understated; it does not include those who give up the job search after repeated experiences of rejection. Too many older women "retire" early, despite the permanent reduction in retirement income that results.

I walked smack into age discrimination in employment at the age of fifty-six. Perhaps I'd been experiencing it and didn't know it because I was content to be underemployed for twenty-five years on the minimum-pay scales of stereotypical female jobs such as typist, nurse's aide, and clerk. After my three older children had received their college degrees, and the youngest was about to start, I closed the house and went to college at the age of fifty-two. I worked as house-mother in a state university. Four years later I received a B.A. in social service and expected to be recognized as a professional. But I was fifty-six years of age, so I took what jobs I could get, and finally at the age of sixty-four, resigned to subtle pressures of age discrimination in the work place, I applied for Social Security as a means of financial survival.

Although a higher percentage of older women than younger women are in the paid work force, older women are even more underpaid as a result of the compounding of age and sex discrimination. Consider the following statistics:

- The gender gap in earnings increases with age. While young women (aged twenty-five to thirty-four) earn 80 percent of young men's salaries, middle-aged women (aged forty-five to fifty-four) earn only 61 percent of middle-aged men's salaries.[13]
- By midlife, men who are going to rise to higher income levels have begun their ascent, while women are left behind—often in traditionally female occupations to face a "sticky floor" of very few and often small pay increases and promotions. Because women often reenter the work force when they are older, they are more likely to face age discrimination at the time of hiring than men.[14]
- Older women workers, and older black women in particular, face pronounced job segregation. Two of every three working women aged fifty-five and older hold jobs in sales and administrative support. These jobs are more likely to be part-time and less likely to provide pension coverage.[15]

In addition to age and sex discrimination, two other factors, the caregiver role and need for training, contribute to older women's dropping out of the work force.[16] Middle-aged and older women may need special training to get into, or return to, paid employment, and should be given priority in job-training programs as compensation for unpaid labor in the home and the community.

Another barrier that some older women workers have had to face is discrimination or lack of access due to a disability. The likelihood of work disability increases with age. Almost a quarter of working women fifty-five to sixty-four years of age have a work disability. Disabled workers earn 38 percent less than nondisabled workers. Today the Americans with Disabilities Act of 1990 (p. xxiv) protects disabled workers from employment discrimination. Disabled women workers can look forward to better opportunities and greater earning potential in the future.[17] However, for some women the effects of discrimination have already set them back in the labor force.

It is difficult to maintain self-esteem while being refused employment or while facing on-the-job discrimination. Getting support from others is very important to keeping your spirits up during the job search and to defending your rights as an employee.

Fighting Back

It is very difficult, either as a job applicant or as an employee, to defend oneself against discriminatory practices and attitudes, but speaking up can go a long way. One woman describes a situation in which her lifelong feistiness got her hired.

When I was sixty-three I applied for a job in a hospital. The woman interviewing me asked me how old I was. I said, "I don't think numbers count. Why don't we race around the block, and if I win then you hire me?" [a ninety-one-year-old woman]

When standing up for ourselves doesn't do the trick, we can exercise our legal rights by filing a discrimination charge through a company grievance procedure or with a governmental agency. Thanks to affirmative-action programs, which put pressure on institutions to advance women and minorities, a few of the many women who had been underpaid and underemployed for decades have begun to reap long-delayed rewards.

I got hold of the figures from the American Association of University Professors (AAUP) and found out that after fifteen years I was being paid two thirds of the very lowest entry-level salary for what was a part-time position in name only. I decided I simply didn't want to put up with this any more and the only way I could think of dealing with it was to say "I am going to retire." At that point there was consternation and "What do you want? We'll give you anything you want." And then I began to get a decent salary, so I stayed on for two more years. But I hope that in another generation women will not wait as long as I did without insisting on being paid for what they are contributing. [a sixty-seven-year-old woman]

Another woman rose to the rank of branch manager and then vice president in the last decade of a long career spent primarily as a teller.

I was doing all the work of an assistant manager without the title and—of course—without the salary. Oh, God, did I argue! And then one year when I came back from vacation I found they had given me a new position, that of Assistant Manager. The former head of the City Division had been a guy who believed that a woman's place was in the home, or if you worked you should be a secretary. When he left, the big boss called me into his office and showed me a note from the personnel department wanting to know why, with the excellent reviews I had and my educational qualifications, hadn't I been promoted? Well, of course I was then, but I was still fuming. [a sixty-six-year-old woman]

If you have reason to believe you have been discriminated against, be careful that you do not speak out *too soon.* "Employees with discrimination complaints often make oral or written complaints which are misconstrued and hurt them later," according to an invaluable booklet published by the Older Women's League. Your first move should be to inform yourself and to gather the evidence. The booklet, *Older Women and Job Discrimination: A Primer,* is a concise, complete, and inexpensive resource that takes you step-by-step through the process of discovering, proving, and fighting discrimination. Every woman should be aware of her legal employment rights and the laws that guarantee equal access to all jobs:

- Title VII of the Civil Rights Act of 1964 prohibits discrimination (including wage discrimination) on the basis of sex, race, color, religion, or national origin. The Civil Rights Act of 1991 provides the right to a jury trial and to money damages.
- The Age Discrimination in Employment Act of 1967 (ADEA), as amended, prohibits employers from using age or pension eligibility as a basis for employment decisions for people forty and older. As of 1991, the act also requires that employers offer employee benefits on an equal cost/benefit basis to all employees, regardless of age.[18]

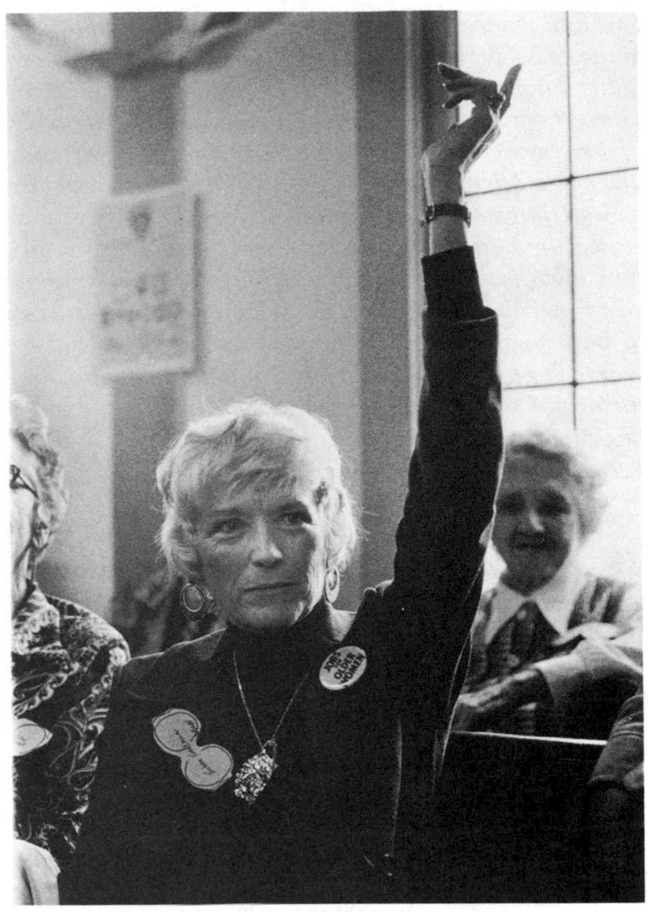

Cathy Cade

To file a charge under Title VII or ADEA you must file with either the local Equal Employment Opportunity Commission field office or with your state or local Fair Employment Practices Agency. The time limits for filing claims are very strict (within 180 to 300 days from the time of the discriminatory act), so contact the agency as soon as possible. If you have missed the time limit of one agency, you may still be able to file with the other.

Proving either age discrimination or sex discrimination alone can be difficult and the procedures complex; it is even more difficult to prove the *combination* of age and sex discrimination that often keeps older women out of jobs. An employer who has many young women and older men on the job may be able to conceal his prejudice against the *older woman.*

Comparable Worth, or Pay Equity

The majority of middle-aged and older women remain trapped in low-paying, traditionally female jobs that offer little possibility for advancement. Pay equity, or equal pay for work of comparable worth, is a tool women can use to collectively upgrade pay in these jobs, usually in conjunction with collective bargaining or court action or both. Women and men often perform different jobs, yet the value of the jobs they do can be systematically compared through job-evaluation studies. These studies often reveal that "men's work" is not intrinsically more valuable than "women's work," even though it is commonly better paid.

One job evaluation study, done in 1973 for the state of Washington at the request of the American Federation of State, County and Municipal Employees (AFSCME), assigned points to each job on four dimensions: knowledge and skills, mental demands, accountability, and working conditions. Points were added across the dimensions to establish the value of each job. Then the wages paid for jobs with similar values were compared. Those jobs held primarily by women paid about 20 percent lower than those held primarily by men. A similar study, done for the state of Minnesota in 1981–1982, again at AFSCME's urging, showed similar results. Overall, women employed by the state averaged almost $5,000 a year less than men.[19] Women's groups and unions organized a political campaign on this issue that resulted in laws mandating comparable worth for all state, county, and municipal workers in Minnesota.

Pay equity is not something you can achieve for or by yourself, but should be accomplished through women's organizations, unions, or other associations. Unions have fought for many comparable-worth cases on behalf of female-dominated occupations such as nursing, library science, teaching, and clerical work. The most successful struggles have been in the public sector. One struggle, waged by the Pennsylvania Nurses Association, resulted not only in comparable pay for nurses who worked in the state prisons, but also in comparable retirement and disability benefits.[20] This suggests that comparable-worth approaches can be used to win improvements in benefits as well as wages. Recently, the school-cafeteria workers in Everett, Massachusetts, won their comparable-worth suit against a school board that paid male-dominated janitorial jobs much higher wages than female-dominated cafeteria jobs.

Despite these triumphs and over twenty years of effort by unions, women's groups, and the National Committee on Pay Equity (see Resources for this chapter), the concept of comparable worth remains controversial. Courts have often ruled against it and most victories in the United States have come through out-of-court settlements and political campaigns. This may be because comparable worth challenges the belief that wages reflect either the demands of the job or are governed by supply and demand. It shows, instead, how biases based on the gender, race, and age of the "typical job occupant" influence the wages and benefits of the job. And in so doing, comparable worth clarifies the grounds on which women and men of color can fight for a fairer deal on the job.

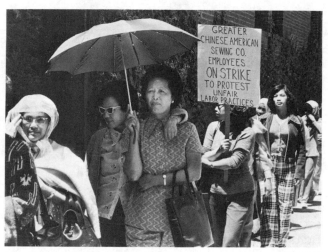

Cathy Cade

Labor Unions

Historically, labor unions have played a significant role in improving working conditions and raising the standard of living for many groups of workers. Regrettably, however, some unions have, over time, developed an "establishment" mentality, catering exclusively to a white male constituency. Today a few progressive unions are moving to reclaim their leadership of the fight for workers' rights by recognizing the significant growth of women in the labor force and trying to meet their needs.

I was the first organizer of women workers for a clothing workers' union in Boston. When I began in 1955, the entire leadership of the union was male while 90 percent of the workers in the shops were female. The union was like a banana republic—women were treated as inferiors. But finally, things are changing. Women are still 90 percent of the membership, but in 1985 three of the top fifteen people in the national leadership are women. [a sixty-three-year-old woman]

Women represented by a union earn 82 percent of men's weekly earnings, while women who are not represented earn only 74 percent of men's wages. Only 15 percent of employed women are represented by a union. However, over a third of labor union members are now women (37 percent).[21] Much of the growth of women in organized labor can be attributed to increasing numbers of union women aged forty-five to fifty-four.[22]

As women begin to enter the higher ranks in our unions they are reaching out to serve previously unorganized workers. Many women's issues have made it onto the bargaining table including the fight for affordable day care, family- and parental-leave provisions, pay equity, reproductive rights, sexual harassment, elder care, and discrimination. Unions provide women with peer support and free legal support, especially when filing charges of sexual, racial, ethnic, or age discrimination.[23]

If you are not represented by a union, and would like to find out more about them, write to the Coalition of Labor Union Women (see Resources for this chapter). Any inquiry is welcome.

Office workers, 99 percent of whom are women, are an important group of unorganized workers. Harvard's Union of Clerical and Technical Workers (HUCTW) was one of the first unions in the country to address the need for organizing around economic issues relevant to the lives of older women workers. Seeing long-term Harvard employees living "a fall away from impoverishment" after retirement convinced older women workers to fight back and join the union. Today, long-term clerical workers are a solid force in the union's campaigns for salary increases, longevity bonuses, and pension benefits.[24]

ENTERING THE WORLD OF PAID WORK IN THE MIDDLE OR LATER YEARS

Many women have worked for pay throughout their adult lives. For single women, women of color, and working-class women, earning money has been a necessity for survival. For a relatively small number of women, commitment to the world of paid work was an early and personal decision, a hard-won struggle against the forces that would deny women's aspirations.

However, many women enter and leave and reenter the work force at times and for reasons that do not fit into male-defined patterns. Rigid notions of a single career beginning at graduation and ending with retirement are breaking down as a growing number of workers exercise options to change careers, go back to school, or continue to work for pay or begin second careers after retirement.

Many women for whom home and family had been a primary focus redirect their energy toward jobs or careers, finding new work, getting more education, discovering new talents and interests, developing their capabilities. Work shifts to center stage in their lives. Those of us who have worked some twenty to thirty years raising children have managed a variety of problematic situations and have learned adaptability and skills that should give us confidence as we face the next challenge—entering or reentering the work force. Yet many of us approach reentry with some secret fears. Do my looks give away my age? Are my skills rusty?

The National Displaced Homemakers Network grew out of a support group for unemployed older women. Today, their programs help women make the transition from the home to the workplace with free sessions on life-skills development (building confidence, setting goals), job-skills assessment, career counseling, preemployment preparation (writing résumés, interviewing techniques), and job referral and placement (see Resources for this chapter).

Many of us have used or developed our administrative skills in volunteer jobs in the community. Indeed, a volunteer position can sometimes lead to a paid position as you become known in a particular organization and make contacts. Volunteer experience *must* be recognized by prospective employers. The federal government already does so. In Massachusetts, a 1986 bill requires employers to include on every application a statement that the applicant may include "any verified work performed on a volunteer basis" as part of her or his work history.

I hadn't worked [for pay] in seventeen years, but I wasn't scared of making the transition. I had done a lot of things in the community, so I felt competent. I went back to work a year after I was separated from my husband. I discovered that the personnel director at a hospital where I volunteered needed some help, so I offered my services and ended up staying nine years. In that situation, being a middle-aged suburban matron was a great plus because the hospital wanted its employees to project the image of being part of the community. So the fact that I lived in the

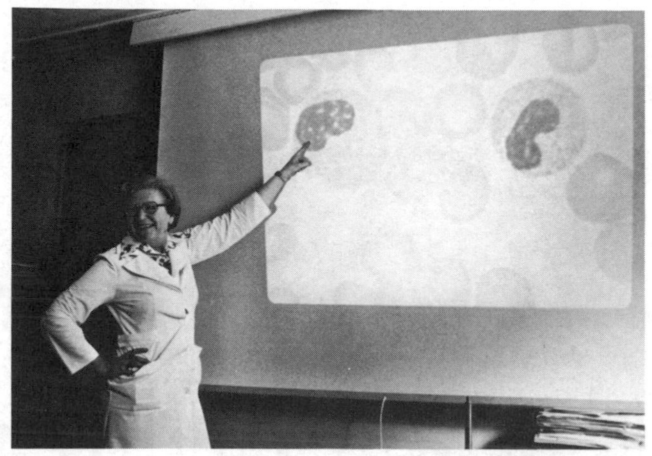

Jerry Howard/Positive Images

community and was active in civic affairs meant to them that I was extending the hospital into the community.

My boss, a divorced woman who had raised two kids alone, was very sympathetic to my working flextime. If there was a school event, I could go and work on Saturday instead. Later I had a male boss who didn't like the arrangement but he said, "What you do, you do very well. I'd have a hard time getting rid of you." [a woman in her fifties]

I reentered the world of paid work at age fifty-five, having been at home for twenty-seven years. The manager of the Wall Street law firm who hired me was amazed at my capabilities. I told him I had been secretary of innumerable organizations and had therefore kept up my steno and typing. Also, while my husband was alive, we often discussed business matters together, so I was aware of what was happening in the business world. Women are constantly learning, even while at home raising a family. [a woman in her sixties]

Since many of us started working late in life and with fairly low career expectations, middle-aged and older women at all levels in the work force express surprise and pleasure in their accomplishments.

I am a reborn person. Widowed at age fifty-five, I had to fend for myself. Having been a homemaker for thirty-five years, I felt pretty inadequate so I went back to night high school for a refresher course in shorthand and typing. When I graduated, I was encouraged to take a clerical test at a bank. With much trepidation, I did. I passed with flying colors and was hired immediately. That was the start of my rebirth. I became a whole person who was appreciated for my labors and liked by my coworkers. The bank subsidized trips abroad for its employees at a very nominal cost and I visited London, Caracas, and Israel. I'm black and blue from pinching myself when I think that I did these wondrous things. The happiest years of my life ended with my forced retirement at age sixty-five. [a woman in her seventies]

When I was divorced at age thirty-seven I went looking for a teaching post. I could do math and general science but when I applied to the school where I wished to work I became a secretary because that was the only job available and I really wanted to be part of that school's community. Strangely, I had an enormous burst of energy—just full of good feeling—even though I was qualified to be a teacher and all I did was secretarial work. Soon they asked me to do some bookkeeping. Then I was asked if I could teach music so I started in the fall of my second year there inventing my own courses. I studied piano to continue to learn more about harmony and I continued to study as I taught. Later on I became the school treasurer. I knew I had managerial ability—I did my tasks well so that the school was never in the red—because I was using everything I had. [an eighty-year-old woman]

As a first step, if you are entering or reentering the work force, take a look at yourself and your own strengths and skills. Ask people who

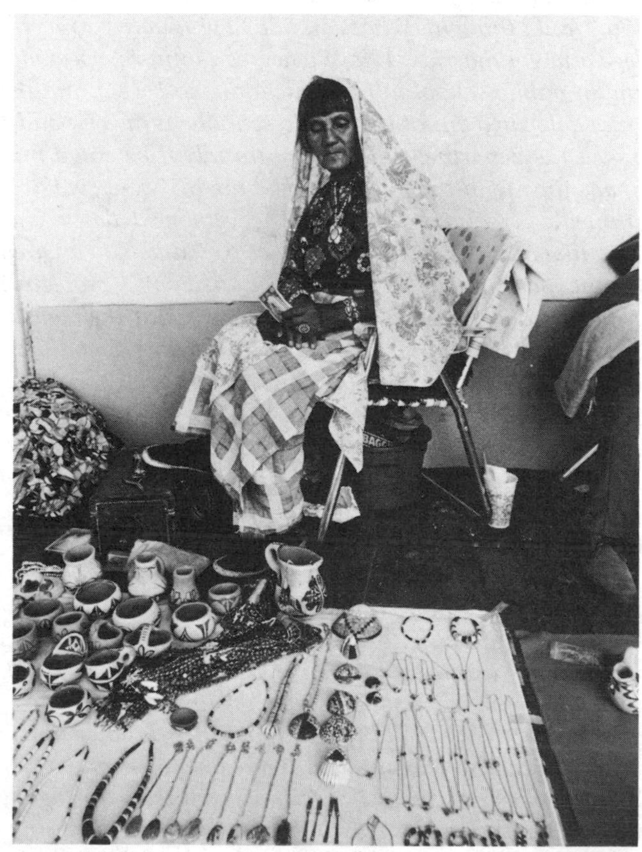

Mikki Ansin

know you well for their opinions of what you are good at. The same qualities that serve you well in your personal life may be the very ones that can give you a sense of career direction. What is it that you like about painting a room or knitting a sweater? Think about what has made you feel most proud and successful in the past, and try to identify some common threads in what you achieved. Did you enjoy organizing the church bazaar because it brought people together in a new way, because it made a lot of money, or because it got you into managing money for the first time? All these are valuable clues as to what you might consider as a future direction.

Some employment counselors can help women reentering the work force put together a "skills résumé," which focuses on abilities and accomplishments rather than a chronological listing of paid employment.

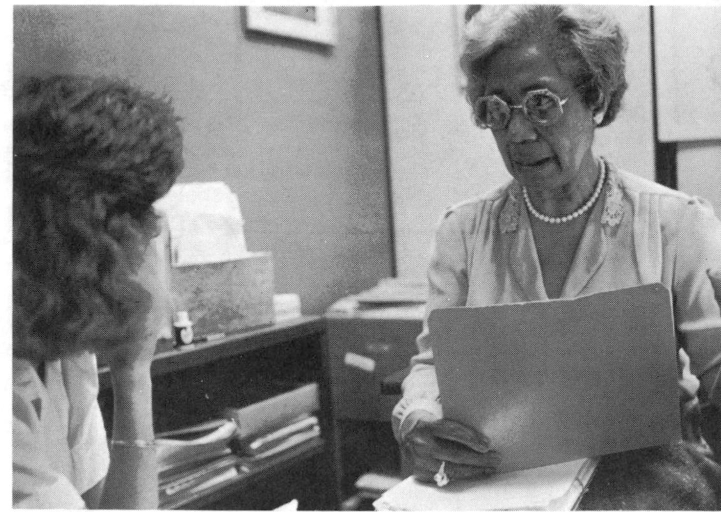

Marianne Gontarz

I was sixty-one when my husband went into a nursing home. At first I stayed with him there every day until I was convinced that it was not like some of the terrible places we had tried before. Then I began to stay home mornings to practice on the piano but I still went every afternoon. One day the social workers got after me. "You can't hang around here so much. This is an institution. You don't belong in an institution. You've got to get a job." And I thought, What can I do? I graduated from college and got married. I have a degree in music, specializing in public school music education, so I went into the music department of the public schools in the city and I asked the department head very timidly if he could find space for me in the fall. He asked me if I were available immediately and I said yes. The very next day I was teaching in a middle school, grades 6, 7, and 8, in an area of the city noted for its school discipline problems. Nobody told me what the kids knew, what their background was, nothing. But the best part was, I could do anything I wanted to. I had high aspirations for them! The place was bedlam. It was wild. My supervisor came in a couple of times and said, "You're doing very well. Just keep on smiling." I was running to all kinds of libraries getting material. And I prepared more than one lesson plan for each class in case one didn't work. I was terribly busy, but very happy. I had wonderful rapport with the kids. I don't think they knew what hit them! I introduced the kids to opera. They had never heard of opera. They wanted only their own kind of music which was loud rock and roll, and each group liked only a certain kind of rock. I didn't eliminate their kind of music entirely because I wanted an inducement for preserving order in the classroom. If no time was wasted during the class, then they could play their records the last ten minutes of the period. The black kids played one kind of rock

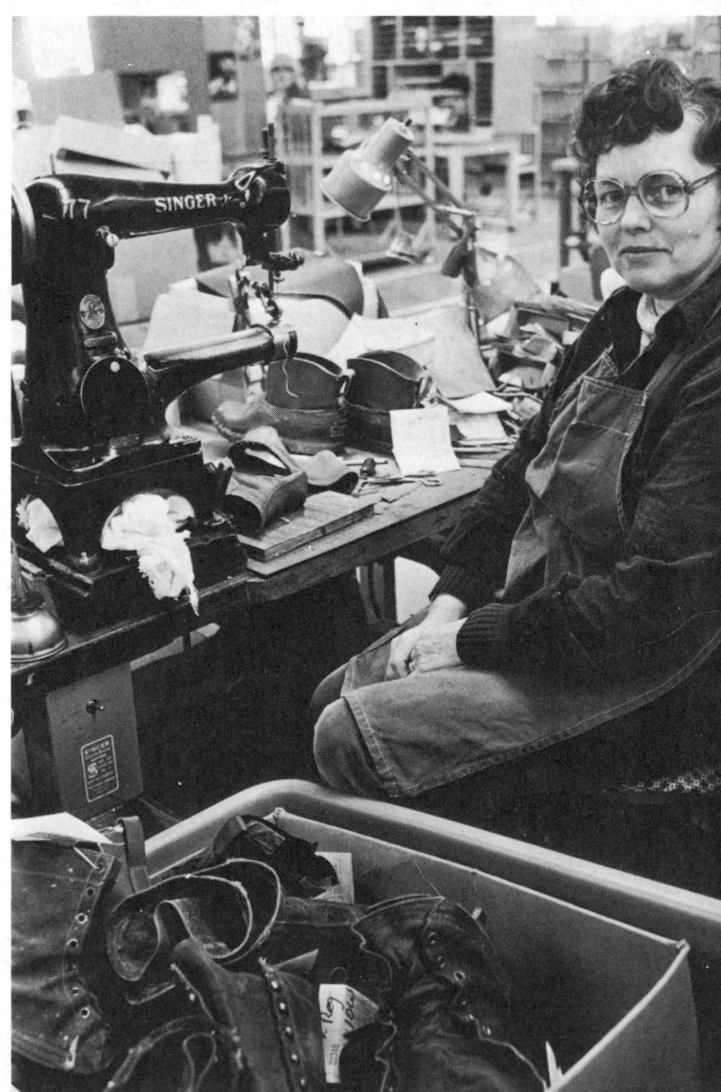

Sarah Putnam

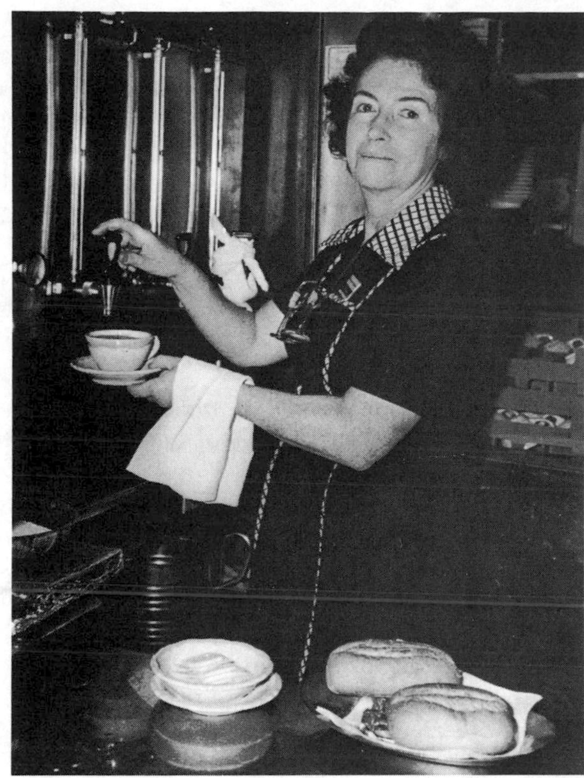

Ellen Shub

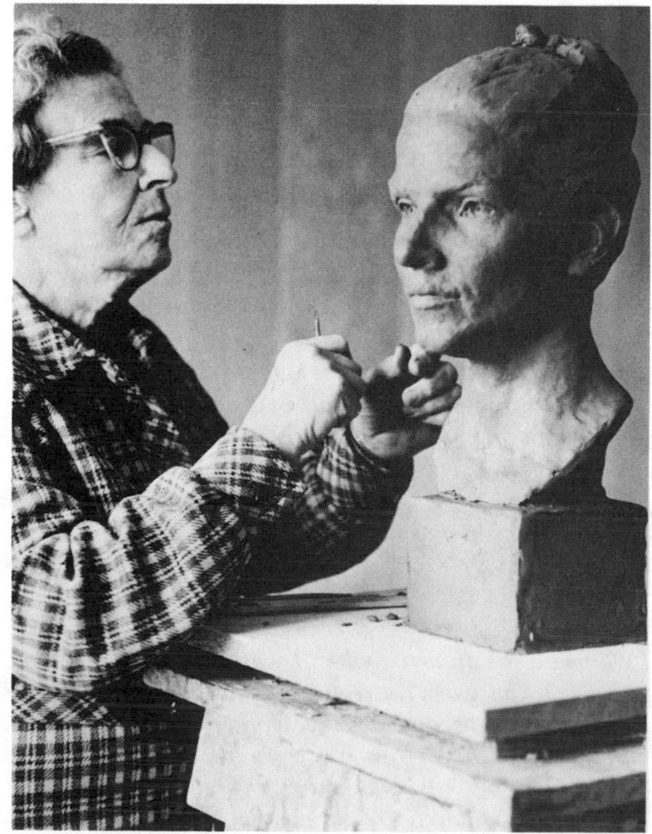

Joan K. Gordon

and the white kids another and they learned to tolerate each other's music. I think the kids felt my vulnerability too and they were sort of protective of me.

I was probably the oldest teacher in the school. I'd be exhausted when I came home from teaching; I'd have to take a nap. And I didn't dare tell any of the younger teachers because they'd say, "Oh, she shouldn't be teaching. She's too old." Then I found out that all the younger teachers did the same thing! I taught on the third floor and I used to take the stairs two at a time to show that I could do it, that I had as much strength as the young people. I just had to prove to everybody that I could do it. When I retired the school gave me a plaque. And I made a little speech. I told the parents that I started teaching there at a time of crisis in my life and that I blessed the kids every day just for being there so that I could infect them with even a little bit of my own enthusiasm for music. [a woman in her seventies]

Education and Job Training

Better access to higher education is one of the key factors in opening up the job market for women and raising women's earnings. Today, continuing education for women has changed the face of many college campuses. We are not as likely to be the only older woman in sight. Many college professors have commented on the determination and commitment of older women students, and on their ability to get good grades and complete demanding programs while still managing family responsibilities.

For information about continuing education, adult education, and special reentry programs for older women, start with your local Department of Employment and Training. Visit your local library to find college catalogs and information about financial aid. If you have been laid off from a job, you might qualify for Dislocated Worker Status, which may help you to get financial assistance toward your tuition. The local Department of Education can help you find a test center to prepare to take the high school equivalency test so you can receive your GED (General Equivalency Diploma).

The statement in the box on page 179 was sent to us by a forty-year-old woman who returned to school after dropping out at fourteen. Embarrassed to resume her education at the same level as her junior high school–aged son, she was advised to take a high school equivalency test, which she passed easily. Armed with her barely dry diploma, she conferred with advisers at the women's center of a nearby college and enrolled in a five-year master's degree program.

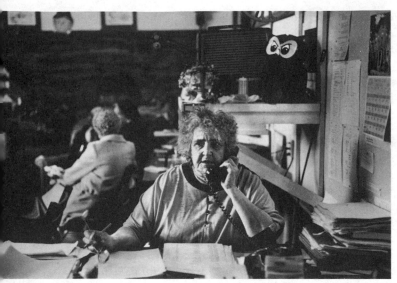

Norma Holt

Obstacles are nothing new to Norma Buchanan, who suffers from a degenerative spine disease. Together with others she spearheaded a campaign to make the campus and its buildings more accessible to students with disabilities. As a student, Norma had to advocate for herself to make special arrangements for exams, since she has a learning disability.

Because education is often proposed as a kind of "therapy," too many women, after completing an educational program, find themselves still unprepared for the job market. Education is not a luxury but a necessity. Remember that a woman needs a college degree in order to earn as much as a man with a high school diploma. According to sociologist Ruth Harriet Jacobs,* women reentering the job market are often directed toward fields in which the wage is too low to support a household. Some career counselors assume that older women are studying for personal growth only and do not really need a decent income.

When employment for pay is an important goal, be sure to inquire about the placement record of the school or department you are considering—with older women in particular. Talk to some recent graduates. Always compare the degree or diploma you will receive with the credentials of those working in the field. Sometimes alternative routes to a degree will not put you in the most competitive position. For example, if most social workers have an M.S.W. degree, will you be able to get the job you want with only a bachelor's degree in social work? If most college teachers hold a Ph.D., will you get a job with an Ed.D.? Also, check the market for the kind of work you plan to do. Government publications available from the Women's Bureau and the Bureau of Labor Statistics tell you about the availability of types of jobs by geographic area. (See Resources for this chapter).

*Center for Research on Women, Wellesley, MA 02181.

If you must start earning as soon as possible, consider a short training program, as this woman did:

I am writing to assure women of middle age or beyond that it is not too late to attend school and begin a career, or to switch careers.

All my life I had wanted to be a nurse, but instead was a secretary. Finally, at age fifty-seven, when the youngest of our children graduated from college, I took a year off from the workaday world to attend school and become a licensed practical nurse.

I made the highest grade in our class on the state board exam. I am not telling this to be boastful but to encourage others who might think they are too old to learn.

Seven years later, at age sixty-five, I am happily employed as an LPN—my lifelong dream.

Many women who aspire to fulfillment and self-actualization through work are more willing to risk a longer period of schooling or a less certain future employment picture than are women who have an immediate need for income. It helps if we have money saved or a supportive partner or family to help us.

I went back to school when I was forty-six; I had ten credits to my name, but I was determined to find a way to do something I liked. My partner was earning a good salary and was willing to help me to go to school. I had four splendid years, and when I graduated I got a job as a group worker with older people in a small agency. Later I began work on my master's degree in an evening program which took five years. It was great because I was able to pick my own courses. I majored in Women's Studies and when I finished I was invited to teach a course at the college. It was very exciting for me. [a sixty-five-year-old woman]

I wanted to be an artist when I was growing up but my father felt that wasn't a realistic aspiration for a Puerto Rican girl, so I became a social worker. I got my motivation for an education from my father but I had to delay my dream. Now my husband is doing very well in his business and the children are old enough that they are not a problem, so I feel now is the time for me to study art.

Because I'm forty-three and not sixteen or eighteen, I feel this pressure to catch up. . . . I don't know whether I will really become an artist or whether I will go back to social work, but right now I am going to art school full time and working very hard at it. It is the first time in my marriage that I haven't earned money, but my husband insisted we can afford it and he really encouraged me to go ahead.

In my fifties I earned an Ed.D. in Sociology, but I found out you need more than the degree to get an academic appointment. You need publications. I wasn't earning enough teaching part-time at a state university, and I had no insurance or benefits, so I took a secretarial job where the pay is decent and the benefits are good. I can't get into the pension plan because I'm too old; nevertheless, I had to take a regular-paying job with benefits for my economic well-being. But it was painful after working so long and hard to give up the dream of an intellectually stimulating job. [a sixty-one-year-old woman]

I reached the point after nine years in personnel that I had no place to advance and the job had become too predictable. I found that about half my time was spent being somebody's listening ear or shoulder to cry on, and that was the part of my job that I got the most gratification from; so I decided to go off and do a social-work internship. But when I graduated, social-work jobs were hard to come by. After a long period of unemployment, during which I struggled with fears that I was not being hired because of my age, I finally got a job as an administrative assistant with a human-services agency. While it's not doing social work as I had planned, it pays more than anything I've seen offered in social work recently, which is a sad commentary. What really lifted my morale is that they called the personnel director where I had been employed part-time for a reference and she told them, "You'd better grab her while you have the chance because we would grab her if there were any way we could afford her and if we could make the job challenging enough for her." So I found out that I was not being rejected because of my age, and that at least two people thought I was not too old to be hired. [a fifty-nine-year-old woman]

Internships and job training can help women learn new technologies and occupational skills for better jobs. The Job Training and Partnership Act (JTPA) is a federally funded employment and training program that provides on-the-job training for people who are unemployed or underemployed. The Perkins Vocational and Applied Technology Act of 1990 provides funding for vocational training pro-

GOING BACK TO SCHOOL—THE DECISION

by Norma Buchanan

Once the thought of returning to school occurs, the roller-coaster ride of your life begins. As you stand there waiting to enter, the questions and doubts begin to haunt you: "Can I afford to go to school? What will my family and friends think? How can I possibly fit into a classroom of youngsters?" Underlying all of these questions is the most fearful of them all, "At my age, can I possibly learn all that is required?" Your own insecurities and self-doubt begin to overwhelm you.

The best answer to all of these questions is YES YOU CAN—if you are willing to ride the roller coaster: the downward plunge into fear of failure; the bottomless pit of frustration; the soaring joy of success; the plateau of tiredness at the amount of work involved; and most of all, the acceptance of the challenge to grow and develop to your highest point as an individual.

You, the returning student, can be your own best friend or your own worst enemy. Don't be afraid to admit that you don't know the answer—seek out those who have been there already, ask for help. After all, you are not alone. Most universities and colleges are staffed with professionals eager and willing to help you through this roller-coaster ride of academia. Fellow students, both younger and older, can be a source of help and insight into this adventure. But most of all, give yourself credit for what you have accomplished and for what you are attempting. After all, you have survived childhood, adulthood, and in some cases marriage and/or employment outside the home—you bring to the academic world a wealth of understanding and knowledge that younger students cannot possibly have. You have the advantage of the experiences of life, organizational skills, and the discipline of reality on your side. The ride is not smooth or calm, but the highs far outweigh the lows.

grams, basic skills remediation, child and dependent care, and transportation. For information about these programs, contact your state Department of Labor or sex-equity coordinator.

For some women, improving literacy skills may be the first step in starting a job-training program. Literacy programs such as English as a Second Language (ESL) may be available through the private sector, community schools, or labor unions. For information, call an organization in your area that provides immigrant services.

Career Change

Those of us who have been in the work force fairly continuously may also want a change in our middle or later years. We may need to earn more money; we may be feeling "stuck" with no opportunity to advance; we may lose a job that we had thought was secure. We may have saved enough money to realize a long-delayed dream of more education or a more satisfying career. Or we may simply want a new challenge.

I had become an administrator and a large part of my job was juggling patient-care demands within the boundaries of a very rigid budget and insufficient nursing staff. I began to feel that I was contributing to the exploitation of the nurses. And so even though it was a "good job," it got to the point where it wasn't satisfying any more.

I sort of eased into studying gerontology, not really knowing that that was where I was going, because I had always had such a good time with my grandmother and I realized I wanted to work with healthy older people. I thought, "I'm getting older and maybe if I get in there and make some positive changes, then things would be generally better for older people and I'd benefit too." [a forty-five-year-old woman]

While there is nothing inherently wrong with staying in a job situation that offers little, it does waste a great deal of time and energy and deprives you of the possible satisfactions that come from meaningful and interesting work. If you are beginning to feel that you would like to move out into something new, but aren't sure what it is, take time to explore your options before resigning from a secure position. You don't have to settle for an unchallenging situation without making an effort to take stock and move in a new direction, but it is wise, particularly if you are over fifty-five, to assess what is available before burning your bridges. Changing careers is especially challenging during times of economic instability or recession.

Even women who have been in the work force continuously and with some degree of success find their opportunities narrowing in their fifties and sixties, especially if they want to change jobs. This is particularly true in fields like human services, where federal cuts in programs have reduced opportunities for advancement. Some of these women are willing to begin again at a lower-level job, but employers are reluctant to hire them, saying that the job would be "demeaning" for them, that they would feel as if they were supervising their mother, and so on. All are variants of that great no-win dilemma: "overqualified."

Take a hard look at the job you have now. Even if you don't like it very much, there are aspects of it that are keeping you there. Perhaps you like the people you work with, the fact that you can leave it all behind at five o'clock, or the satisfaction of producing a few finished products every day. Think about what you would miss if you left that job, and how it would affect you. What would change in your life if you were working somewhere else instead? On the other hand, what would you be glad to leave behind? A thorough analysis of your likes and dislikes should help you decide what would and would not work for you in a new situation.

Next, start investigating the alternatives. Perhaps simply a change of setting rather than occupation would accomplish what you want. If you're working as a nurse in an inconvenient location miles from home, with a shifting schedule, you may be able to take the edge off your dissatisfaction merely by moving to another kind of institution, or one in another part of town.

For most women, further exploration will be needed. The technique of "informational interviewing" has become commonplace in the last fifteen years. Ask anyone whose work you are interested in whether they would be willing to talk with you to tell you about what they do, how they got into the field, and why.

In considering options, remember that you don't have to make drastic changes. Try the modest and attainable first. Don't push yourself toward inappropriate or unrealistic goals, but don't avoid an unorthodox path solely because of your age.

An increasing number of women have moved into blue-collar jobs,[25] where they face enormous prejudice, not only from employers but from their fellow workers. Yet women who have been able to break into such jobs have enjoyed the physical freedom from sitting at a desk and have dramatically increased their earning power.

Some women who are dissatisfied with their jobs have decided to stay put and concentrate on trying to make the job more rewarding.

I'm a little bored at work because I feel that I'm not working at the right level, but I would not leave unless someone tapped me on the shoulder and offered me a job, because the last time I made a change (from a university job back to industry) it took me nine months. Instead I am focusing on making some changes in my present job so that I can move up. [a fifty-five-year-old woman]

For women who want to advance within their present organization, a support system can be enormously helpful. Find at least one supportive person to help you feel less isolated. Start a "women and work" group in your community. Check out networks of women who work in your field.

We spoke with many women who felt stymied in their growth and creativity but were reluctant to risk accumulated benefits and pensions. For women at or near their sixties, this is a particularly prevalent problem. Some women who enjoyed part-time or free-lance work in their younger years now want the security of a full-time salary and benefits, and the daily structure and companionship of colleagues in the same office. During times of recession and economic hardship it is increasingly difficult to move into the full-time labor force. In fact, there's a growing trend in the United States toward "permanent temporary" employment, an oxymoron that in essence means that workers are hired on a per-project or temporary basis, and then may or may not be "rehired" after a period of time. Such workers become part of the contingency work force.

If you are just a few years from retirement you may prefer not to "rock the boat" but instead to put your energy into exploring community activities and hobbies that may develop into satisfying retirement pursuits. We interviewed one woman in her sixties who turned a part-time avocation into a business, leading to a more satisfying work life after rather than before retirement!

Starting a business of one's own may be a good option for older women whose accomplishments are less likely to be recognized in the conventional workplace. Entrepreneurial opportunities have improved under The Women's Business Ownership Act of 1988, which provided funding for financial, management, marketing, and technical assistance for women business owners.[26] It can be an advantage to create one's own structure rather than to try to fit into someone else's. Yet this can be a particularly strenuous option. Consider carefully whether you have the health and energy to put in lots of extra hours, and the self-esteem to cope with the risk of failure.[27] Some women enjoy the convenience and economy of running a business out of their home, but may begin to feel isolated. For these women, networks of home-based entrepreneurs have been helpful in providing emotional support and exchanges of practical information. For information about long-term training and counseling programs, mentoring relationships, and networking contact the Women's Network for Entrepreneurial Training (WNET) through the Office of Women's Business Ownership in the U.S. Small Business Administration (SBA).

Getting Help

Recently, some career-counseling agencies have come under fire for charging excessively high fees and/or not delivering on promised services. Unlike employment agencies, which arrange interviews with prospective employers, career counselors offer only counseling and support while the applicant pursues the job search on her own. It can be immensely helpful to talk with an experienced, objective outsider on a regular basis, but consider carefully: Are you unemployed or working in a low-paying job and not in a position to pay large fees? How will you feel if counseling does not lead to a better job? Frequently, the value of counseling is overstated and made to seem essential to the process of change. Can you go through the same decision-making process on your own, or by talking with friends and colleagues? Job seekers are advised to check a counseling firm's reputation with the Better Business Bureau.

Some of the services offered by career-counseling firms are available free or on a sliding scale through the YWCA, the Department of Employment and Training, the Urban League, and Women's Educational and Industrial Unions. Books about job seeking and résumé writing are available in public libraries, as are reference books that list facts about corporations and names of personnel directors. You can take occupational-aptitude tests at colleges and other community centers and organizations.

Talking with friends and acquaintances, especially those who have good jobs, can help you find what you are looking for. Don't let pride stand in the way of letting people know you are looking for a job. A good contact alone probably will not get you a job, but a recommendation can get your résumé noticed.

RETIREMENT

RESISTING RETIREMENT

As of 1986, federal legislation made it illegal to force anyone to retire because of age, but compliance and enforcement are poor and litigation challenging forced retirement too long and too expensive for most women. Abolition of mandatory retirement provides us with the opportunity to make our own choices about whether or when to retire. Yet given the weight of custom and ingrained prejudice against older workers, compounded by the economic pressures of a society facing recession, those of us who want to remain employed well into our later years had better be prepared to fight for our newly won right.

Mandatory retirement policies and laws were based on the ageist assumption that our abilities decline with age. In fact, most abilities stay the same or improve; only those involving speed or great physical strength or dexterity tend to decline. Older workers are contributing important skills in many organizations.

A person's psychological need to find fulfillment through work does not end at sixty-five or seventy or any other age. Many older people feel oppressed by the forced inactivity of retirement and enjoy the mental and social stimulation of working. Furthermore, few women have earned enough or accumulated enough pension credits to feel assured of an adequate retirement income.

I was getting to the age when people expect you to retire and [was] getting a lot of messages that younger workers were more valuable. It was not easy to cope with. Leaving was traumatic, but I was delighted once I got out. I would have left sooner had I realized how well my free-lance work would go. I left with a decent pension, but only half what men in my position would get, because I had been paid less all those years. It is scary to retire, and I wanted to get all the benefits I could get. [a sixty-six-year-old woman]

Three quarters of Americans approaching retirement would prefer to reduce their hours rather than retire completely.[28] Some companies have begun to offer the option of part-time work to their retirees who wish to return. For the company, increasing their contingency work force provides a flexible, less costly pool of experienced workers on an as-needed basis. For the retiree, it provides an opportunity to maintain contact with former coworkers and to earn a partial income, meanwhile enjoying a less structured life, more freedom for recreation, or more time to attend to family responsibilities (e.g., elder care, spousal care). Women who work part-time may not be eligible for pension plans and other benefits, so be certain of what you are getting into if you are asked to participate in such a plan.

Some of us who want to continue working face pressures from employers to cut back to part-time work or to retire simply because of age.

They encouraged me to retire and work part-time running one of the elder programs I introduced, but part-time means no benefits and half salary. Then they treat you like a flunky instead of a professional. They've just introduced an early-retirement benefit for workers who retire within the next three years and I plan to go for it even though it's not early for me. With that additional benefit I'll have a decent retirement income. [a seventy-eight-year-old woman]

Eight years ago I was forced under protest to retire because the state office I worked for said I was too old and too disabled to work anymore. Since then I have served three terms in the Silver-Haired Legislature (see General Resources, page 444) and attended the White House Conference on Aging. I teach two classes a week at a community college, serve on two committees for a transportation system for the elderly and disabled, and volunteer five afternoons at the Department of Elder Affairs. But I am too old to work!!! [a seventy-six-year-old woman]

We have good reason to fight against the forced inactivity of retirement. A study of 229 older members of a health-maintenance organization found that of those whose inductive reasoning and spatial orientation skills had declined since first measured in 1970, about 40 percent were able to recoup the losses after only five one-hour training sessions. The researchers recommend that older people "flex their mental as well as physical muscles for better health" and offer suggestions such as working crossword puzzles or playing word games to improve inductive reasoning, and doing woodworking, assembling objects, reading maps, or doing needlework to improve spatial orientation. Especially if you are no longer working at a job, it is important to have hobbies, activities, and volunteer work that are mentally stimulating. Most important is to do something you really like and are interested in.[29]

Choosing Retirement

On the other hand, some of us *want* to retire. We may want more time to be with a retired partner, family, or friends, to start our own business, or to pursue the arts. Increasing numbers of women will choose retirement in the future because more women are working for pay and will have more adequate retirement incomes.

The Tower

She struggled
heart pounding
inched up the tower
tested each rung
gay voices higher
mocked fear.

Halfway up,
a rung missing,
she froze.
Then—
"Why am I climbing
this tower?"

She danced down.

Lois Harris

When the chairperson of my department asked me to reconsider and stay on, to my surprise I found myself saying, "I'm tired." The more I did, the more things would open up for me to do. I felt I was giving a lot more than I was getting paid for. Part-time jobs tend to be exploitive, and I felt that over the years I had been taken advantage of. [a sixty-seven-year-old woman]

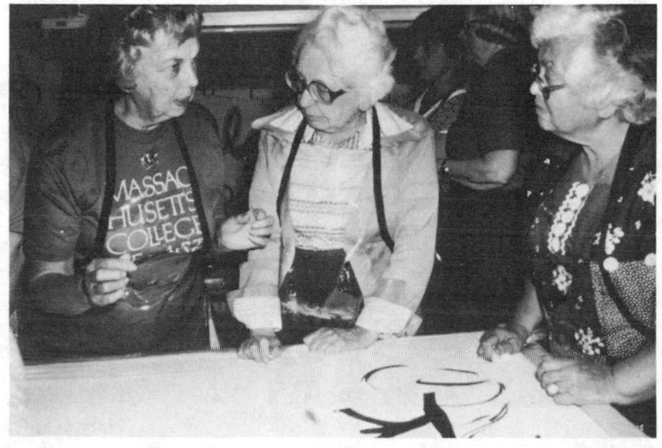

Ellen Shub

One trivial reason I retired was that my work hours were changed. All of a sudden I had to be at work at 8:00 in the morning and I found that waking up a half hour earlier was a great burden. So today, eleven years later, I awaken in the morning and look at the ceiling and say I don't have to get up—and I get up! [a seventy-six-year-old woman]

My poor husband had this terrible back operation. I worked right through the whole time and then I thought, "We have to spend more time together. We have a place in Vermont which is a sheer delight, and our grandchildren live there. I want to see more of them, to really know them. We have a son in California. When do I get to see him?" [a sixty-seven-year-old woman]

I haven't regretted retiring. I didn't quit my job through any dissatisfaction with the job or the people, but I just felt that my life needed a change. I noticed that after working an eight-hour day I didn't have much steam left for social life and fun. It's been pleasant spending these years doing what I want to do because I spent so many years accommodating myself to other people's needs and plans. [a woman in her seventies]

When I retired and walked out of that place for the last time I felt so relaxed, so free. It took me about a year to finally believe I didn't have to hide. I had been so afraid that the people I worked for and those who worked for me might guess my secret. No matter where my lover and I went as a couple we held back. Only lately, now that she is sixty-two and I am retired, did we go to a party where we knew there were others like us and we danced together for the first time publicly. I don't flaunt it anyway, so I never had any problems, but now I feel much better not having to worry about being found out. [a woman in her sixties]

After Retirement

Those of us who find a feeling of self-worth in work may be willing to retire if we can find an alternative way to make a meaningful contribution to society.

I had to begin a whole new life! I tried several different things. I worked for a U.S. Senator, not for money. I never worked for money after I retired, because I didn't need to earn money. But I could not live without work. I cannot

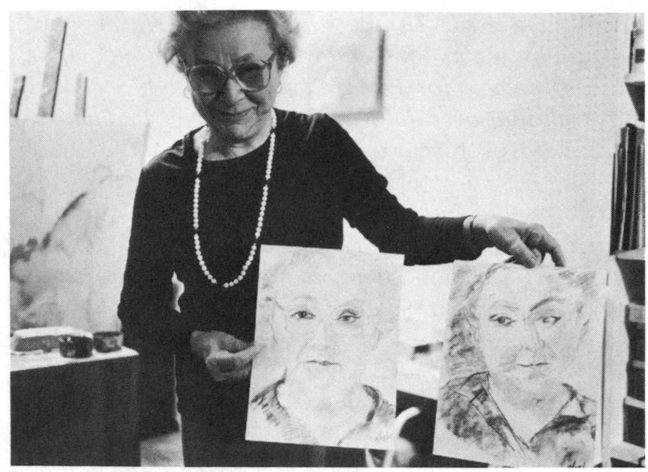

Marianne Gontarz

live my life without a purpose, a humanitarian purpose. [a seventy-five-year-old woman]

I resented having to retire. Reorganization forced me out. For two years I did not know where to turn. I did small jobs; my years as an information and referral director had given me many contacts. As I got involved in community action—hearings on the Hill (i.e., Congress), work on many D.C. committees (Ambulatory Care, Nursing Homes, Health Advocacy), and national and local work with the Gray Panthers—I find myself almost busier than I was when I worked. I manage to keep time to spare for my great-grandsons; one is six months, the other is two. [an eighty-two-year-old woman]

After I retired at age sixty-nine, I tried to sign up for some classes I thought might be interesting. To my dismay I discovered they were all evening classes. The only daytime choice that interested me at all was a beginners' class in oil painting. I decided to sign up although I was sure I couldn't draw a straight line. My first attempt was a still life of a fruit basket flanked by colorful straw-bottomed bottles of wine. Surprisingly, the fruit turned out lifelike and the whole painting was in good perspective, although very crude. I have now progressed to beautiful portraits with excellent likenesses. [a woman in her seventies]

All I could do when I worked was work. I always wanted to be involved in the community. Now that I am retired, I belong to a senior advocacy group, I work with kids in school, I live in subsidized housing that has a wonderful mixture of people of different ages, different races, various disabilities. I am one of their representatives on the neighborhood development association which is building more houses for sale and more rental apartments for low- and middle-income people. I also get paid for role-playing with students at a local college of optometry to help them learn to relate better with patients. My daughter asks me why I am so busy and I tell her that I am spending my time the way I want to. [a seventy-one-year-old woman]

I do as I please with more freedom than when I was younger; I can decide how to occupy my time and what people I want to know. Sometimes I feel like a street-smart kid. I plan to continue to work on my memoirs, a book that is one third completed. My book of poems is in the process of its second edition. My plans for more poetry are as varied as the issues that move me. [a ninety-one-year-old woman]

Retirement gives a growing number of older women the opportunity to pursue higher education through enrollment in college or in a short-term adult education or Elderhostel program (see Resources for this chapter). The large number of older people, mostly women, who go back to college testifies to their desire to remain mentally sharp. Evidence shows that older persons do just as well or better academically than their younger peers. Short-term memory may recede, but judgment is enhanced. "Use it or lose it" applies to both our bodies and our minds.

Volunteer Opportunities

Good volunteer opportunities are available in hospitals, schools, libraries, art museums, and numerous nonprofit organizations. Contact your local Council on Aging, Office of Elder Affairs, Area Agency on Aging, or Voluntary Action Cen-

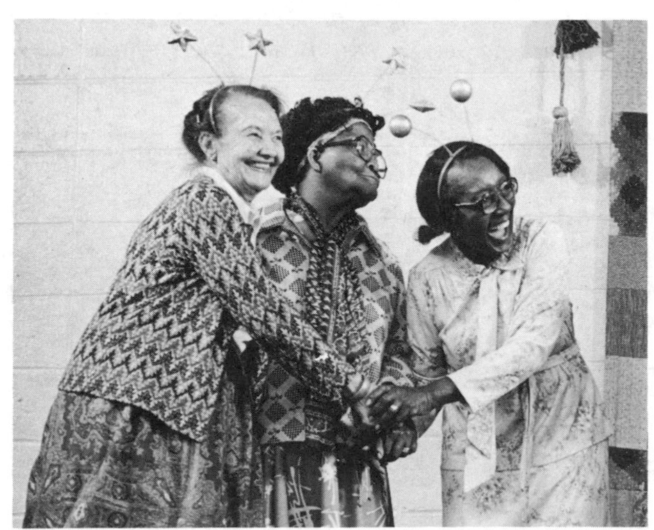

Deborah Kahn

ter to find out about volunteer programs. Call your state house of representatives or city hall to find out which agency administers volunteer programs for elders in your community.

Before going to bed I plan my next day. The priority things I do first; then if I have time I do the rest. I find keeping busy keeps you alert and young. I belong to several organizations and always offer my services, such as being a corresponding secretary, getting ads for the calendar, helping arrange programs, etc. I have many friends who can rely on me for a ride to the doctor or shopping or just company. I taught remedial reading for several years and worked as a volunteer in the hospital. I'm enjoying my retirement. My grandson said to me he can't wait until he is a senior citizen so he can have as much fun as I do. [a seventy-eight-year-old woman]

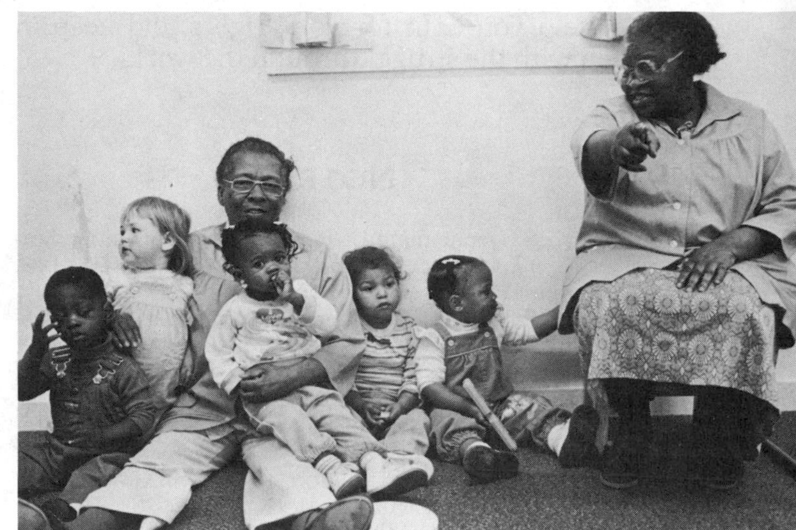

Marianne Gontarz

Several federally funded volunteer programs for older Americans are available in most communities, such as Elder Service Corps, Foster Grandparents, Retired Senior Volunteer Program (RSVP), Service Corps of Retired Executives (SCORE), and Vista. Other paid opportunities, such as Senior Aides Programs and Senior Companion Programs, are available through the Senior Community Service Employment Program (SCSEP) funded by Title V of the Older Americans Act.

Many of these programs enable women to use their skills, participate in job training, or explore new interests while serving their community. Some of the programs provide small stipends, meal and travel allowances, and accident insurance. Participants may have to qualify by meeting minimum age requirements and specific income guidelines. If you receive Supplemental Security Income (SSI) or a housing subsidy, such programs may be more advantageous for you than a minimum-wage job, since they are not counted as income and thus will not affect your eligibility for such assistance.

I don't worry. If I have no money, I'll go on welfare. I worked until I was sixty-nine at everything from factory work to the office at the shipyard. When I retired I stayed home and brooded. After I was home nearly a year I found the foster-grandparent program. It's been great. It's made a new life for me. [a seventy-two-year-old woman]

There is definitely a changing attitude toward older people. When I became director of the foster-grandparent program in 1976 I had to convince the directors of a day-care center that a foster grandparent could help the children. Now I have so many centers waiting for foster grandparents that I can't fill all the requests. The day-care teachers tell me that the mixing of the young and old creates a magic atmosphere, something they had never dreamed of. Now the foster grandparents also work (volunteer) in public schools, hospitals, and battered women's shelters. Everybody wants them. [a sixty-five-year-old woman]

The work I do now as a volunteer is very important. I feel that each of the three organizations I work for is important in a different way. One group does education, another does direct-action political work, and the third works for passing legislation. In each of these organizations work is saved for me, so I know that they rely on me for specific tasks. They used to have lots of women whose children were off at school, but now women are in paid jobs and so I am an important volunteer. [a ninety-year-old woman]

Work and retirement are two areas where we must expand choices for women of all ages. We must fight sex, age, and other types of discrimination and join together in women's organizations, labor unions, elder and other advocacy organizations to fight the gender gap in earnings and to enforce our right to decide when and whether we want to retire. We want retirement to mean that we have chosen to leave paid work for something else, and not survival on a pittance because we are no longer welcome at work. To accomplish all this we must keep informed and connected with movements for equal rights in the workplace. See Resources for this chapter for names of organizations and publications that can help you fight for your rights and keep in touch with the struggle around the world.*

Notes

1. U.S. Department of Labor, Bureau of Labor Statistics, *Employment and Earnings*. Washington, DC: U.S. Government Printing Office, December 1992.

2. U.S. Bureau of the Census, Economics and Statistics Administration, "New 1990 Census Report Shows Occupational Shifts for Nation's Work Force." *United States Department of Commerce News*, Jan. 29, 1993.

3. U.S. Department of Labor, Bureau of Labor Statistics, *Employment in Perspective: Women in the Labor Force*, Report 834, Washington, DC: U.S. Government Printing Office, Third Quarter, 1992.

4. U.S. Bureau of the Census, Economics and Statistics Administration, U.S. Department of Commerce, "Money Income of Households, Families, and Persons in the United States, 1991." *Current Population Reports, Consumer Income*, Series P-60, No. 180, Washington, DC: U.S. Government Printing Office, 1991.

5. AARP, "The Contingent Workforce: Implications for Midlife and Older Women." *Women's Initiative Fact Sheet*. Washington, DC: AARP, 1991.

6. Paula Rayman, Kimberly Allshouse, and Jessie Allen, "Resiliency Amidst Inequity: Older Women Workers in an Aging United States," in Jessie Allen and Alan Pifer, eds., *Women on the Front Lines: Meeting the Challenge of an Aging America*. Washington, DC: The Urban Institute, 1993, pp. 133–65.

7. U.S. Bureau of the Census, "Money Income of Households," op. cit.

8. Older Women's League (OWL), "Paying for Prejudice: A Report on Midlife and Older Women in America's Labor Force." *1991 Mother's Day Report*, Washington, DC: OWL, 1991.

9. U.S. Department of Labor, Women's Bureau, "Women of Hispanic Origin in the Labor Force." *Facts on Working Women*, No. 89-1, Washington, DC: U.S. Government Printing Office, August 1989.

10. Jean Dresden Grambs, ed., *Women Over Forty*. New York: Springer, 1989.

11. U.S. Bureau of the Census, Economics and Statistics Division, U.S. Department of Commerce, "Sixty-Five Plus in America." *Current Population Reports, Special Studies*, P23-178, Washington, DC: U.S. Government Printing Office, 1992.

12. U.S. Department of Labor, Bureau of Labor Statistics, Employment in Perspective: *Women in the Labor Force*, Report 831. Washington, DC: U.S. Government Printing Office, Second Quarter, 1992.

13. U.S. Bureau of the Census, "Money Income of Households," op. cit.

14. Rayman, et al., op. cit.

15. OWL, op. cit.

16. Testimony of the Older Women's League on "Older Women and the Labor Force" before the Joint Economic Committee, June 6, 1984.

17. U.S. Department of Labor, Women's Bureau, "Women with Work Disabilities." *Facts on Working Women*, No. 92-2, Washington, DC: Government Printing Office, March 1992.

18. U.S. Department of Labor, Office of the Secretary, Women's Bureau, *A Working Woman's Guide to Her Job Rights*, Leaflet 55. Washington, DC: U.S. Government Printing Office, August 1992.

19. Sara M. Evans and Barbara J. Nelson, "Comparable Worth for Public Employees: Implementing a New Wage Policy in Minnesota," in Peggy Kahn and Elizabeth Meehan, eds., *Equal Value/Comparable Worth in the UK and the USA*. London: Macmillan, 1992, pp. 230–58.

20. Roslyn L. Feldberg, "Comparable Worth and Nurses in the USA," in Peggy Kahn and Elizabeth Meehan, eds., *op. cit.*, pp. 181–214.

21. U.S. Department of Labor, Bureau of Labor Statistics, *Employment and Earnings*. Washington, DC: U.S. Government Printing Office, January 1991.

22. U.S. Department of Labor, Women's Bureau, "Women in Labor Organizations." *Facts on Working Women*, No. 89-2, Washington, DC: U.S. Government Printing Office, August 1989.

23. Joyce Miller, "Women and Unions: The Perfect Match." *Charlotte Observer*, Jan. 23, 1992.

24. Mark Feinberg, "Long-timers Join Fray at 'McHarvard.'" *In These Times*, Vol. 11, No. 30 (1987).

25. U.S. Department of Labor, Women's Bureau, "Women in the Skilled Trades and in Other Manual Occupations." *Facts on Working Women*, No. 90-5, Washington, DC: U.S. Government Printing Office, January 1991.

26. U.S. Department of Labor, Women's Bureau, "Women Business Owners." *Facts on Working Women*, No. 89-5, Washington, DC: U.S. Government Printing Office, December 1989.

27. Mary D. Fillmore, *Women MBA's: A Foot in the Door*. Boston: G. K. Hall, 1987, p. 177.

28. F. Thomas Juster, Institute for Social Research, University of Michigan, reporting on first wave of a five-year Health and Retirement Study. Quoted in *The Boston Globe*, June 18, 1993, pp. 6–7.

29. Sherry Willis and K. Warner Schaie, "Can Decline in Adult Intellectual Functioning Be Reversed?" *Developmental Psychology*, Vol. 22, No. 2 (1986), pp. 223–32.

*Increasingly, as corporations become global we need a worldwide perspective to understand trends in work, employment practices, and unemployment. See Vilunya Diskin, "Developing an International Awareness," in Boston Women's Health Book Collective. *The New Our Bodies, Ourselves*. New York, Simon & Schuster, 1992, Ch. 27.

14

MONEY MATTERS: THE ECONOMICS OF AGING FOR WOMEN

✦

BY GILLIE CAMPBELL AND CAROLINE T. CHAUNCEY

SPECIAL THANKS TO MARILYN ROGERS AND NAOMI B. ISLER

1994 UPDATE BY GILLIE CAMPBELL WITH SPECIAL THANKS TO LYNN BURBRIDGE, JOAN CHASAN, AND FRANCES LEONARD

RESOURCES FOR THIS CHAPTER ON PAGES 477–79

The middle and older years are a time of many changes in our lives, some of which will be reflected in our financial situation. Some of us may have more money on hand as children leave home and household expenses diminish. Advancement in our work may bring us new resources to manage and to enjoy. Or we may receive an inheritance or insurance settlement and want to learn how best to manage it for our future security. For far too many of us, however, an illness—ours or our partner's—can create overwhelming medical bills; divorce, widowhood, or employment discrimination may leave us vulnerable financially. We may need to apply for public assistance for the first time. Whatever happens, we may find ourselves facing more complex financial decisions.

THE ROOTS OF POVERTY AND DOWNWARD MOBILITY

Economic discrimination based on sex and race affects us, as women, throughout our lives. As we get older, age discrimination compounds and deepens the inequality of resources. The poorest groups in the United States are women over sixty-five living by themselves and women raising children alone. These two groups make up 70 percent of all poor people.[1] Consider these facts:

- 53 percent of children who live with their mothers are poor, compared with 10 percent of children who live with both parents.[2]
- Over 15 percent of older women are poor, compared with less than 8 percent of older men.
- 38 percent of older black women are poor; 25 percent of older Hispanic women are poor.
- 27 percent of older women who live alone are poor.
- 20 percent of women aged seventy-five and over are poor, and another 30 percent are near poverty. Men aged seventy-five and over, by comparison, have poverty rates of 10 percent, and near-poverty rates of 16 percent.[3]

We who are in our forties and older are caught in the dilemma of meeting contradictory social expectations. Growing numbers of us need to support ourselves, to provide for children or dependent relatives, and to take responsibility for our own financial futures. Yet employers still perceive women as dependents of men. Because of low earnings and the pressure to interrupt paid jobs to care for families, women face a tremendous risk of poverty—especially when we do not accept or have access to financial support from men.

My situation has really changed. I was married to a professional in a high-paying field, but I worked with low-income people. It was as if I had one life by day and another by night. Now that we are separated, I'm poorer than I've ever been—more like the people I used to work with. [a woman in her forties with children still at home]

The risk of poverty for independent women is nothing new; what is new today is the rapid growth in the number of women who fall prey to this poverty.

- An increasing number of all families, 17 percent in 1989, are now supported by women.
- 53 percent of all poor families are maintained by women.
- 76 percent of poor black families, 48 percent of poor Hispanic families, and 44 percent of poor white families are headed by women.[4]

At midlife, many women experience a sudden loss of income, often precipitated by divorce or the death or disability of a partner. Women who have never worked outside the home may suddenly find themselves with no income and little or no experience to aid them in earning a living.

I have no home, no job, poor health, and no health insurance. I married at eighteen and spent thirty years raising six children. I graduated first in my class in high school and wanted to go to college, but I didn't have the money. My husband threatened to throw me down the stairs, and he hit me twice. There were no transition houses in those days, and when things were really bad I ran out in the woods and slept in the leaves. Today I realize that by staying I harmed my children. I shouldn't have tried to keep us together for financial reasons. It's incredible that I lived through it. [a woman in her fifties]

A woman who does unpaid work in the home has no personal benefits such as disability insurance, unemployment compensation, pension plans, or health coverage. Her financial security is tied to her husband's earnings and benefits.

When a marriage is dissolved, the woman who has been a housewife is like any other displaced worker—she needs a new source of income and new skills. But there are few sources of support to help her make this transition. Few widows can reinstate lapsed medical insurance, and those below the age of sixty-two cannot draw Social Security benefits. Only a small percentage of divorced women ever receive alimony or child-support payments. One study found that only 15.5 percent of divorced or separated women were awarded alimony in 1990. When child-support payments were awarded, only half of women awarded child support had received full payment in 1989.[5] Fathers must be forced to meet their child-support responsibilities. Some states now require middle-class and affluent fathers to pay child support, not just families applying for welfare.

Changes in divorce laws have dramatically affected many older women. As Ellen Goodman observes, "Courts have treated husbands and wives, fathers and mothers . . . with an evenhandedness that is, in effect, unfair. Property has been divided both equally and inequitably."[6] For women who have devoted themselves to family and homemaking, who have put husbands through school, and whose own employment experience is either limited or paid at a much lower level, an equal division of assets is unfair. This is especially true when children are still at home or in school. And many women get even less than half the assets.

The overwhelming majority of states now permit "no-fault divorce," divorce that is granted without the necessity of finding a spouse guilty of some marital misconduct. The most common no-fault ground is voluntary separation for a period of time. Prior to the enactment of no-fault divorce statutes, there had to be a specified fault, a wholly innocent plaintiff spouse, and a wholly guilty defendant spouse.[7]

No-fault divorce has made it easier to get a divorce, but it has reduced women's bargaining power toward winning a fair settlement. States vary, however, in the factors they take into account in determining alimony and assets settlements. In many states such factors as length of marriage, health of the parties, and ability to earn income and acquire assets in the future may be considered. In a very few states, conduct of the parties may be considered for purposes of the settlement, though not in granting the divorce. All states have laws concerning support of minor children.

One of the consequences of the spread of no-fault divorce has been a rapid rise in the number of lengthy marriages (fifteen years or more) that have dissolved.

Suddenly my (I thought so good) husband said, "You don't deserve this—I couldn't have a better wife, or a better mother on this earth, and certainly wouldn't be where I am without you—but I have to leave and think." I truly was my husband's buddy and helper. How I wish I could talk to the people who passed the [no-fault divorce] bill. Please forgive me for sounding bitter, but I got the bills today and where are the dollars for me to pay them? I do not deserve this kind of life, as hard as I worked. [an Indiana woman][8]

Divorce "reform" has been a financial disaster for women—especially older women—and for children. A recent study shows that following a midlife divorce, a woman's income can drop by $10,000 to $15,000 one year later.[9]

New approaches are needed to strengthen women's chances of gaining an equitable settlement in divorce proceedings. The following factors should be taken into account. Many middle-aged and older women have not worked outside the home consistently enough to qualify for a job that pays enough to live on. Alimony should not be seen as a stopgap measure, since the gap between work in the home and paid work may be a difficult one to cross in the middle and later years. Spousal support (alimony) in such instances should be approached as compensation for past unpaid work in the home and for the cost of having dedicated oneself to a husband's career. There is a recent trend to award alimony to older women who have been in long-term marriages where there is an extreme imbalance between the partners' incomes. This trend primarily benefits white women over forty who have no children present, and whose unpaid support has helped their husbands' careers. A substantial cash settlement instead of, or in addition to, monthly payments can protect women against the common practice of nonpayment and will provide funds for the divorced woman to manage and invest. Finally, the husband's pension—a product of his earning capacity—reflects our investment in his career, and so represents an asset that we have a legal right to share or to use as a bargaining chip in negotiations.

Some husbands, especially those who are self-employed, will intentionally limit, defer, or even deliberately misstate their income in order to appear less affluent during the divorce negotiations. Frequently, in the years following the divorce a former husband's income may sharply increase, but his former wife, during the divorce negotiations, may have bargained away her right to an increase in alimony. Even if she did not do so, it will require tremendous effort on her part and significant lawyers' fees to try to modify her divorce judgment in order to increase the alimony or child support to share in her ex-husband's increased income. Sometimes the high cost of getting a fair settlement forces women to drop their legitimate demands.

My husband is self-employed and has always had total control of the flow of income from the business, even though it was jointly owned by both of us. He has been consistently secretive about the amount and location of funds and property. In the settlement, my husband got the business and I got the house. My husband offered $10 per week in support to the child who is under eighteen and it cost me $10,000 in legal fees to get him to agree to $40 per week. [a fifty-two-year-old woman]

You have a right to sue for failure to pay court-ordered alimony or make child-support payments. You can also sometimes reopen divorce-settlement cases because of changed circumstances, though this can be very expensive and time-consuming. Check with your attorney or a Legal Aid office. (See Resources for this chapter for helpful books on divorce.)

The Economics of Retirement

Traditional wisdom has it that sound retirement finances are like a stool with three legs. The three legs of the retirement stool are assets (such as savings or a house), pension payments, and Social Security benefits. However, because of economic discrimination, all three legs of the stool are rickety for older women.

Assets are the most obviously wobbly leg. Since women earn less than men, it's no surprise that we have little chance to accumulate savings. Very few women over sixty-five are receiving income from savings accounts, and even fewer have income from investments. For many of us, our sole asset is our house. Not only is it difficult to cash in this asset but it costs money to keep it up. Reverse mortgages have been one way for women to get out of this financial bind. There are pitfalls in these agreements, however, and in recessionary times banks are reluctant to lend on this basis (see Housing Alternatives and Living Arrangements chapter).

Women who are widowed are no better off economically than divorced or never-married women. According to a 1990 report, widows are often the poorest of all elderly people living alone. A woman may not have been poor before

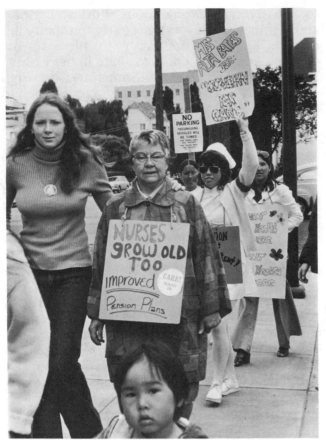

Cathy Cade

her husband's death, but the expenses of his illness and burial may have used up savings, and the loss of his pension may leave her newly poor.[10] Yet widows go on to live an average of eighteen and one-half years after their husbands' deaths.

Only 22 percent of all women over sixty-five receive any income from public or private pensions—the second leg of the stool—as a spouse or as a retired worker; 78 percent receive nothing.[11] Only 15 percent of black women and 7 percent of Hispanic women receive any pension income.[12] Most employers require that workers stay in a job at least five continuous years in order to qualify for a pension. But middle-aged and older women often have interrupted employment to take care of children, to accompany partners whose careers demand a move, or to take care of elderly parents or ill partners.

Those of us who stay home to raise children have fewer years in which to accrue pension benefits; special bonuses, such as those offered for more than twenty-five years of continuous service, are out of our reach. In 1986, the average annual pension income was $7,384 for men and $4,383 for women.[13] Sections 401(k) and 403(b) of the federal tax code allow employees to shelter income from taxes and have it matched by their employer. But this primarily benefits those who work for corporations large enough to participate in these plans and those who earn enough to set some earnings aside for the future.

A statement about my pension came the other day. If I work until I'm sixty-five, I'll get $125 a month. My boss's came also—he'll get $900 a month. He has had the resources from his high salary to contribute to that fund over the years, but I have not. [a sixty-one-year-old woman recently employed]

Some of us who do not have pensions of our own qualify for benefits on the basis of our husband's earnings. Nonetheless, women are often left without these benefits through divorce or the death of their husbands before retirement. Many older women are struggling today because until recently an employed husband could elect to receive benefits for his lifetime only. Though the pension checks received by the retired husband were larger under such an arrangement, the surviving wife was entitled to no benefits upon her husband's death. The 1984 Retirement Equity Act requires the written consent of both spouses before survivor benefits can be waived.

In the absence of income from pensions or assets, most older women find themselves relying on Social Security—the third leg of the "retirement stool." Thirty-three percent of older single women depend on Social Security for 90 percent of their income.[14] And it's not much income. The average benefit paid in 1992 to retired women, based on their own earnings, was $562 a month;[15] the poverty threshold for a single person over sixty-five was $561 per month,[16] and 15 percent of women over sixty-five live below it.

Like pensions, Social Security discriminates against women in a number of ways. Benefits are based on earnings averaged over a period of years, including years when we may have left the labor force and earned no income. Payment of benefits based on a low level of earnings extends the discrimination that kept them low in the first place. Most important, Social Security does not give recognition to the value of our unpaid work in the home. Those of us whose husbands' earnings exceeded our own may find that we receive more money if we draw benefits based on our husbands' earnings—as if we had never worked outside the home at all. In this case we forfeit all the money we paid into Social Security during our working years.

The association of poverty and old age for women seems inevitable if we look at the whole social structure and a woman's subordinate place in it. Yet growing poorer as we age comes as a bitter shock to many of us. Some of us may feel ashamed, as if our economic problems reflect personal failure; others feel angry.

In fact, our poverty is the result of social pressure to be dependent on others, to put our families first and ourselves and our work second. For those of us who raised families, saving for our own retirement may not have been a priority during the busy years of paying for children's education or covering immediate costs of living. For those of us who worked all our adult years, with or without families to raise, retirement may have seemed far away. Few of us envisioned ourselves alone and poor.

Legislation must be passed to provide benefits that recognize women's unpaid labor contributions, support during transition periods from homemaking to the labor force, and security for widowhood in old age. Employers must be encouraged to provide part-time work for all women, from young mothers and students to elders. Adequate retirement and disability benefits should be available to all, including women who have been homemakers all or most of their lives.

MANAGING OUR FINANCES WHATEVER OUR MEANS

MAKING ENDS MEET

Despite our best efforts, few of us can expect to live without having to worry about making ends meet. The accumulated obstacles that women confront in working for financial self-reliance take their toll even among those who plan thoroughly and save diligently.

I'm on Social Security and SSI. I have no savings. I get two checks a month—one for $235 and one for $238. I have to pay $233 in rent. I get $10 in food stamps—that's gone in one minute. How am I supposed to survive on $250 a month? [a woman in her seventies who lives alone in subsidized housing]

Learning to cope with a lowered or inadequate income requires a creative outlook and a flexibility we may not have realized we possessed. Making a budget is one of the most important tools in knowing where money is going and altering or cutting expenses.

Here is one budget strategy. First, list monthly costs for survival expenses: food, rent or mortgage payments, utilities, taxes, loan repayments, transportation to work. Next, list flexible expenses: savings, clothes, entertainment, travel, and gifts. Flexible expenses can also be the ones we don't notice until after the money is gone, and a budget can serve to make us aware of these unconscious, sometimes expensive, spending patterns.

For most of us our largest expenditure is housing. Housing costs are difficult to reduce unless we are open to changing the way we live (see Housing Alternatives and Living Arrangements chapter). Expenses can also be reduced through senior-citizen discounts in most communities. The American Association of Retired Persons and other groups have obtained discounts for members from fast-food chains, hotels, car-rental agencies, and bus and train companies. Entertainment costs can be cut by joining community groups that may get discounts on group activities or provide free social events for elders. Some women barter skills and services with friends to conserve money. Each of us is the best judge of where we do or do not want to economize.

When I retired, I cut down on a lot of my expenditures. I stopped going to the hairdresser every week—you'd be amazed how much that amounts to over the course of a year. I no longer bought expensive clothes, because I didn't need them for my job. I could dress any old way I wanted. I mowed my own lawn and shopped for food carefully so my money would last. But I kept my symphony tickets, even though they were expensive, because it gave me pleasure. [a woman in her seventies]

I am supporting myself and two children on $13,500, which is close to poverty level by government standards. To make ends meet, I have yard sales when the weather is good, and I sell household items, used clothing, and plants. I never buy magazines or extras, to avoid anxiety about paying bills on time. [a fifty-two-year-old woman]

After I've paid the rent, I pay the phone bill. My burial plot is all paid for, and I have just a little insurance for my grown children. Then there's my health. My doctor refused Medicaid—after fifteen years—and now I have to pay him $27 out of every check. Then it takes $2.50 to do the laundry—you've got to keep your linens clean. I try to

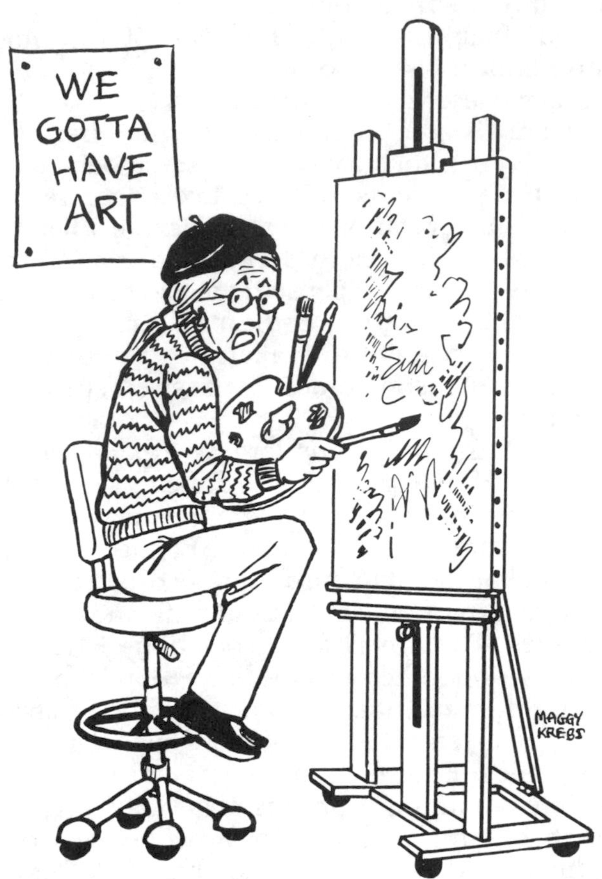
WE
GOTTA
HAVE
ART
MAGGY
KREBS

"I'm finally old enough for Social Security. Now I can be a subsidized starving artist." ©Maggy Krebs

buy the cheapest things. I always make my own milk from powder. I only buy bread and chicken, and those no-name paper articles, but it still adds up. If I need clothes, I go across the street to the thrift shop. I watch for yard sales—if you see something for half a buck, there's a Christmas present. If I have 80 cents I can go to the Council on Aging for a hot lunch. But the last two weeks of the month are always hard. You just can't make it. I'm down to my last $10, and I've got more than two weeks to go. [a woman in her seventies]

Applying for Benefits

Many older women do not sign up for Supplemental Security Income (SSI), food stamps, or Medicaid benefits because they don't want to take "welfare." Seventy-five percent of those eligible for SSI but not receiving it are women.[17] We need to realize that we earned those benefits through the taxes we paid on our earnings or by doing unpaid work while our husbands worked and paid taxes. We should not hesitate to apply for and receive whatever benefits we may qualify for. For many women, such benefits spell survival.

Supplemental Security Income is a cash-assistance program designed to meet the needs of the long-term disabled, the blind, and those elders whose income and assets fall below certain limits. Some states supplement the low SSI federal payment. SSI eligibility may, in some states, also qualify you for Medicaid, food stamps, and other noncash assistance such as fuel assistance. Programs vary from state to state, so you should check. The program is administered by the Social Security Administration and funded by the federal and state governments.

We may find it difficult to apply for these programs and to persevere in spite of bureaucratic indifference or hostility. Often it is necessary to reapply or to appeal adverse decisions.

It's very difficult to make an application for all these kinds of things when one has been financially and personally independent, but if you get scared enough and hungry enough and desperate enough, you'll swallow your pride and go through it. The frustration of dealing with most of the agencies is indeed enough to deter most.

A piece of advice I have learned from people in the know: appeal absolutely everything. Don't ever accept no for an answer. In making applications and in making appeals, always smile and be gracious; be assertive without being aggressive. I have learned that little things help, like not blaming the person who must carry out a policy set by the government. Most of us, when we apply, are naturally focused on ourselves, and I think it helps to acknowledge your interviewer as a human being, too. I say things like "Your job must be distasteful at times," "Gee, Susan, you seem rushed today," or "You're looking a little tired today, Linda. Has it been a rough day for you?" These kinds of things I think make a big difference. [a woman who applied for Social Security Disability Income (SSDI) when she became disabled at age forty-five]

I didn't have to work until after the divorce. My husband was a construction worker and made pretty good money—at least it seemed so at the time. We had a joint bank account, but he took it all and I worked for thirteen years as a practical nurse just to pay the bills. Then my health went. If I wasn't sick, I'd still be working. I didn't know where to go. I had to go on welfare in the beginning. Eighty-seven dollars a month—I don't know how I lived on it, but I did. It took me five years to get on SSI, but finally I did. Your forties and fifties can be a bad time. Once you're sixty-two and eligible for Social Security, you get a little more understanding. [a woman in her seventies]

Life was never easy. My husband was an alcoholic who worked when he felt like it. I wouldn't see a penny of his pay—he'd go down to the bar and cash his check there. I wasn't able to work—I have arthritis of the spine and diabetes. When we separated, I went on welfare. Now that I am on SSI, things have picked up a little. [a woman in her sixties]

For these women, one solution to their financial dead end has been to become politically active—pressing doctors to accept Medicaid, lobbying to protect Social Security, and fighting for fair treatment of women on welfare.

We're not sitting back and letting others walk all over us anymore; now we're fighting for the elderly. We've been on TV and in the papers and I've learned to chair meetings. It's encouraging to see things being accomplished. [a woman in her seventies]

PLANNING FOR THE FUTURE

It is not unreasonable for women in their middle years to prepare for living alone. It is no less necessary than preparing for illness by carrying a health-insurance policy. The massive obstacles we face as women make economic survival a difficult task. It would be a lie to pretend that, for the vast majority of women, saving for retirement on our low earnings is easy or even possible. But the key to a positive and self-reliant future is the ability to confront the financial issues of our own survival now.

I wish that from the age of eighteen I had had a really knowledgeable attitude about money. My God! It determines the quality of your life. Women should become aware of money as a power. If you are a middle-aged woman and you haven't got a pension plan, you'd better start thinking. So much of your future is going to depend on economic resources. [a fifty-six-year-old divorced woman]

No matter what the circumstances, we must have effective control over our financial affairs. Money, after all, is not only essential to survival in our culture, it is a crucial part of our personal lives affecting our most significant relationships. To *expect* to understand it and use it effectively is the place to begin. This means educating yourself about your financial position, knowing exactly what would happen if your partner died or left, and setting priorities for the future. This can be done whether you are alone, in a marriage, or in another kind of partnership.

Many women, especially middle-class women, have grown up with some disabling assumptions about money: It's not nice to talk about it; I'll be cheated if I take a risk; men know more than I do; someone will show up to take care of me. Working-class women often grow up expecting to take care of themselves, but may have another set of disabling assumptions: Men are unreliable; I'll have to shoulder all the burdens myself; I'll cope with today—tomorrow will take care of itself; planning won't make any difference. All of these assumptions can have devastating results.

I started an advocacy organization. Because funding is so tight the last thing that gets addressed is providing benefits the staff need. As I get older I'm more aware of pension and disability insurance, and of paying a price for doing work I love. I had no other source of income than my salary so I called the board together and created a personnel committee to address the range of issues relating to providing benefits for staff. [a forty-nine-year-old woman]

Many women take charge of the financial record keeping for their household, paying the bills and balancing the checkbook. They are more knowledgeable about the day-to-day financial picture than women who are less involved, yet they may still defer to a man to do the long-term planning, or they may rely on fate and hope for the best.

We *are* capable of understanding and managing our finances. Both self-supporting women and those supported by a partner are responsible for running a household at a given level of income. Much of our experience and expertise has been focused on knowing how to stretch a limited amount of money. We know how to "squeeze a dollar till the eagle screams," clipping coupons, buying at sales, and so forth. But when it comes to managing money and *making it grow*, many of us feel at a loss.

Until I was divorced at age forty-eight I never gave a thought to my old age, except to say that I didn't want to end up like my mother, who outlived my father by twenty-three years. But my marriage seemed solid and we were the same age, and my husband expected a sizable pension besides Social Security benefits. Who thinks that far ahead? The divorce was an awful shock and the lawyer (also my husband's) wasn't any help at all. I ended up with very little except my low-paying job and half a house. No pension for me and not much Social Security. It took a while to get myself going again, but thank God I did. I went back to school part-time and decided to go into financial planning for women. I've not only done quite well for myself, but I've helped a lot of other women who were just as lost as I was. It was just like starting all over again, but worth it.

We should begin thinking of ourselves as independent financial entities, keeping some portion of our finances separate from our partner's if our budget allows—our own savings, checking, or investment account, or our own retirement plan. If we do not earn a salary of our own, we can look on this separate account as compensation for the unpaid work we do at home.

While having separate finances can contribute to a sense of self-respect, keeping our money totally separate can in some cases prevent a productive partnership from developing. A relationship deepens by considering both our independence and our interdependence. Competence with money should support us, not isolate us, in all of our relationships.

Managing money effectively means paying attention to cash, credit, investments, benefits, taxes, insurance, and estate planning. Although these matters may seem unrelated, they fit together in a holistic pattern. We should come to view finances holistically, just as we do health and the body. Change in one area affects the other areas, and they must combine effectively in order to provide for overall financial security.

Information Roundup

A simple but essential step toward financial competence is to set aside one day a year for a financial roundup. The best time is usually at the beginning of the year, as you're getting your tax information together. Sit down, by yourself or with your partner, and go over all your sources of income and all your outstanding debts. Use this information to determine your household's net worth—that is, the sum of all your assets minus the sum of all your liabilities. Your assets include cash on hand, investments, real-estate holdings, life-insurance policies, personal property (such as automobiles and furniture), and money owed to you by others. Liabilities include outstanding debts, payments due on loans, bills, living expenses, and taxes. Once you have determined your net worth, you have a comprehensive picture of where you stand financially over the next year or so.

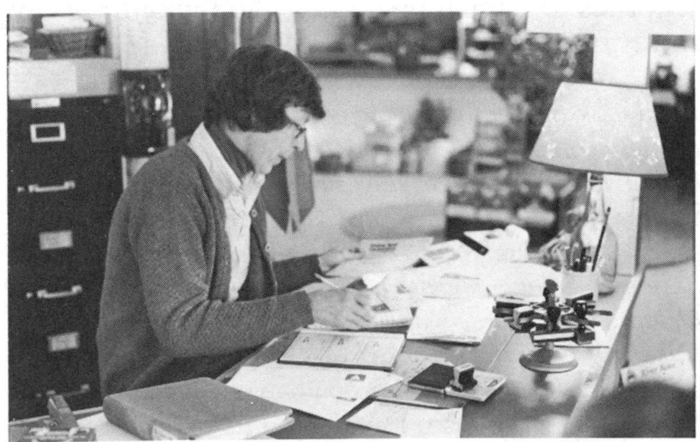

Jerry Howard/Positive Images

Cash and Credit

Budgeting is the most effective tool to help you handle cash and make decisions about credit. You can use the budgeting strategy described earlier to support you in using cash and credit appropriately.

Each of us should have a credit record in her own name. Department-store credit cards are usually easier to obtain than bank credit cards if you are a first-time cardholder. Another way to establish a good credit rating is to take out a small loan from a bank or credit union that you don't really need and deposit it in a savings account, paying it back month by month.

Credit can be an important part of financial health when used carefully. Keep safe limits in mind. One guideline is that the total amount you owe (excluding a mortgage) should not exceed 8 percent of your income. Another rule of thumb is that one should borrow only to buy a major, permanent asset. Borrowing money at 18 percent annual interest and more for clothes, entertainment, or travel is not wise, even though it is tempting to use credit to cover everyday expenses when money is tight. If you do borrow, it is wise to shop for the lowest interest rate available.

If your debts get too high to manage, you can get help. Most cities have branches of the nonprofit National Foundation for Consumer Credit (see Resources for this chapter) whose advice is free. They can help you develop a workable budget and reschedule your payments so that you can reduce your debts.

Many women are afraid of any form of credit other than charge cards and mortgages, but we can all learn when and how to use credit *financing* to advance our own goals. Self-employed women and entrepreneurial women have to learn to deal successfully with lenders. Taking a financial risk requires us to look at ourselves as fiscally competent and capable of making commitments to meeting our own financial goals.

Insurance

Insurance should be carried to cover the financial cost of a major loss—earning power, health, property, or life. Without adequate insurance, assets we need for the future—savings, homes, investments—are very vulnerable.

Make sure you are insuring for the needs you actually still have. For example, if you no longer have dependents you don't need life insurance and may want only a small amount to cover final medical and burial expenses. However, life insurance is important when family members are dependent on your income, when business partners are dependent on your work contribution, or vice versa. The type of policy you buy should fit your circumstances:

- Is the size of the death benefit appropriate?
- Do the premiums fit your budget?
- Is the insurance company sound? (Choose only companies with an A+ rating from A. M. Best, Moody's, or Standard & Poor. Choose a company with a top rating from more than one rater.)

To calculate how much life insurance your partner should carry for your benefit or you should carry for your survivors, make a "survivors' budget." First, total the value of all liquid and convertible assets (savings, investments, other insurance). Then subtract all immediate expenses attendant to death (burial, estate tax, and settlement fees). If you have a deficit, you know you need to have at least that much insurance available immediately. Second, go on to add regular living expenses (including the costs of new health insurance, long-term health care, and paying for caregiving, housework, repairs presently done by you or your partner). Then add up any sources of income (survivor pension benefits, Social Security, wages). If your income is lower than your expenses, calculate what lump sum (i.e., insurance settlement) will yield that much in dividends annually, expecting (in 1993) a 4 percent return; $50,000, for example, will pay out $2,000 annually. Add the first and second figures to see how much your life-insurance policy should be worth. These figures should be revised as interest rates and your circumstances change.

Health costs are very high and usually increase as we get older. (See Women's Health and Reforming the Medical-Care System chapter for discussion of health insurance and related issues.)

Many people don't think of taking out disability insurance, but it is a fact that between the ages of forty-five and sixty-five you have a three times greater risk of being disabled than of dying. Though it is expensive to replace homemaking services when a homemaker is disabled, homemakers cannot get disability coverage. Look for a policy that is guaranteed renewable and that pays if you are unable to work in *your current occupation,* rather than only if you are unable to do any work at all.

Your home and its contents can be insured against fire and theft through a home-owner's or renter's policy. According to insurance-company requirements, a home-owner's policy should insure your house at 80 percent of its replacement (not current market) value. You can then collect 100 percent of partial claims. Many agents are lax about this provision, and you may need to check to be sure your house is covered adequately and that you periodically raise the coverage to keep up with inflation.

Savings and Investments

After getting the day-to-day issues of cash and credit under control and *after* insuring against major losses, you can start building a nest egg for the future. Most financial advisers suggest saving at least 5 to 10 percent of your income every month, or more if you haven't saved before. This money should be put into a separate account for emergencies. You should build up that sum until it is equal to three to six months' income. It should be easily convertible into cash. You can keep it in a money-market fund or a conservative mutual fund, and/or consider cash values of life-insurance policies as part of your emergency fund. Once that emergency fund is built up, you can move on to other kinds of investments.

Getting in the savings habit takes some doing—especially when you are not earning much. Our culture is no help either. Every day we face pressures to buy, buy, buy. We're told that our identity depends on our possessions. Our jobs may demand that we wear expensive clothes; our children may pressure us for cars, stereos, trips, and luxuries that "everyone else" has. Often, the less money we have, the more we may feel that it's important not to let it show nor to let our children feel "different." We are so quick to put money into everyone else's pocket—the grocer, the landlord, the store owners—yet we find it hard to put money into our own.

One way to approach savings is to think of it as paying yourself. Consider it a bill to be paid. Some people put a bank-deposit envelope in with their other bills—rent, utilities, phone—and "pay themselves" at the beginning of every month. Consider it a debt you owe to your own future.

Money saved should not sit around in a low-interest savings account. Except for emergency funds, any time you have money on hand that you know you won't need for a month or more, put it in money-market accounts, certificates of deposit, treasury instruments, or other higher-yield investments. *Always* use a bank that is a member of the Federal Deposit Insurance Corporation (FDIC); your account will be insured up to $100,000.

The amount of interest and the frequency with which it is paid (or compounded) is the key to making savings grow. The more frequently interest is compounded, the faster your money will grow. Make sure you find out about all service fees, minimum-balance requirements, and early-withdrawal penalties that may drastically reduce apparently high interest rates.

Shopping for the best interest rate is like comparative grocery shopping. A few percentage points, like a few pennies per item, can make a big difference. For instance, if you put $50 each month into an account earning only 2½ percent, the amount after ten years would come to $6,808, but an interest rate of 6 percent paid on the same deposit would generate $8,194 after ten years (compounded monthly, not counting effects of inflation and taxes).

To estimate how fast your money will grow at a certain rate of interest, use a handy tool called the "rule of 72." Divide 72 by the interest rate—the result is the number of years it will take your money to double. For instance, at 4 percent interest, a given deposit will double in eighteen years.

Some women have developed considerable skill in investing, while others regard the process with dread and fear of failure. We need to develop a sense of taking the right risk. As women, we have often been trained not to take risks with money. The truth is that we are always taking risks with money, whether or not we are aware of it. Keeping money in a savings bank is a risk—the combination of inflation and low interest was not anticipated by many investors. We may think that by making conservative decisions we are protecting ourselves from loss, but that isn't always the case. It is important to inform ourselves about finances so that we can take the appropriate risks to meet our goals.

One way to begin learning about investments is to spend a few months tracking the stock market on paper. Pretend that you have bought some shares in stocks that you are interested in, then follow their performance in the newspaper. At the end of a period of time, you can see how well your choices worked out for you.

Some women have found it helpful to join or form investment clubs with a group of friends as a way of getting their feet wet without risking much money. Beware of those run by someone selling a particular stock or fund.

The Ethics of Investing

Owning a share or a bond in a company is a way of taking part in that company. A growing number of investors look at the products and practices of companies they invest in from an ethical point of view. They consider the companies' practices concerning environmental protection, occupational safety, and treatment of minorities and women. They shun companies that produce harmful products, from weapons to cigarettes.* The Social Investment Forum (see Resources for this chapter) is a nationwide network of financial advisers and institutions that supports ethical investing by both individuals and organizations.

Some women in relatively comfortable financial circumstances are putting their money to work for those who have less.

My parents left me a farm in Indiana. During their lifetime it wasn't worth much, but in the 1970s, when land values tripled, it became more valuable. If I hadn't had that farm, I would be in far more severe straits today. But what did I do to earn that money? I believe that land is a natural resource that ought to belong to all of us. Since I

*Institutional as well as individual investors are using these criteria, so we are seeing public and private pension funds, college endowments, and other large funds subjected to ethical investment standards. College students took the lead in pushing their schools to divest themselves of investments in companies doing business in South Africa. At any age investors concerned with fairness and justice may also want to avoid such investments and to find additional ways to use their financial power individually and collectively toward a more economically just society.

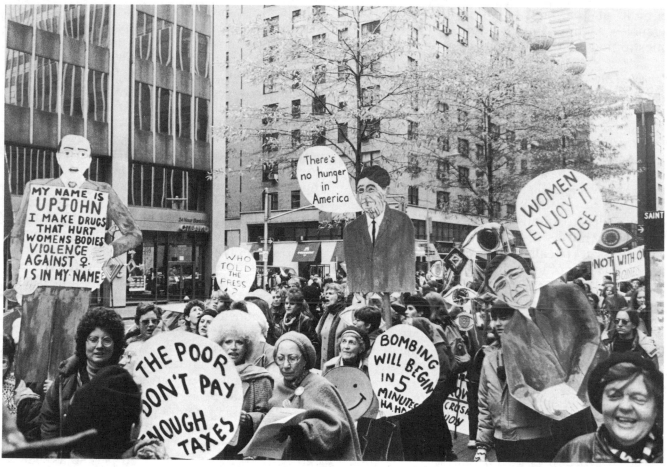

Ellen Shub

now have money that I didn't earn myself, I set some aside for my "sisters," women who through no fault of their own do not have enough money for old age.

One woman who has inherited a considerable fortune chose to give away half her total income to what she terms "socially responsible community investments." Recognizing that women with wealth experience a sense of isolation, she started conducting seminars on "Managing Inherited Wealth," and organized a support group for women in this situation. The meetings are offered in conjunction with The Women's Fund (see Resources for this chapter), which provides grants to low-income women's groups. By bringing these women together, she also provided a role model for responsible management of economic good fortune.

I get calls from women all over the country. Women face unique problems with inherited wealth that have mostly to do with being left out of the decision-making process. The older men and brothers in the family have traditionally been given the responsibility. Men have tended to be much more involved in the family business than women. We're sort of kept in this "you needn't worry about this, dear" posture.

INCOME FOR RETIREMENT

Those of us who want to retire or have retired must plan to earn enough money to live on and make it last. The assumption that "somehow it will work out" can have devastating consequences. Instead, we must look ahead to get a good sense of where we will stand financially at the time of retirement.

Pensions and Benefits

The first step is to review the financial benefits that we have coming to us, both public benefits, such as Social Security and Supplemental Security Income (SSI), and payroll benefits, such as savings and retirement plans and life, health, and disability insurance. Whatever the sources, we can take full advantage of them only if we know what they are. Often this takes aggressive pursuit of the facts—writing to government agencies, asking administrators for information, questioning their answers if necessary.

I checked my Social Security earnings record for the first time at age fifty-two and panicked when the report came back that no earnings were found under my Social Security number. Upon further investigation, I found that my deceased husband's number had been put on my earnings when I collected survivor's benefits. I was glad I had the opportunity to straighten out my account then instead of facing a scary surprise at retirement.

In order to qualify for Social Security on your own (not as a spouse), you need to have worked for forty calendar-year quarterly periods (the equivalent of ten years) in employment that is covered by the Social Security system. You can find out what your current coverage is by sending in Form SSA-7004 (PEBS) to the Social Security Administration (get the form from your local office). Those who work part-time or freelance for several employers must contribute, and their employers are required to contribute too, yet many do not. Many low-paid women, especially those who work as domestics, are left out of the Social Security system and also left without medical coverage. *You need to be covered by Social Security or pay your own Medicare share during your working years in order to be covered by Medicare.*

While you are still employed, you should get an annual statement from your employer telling you what your current pension and insurance benefits add up to. If you have questions, speak with the plan administrator. Always make written notes and keep them on file, especially if you are challenging a decision.

To know how much you need to save for retirement, calculate your yearly expenses and multiply them by the number of years you expect to be retired. Calculate your years of retirement by estimating your expected longevity and subtracting the age at which you expect to retire. If you are already sixty-five or over, it is wise to give yourself a generously long life expectancy, because you have already avoided or survived the health hazards of the middle years. While average life expectancy is seventy-nine years for women and seventy for men, it is prudent to plan for your money to last until age eighty-six for women and age eighty for men. You may want to throw in a few more years if your parents were exceptionally long-lived for their time, or if you are in excellent health.

Suppose your expenses add up to $15,000 per year, you have a private pension that will provide $5,000 a year, and you expect to receive about $3,000 per year in Social Security benefits. If you expect to be retired for fifteen years, you can estimate that you need to save $7,000 for each year of retirement, or $105,000. If you have another ten years before retirement, you need to save $10,500 per year to meet your goal. Before you panic, remember that this rough estimate does not take into account the interest your savings will earn over this ten-year period. You can go to your local bank for help in calculating how much you need to save, given current interest and inflation rates. Also, remember to subtract whatever money you have already saved from the lump sum you need to accumulate. If you still do not have enough, you may want to postpone retirement, work part-time after retirement, or consider ways of reducing your living expenses.

A good alternative to employee pensions are IRAs, SEP-IRAs, and Keogh plans. All of these plans allow money to grow, untaxed, until you withdraw it at retirement. Funds up to $2,000, plus $250 for a nonemployed spouse, may be put in an IRA account annually in your own name. A SEP-IRA (Simplified Employee Pension IRA) can be used by self-employed people as well as by employees of a company; a SEP-IRA can accept employer contributions and can take up to 13 percent of your income. Keogh plans involve more paperwork but can accept up to 20 percent of your self-employment income. Whichever plan you do, and you can do several, don't miss saving like this. Remember, there are penalties for withdrawing the money before you reach fifty-nine and a half.

Under the 1986 Budget Reform Act, limitations have been placed on these accounts that have serious consequences for women who need to be saving in their own names for retirement. As of this writing, contributions to IRAs are fully deductible only as long as adjusted gross income does not exceed certain limits: $25,000 for a single person; $40,000 for a married couple. Deductibility is also limited if either the taxpayer or spouse is an active participant in a workplace pension plan. In place of these limitations, Congress should implement tax-deductible means for everyone, especially women, to save for their retirement years.

IRAs still offer some tax advantages. Even when you cannot deduct your contribution from your taxable income, you defer taxes on the

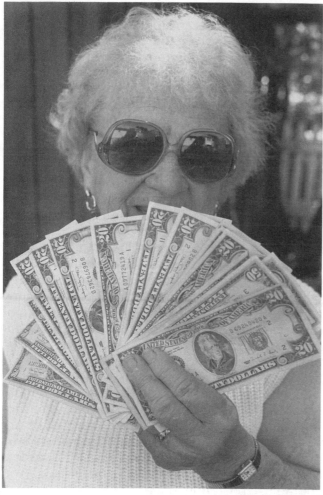

Marianne Gontarz

interest and dividends your money earns until you withdraw it—when you will presumably be in a lower tax bracket. So, every year, you are accumulating interest on a larger and larger sum. By the time you retire, the savings from an IRA can be substantial. The sum of $2,000 invested at the beginning of every year, earning 6 percent interest compounded annually, would be worth $46,552 at the end of fifteen years. Like all tax advantages, these plans benefit the affluent disproportionately; however, middle-income women can also use them to advantage in planning for retirement. It is a good way for married women to accumulate assets in their own name. New legislation must be developed to assure economic security in old age for low-income women. SSI has helped, but it is not enough.

Using Savings

As we grow older, we become so concerned about the future and the need to maintain independence that we may find ourselves living marginally and denying ourselves pleasures and even necessities at a time when we can afford to be living off what we've saved. Some families assume that the principal is really there to be inherited by children and that parents are not entitled to it. This is fine for those who have ample funds. But with increasing life expectancies and major medical expenses facing us, this assumption must be reexamined. Just as we need to plan for accumulating savings, we need to plan for withdrawing money when we reach a certain age.

Getting Help

As we take more responsibility about finances, we may be working with brokers, bankers, agents, attorneys, accountants, and financial planners in a new capacity. Many of us have found our financial advisers in haphazard ways. "He was my husband's lawyer." "She was just getting started selling insurance and seemed so nice." You don't have to be afraid of hurting anyone's feelings by changing advisers. If you feel awkward at first, especially if you are not accustomed to acting on your own behalf, remember that *you* are employing this person to support *you* in taking care of *your* finances. You should come away from such meetings with an enhanced sense of your own competence and increasing sureness in the financial world. Keeping good records and knowing your actual income and expenses enable you to deal realistically with financial professionals.

Find advisers who respect you, are competent, and will help you educate yourself about money and finances. A good adviser will explain new concepts clearly, without hurry or condescension. You should be comfortable saying, "Would you explain that again? It's not making sense to me." Take your time, and take notes, or use a tape recorder if that makes you more comfortable. Our best learning takes place in a setting where it is safe to ask all the questions we have been afraid to ask and where we have classmates with whom to learn. Seminars and courses may be available at community colleges and adult-education centers.

Be wary of an adviser who pressures you to insure or invest in only one way or only through them. Financial planners are paid by fee, commission on sales, or both. They may charge a fee for their planning services, and also collect commissions on any investments or insurance you buy. Make sure the advice you get is at "arm's length"; that is, you should be able to implement financial recommendations through any qualified broker.

When you are starting out with a new adviser, ask for references such as former or current clients or other financial professionals. You want someone who's already done a good job with work similar to yours. We wouldn't ask a dermatologist to perform an appendectomy, yet we're often willing to let financial advisers do tasks for which they aren't qualified.

Taxes

It is important to consider your tax situation when you plan for retirement. Always base figures on your after-tax income when planning what you have to live on and invest.

You can take some of the mystery out of taxes by filling out your tax return yourself. You can get help by calling the local IRS office or your state tax bureau. Your call is anonymous, so you need not give your name. Senior centers and other community agencies sometimes bring in tax experts to offer help and answer questions.

If your financial situation is more complex, it is wise to get professional help in preparing tax returns, but you can learn a lot about your finances and save money by keeping careful records for the tax preparer.

If you file a joint return with your spouse, make sure you understand everything you sign your name to, since you are probably liable for your husband's errors, whether willful or accidental and whether or not you are still married when the return comes up for audit. There is an "innocent spouse" statute that can help some women in such situations. Ask your lawyer or accountant whether you qualify in the event that the Internal Revenue Service demands payment from you for taxes on a husband's or former husband's income.

Estate Planning: Wills and Trusts

For those of us with dependents, whether children, aging parents, disabled partners, or others, planning our estate and making a will to protect these dependents in the event of our death should be a top priority. Fortunately, this most important step costs very little.

If you're nervous about making a will, you're not alone. Seven out of ten Americans die without a will.[18] If a person dies without a valid will, the state's laws determine where that person's property goes and who the guardians and executors will be. This will happen even if the person's wishes and the needs of her or his dependents are well known. For couples in relationships with no legal standing, a will is especially important. The fact that you and another person have been lovers or friends or simply shared a house and lives for years does not establish a legally binding relationship. So it is especially important to have agreements or wishes for care and financial settlements in writing. If your finances are substantial and your relationships complex, it is risky to make a will without a lawyer, although many states may allow you to do so. If the wording is ambiguous or the will was executed under questionable circumstances, the will is useless and may lead to litigation. Many states are very particular about questions of duress, fraud, or incompetency of the testator (the person making the will). A will that accomplishes your purposes effectively is a loving gift to your heirs and community.

Before you make your will, you must choose someone to be its executor (to oversee distribution of your property and make sure taxes are paid properly). Banks, attorneys, and financially knowledgeable friends or relatives can be executors. The executor may charge a fee, and you should establish how the fee will be determined. Your executor should be given the power to hire legal, accounting, or financial services if necessary. It is wise to make sure that that person knows the provisions of the will, and also wise to tell her or him where all your financial records, the will itself, various insurance policies, tax records, bank statements, deeds, stocks, and so forth are kept.

When you choose an executor, you should also name guardians for any minors or developmentally disabled adult dependents, and trustees for any trusts that will be created. These precautions may sound depressing, but they can help your survivors avoid a great deal of confusion, worry, and trouble.

My cousin died five years ago, and nobody wanted to step in and settle her estate. I was the one who finally got stuck doing the job. We thought she died without a penny, so I had to pay for her funeral expenses. After we went through the mass of rubble in her apartment, we found this little black book where she had written down everything. It turned out she had three bank accounts stashed away and had two different kinds of pensions. If I had found that little black book right off the bat, things would have been a lot simpler. . . . She lived in an apartment, and when she died, they wouldn't let anyone in without the proper legal papers. I couldn't get the papers, so we had to keep paying the rent on the apartment for four months. [a woman in her seventies]

Some of the estate-planning methods described here are extremely simple. Some can be done without a will, such as opening a joint bank account. Wills and trusts and some powers of attorney should be drawn with competent legal advice. Lawyers do cost money. However, money spent on a good lawyer can save untold grief and financial loss and can result in enormous savings. You can save some money by gathering all your records and writing out your wishes and intentions in your own words before meeting with an attorney. Local councils on aging or social-service agencies may be able to recommend agencies where low-cost legal assistance is available. Your state or county bar association can provide a list of lawyers with the kind of background you need (look for several years of estate-planning experience). Some banks do estate planning but they cannot draw up wills or trusts. Banks can, however, manage funds for a large estate or trust. If you are interested, ask about the minimum net worth requirement, and the type of accounting they will provide your heirs.

Estates go through a court process known as probate. Probate is the process used to make an orderly distribution and transfer of property from someone who has died to a group of beneficiaries. The probate procedure involves court supervision of property transfers, filing of claims against the estate by creditors, and public notice of a last will and testament when there is one.[19] It can never be totally avoided, but you can sometimes reduce the time and expense of the probate process by using some of the tools of effective estate planning. You should consult an attorney about how your property should be held to minimize financial loss.

Some people use joint ownership of property as a means of planning for its transfer immediately at their death. By holding property jointly, you can retain ownership of your asset(s) and be assured that when you die, the jointly owned property will pass directly to the joint owner or to heirs designated by you, depending on the type of joint ownership.

The cost of ill-advised probate-avoidance devices can be very high, however. For purposes of Medicaid eligibility, for example, joint property may be construed to be the sole property of the applicant, leaving a spouse without funds for support. Joint property may also be attached or frozen by creditors of one owner, whether or not it was the other owner who contributed most of the assets in the account. Thus, a mother may lose her own savings in a son's or daughter's bankruptcy proceedings just because she put that child's name on her account.

There are three ways to hold property jointly with others:

1. **Joint Tenancy with Right of Survivorship (JTWROS).** This arrangement provides for two or more people to own property together. When one person dies, all the property goes to the other(s). The property can be real estate, securities, or bank accounts. This provision cannot be changed by a will, and property in such an account is not probated.

   Bank accounts, securities accounts, or real estate held as JTWROS can require either one signature *or* the other, or one signature *and* the other to make a withdrawal or sell the property. Be sure the person with whom you share the account is completely trustworthy, especially if you share an account that requires one signature *or* the other to make a withdrawal or sale. Many older people share ownership of their assets with a relative, thinking they will avoid probate or taxes and tacitly asking for emotional support, only to find that they have no assets left to live on.

I'm almost ninety years old . . . and I've been here between three and four months. How is it? Don't even ask. I can't go back to Florida because my son has tied me up here by taking all my money out of the bank and by making arrangements with the nursing home. I had all my money in joint accounts with my son. I've always kept my money in joint accounts, first with my husband and then with my son, because it avoids probate and inheritance taxes. But I wouldn't advise any older women to do that after my experience.

2. **Tenancy by the Entirety.** This works much like the above arrangement, except that it is available only to married couples in noncommunity-property states. One tenant is not permitted to sell any of his or her interest in the property without the other's consent, and the

arrangement automatically ends if there is a divorce. If one party dies, the survivor automatically inherits her or his spouse's share. The survivorship rights can be terminated only by mutual consent.

3. **Tenancy in Common.** Under this arrangement, ownership is measured in shares that do not necessarily have to be equal. These shares can be bequeathed to one's own heirs, not necessarily to the other tenants. If two or more people own property together, but want their *own* heirs to inherit it (as in a second marriage, for example), they should hold the property as tenants in common.

   Do not assume that property held by husband and wife is automatically jointly owned. Except in community-property states (Arizona, California, Idaho, Louisiana, Nevada, New Mexico, Texas, Washington, and Wisconsin), only property explicitly held by joint tenants with right of survivorship or tenants by the entirety is actually considered to be held jointly.

Other alternatives to joint ownership are available for sharing responsibility while continuing to direct the management of your property. Here are two examples:

1. **Power of Attorney.** This is a useful tool for sharing responsibility for assets. It is a document in which you authorize someone to handle specific things for you, such as managing a piece of real estate or even all of your financial affairs. A power of attorney becomes invalid if the grantor should become mentally incompetent. All states have a "durable power of attorney," which remains in force if the grantor becomes incompetent, or a "springing power of attorney" for the purpose of having someone act in your name in the event that you *become* mentally incompetent. These are more thoroughly discussed in the chapters on Caregiving and Dying and Death.
2. **Trust.** A *trust* is a legal entity, like a person or a corporation. It can provide a way to transfer ownership of assets while still making sure they are held according to your wishes. For example, a trust can own and manage property for someone who no longer has the energy to do so; it can allow an elderly mother to provide care and spending money for a disabled child after her death; it can provide income for the person establishing it while she is alive, and then give the money to a relative or a charity after her death. Putting assets in trust can also reduce estate taxes.

   Depending on how it is created and what it provides, a trust can affect your Medicaid eligibility. If you think a nursing home could be in your own or your husband's future, you should do Medicaid planning with the help of a competent attorney familiar with your state's Medicaid requirements.

   There is no such thing as a do-it-yourself trust. You will need a skilled, experienced attorney. This is a complicated area, and a person with good intentions but imperfect knowledge can make a complete mess of things.

My husband left close to half a million dollars in a trust fund—I was to get the income. Every time I asked for money I was sent a check, so I never questioned it. Then my son-in-law said I should get an accounting of it—and when we looked we found that there was only about $80,000 left—the trustee had been gambling in the stock market and losing; when I asked for money he didn't send it to me from the income but from the principal. So it's almost all gone now.

Whether you create a trust or are the beneficiary of one, you should watch it carefully to make sure that it functions as intended. A trustee should be required (in the terms of the trust) to give an annual accounting to the beneficiaries. If you have a trust, make sure the trustee gives you an annual report.

Passing On the Responsibility

A last step to protect our own financial health is to be prepared for the time when we will want to hand over our financial affairs to someone else. The plan doesn't have to be based on chronological age. Instead, it may be made effective at the point at which we no longer feel up to coping with balancing a monthly statement or making decisions on reinvesting money.

Those of us who have worked hard to learn about money matters find that giving responsibility for them to our children is a good way to pass on some of our financial acumen—especially to our daughters. We shouldn't assume that our sons will take care of our finances and our daughters will take care of our personal needs. It is a good idea to prepare for this time by keeping our affairs in order and by making sure that a responsible person understands our wishes.

Most of us were raised with the expectation that our work, in and outside the home, would be rewarded in our old age. Yet most women find that in their older years they must rely on their own ingenuity to supplement their often meager savings and pensions. Our learning, efforts, and struggles should go beyond our own survival to teaching younger women the skills we have so painfully acquired, and to urging them to carry on the battle for a more secure economic future for older women.

NOTES

1. Martha Avery, "Prime Proposal." *New Directions for Women,* November–December 1984.

2. U.S. Bureau of the Census, "Family Disruption and Economic Hardship." *Current Population Reports,* Series P-70, No. 23, Washington, DC: U.S. Government Printing Office, January 1991.

3. "Facts About Older Women: Income and Poverty," AARP Women's Initiative Fact Sheet, 1991.

4. U.S. Department of Labor, Women's Bureau, *Facts on Working Women,* September 1990.

5. U.S. Bureau of the Census, "Child Support and Alimony: 1989." *Current Population Reports, Consumer Income,* Series P-60, No. 173, Washington, DC: U.S. Government Printing Office.

6. Ellen Goodman, "The Post-Modern Divorce—Another Way to Divvy Up the Assets." *The Boston Globe,* Jan. 2, 1986.

7. Steven H. Gifis, *The Law Dictionary,* 2nd. ed., Woodbury, NY: Barron's Educational Series Inc., 1984.

8. "The Disillusionment of Divorce for Older Women," OWL Gray Paper. Available from Older Women's League. See General Resources, pages 443–44.

9. Christopher L. Hayes, *Our Turn: The Good News About Women and Divorce.* New York: Pocket Books, 1993.

10. Karen Davis, Paula Grant, and Diane Rowland, "Alone and Poor, the Plight of Elderly Women." *Generations,* Vol. 14, No. 3 (Summer 1990), pp. 43–47.

11. Jill Quadagno and Madonna Harrington Meyer, "Gender and Public Policy." *Generations,* Vol. 14, No. 3 (Summer 1990), pp. 64–66.

12. Frances Leonard, "Older Women and Pensions: Catch 22." OWL Gray Paper, 1988.

13. Ibid.

14. Marie Smith. *Statement of the AARP on Women and Social Security before the Subcommittee on Social Security, Committee on Ways and Means, U.S. House of Representatives,* April 8, 1992. Washington, DC: American Association of Retired Persons.

15. U.S. Department of Health and Human Services, Social Security Administration, *The Social Security Bulletin Annual Statistical Supplement,* August 1993, Table 5, A-16.

16. U.S. Bureau of the Census, Current Population Reports, Series P60-185, *Poverty in the United States: 1992.* U.S. Government Printing Office, September 1993, p. vii.

17. Lucy Freeman, "Anatomy of a Project: SSI Outreach." *OWL Observer,* March–April 1986, p. 9.

18. *Consumer Reports,* February 1985.

19. Paul Cochray, *The Financial Planner's Guide to Estate Planning.* Englewood Cliffs, NJ: Prentice Hall, 1986, p. 265.

15

CAREGIVING

✦

BY LOUISE FRADKIN AND MIRCA LIBERTI

SPECIAL THANKS TO TISH SOMMERS

HELPING PEOPLE WE CARE FOR TO MANAGE MONEY BY NAOMI B. ISLER

1994 UPDATE BY PAULA B. DORESS-WORTERS, LOUISE FRADKIN, AND JOAN DITZION WITH HELP FROM SHARON TENNSTEDT AND JANE ECKERT

1994 UPDATE OF *HOME CARE AND COMMUNITY SERVICES* BY JOAN DITZION AND MICKEY TROUB FRIEDMAN

RESOURCES FOR THIS CHAPTER ON PAGES 479–81

CAREGIVING IS A WOMAN'S ISSUE

Because so many people are living to older ages, it is crucial that the broader community take on a greater share of caregiving for elders. Such support can help family members who provide caregiving, and elders who have no family members to help them. Caregiving has traditionally been a woman's role. Women have always cared for dependent members of the family and community*—infants, children, the infirm, those with disabilities, and the frail elderly. Societal pressures and expectations have trained generation after generation of women to put others' needs before their own. Women constitute 72 percent of family caregivers;[1] they are "the invisible laborers without whom neither the health system nor the patient could survive."[2]

*Though we are focusing on the unpaid caregiver here, we do not wish to overlook the work of paid caregivers in hospitals, nursing homes, and private homes. Paid caregivers are also predominantly women, and are underpaid and undervalued in society. We feel that recognition of the importance of caregiving will contribute to better quality of life for all caregivers, paid and unpaid, and those they care for.

It is imperative for all of us to take a hard look at the unthinking way women are simply handed the job of taking care of whatever dependent person happens to be in their home or even outside their immediate home and family. I have a forty-five-year-old daughter who has been disabled by an obscure form of epilepsy since birth. When she is not institutionalized I take care of her and when she is, I am constantly doing errands to make her stay in the hospital more bearable. With a great deal of prodding from her professionals, my daughter is trying to be more independent at last. My mother lived to be ninety-eight, the last twenty-one years of her life as a widow. I became her principal caregiver in my early forties. Now my husband suffers from memory loss and has been diagnosed as having Alzheimer's disease. Again I am the principal caregiver. I have given this kind of care without questioning it since the beginning of my marriage. [a sixty-six-year-old woman]

For the last four years of her life, I saw my grandmother every day on my way home from work. I did her shopping, her laundry, and anything else she needed. I now volunteer at Rosie's Place [a Boston shelter for homeless women], where I continue to give direct care to women. It's a way of acting on my need to be part of a community of older women who, in allowing me to be part of their lives, have given me immeasurable gifts—love, laughter, warmth, and occasionally tears. [a divorced woman in her fifties]

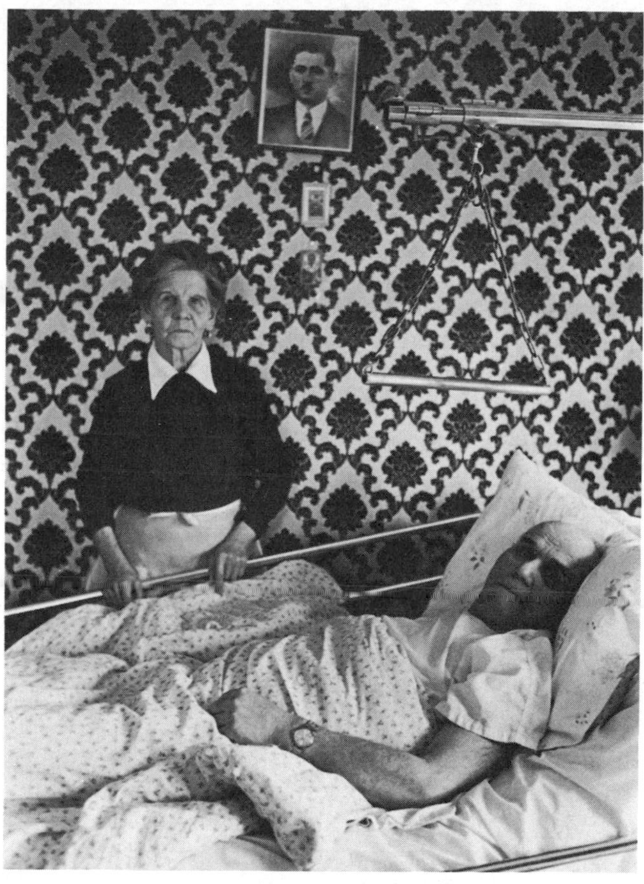

Marianne Gontarz

CAREGIVING WIVES

Remember the poem that says, "Grow old along with me, the best is yet to be"? Unfortunately, many couples plan their retirement years with this in mind only to have their dreams end in a nightmare when one partner becomes disabled or chronically ill—a victim of Parkinson's disease, Alzheimer's disease, a stroke, or cancer.

I'm glad now that we did so much traveling before my husband became ill. I try to think of those times now and relive them. We had so many things planned for after the children had grown, but that's not the way it turned out for us. Because of my husband's illness, we never go anywhere. We're caged in, the two of us. [a woman in her seventies]

A familiar pattern is that when a man becomes ill or disabled, his doctor will send him home, commenting that he is lucky to have a wonderful wife to care for him. When the same thing happens to a woman, however, the doctor will recommend a nursing home. (In some cases, men *are* caregivers for their wives, and of course those who are certainly deserve the same relief and support argued here for women.) As medical science prolongs lives, women, who are frequently younger than their husbands and also tend to live longer, will more and more often find themselves facing the difficult task of caring for their husbands.

I cry a lot because I never thought it would be this way. I didn't expect to be mopping up the bathroom, changing him, doing laundry all the time. I was taking care of babies at twenty; now I'm taking care of my husband.[3]

Wives usually have no special preparation for caregiving, and little choice about offering it. In many communities, when a husband needs constant care, the only alternative is a nursing home. Many women prefer to keep their husbands at home when faced with this alternative,[4] feeling that the separation would break the vow "Till death do us part." Also, both husband and wife may recoil from a nursing home because of horror stories heard from family, friends, and the media. Both partners may want to remain together without realizing what a physical and emotional strain will eventually be placed on the wife.

Caregiving wives carry a heavy emotional load. They often have no one to tell them how well they are doing or how to do the job better, and no one to help when a difficult situation arises. They usually put aside their own lives and aspirations to give their husbands' needs top priority. On top of all of this, they may have their own physical ailments, which may be aggravated by the work they have to do.

I'm seventy-three years old and use a walker. Last year I had a hip replacement. My husband is a paraplegic. When I'm helping him in the bathroom, I have to get into positions that hurt my hip. He doesn't want anyone else to help him.

Caregivers often talk about being isolated, of losing companionship and social contacts. Friends and family who are upset by seeing changes in the husband tend to stay away. Sons and daughters—especially sons, who may see their own future in their father's illness and be unable to face it—may have difficulty coping with the new situation. Sons and daughters may also view their mother as the one who always holds things together, and may continue to expect her to keep this role in the family despite the change in circumstances.[5]

People tell me that he deserves all the care I can give him because he's such a nice person and was always so good to me. Well, I'm a nice person and have always been good to him—what do I deserve? [a seventy-three-year-old woman]

Wives feel isolated as caregivers because they have lost the support of their husbands—often the one with whom they had their closest relationship. This is especially the case when a husband is mentally impaired, since the wife has then essentially lost the man she married. He is still alive, but their relationship, with its shared memories, humor, hopes, and dreams, slips away as his illness progresses. Some caregivers in these circumstances experience apathy, nervousness, irritability, a decrease in vitality and mental energy, and a prevailing sense of depression. Many husbands are aware of the burden that their illness has created for their wives, saying, "This illness has been as much my wife's as it has been mine."[6]

Caregiving may mean taking over affairs that the husband took care of before. Such a change in roles may cause anger, pain, conflicts, and confusions for *both* husband and wife, adding even more stresses to an already stressful situation. In a marriage, spouses often act as loving fathers or mothers to one another during times of stress, uncertainty, or illness. When the husband becomes so ill that he cannot share in making decisions, the wife's sole responsibility becomes permanent.

He was such an intelligent man, an engineer, used to giving orders. Now he has no memory, I have to tell him what to wear and what to do, and he resents it. He doesn't really know who I am. For the first year or so he thought I was a housekeeper; now he must realize that I belong with him. If he had a moment of clarity and saw what has happened to him and to us, he would want to die. It would have been a blessing if he had died in the hospital. [a sixty-eight-year-old woman, with an eighty-one-year-old husband]

Wives may feel guilty if at times they wish for their husbands' or a parent's death and resent the continuing need for care. For those women who have stayed married despite unhappy marriages, caregiving is even harder. To all the other stresses are added resentment over wasted years and dislike of their husbands.

Some wives caring for husbands are helping an elderly parent at the same time. The parent may not be able to understand the extent of care that the son-in-law requires and thus resent the time that the daughter gives to him, or the husband may resent time devoted to caring for the parent. This situation places extraordinary stress on the caregiver.

DAUGHTERS AS CAREGIVERS

We live in a time when many of us are fortunate enough to see our parents live until they are quite old. The challenge of longevity is that older parents may need our help, not just occasionally, but on a continuing basis and at a time when we may be working outside the home and/or still caring for children. Moreover, we ourselves are getting older. It is not uncommon today to hear of a seventy-year-old woman who is concerned about and responsible for her ninety-year-old mother.

Those of us who take on caring for parents often have to make major adjustments. Both caregiver and parents lose freedom and privacy and may have to give up or defer plans for the future. It is not easy for either the daughter or the parent; both feel resentment and frustration. Caregivers often feel caught between their parents' needs and their own. Women who still have children at home feel the additional squeeze of being "sandwiched" between generations.[7]

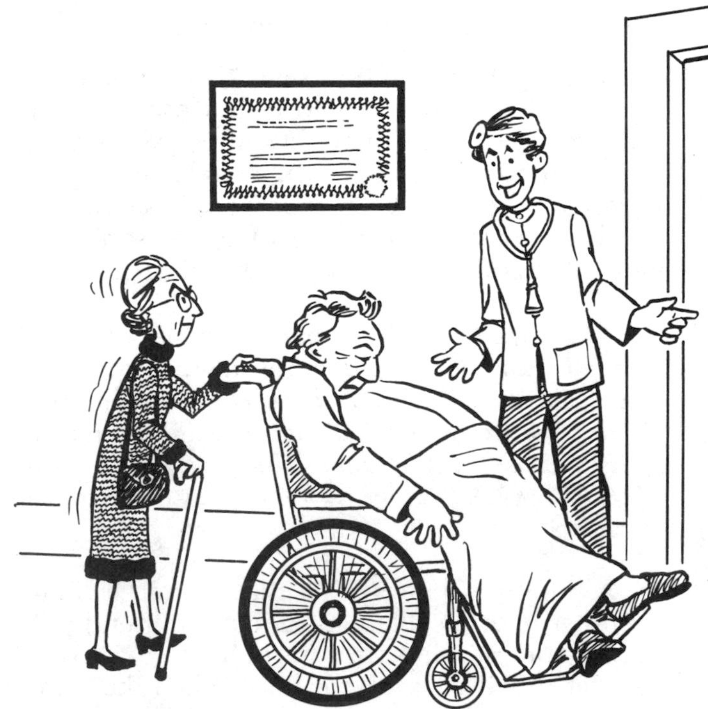

"Your husband is lucky to have you to take care of him at home, Mrs. Jacobs." Maggy Krebs

The Bath

My mother's eyes are tranquil.
She shreds bits of paper.
I give her more paper, more—
napkins, tissues, a forest.
She says, Yes, I'm grateful,
I'm so fortunate in my daughters.

I run the tub.
I bathe her.
I scrub the shadowed place beneath her breasts.
She says, Thank you my darling
you're so kind I love you.

In the moist, closed room
I see she is my grandmother,
the grandmother I never had:
a brand-new lady, dripping with gifts,
arrived in time for me to play with
like a baby

or a mother—
that unknown grandmother
who ripped the lining from her coat before she died
and gave this child who nursed her through the nights
all she had left to give:
a saved-up envelope of money.

I kneel on the mat.
The room dissolves me.
I become a pool of children, mothers, babies.
We pluck at coats.
We dip our hands in secret pockets.

The commandment floats, buoyant in water.
My daughter watches with her radar eyes.

—*Kinereth Gensler**

Most caregivers have very little understanding at first of what the job will entail. Many agree to take care of a parent when she or he is still somewhat self-sufficient, and are unprepared for what happens when the picture changes.

I decided I would take care of my father when he could still stay by himself and get snacks. But by the time he actually came to me (only a few weeks after I made the original decision) he was partially paralyzed and needed help doing everything. [a woman in her late thirties with two preschool children]

My father had a heart attack and my parents came to live with us when we still had children at home. Then my mother had a series of strokes. She died when my oldest was eighteen. I would really tell anyone in that situation not to try to care for parents in your home—to make other arrangements, have your family life less conflicted and better balanced. It was a very difficult period. My father was very nervous from his illness. He was a helpless person who was taught that the woman did everything. [a woman in her sixties]

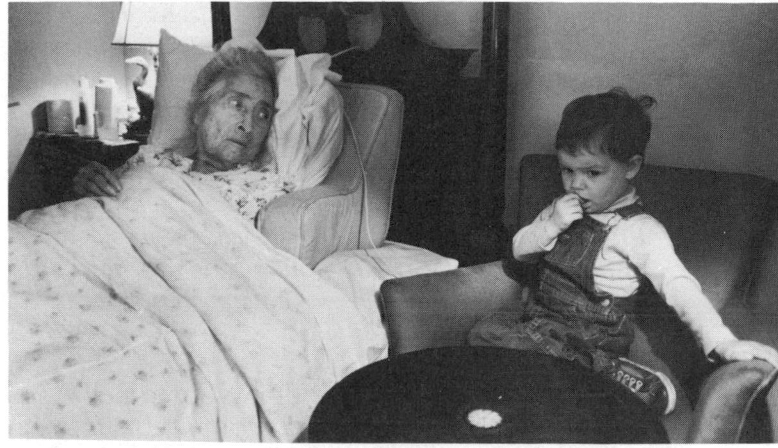

Jerry Howard/Positive Images

Helping an older parent stay in his or her own home often requires extensive logistics and support systems.

I help my eighty-eight-year-old disoriented mother stay in her own apartment through a system of phone calls and hired help coming in four times a day. They give my mother her meals, bathe her, and dress her in the morning and help her get ready for bed at 10 P.M. I've accident-proofed the apartment and constantly modify the support system as my mother's condition changes. I drive fifty-eight miles round trip to do the laundry, the shopping, and pay the bills. In effect, I run two households and I also have a full-time job. This is a ten-year-old routine that is demanding but has worked for us both up to now. [a fifty-seven-year-old woman]

Despite the difficulties, however, keeping a parent in her or his own house may be preferable from the standpoint of preserving both the parent's and the daughter's independence.

Elderly parents often expect their daughters—rarely their sons—to care for them. Parents may not approve of their daughter's working (or of her involvement in outside activities if she does not have a paid job), as these take up time that parents may feel belongs to them.

My mother, a feisty, proud immigrant woman, always looked to me for her primary emotional support. My

*From *Threesome Poems*, Cambridge, MA: Alice James Books, 1976. Copyright © by Kinereth Gensler.

brothers were devoted to her but she rejected a good deal of what they offered because traditionally daughters are expected to be the primary caregiver. When I returned to college while my children were growing up, my mother was often hostile toward my pursuits, making my visits with her very uncomfortable. However, when I graduated, she insisted upon having her picture taken with me after the ceremony—a frail eighty-eight-year-old immigrant lady with a face full of pride posing with her daughter, the college graduate. It was a moment of pride for us both. [a woman in her forties]

Some parents believe that women belong in the home and that taking care of parents is a logical extension of that. Many daughters place themselves in the caregiving role in their own minds, subjecting themselves to internal as well as external pressures. Their brothers, husbands, and male friends do not feel the same pressures. Most men are able to separate themselves both physically and emotionally from their parents, and experience less guilt about doing so.[8]

I live near my parents and take care of them. I do the shopping, cooking, cleaning; you name it and I do it. My sainted brother lives in Florida. Once a year he flies up, takes them out for dinner and a show, then he's off again for another year. My parents think he's great and I get all the complaints. [a woman in her forties]

I am basically the only child for all practical purposes; my brother lives twelve hundred miles away and only comes home about once a year. My mother is in a nursing home and has had seven strokes as well as suffering from innumerable other cardiovascular problems. My dad has had one CVA [cerebral vascular accident—a stroke] and has other medical problems and is getting quite senile. He lives with me and basically I have very little family support. I am single, which makes it doubly hard. At times I think I'll be the third stroke victim. [a forty-five-year-old woman]

In traditional families, if the sons provide financial help, mend a broken door, visit, call, or send flowers at the appropriate times, then they are "good sons" and meet their parents' expectations. Some men do care for parents, and provide substantial help, although less often;[9] when they do they are usually not torn by the same conflicts as women. Most often, sons expect to hire help or delegate other people (fill in wife, sister, aunt, some female relation) to do the actual caregiving.[10]

My brother does most of the work of coordinating home care and medical appointments for my parents. We try to share the calling, errands, and visiting as much as possible, but I am a divorced parent with a full-time job, including some evening meetings, while he is married, without children at home. Though his job is also demanding, he has more time and energy to give at this point in our lives. When I hear some of the horror stories other women tell, I feel lucky that my brother is so responsible. [a forty-five-year-old woman]

Daughters may feel a nagging guilt over putting their own needs first. Some parents find it scary or difficult to make new friends and to be in new social situations, and thus rely heavily on their daughters to meet all of their needs.

My mother is eighty-two and needs assistance because she is partly deaf and has severe cataracts. She lives alone and spends most of her time by herself. She is nervous but very independent and I wouldn't consider a nursing home or an old age home for her. She is in fine health otherwise, but really needs a little more companionship. I don't have a lot of time to spend with her, since I work full-time and have two children at home. She refused any help that I could get and will not go to a group in her church or join a senior citizens' center. She wants me to be there. [a forty-eight-year-old woman]

I usually call my mother every day to check on her. Sometimes I get busy and a day or two will go by and I forget to call. The calls are repetitious, we don't have much to say—she usually complains a lot. But what really riles me is that when I miss a day she calls me and starts out with "I thought your index finger was broken and you couldn't use a phone—how are you?" I can feel the hair on my body rise, but I ignore the moment and just say, "How are you?" [a fifty-five-year-old woman]

My grandmother lived to be almost one hundred and two years old, and my mother cared for her until she was ninety-seven and had to go into a nursing home. Now my mother obviously feels it is her turn, which it is. I am the real problem here, for I have led a very active life and cannot seem to adjust to this demanding and devastating situation. I do not know what to hope for and am almost overcome with the inevitable guilt at my resentment and anger. I have no one to talk to. [a seventy-two-year-old woman]

Some of us may have parents who were never happy or content with life. To maintain a sense of balance and sanity, we have to face the fact that we may not be able to make them happy and that their unhappiness is not our fault.

People who have lost eyesight, hearing, or mobility and are undergoing a lot of pain have legitimate reasons for being unhappy. Parents may also be angry about not being able to do things for themselves. It's important to recognize that they aren't angry at you, just as you aren't angry at them; it is what has happened to them that is the source of the anger.

If we have unhappy childhood memories of parents and believe that they wronged us, we may feel resentful and angry at having to care for them.

My mother left me when I was two and my father moved us into his parents' house. My grandmother actually raised me and I loved her. I rarely saw my father—he ran around and was not part of my life. After I had children, he and his new wife grew close to us because of the grandchildren. Now he's a widower and sick, so he moved in with us eight years ago. Our children are grown and we finally had the house to ourselves, but now he's here. We have no privacy. He expects me to wait on him. He was a lousy father, but I can't throw him out. He has no money and where would he go? Inside I'm angry at him and I resent him all the time. [a fifty-six-year-old woman]

Some of us may feel that we *want* to be the caregiver of a parent or close relative.

My aunt was still very active into her nineties. I felt as though she was almost like my mother. But she kept having these little "occlusions"—the blood wasn't getting through the arteries to the brain and she would pass out. Finally the doctor said she could never be left alone again. So I took care of her at home for five and a half years. I made the garden for her and cooked the best food in the world for her. She had taught me how to cook. She was a dear wonderful person. She gradually got worse. When she couldn't go down the stairs, I would carry huge pots of flowers to show her because she loved plants and flowers so much. She gradually got weaker and weaker until one day she said, "I'm just all tired out." She was just like a clock that had run down. And I was with her. So I felt that I had done all I could. I really loved her more by the time she died. It was a hard job but I'm glad I was able to do it. I feel very good about it. [a single woman in her fifties]

My mother never had any joy, only hard work and struggle. I tried to make it up to her, to do things for her and give her things, and felt guilty because I couldn't take away the old pains and troubles or make her into a happy person. But at least I was able to take care of her in her old age. I have no guilt about that. And she died at home, in my house, where I could say goodbye to her in my own way and in my own space. That was five years ago, and as I get older I see more and more of my mother in myself, and that's okay because she was a wonderful mother and I love her. [a mother in her fifties]

Sometimes siblings reopen old wounds and feelings when discussing how and who should help care for the parents. You hear statements like "You were always Mom's favorite," or "You always got what you wanted, so you take care of them now."

I have six brothers and I'm the only daughter. None of them wants to help out at all, they all feel it's a woman's job. So do my parents. After my parents die, I never want to see any of my brothers again. [a fifty-two-year-old woman]

We feel helpless as we watch elderly parents become more dependent and frailer. We may be afraid and sad, fearing our parents' death or our own old age. Deep inside we still think of our parents as dependable and strong, the way we saw them when we were children; and the child inside us still wants it that way. We may still want their approval and their wise, loving care.

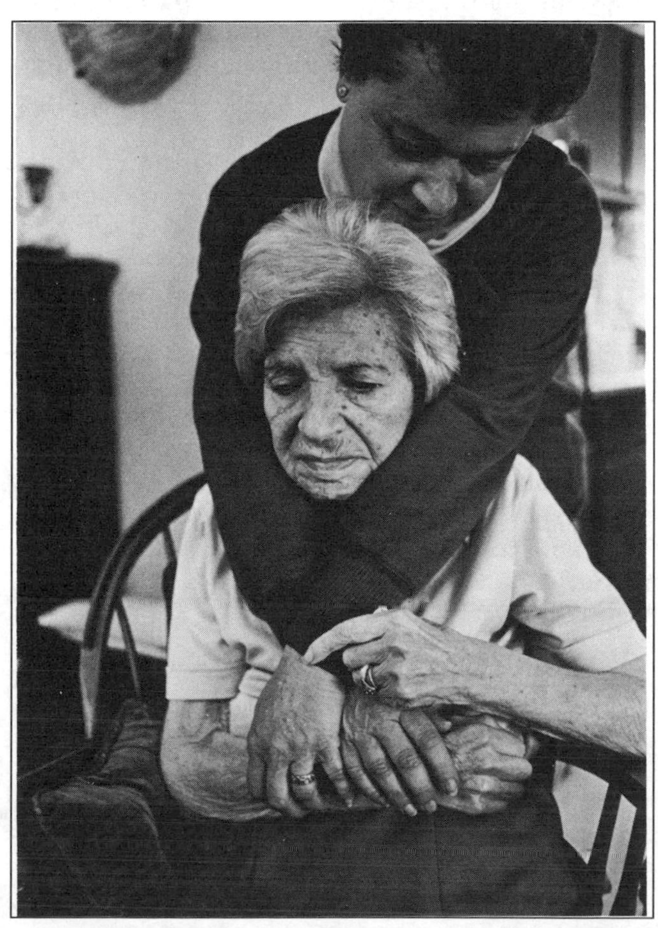

Marianne Gontarz

I take care of my mother, who is physically well but has no memory and is disoriented. Several years ago my oldest daughter went into the hospital for a biopsy. I made arrangements for someone to care for my mother and I told her where I was going. For one moment she understood and said, "I hope everything goes well"; then she lapsed back into her usual state, and I wanted to cry. I realized that I wanted my mother; I wanted her to comfort me and tell me it would be all right like she did when I was a child. But she's like a child now and I'm her mother. [a fifty-eight-year-old woman]

The nature of the parent-child relationship changes in late life, but it is not role reversal. The caregiver's challenge is to know when to step in and provide help without thinking of frail elders as children; the challenge for those receiving care is to be able to accept help without feeling diminished.

It is difficult for caregivers to find time for themselves. Most try to maintain their family obligations and perform well on their jobs, but may overlook their own personal needs, especially time for fun, exercise, and relaxation. It is not surprising that caregivers often develop physical manifestations of internalized emotional stress. We may have to set limits on the time we have available, and encourage our parents to make use of community services.

My father had a stroke and has gotten continually worse since. I quit my job two years ago to take care of him and my mother at their house. But it became too much for me so I moved him to my house. The living room is set up like a hospital—the house is small so we had no other place for him. We have looked into nursing homes but my parents have so little savings that they can't even afford one year. We are living day to day but I do not know how long I can do it. It's like having a 175-pound baby. He gets me up three to four times a night. He wants constant care. I pray for patience every day. But I am afraid that I am going to end up with an ulcer. We don't go out, and we've no place for friends to come visit. My husband is very helpful and understanding but our life isn't our own. [a forty-five-year-old woman]

No one should have to give up her own life or risk her health to the degree described by this and other women who care for family members at home. Family caregivers need a variety of support and respite services.* We must get together and fight for universal availability of such services, and for the funding to keep them going, so that we can keep going. Family caregivers who want to keep their family member at home need help to do so. The nursing-care system in this country depends on the in-home caregiver and threatens to move even further in this direction. More nursing-home beds are needed nationwide as well as a universal system of coverage for nursing-home care.

*See below, Home Care and Community Services Caregivers Should Know About.

Exchanging Caregiving

Some of us have been able to turn to friends and relatives for help that should be forthcoming from the health-care system.

For many years after my mother's death, my father and I shared an apartment. The landlady lived upstairs with her elderly mother, who also needed someone to be around. So the landlady and I alternated taking weekends off. Both parents would leave the back door open so they could be in touch. I also had a "temporary" roommate, who was helpful in doing things with my father such as watching the ballgame or taking him for a ride. I in turn would get the meals.

After my father died, my roommate and I just kept living together. We each have had some illnesses and have recently developed a bond that has a different dimension. Now that we need each other, we do more things together, and our caring has grown. We still have our usual disagreements but we learned how to resolve them long ago.

The landlady and a friend who bought a share of the house are both older than we are. I heard one of them fall at 3 A.M. and we took her to the hospital. We shop for them often and they feed the cat for us, and vice versa. There's a reciprocal feeling of caring. [a seventy-two-year-old single woman who has lived with her roommate for twenty years]

A retired librarian who works as a volunteer for the Gray Panthers and is connected with others in a "family of choice," as Maggie Kuhn has called it, reported:

Don't forget—the only way you achieve independence is through interdependence—when you do things for each other. I remember many years ago when I broke my arm and my neighbor had an eye operation. I had one arm and she had one eye. I would go in and give her breakfast. Then she helped me with things I could not do.

A seventy-year-old woman, a leader in the Older Women's League, describes a mutual caregiving arrangement:

"WOMEN'S WORK"—BALANCING JOBS AND CAREGIVING

by Paula B. Doress-Worters

Today more than 50 percent of married women work in paid employment compared with 4 percent at the turn of the century, and a growing number of single mothers are the sole providers for their families. Yet the demands of the women's movement for child care and maternity leave have been ignored in this country, forcing women to use inadequate child care or give up their jobs in the early child-rearing years.

In our middle and later years, many of us care for an older or infirm family member, and as a result fall even further behind men in our careers and retirement benefits. Elder-care responsibilities are one of the major reasons middle-aged women take time away from the workplace or retire early.[1] When we do so, we increase our risk of poverty in our older years.

As women, we must recognize that elder care, like child care, is expected of us throughout our lives. We need help from other family members, and supports provided by employers and government to level the playing field for women in the world of paid employment. In countries where women have these supports, their pay is higher relative to men's.[2]

The Medical and Family Leave Act, signed into law by President Clinton upon taking office in 1993, mandates that companies with fifty or more employees provide career continuity in the form of a right to return to employment at the same level following a caregiving leave, and uninterrupted health benefits.

Yet most women are employed in smaller companies, and the leaves mandated are unpaid, which may not be of much help to low-income workers who lack savings or other means of economic survival. In effect, "we get unpaid leave to perform unpaid labor."[3]

We need an expanded Medical and Family Leave Act that will protect the jobs of *all* workers with caregiving responsibilities and will provide income and pension credits when employment is interrupted. We need universally available caregiving supports, including at-home care, and community-based and workplace care centers for children and for frail elders.

1. Lou Glasse, President, Older Women's League. Statement before the Senate Special Committee on Aging, August 2, 1991.
2. Sylvia Hewlett, *A Lesser Life: The Myth of Women's Liberation in America*. New York: Morrow, 1986.
3. Norma Meras Swenson, coauthor, *The New Our Bodies, Ourselves,* in an address to the Women's Initiative of the American Association of Retired Persons, January 15, 1993.

The maxim "the blind leading the blind" usually suggests poor leadership, but why shouldn't two people with disabilities help each other? We both have cancer, but of different degrees and with different ups and downs. We share a home and help each other in every way. To assure that the medical citadel doesn't try to take over beyond our wishes, we have "durable power of attorney for health care" for each other so that our wishes will be respected even if we're not in a position to protest against "heroic measures."*

Some women have figured out a way to make informal exchanges of help more available. The San Diego chapter of the Older Women's League found an enthusiastic response from members who were willing to respond to SOS calls from sister OWL members with help such as filling in for an in-home-care worker or lending a wheelchair.[11]

CAREGIVING IS STRESSFUL

Though each caregiver has her own set of problems and her own ways of coping—and sometimes her own ways of falling apart—all caregivers experience emotional, physical, or economic stress, and sometimes all three. All experience feelings of frustration and isolation. To add to these stresses, many caregivers are the only breadwinners in the family. Some hold demanding jobs outside the home in addition to the demanding job of caregiving.

I've been caring for my father for over eight years. The first few years were good ones. He'd been a chef and con-

*See pages 422–23, *Advance Medical Directives.*

tributed to the family by making all our meals. Now he is blind, confined to a wheelchair, and needs a lot of help. I am a special education teacher and love my work. I have hired a woman to stay with my father during the day, but from the moment I come into the house at 4 P.M. until he goes to bed around 8, I am the one who gives him all the care. I get up with him several times a night and I get up at 6 A.M. and get him ready for the day. One day my neighbor told me that if I really loved my father I'd quit my job and stay home to care for him. I was angry and hurt and asked her if she would have told me that if I were a man. My work is very important to me and it keeps me sane. [a fifty-seven-year-old woman]

No one can be a full-time caregiver without help. Think about friends or relatives who could sometimes fill in for you. One woman had a good idea.

I have often been at a loss when people offer to help, so I made a list of tasks I would like help with. Now, when friends offer, I say, "Would you like to come on Tuesday afternoon and help Mom write some notes while I go out to do some errands?" or "Would you help me take Mom to the shopping mall to buy some new clothes?" Sometimes, when I'm not sure what the person's preferences and scheduling are like, I just show them my list of "rescue coupons" and ask them to pick something they would like to do. [a woman in her fifties]

For the first time, only recently, after attending a self-help group, I was able to really hear my daughter when she offered to come home and stay with her father for a week or two so I could get away. [a sixty-six-year-old woman]

One third of caregivers are in fair to poor health themselves.[12] If you find yourself frequently feeling unwell, don't excuse it by saying, "Well, I had a bad night," or "The weather is damp." Take time off to go for a complete physical exam. Explain to your health-care practitioner not only your symptoms but also your role as a caregiver so that she or he fully understands the stresses you are under. Beware of a doctor who dismisses your concerns or feels that the answer to all your aches and pains is a tranquilizer—which will make you feel groggy and only add to your problems. If your blood pressure is high—a common symptom among overworked caregivers—your body is sending you an important message. You have to learn how to reduce your stress level to help bring down your blood pressure. (See Hypertension, Heart Disease, and Stroke chapter and the section on stress management in Aging and Well-Being chapter.) Caregivers also often experience nausea, fatigue, and difficulty in sleeping. If your health-care practitioner has determined that you don't have an underlying medical problem, you'll want to go beyond the medical community to get help and relief.

Mutual-Help and Support Groups

Those of us who are caregivers have found mutual-help and support groups a valuable source of comfort, advice, and understanding. Among other things, sharing experiences provides a safety valve for pent-up anger and frustration.

I need someone out there who will listen to me and not say, "But they're old, they need you." I already know that—boy, do I ever. I have eighty-two-year-old parents; my father is in a nursing home getting along pretty well, but my mother is another story, which would take too long to tell. I feel sometimes as if I'm handling things pretty well, but some days I want to pack my suitcase and leave forever! [a woman in her fifties]

These groups offer a supportive and nonjudgmental atmosphere where members can openly express their innermost fears, discuss problems, and share coping skills. Joint problem solving is far better than what most of us can do on our own, especially because it's often difficult to keep a perspective on problems when you're alone. Members share their knowledge of community resources and services. New members often say, "It's great to learn I'm not alone. All of you understand what I'm going through." Members sometimes develop a buddy system, so each has someone to call in times of crisis. A member of Women Who Care, a support group in Marin County, California, composed of women who care full-time for their severely disabled husbands, writes:

The best thing about it was that we found out we were not alone. I guess burdens are easier to bear if you know other people going through what you are, or even worse. We open up to each other more than we can to anyone else. We share our fears and our sorrows, our feelings of guilt and our occasional joys. Sometimes we cry, but it's amazing how much we laugh. We also trade ideas on how to make the job easier and we share resources that we've found useful. Some of us make pacts to call each other when things get too heavy. And knowing you can help someone else in the same spot you are in lightens the load.

Support groups can be self-run by members. They can decide on their own format, arrange for outside speakers such as social workers or pharmacologists, and organize fund-raising activities. Such groups require a lot of work from dedicated volunteers—they do not happen overnight.

Professionally led and organized support groups have been developing over the past several years as health, mental health, and social service agencies have begun to respond to the needs of caregivers. Some of these groups meet over a period of only six to eight weeks with a specific format and focus on a determinate set of issues; others run continuously, with people joining and leaving according to their needs. Religious organizations are also starting professionally led and self-run support groups. Each caregiver can choose the kind of group that answers her needs and in which she feels comfortable.

CARING AND CAREGIVING

by Lois Harris

This chapter devotes considerable attention to the problems faced by caregivers. However, *caring,* in the sense of loving concern, can be expressed by those receiving care as well as by those providing it. Examples abound of serenity despite pain, gallantry and thoughtfulness despite discomfort.

Several years ago in my late seventies I took up cross-country skiing. I remember an exercise that was scary. We took turns going down a hill. Only when we approached the instructor did we learn in which direction we were to turn. I thought of this recently as I was musing about aging and caregiving. I realized that most of us do not know whether later in life we will have to join the caregivers' group or the care receivers'. We may experience both roles at different times. So all of us need to do some advance thinking about both.

PLANNING AHEAD

Ideally, families should plan ahead for various crises before they actually happen. Even though you can't anticipate everything, everyone in the family should have a turn to voice her or his feelings without the pressure of an imminent emergency. It is best to do this when your parents are still living active, independent lives, and are in relatively good health. Preplanning takes effort and thought on the part of everyone in the family, but can prevent irreversible or long-lasting errors of judgment, such as selling a house or furniture in the midst of a crisis and regretting it later. Though sisters and brothers who live far away can be part of the dialogue through phone calls or letters, it's best when a whole family can get together.

My brothers and I sat down one night with our mother and decided who would do what to care for her. My two brothers and I have been sharing the care of our mother for several years now. Mother is eighty-five and lives in a retirement apartment building that is convenient to all of us. I do her food and clothes shopping and the laundry, and sometimes my sisters-in-law help me. One brother handles the financial matters, pays the bills and so on, and the other brother takes her to the doctor, gets her medicines, and watches over her health. My brothers and I and our spouses meet for dinner once a week and then visit our mother. We all enjoy getting together—it keeps us close as a family. Mother enjoys having us all as guests once a week. So far it's worked out well for us. [a fifty-eight-year-old woman]

Preplanning does *not* mean making promises that can't be kept. Sometimes, out of love and with the best intentions, we say, "I'll never put you in a nursing home," or announce some other "never" regarding something we have no control over. These "nevers" may come back to haunt us. None of us knows what the family situation will be in the future. Nevertheless, we can try to plan for a range of contingencies by asking our parents what kinds of plans they have or would prefer.*

Planning discussions should be open and loving, with no secret pacts between family members. Unfortunately, even talking about caring for a parent can cause hard feelings and bitterness among brothers and sisters. If your family meetings deteriorate into fighting and recrimination, or if it has always been difficult for your family to communicate well, you may want to ask a third party, such as a social worker or member of the clergy, to join you. This person should be someone everyone respects and will listen to. It is ideal if she or he has had experi-

*We can plan for ourselves by designating a health-care proxy and encourage them to do the same. See Advance Medical Directives, pages 422–23.

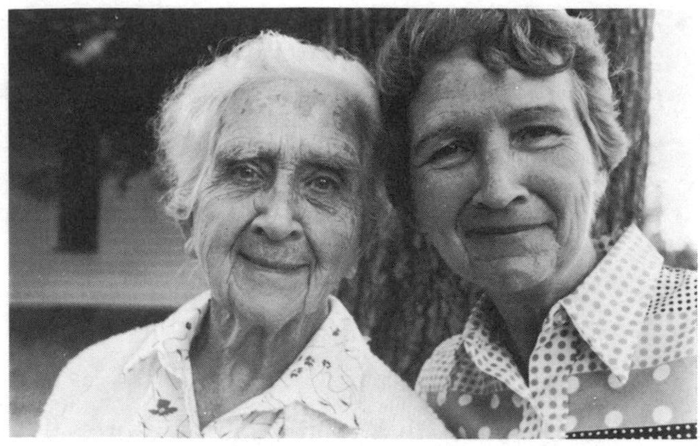

Marianne Gontarz

ence with the problems you are discussing. An understanding outsider can dispel family hostility, keep the discussion going in a productive way, and allow everyone to voice feelings and opinions.

Preplanning is easier to write and talk about than to put into practice because most people avoid discussing growing old or getting sick. When parents are healthy and leading active lives, we may feel uncomfortable bringing up such a "morbid" subject. Try putting it this way: "Mom and Dad, we hope that you have many more healthy years. We'd like to talk together about what could happen in the future and ask what you would like us to do in the event of disability or illness. Do you have any plans that you'd like to discuss with us? We want to do what is best and what you think would be right for you." Your parents may be thankful that you took the initiative.

Helping People We Care For to Manage Money

Whether or not any long-range planning has been done, there may come a time when an ill or confused person is managing financial affairs so poorly that it becomes necessary to intervene. Deciding when this should happen may not be easy. Some people live their entire lives missing appointments, losing keys, and paying bills only after they get threatening notices. Nearly everyone occasionally forgets a meeting, gets locked out, neglects a bill, or leaves the burner on under the teakettle. However, a developing pattern of such habits in someone who has not previously had them is a sign of trouble. People who suffer from disorientation, memory loss, or other conditions that make their handling of money erratic and unreliable may dissipate assets, become victim to frauds and swindles, or become poor credit risks subject to eviction and utility shut-offs. Families or other caregivers must step in to prevent such a person from harming himself or herself further.

My mother lived in Florida for years. She had started to slow down a little and was beginning to forget things, like when I was coming from Boston to visit, or the names of some relatives. The kitchen table always seemed to be piled up with stuff—papers she said she was sorting through, charitable appeals she couldn't throw out. She was always a saver, so even though this looked unusual, it didn't worry me too much until I found the overdue rent and Blue Cross notices. I took one of her checkbooks (she had my name on her checking account) and got the bills sent to me. It took her three months to notice this—and then she wasn't pleased about it. [a fifty-year-old woman]

Staying in contact with friends or neighbors who live near your parent(s) is useful. Case-management services (see page 216) have visiting services that, for a fee, will check on elderly people living long distances from their families.

It is important not to do more than the situation really requires. A person who needs help with paying rent or utility bills may still be perfectly capable of shopping and paying for her or his own groceries and toiletries. Your help should be designed to recognize and support a person's abilities as well as to compensate for weaknesses.

If the person being cared for should become mentally incompetent, the caregiver can act in her or his name if a "durable power of attorney" has been set up in advance.

Remember that in some cases confusion and memory problems may be reversible, so assistance may not have to be permanent.

If you are now entering into a caregiving relationship with someone who is mentally competent, it is important to talk over money matters at the beginning. This is especially important if you begin sharing living quarters with a parent. For example, a parent who moves in with an adult daughter or son may lose eligibility for subsidized home-care services she or he was previously receiving. This is because total household income, rather than just the parent's own, is considered for eligibility for home care and other services in many states.

If you are caring for a spouse, financial matters become much more complicated. If a husband's illness occurs before either partner reaches retirement age, for example, a couple may lose virtually all of their income. Early retirement due to illness may mean lower pension benefits. Wives who realize they will probably outlive their husbands fear for their own future. Couples are now offered financial protection under the Community Spouse Maintenance Allowance permitted by most states under Medicaid. See the Money Matters chapter for a fuller discussion of the financial and legal issues faced by older women.

Following are various legal devices available to caregivers. Others, such as joint bank accounts, trusts, and power of attorney, are described in the Money Matters chapter.

Durable Power of Attorney

This is a form of power of attorney that continues to be valid despite the physical or mental incompetence of the grantor. It terminates only upon the death of the grantor or if revoked by a legally appointed guardian. The grantor, however, can revoke it at any time as long as she or he is competent. A *springing durable power of attorney* goes into effect only if the grantor becomes incompetent.

These arrangements can enable your wishes to be carried out even if you are no longer able to speak for yourself, owing to a coma or some other incapacitating condition. Most people would feel more secure knowing that, in the event of incapacity, a trusted person rather than the courts will be making decisions for them. If you decide to give someone a power of attorney, you should be sure that person understands how you want things managed and agrees to it before you sign the document.

Simple and limited powers of attorney can in many cases be drawn up without a lawyer. However, because of the far-reaching nature of the document, it is best to consult a lawyer before entering into such an agreement.

Social Security Representative Payee Status

My dad is competent but blind, and with his arthritic hands he cannot handle a pen. When checks come in he can't even mark an "X" to endorse them. [a woman in her fifties]

In situations such as the one described above, it may be helpful for the caregiver to become a representative payee. In this arrangement, the Social Security office appoints a person, institution, or community association as representative payee. The name on the check is changed from the direct beneficiary's to the payee's. The payee is then responsible for distributing the money on behalf of the beneficiary. Periodic accounting statements must be filed by the payee with the Social Security office, so if you are a payee, keep careful records of your expenditures. This is a relatively simple way of dealing with physical or financial incapacity that works when the beneficiary's income is basically limited to that one pension check.

Guardianships or Conservatorships

These arrangements are useful when for whatever reason a person is not capable of managing financial and/or personal affairs, *and* does not know that she or he is managing poorly, *and* that incapability poses a major threat to her or his well-being. You must have an attorney arrange these.

My mother gives money away to anyone who comes into the house. She doesn't understand her finances. All she cares about is seeing the dollar bills and sharing them. I know she's incompetent, but how can I subject her to a courtroom? If only I had known, I would have planned something. [a woman in her forties]

All guardianships must be granted by a court. Actions taken by a guardian, who may be a relative, friend, or community agency or institution, are often subject to the court's prior approval. The strictness of supervision varies among courts.

In most states, guardianship can be of a parcel of property or of a person. The former is generally granted when financial management is a problem but other areas are not.

Guardianships and conservatorships, for all intents and purposes, prevent an individual from acting on her or his own behalf. The person placed under guardianship bears the stigma of having been judged incompetent. She or he may lose the right to vote, to decide where to live, to sign checks, to spend money, to make decisions about medical treatment, to enter into contracts, or even to get married. The court gives the guardian the ultimate responsibility for making decisions for another person.

It is important to remember that if an older person disagrees with her or his relatives about how to handle a situation, this is not in itself a sign of incompetency. People may knowingly refuse a medical procedure that will prolong life

Home Care and Community Services Caregivers Should Know About

Increasingly, communities are recognizing that elders need a continuum of services, including preventive care and health promotion for healthy elders; community and home-based services to support frail elders to live on their own or with relatives or friends who are their caregivers; and institutional or home care for those who need twenty-four-hour care. We hope that the full range or continuum of elder services will be integrated into a national health-care system. All caregivers need help in the form of time off, emotional and social support, and financial assistance, including federal and state aid for home care. Many communities have such services but face problems of funding programs and training workers.

Locating services and getting to the right contact person can be complicated and challenging for the caregiver. A good place to begin is by calling the Eldercare Locater (1-800-677-1116), a national referral hot line, which will give you access to a network of national, state, and community organizations in your parent's community. Alternatively, every state has a statewide agency on aging, though the names of these vary. Consult your telephone book. Many directories have a separate section listing human services and some are adding "silver pages," listing services for the elderly. Look under Area Agency on Aging (AAA) or Council on Aging, Home Care services, Visiting Nurse services, or under Aging, (State) Department of; or try Family Services, Jewish or Catholic Family Services, or Catholic Charities. You can also try local churches and synagogues, or the social services department of a local hospital or nursing home.

Licensed practical nurse programs, in either community colleges or technical high schools, may have students who take part-time positions to help pay for their schooling. A youth employment service for high school students can be a reasonably priced source of chore services or companion sitting. Organize family, friends, and services into a rotating schedule so that each person has a specific time slot and assignment. Caregivers need to know about the range of services available in the home and in the community.

Case-Management Services

A health-care professional or social worker evaluates, plans, locates, coordinates, and monitors services selected to meet the needs of a particular person. Fees vary; the agencies may be either private or public. This arrangement is particularly useful for working adult children and long-distance caregivers, and especially helpful when you start planning for services you know nothing about. Elderly persons can engage a case-management worker for themselves.

Adult Day-Care and Day-Health Centers

These centers offer social, recreational, and therapeutic activities to older people who need supervision during the day. Day-health centers provide some nursing services. The centers are approved and staffed by professionals and may be subsidized by a government agency. They provide more personal attention than a senior center. They are for individuals who are too dependent to manage alone and too independent for a nursing home. Some provide transportation.

Respite-Care Service

Short-term institutional care is provided to give temporary relief to family caregivers who may need a vacation or medical care for themselves. Overnight, weekend, and longer respite care may be offered by some nursing homes. Expanded facilities for respite care could be developed using underutilized rooms, wings, or buildings in hospitals, live-in residential schools, and other medical facilities where round-the-clock staff and a physical plant already exist. Such programs have already been developed in some communities. Costs, hours, and availability vary.

Respite care may also be arranged at home on an occasional or regular basis to provide a short-term break for the caregiver.

Home-Care and Community Services

If you are the caregiver for an older person—or if you yourself could use some additional care, there are a variety of services available.

- **In-home care services** may include skilled nursing care, physical, occupational, and speech/language therapy, social work, case management, mental health assessment, and the provision of certain medical supplies. Agencies that provide such services usually operate under the direction of a social worker, nurse, or other health professional and may be licensed by the state. There is a service fee, sometimes sliding or adjustable; some agencies take third-party payments, Medicare, and Medicaid.
- **Home health aid catalogs (see Resources p. 481)**
- **Homemaker services** These agencies provide personal care for the invalid and perform household tasks related to maintaining individuals in their own homes. Some services allow volunteers to "bank" hours so they can receive services when they are in need.
- **Chore services** Community organizations sometimes offer the services of an individual who will perform minor repairs or housecleaning tasks for the infirm elderly. Their services are usually free if the resident pays the cost of materials.
- **Friendly visitors** Paid or volunteer visitors offer to write letters, make phone calls, play cards, chat, and generally provide human companionship for homebound people.
- **Attendant care service** is available in some states to help disabled adults live independently. It is for those who know exactly what services they need, who can interview helpers, and who can pay, supervise, and, if necessary, fire a helper.
- **Hospice services** provide care and support for the terminally ill and their families (see Dying and Death chapter).
- **Meals on Wheels** delivers one hot meal each day to those homebound elderly who are unable to cook for themselves and who have no one to provide meals for them. It is usually funded and operated by local volunteer organizations or area agencies on aging. Ethnic, kosher, or vegetarian meals may be available. The program may charge fees on a sliding scale or may be completely subsidized. This program also serves as a checking system in case of a fall or a sudden illness.
- **Emergency alert/emergency screening** is offered by many hospitals and private companies under various names. A person wears a button that she or he can push when an emergency occurs. This button sends a signal to the hospital or "response station," which calls the neighbor who has agreed to be the support person. If there is no answer, the hospital will send an ambulance with a medical team. Prices vary. Call your local hospital or your state hospital association for information.
- **Telephone reassurance** is a volunteer program in which daily telephone calls are made as a "safety check" to homebound elders. Calls may be made on weekends and holidays as well, if requested.
- **The American Red Cross** lends medical equipment, such as wheelchairs, crutches, and walkers in some areas.
- **Protective services** These services are designed to protect severely disabled elderly people who are subject to abuse, neglect, and exploitation. Protective service agencies optimally provide 24-hour coverage and are connected to a police radio.
- **Transportation services (Dial-a-Car, Wheels, Dial-a-Bus)** Reduced transit fare for "senior citizens" during off-peak hours is available in many states. Some states even operate private limousines and special vans for elders. Reservations are needed one day or more in advance; charges are minimal for people over sixty-five. Need is greatest in suburban and rural areas. School buses might be used after they finish their regular routes.
- **Congregate meals** are often available at schools, senior centers, or housing complexes. When combined with community-based transportation, they can provide a hot meal, independence, and companionship.
- **Mental health and counseling services.** Social workers can help individuals and families with stresses of aging, caregiving, and other intergenerational issues.
- **Senior centers** provide social, physical, recreational, educational, and cultural activities for older persons. Other services that may be provided are legal and financial assistance and support groups.

simply because they do not wish to live the way the procedure will require. A mother who decides to sell the family silver to take a trip to Paris before she dies is not necessarily incompetent. She may just want to go to Paris, and she has a right to do so even if her daughter wants to inherit the silver.

Some states are experimenting with limited guardianships for specific purposes, such as representation in the sale of property or in medical decision making. In some states, the power of the guardian is limited to the areas in which the individual is incompetent to act, or to a specific period of time, after which the guardian must show that the incapacity continues in order for the guardianship to be extended.

ADVOCACY FOR THE SERVICES WE NEED

The aging of the population has made elder care a national issue. Caring for frail elders and others who need caregiving should be society's responsibility as well as the family's. More public support for caregiving will not weaken the family structure, but will instead strengthen it by making it easier for family members and friends to provide for each other.

In addition to universal national health care, a variety of legislation is needed at the state and national levels to meet the needs of caregivers for support services, respite care, and financial compensation. Grass-roots local action has been a way for many caregivers to begin to create institutions that respond to their needs.

Children of Aging Parents in Levittown, Pennsylvania, began by offering support groups for caregivers and went on to found an organization that has collected and compiled information about caregiving services and legislation locally and nationally. The founders have appeared on national television news shows, have been interviewed for national magazines, and have testified before state and federal legislative communities regarding the need for support and respite for caregivers.

Women Who Care, with the help of personnel from an adult-care center, devised and funded a program to give each woman some relief. Then they told their story on a national television network, which sparked other support groups and growing national interest in respite-care programs.

In several states, activists working with organizations such as the Older Women's League are introducing bills to provide for respite and support services for caregivers.

As part of our own long-term planning, we must all get behind these and other efforts to improve the prospects for those in need of care and those providing it. The Older Women's League is now spearheading the Campaign for Women's Health, a broad-based coalition working for women's interests in national health care reform (see Women's Health and Reforming the Medical-Care System chapter) including home care and long-term care. As long as caregiving is viewed solely as a woman's concern, it risks being overlooked by legislators and policy makers and being left out of a new national health-care system unless we become active, vocal advocates for change. (See Changing Society and Ourselves chapter.) When legislators, bent on balancing budgets, romanticize *family* care, we must remind them that *women* who care for family members need a continuum of support services in order to provide help to elder family members. We must advocate for government to recognize the contribution we make as caregivers to our families and communities. We must have policies that protect our jobs and our health and retirement benefits when we take time off for caregiving, and that protect our health and economic security in our older years.

NOTES

1. Robyn Stone, Gail Lee Cafferata, and Judith Sangl, "Caregivers of the Frail Elderly: A National Profile." *Gerontologist,* Vol. 27, No. 5 (1987), p. 616.
2. Elinor Polansky, "Take Him Home, Mrs. Smith." *Healthright,* Vol. II, No. 2 (Winter 1975–76).
3. Alfred P. Fengler and Nancy Goodrich, "Wives of Elderly Disabled Men: The Hidden Patients." *Gerontologist,* Vol. 19, No. 2 (1979), p. 178.
4. Vanda Colman, et al., *Till Death Do Us Part: Caregiving Wives of Severely Disabled Husbands,* OWL Gray Paper No. 7 (1982), p. 4. Available from Older Women's League. See General Resources, pp. 443–44.
5. Linda Crossman, et al., "Older Women Caring for Disabled Spouses: A Model for Supportive Services." *Gerontologist,* Vol. 21, No. 5 (1981), pp. 464–70.
6. Fengler, op. cit., p. 182.
7. Elaine M. Brody, *Women in the Middle: Their Parent Care Years.* New York: Springer, 1990.
8. Amy Horowitz, "Sons and Daughters as Caregivers to Older Parents: Differences in Role Performance and Consequences." *Gerontologist,* Vol. 25, No. 6 (1985), pp. 612–17.
9. Stone et al., op. cit., p. 623.
10. Horowitz, op. cit.
11. "Owls Fly to Help." *OWL Observer,* May/June 1985.
12. Stone et al., op. cit., p. 621.

Understanding, Preventing, and Managing Medical Problems

✦

16

WOMEN'S HEALTH AND REFORMING THE MEDICAL-CARE SYSTEM

✦

BY DIANA LASKIN SIEGAL

SPECIAL THANKS TO NORMA MERAS SWENSON, ALICE QUINLAN, AND EVE NICHOLS

1994 UPDATE BY NORMA MERAS SWENSON WITH HELP FROM DIANA LASKIN SIEGAL AND PAULA B. DORESS-WORTERS

SPECIAL THANKS TO NAOMI COTTER, JOAN DITZION, ARTHUR MAZER, AND WENDY SANFORD

GENERAL HEALTH RESOURCES ON PAGES 482–84

RESOURCES FOR THIS CHAPTER ON PAGES 484–86

Women are treated with less respect within the health-care system and receive poorer medical care than men. As we age we are in double jeopardy because the widespread bias and discrimination against older people that is so deeply ingrained in our culture exists even among the people and institutions we turn to for help and support.

Ageism manifests itself first and foremost in the attitude that aging is a disease. Gerontology, meaning the study of the aging process from maturity into old age, as well as the study of older people as a special population, is often confused with geriatrics, the medical treatment of old people. Because of male domination in medicine, researchers have emphasized general problems or male problems, without noticing that women experience aging and illness differently.

AGING IS NOT A DISEASE

There is a crucial difference between aging and disease. Both happen at all ages but health care providers and researchers don't always distinguish between the signs of aging and symptoms of disease.

If we recognize that a particular problem is probably a symptom of disease rather than a normal part of aging, we will be more likely to seek solutions for it. Even if a cure for the disease is not available, specific interventions may help us live more comfortably.

Recognizing the distinction between aging and disease also helps us identify the effects of environmental and social factors on aging. Industrial laborers experience certain health problems earlier than white-collar workers. Similarly, poor women are more susceptible to diseases associated with old age than middle-income women, who have more opportunities to take advantage of preventive services and to deal with health problems before they interfere with daily life.

On television, treatment of injuries and acute illness is portrayed as a drama with heroic doctors winning a life-and-death battle. Western medicine emphasizes trauma and acute conditions, not care for chronic conditions. In reality, by age sixty-five most people have developed at least one chronic health problem; these rarely limit mobility or functioning but often require long-term management to prevent them from becoming worse. Our personal attention and

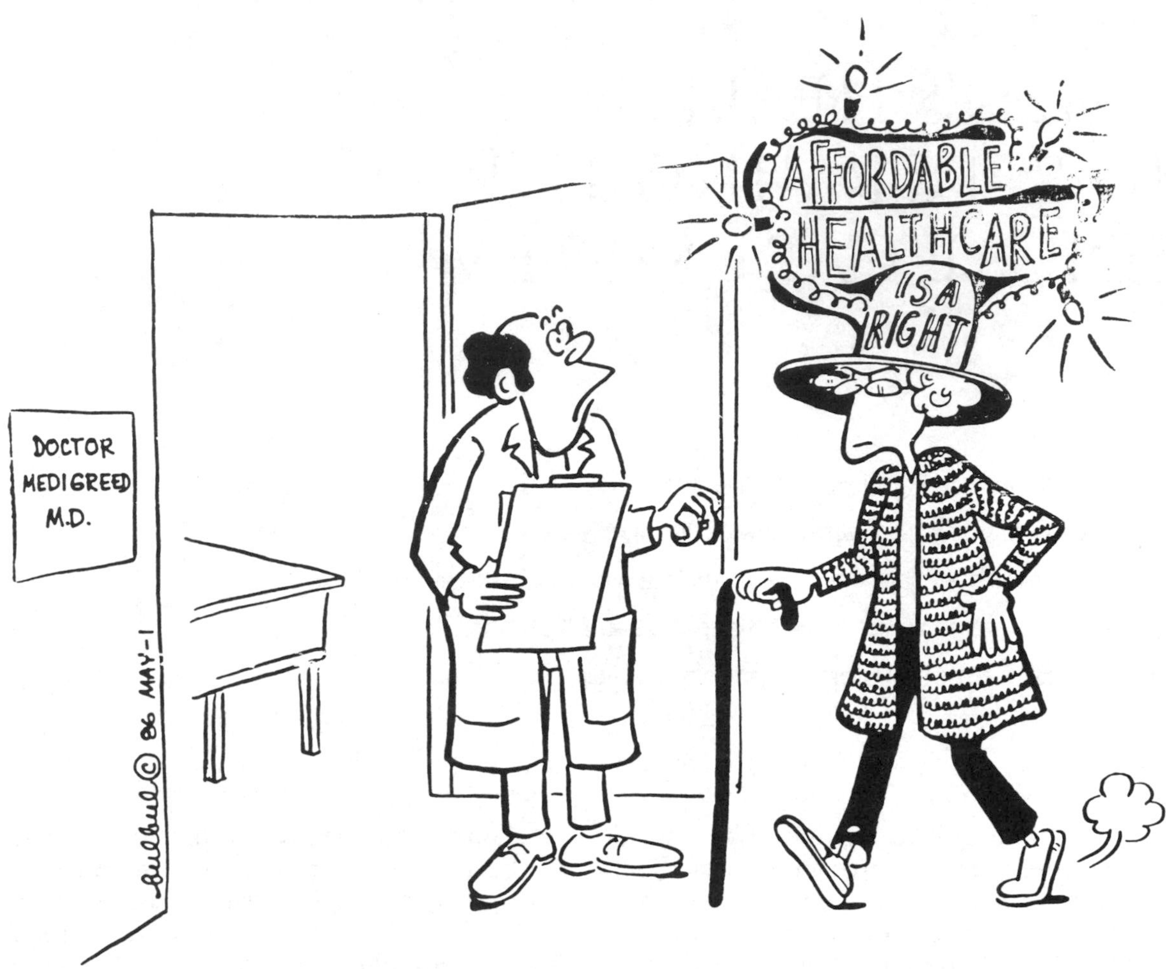
AFFORDABLE HEALTHCARE IS A RIGHT
DOCTOR MEDIGREED M.D.
Bulbul © 86 MAY-1

Bulbul

much of the resources of society would be better spent on prevention of disease, on the reduction of complications from disease, and on rehabilitation and continuing care. Many health-care practitioners dismiss older people's complaints with the classic put-down: "What can you expect at your age?" Equating aging with illness and pain often causes physicians to overlook manageable complaints and problems.

Four years ago, after a coma from a virus, I couldn't walk. Neither my doctor nor the physical-therapy department knew how to help me. The doctor wanted to put me in a nursing home. When I insisted on a referral to a rehabilitation hospital, the social-service department helped me find the best one in the area. After five weeks of special physical therapy I could walk again—not as well as I used to, but I am walking. If I hadn't insisted on rehab I'd be immobile in a nursing home today. [a seventy-six-year-old woman]

Women's Health and the Medical-Care System

Women are central to both the formal and informal health- and medical-care systems. At the same time women's own health- and medical-care needs are quite different from men's. Thus any changes either in the insurance or health- and medical-care systems will affect women the most, especially women over forty. For these reasons alone it is crucial for women to study carefully all proposals to reform health and medical care, whether at the national, state, or organizational level. We need to become more active politically to make sure whatever changes are enacted do not disadvantage women or those we care for.

As we go to press, national reform of both the private health-insurance industry and the major government health-insurance entitlement programs (Medicare and Medicaid) is a high and long-awaited priority of the American people. So some change appears inevitable. However, because reform is a political process it is likely to take a long time. The longer national reform takes, the weaker that reform is likely to be, making it more likely that changes will be taking place at the state level, in our institutions, in our own health plans, and among the health industries nationwide.

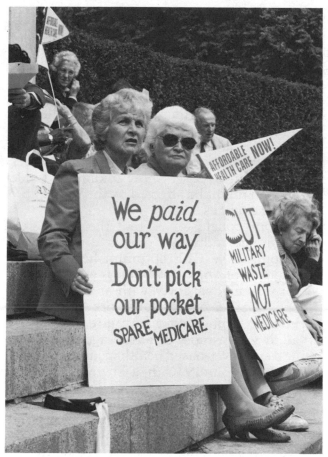

Marilyn Humphries

Issues, Problems, and Prospects for Change

Women are much more centrally involved in the health- and medical-care system than society has recognized. We are half the population, have health needs of our own, and interact with the system twice to three times as often as men.[1] Women have been shown repeatedly to be both overtreated and undertreated, depending on their insurance status, income, age, and race. We have been discriminated against in treatment settings and excluded from research in ways that have been dangerous to our health and survival.

We are the overwhelming majority of health-care workers: 85 percent in hospitals, 75 percent in the overall system.[2] We may also be members of groups working for improved recognition of the health needs of people of color, the elderly, and people with disabilities. We spend tremendous amounts of time, energy, and money on the health needs of others. We advocate for family members, functioning as unpaid administrators, arranging for their care, and accompanying them on medical visits. We frequently organize and manage follow-up care at home after these visits, keeping track of medications and special diets, supervising exercise programs, and being available for therapists and other health workers who visit at home.

Finally, we are central to the physical and mental health of communities and families, through personal support and caregiving, companionship, volunteer labor in organizations, and acting as citizens in the public interest. We may give as much in unpaid labor caring for elderly, infirm, or dependent spouses or parents as we once did caring for dependent children. We frequently sacrifice earning potential and economic security in retirement in order to do so. We take on life-and-death responsibilities without adequate support or resources. Although women are the backbone of the existing health- and medical-care system in many different ways, we get very little in return. Though more than half the population, women have almost no say in how this system works, in spite of how much influence it has over our lives.

Unfortunately, the system and much of society have not fully appreciated the reality of women's situation and how much women are taken for granted throughout all parts of the health- and medical-care system. It is assumed in many families that all this activity is "women's work." Women's groups and consumer groups, small and underfunded, are usually not taken very seriously on health issues, and are assumed to be complaining, looking out mainly for their own interests and needs.

One problem is that the terms *health care* and *health insurance* have become common usage instead of the more correct *medical care* and *medical insurance.* Health care includes personal, public, preventive, and environmental efforts not usually included in medical care or covered by insurance. We have a broader view of health and so will use *health- and medical-care system* to refer to the whole system.

AUTHORS' STATEMENT

by Norma Meras Swenson, Diana Laskin Siegal, and Paula B. Doress-Worters

The authors of this chapter have spent many years studying the American health- and medical-care system and its effects on women. We have made an intensive study of the contemporary national health-care reform movement to assess how midlife and older women might be affected by the various proposed changes.

Our conclusion is that the commercial insurance industry's role is fundamentally incompatible with optimum health for the majority of Americans. This is especially true for women over forty, with or without families, whether or not they work outside their homes. Women over forty are, in fact, the adult group most disadvantaged by private and employer-based health insurance.

In a country with a stagnant or slow-growing economy, and with a rapidly growing aging population, we believe that women's disadvantaged situation will not improve and may even grow worse. Most women continue to earn consistently less than men for the same work. Jobs are scarce and government-funded "entitlement" programs will continue to be cut, forcing more midlife women to take up the caregiving slack as volunteer and unpaid health workers in their families and communities. Many women approaching retirement today have moved in and out of the work force, often as low-paid, part-time, or temporary workers, because of family demands. Therefore, their Social Security benefits will be low, their pensions and retirement benefits will likely be nonexistent.

We believe it is *morally* unacceptable for women to be obliged to continue to contribute from their meager earnings to the excessive profits of the very same "health" industries that now obstruct women's access to reasonably priced, good-quality health and medical care.

As much as we admire and support the Clinton administration's efforts to achieve universal coverage, we believe managed-competition schemes (see "Reformspeak" box, pages 230–31) would be a detriment to women, would cost more than most women can afford, and because they preserve the role and profits of insurance companies, would not reduce costs enough to pay for universal coverage. It is vital that we inform ourselves about all aspects of reform proposals so we can work to correct the double jeopardy of sexism and ageism that is built in to the present system and is still in most reform proposals.

We believe only a single-payer system financed from general revenues can actually save money, extend coverage, and provide best for women's needs. We urge all women to support the single-payer option, to oppose those who would exclude it from debate, and to examine carefully all features of any reform bill at either the state or national level.

Women's Health

This subject has been in the news during recent years since Dr. Bernardine Healy was appointed the first woman director of the NIH (National Institutes of Health), and created the Office of Research on Women's Health at NIH, charged with looking at women's health research in each of the Institutes. She called for the largest series of clinical and community research trials ever conducted on women, costing $500 million (see box, page 226). Responding to clear evidence that women were being ignored in research on chronic diseases, and that results on men were being applied to women incorrectly, this research program will try to close that gap and correct these errors. The NIH program also calls for incentives to involve more women in performing the research. Finally, portions of the Women's Health Equity Act of 1992 were passed by Congress, providing a major package of research, services, and education.

However, the existence of this massive focus on women's health research at the federal level may serve to reinforce the notion that women's health is only about what goes on inside women's bodies. This "biomedical model" approach may further delay the understanding of the economic, racial, and cultural determinants of women's health. This disease-research focus also helps obscure recognition of women's large role in relation to the functioning of the health- and medical-care system as unpaid workers.

GOVERNMENT RESEARCH IN WOMEN'S HEALTH

Although the federal government has never attempted to direct or plan the entire health system, it does spend funds to study many different aspects of health and disease, and how the system works. Listed on the next two pages (see box) is a selection of federal agencies currently involved in some aspect of health research affecting midlife and older women. Several women's health groups regularly monitor their activities and decisions. (See Resources for this chapter.)

The federal government spends billions each year on health and medical care. Even with the massive planning efforts that resulted in the publication of *Healthy People 2000,*[3] most actual appropriations and funding decisions are made by a political process in Congress. Those with the most powerful voices or influence will dominate that process. The result is that less than 3 percent is spent for research on health care of midlife and older women, and on the aging process itself.

As mentioned, women have succeeded recently in calling attention to our needs and in identifying errors and gaps in women's health research,[4] with the result that almost every federal agency, at long last, is including something of concern to women. Some of the research is excellent. Unfortunately, some of the research is of dubious quality and some may be actually harmful to women.[5] Results may be gained at the expense of exposing some women to known risks, for example, breast or uterine cancer from hormone therapy. Another research project (not part of the NIH Women's Health Initiative) that has received nationwide attention is the decision to give tamoxifen, a highly potent anticancer drug, to healthy premenopausal women. The purpose is to test whether this exposure will reduce their chances of developing breast cancer.* (See Cancer chapter, pages 364–65.)

*Many ethicists and women's health groups protested this research because it exposes healthy women to substantial risks even after the informed consent materials were improved because of the protestors' pressure. See Susan Rennie, "Tamoxifen: What Are the Risks?" *Ms.*, Vol. III, No. 6 (May/June 1993), p. 46.

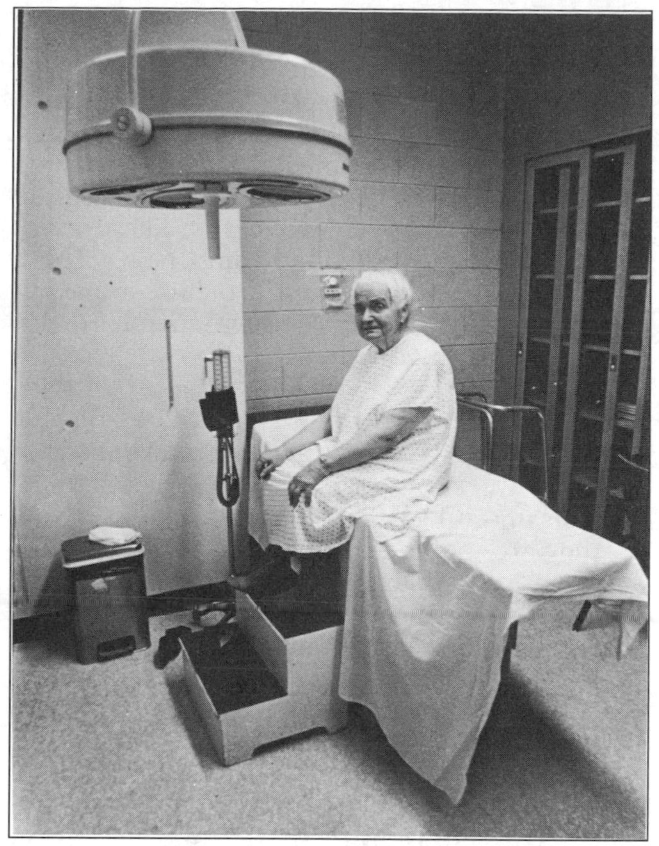

Marianne Gontarz

Another danger of so much publicity about women's health research is that we will be lulled by enthusiastic media reports into assuming everything is going well. We must keep involved in monitoring research quality, determining its relevance for various groups of women, and making sure research reporting includes full disclosure to the public. We must ensure that research results are translated into action. Finally, we must make sure the public realizes that research is only one of a number of tasks necessary to improve health for women.

WOMEN'S STAKE IN CHANGING THE SYSTEM

National health reform may not address issues most crucial to women's health, especially those affecting midlife and older women, unless we become much more active on our own behalf. In fact, basic structural reforms to the system, needed most by women, were not addressed by either the NIH research plans or the Women's Health Equity Act of 1992. Women are bearing the greatest burdens in many instances.

SELECTED AGENCIES CONDUCTING WOMEN'S HEALTH RESEARCH

The Agency for Health Care Policy and Research (AHCPR) conducts research on a wide variety of subjects designed to help practitioners to be more effective in dealing with many different concerns, like urinary incontinence and managing pain. These guidelines and a patient brochure are available to consumers. (See General Health Resources, page 482.)

The Centers for Disease Control and Prevention (CDC) conducts studies and produces weekly reports on public health problems and infectious diseases like AIDS. Now they are looking at quality of life as well as disease and death, including the chronic diseases affecting older women. Now that smoking, breast and cervical cancer, tuberculosis, violence, and other life-threatening conditions are increasingly becoming problems for older women, CDC is expanding its activities.

The Food and Drug Administration (FDA) has many scientific advisory committees charged with evaluating new and existing treatments, primarily drug therapies and new devices, many of which directly affect midlife and older women. These committees are usually appointed and include consumers as well as clinicians. They review research and practice and make recommendations to the FDA Commissioner about which drugs to approve and/or remove from the market, as well as what information should be available to practicing physicians and to consumers.

Watchdog groups like the National Women's Health Network are constantly monitoring the activities of these committees, often help identify knowledgeable clinicians and consumers, and regularly give testimony at the FDA's public hearings. The Network reports its findings and analysis to press and public. (See Resources, page 482.)

The Public Health Service (PHS) is the major agency concerned with issues affecting the public health system as a whole, especially how services are organized. They have proposed a "PHS Action Plan for Women's Health," thirty-eight goals for prevention, services, treatment, research, education, and policy, to be monitored by the Office of Research on Women's Health in NIH.[1]

The Indian Health Service is supposed to establish at least one major Indian Women's Health Center in each of its regions.

The National Cancer Institute (NCI) has focused on breast cancer as the death rate remains unchanged and the number of women diagnosed continues to rise. However, it also studies lung cancer, which now surpasses breast cancer as the most frequently fatal women's cancer (mainly due to active or passive smoking), as well as reproductive cancers like cervical cancer, still prevalent in older women, and ovarian cancer.

The role of U.S. women's diet in relation to breast cancer is being studied at last, following years of effort by health activists pointing to worldwide reports linking breast cancer rates to fat in the diet. Also, funds from the **Department of Defense (DOD)** were recently allocated for breast-cancer research.[2]

More recently, activists have begun raising the issue of the contribution of pesticides, radiation, and other carcinogens to U.S. breast-cancer rates (and likely ovarian cancer rates as well). So far, the NCI has not undertaken any studies to investigate environmental causes of cancer in women.

National Institutes of Health (NIH). An increased amount of NIH research dollars are now allocated through the **Office of Research on Women's Health (ORWH)** mainly for three major areas of chronic disease: heart disease, breast cancer, and osteoporosis. Programs in communities will attempt to encourage healthy habits in women of all ages and backgrounds by helping them to decrease smoking, improve diets, increase regular physical activity, and maintain optimum weight.

Most of these research trials are now under way, but the results will not be available for many years. Critics of these studies, however, suggest that their design is flawed and prepared without adequate peer review; they may not be able to "prove" what they set out to show. What most women need to know—how to prevent these diseases in the first place, and how to make treatment decisions once a disease is diagnosed—may not necessarily be forthcoming.

The second prong of the ORWH program is to get more professionally trained women onto the staffs of research projects at NIH and elsewhere. This will surely be helpful to the women researchers. But it is critical that we not confuse their increased involvement with improved participation of community women, and users of the system, in planning, decision making, and accountability in the health- and medical-care system.

In the past, the NIH has held a number of **Consensus Development Conferences**, many of them on women's health issues, but critics say these meetings have been too easily dominated by the drug industry and researchers' viewpoints, which emphasize particular treatments more than prevention or alternatives.

The Office of Alternative Medicine at NIH was established in 1992 to study, gather, and disseminate information about "alternative" therapies of all kinds in the United States.[3] Widespread national use of these therapies was recently revealed.[4] While this office has no special focus on older women, the fact that chronic diseases are more common in older women and are less effectively treated by conventional medicine makes this development important to watch. Many women have already discovered the benefits of acupuncture, massage, and chiropractic treatments for long-term management and comfort as alternatives to drugs and surgeries.

The National Institute on Aging (NIA) is studying issues like frailty and through pilot programs is developing a set of guidelines that could potentially help reduce some of the falls and fractures to which women are especially vulnerable. (Not all fractures are a result of osteoporosis.) Without vigorous, community-based programs to implement these recommendations, however, women will receive little benefit from them.

The Office of Technology Assessment (OTA), an arm of Congress, has conducted a number of studies and reviews on key women's health issues, most recently an excellent report on hormone treatments at menopause. (See Resources, page 468.) Key among its findings was the lack of adequate information available to women making treatment decisions. OTA's work is more objective and critical than some other federal agencies', but it is less well able to publicize its work, and often is under heavy attack from special interests.

Many of the other Institutes have programs of interest to women. One example is the **National Institute of Diabetes and Digestive and Kidney Diseases (NIDDKD)**, which studies a variety of chronic diseases affecting women such as osteoporosis, urinary incontinence, gestational diabetes, obesity, interstitial cystitis, urinary tract infections, gallstone disease, and nutrition deficiency anemia, especially in the elderly.[5] (See Resources for this chapter.)

1. James O. Mason, "From the Assistant Secretary for Health, US Public Health Service." *Journal of the American Medical Association,* Vol. 267, No. 4 (Jan. 22/29, 1992), p. 482.

2. "Effective Lobbying Increases Federal Funds for Breast Cancer." *The New York Times,* Oct. 19, 1992.

3. "Exploratory Grants for Alternative Medicine." *NIH Guide,* Vol. 22, No. 12 (Mar. 26, 1993).

4. David N. Isenberg, "Unconventional Medicine in the U.S.: Prevalence, Costs and Patterns of Use." *The New England Journal of Medicine,* Vol. 328, No. 4 (Jan. 28, 1993), pp. 246–52; also see Editorial, pp. 382–83.

5. "Women's Health Issues." *NIDDKD,* August 1991.

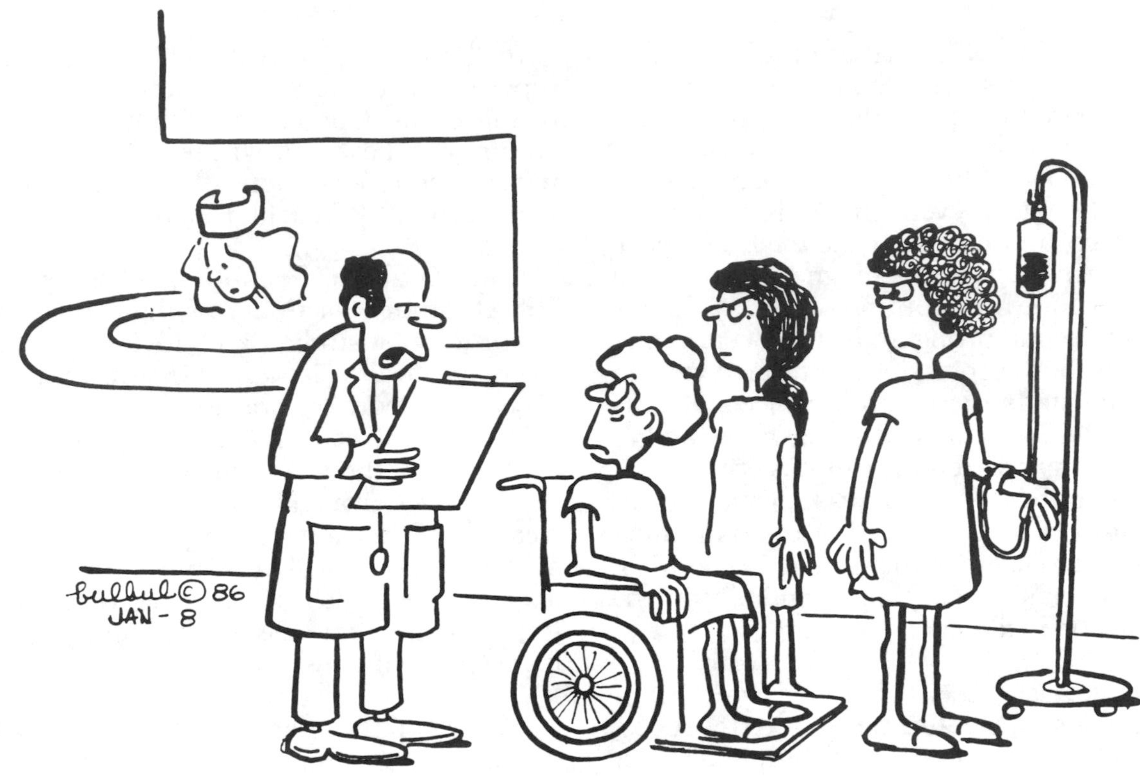

We're releasing you from the hospital early. You're cutting into our profit margin!

- **Costs.** Because of the growth of female-headed households and the "feminization of poverty," low-income families pay more than twice their share of income for health care compared with high-income families. Poor families pay a greater share of earnings for both personal and family insurance premiums, and eight times more for out-of-pocket, unreimbursed medical expenses for office visits, drugs, and other services.[6]
- **Insurance.** Women are both uninsured and underinsured. The existing financing mechanisms are built around assumptions that we will be dependents of wage earners rather than workers or heads of households. The services women need most—reproductive health, screening, and preventive services—are frequently not covered.
- **Basic Health Care.** Even when insured, women lack access to quality medical care.[7] True primary care (see definition, page 230) for women is almost nonexistent. Female-headed households—women and their children—are much less likely to have access to care, especially primary care.[8]
- **Information.** Women have an extremely difficult time obtaining good health- and medical-care information crucial for decision making, for themselves or for family members. Frequently they feel frustrated and dissatisfied by the conflicting information they receive or the poor quality or inadequate amount of that information.[9]

We are obliged to use and learn about a system that is not designed by us or for us and frequently does not have our needs, interests, or communciation requirements in mind. It is too difficult to get crucial information about technology and drugs, or about the true benefits of procedures and therapies—especially for women, older women in particular.[10]

More women than ever before are involved in the medical-care system at the professional level as physicians, researchers, and administrators, but most women are still clustered at the bottom of that system, doing underpaid practical, clerical, or housekeeping work in hospital systems.[11]

The NIH program and many women's groups call for more professional women to be involved in policy and high-level decision making in the health system as a way to improve the system's

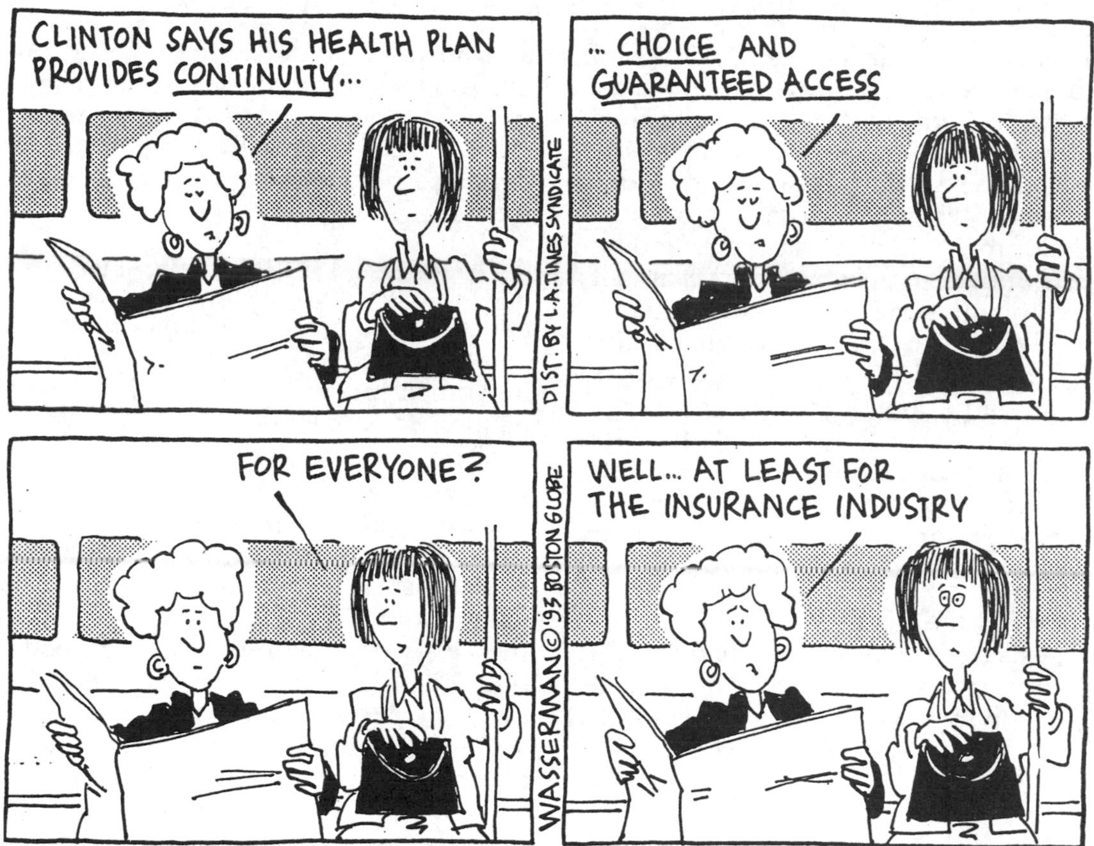
CLINTON SAYS HIS HEALTH PLAN PROVIDES CONTINUITY...
... CHOICE AND GUARANTEED ACCESS
FOR EVERYONE?
WELL... AT LEAST FOR THE INSURANCE INDUSTRY
DIST. BY L.A. TIMES SYNDICATE
WASSERMAN © '93 BOSTON GLOBE

accountability to women.[12] Including the talents of trained professional women can never be a substitute for the input and direction that the health- and medical-care system needs from community women of diverse races and cultural backgrounds. Rarely do we hear a call for more women to be involved at the community and citizen levels.

We will have to *demand* those better systems of accountability, planning, evaluation, and information to be available to us as individuals, families, and community members. We will have to insist that a powerful community and citizen role for women be an integral part of any new system and all patients' rights.[13] Otherwise, we will be obliged to rely on experts, female or male, who have not been trained to see the situation from a laywoman's point of view, and who frequently identify primarily with professionals and special interests.

Assumptions About Women

Women ages forty and over have the most to gain from changes in the way health and medical services will be financed and delivered, but only if those changes are designed to benefit us. Unless women get involved in fighting for what is needed, the new programs once again will be built around the old assumptions about women, namely that:

- Our labor is available free or at low cost, especially as midlife caregivers of ailing spouses or parents.
- We must be dependent on spouses/partners or employers for access to insurance and care even though working women pay into the system.
- Poor women and women of color are liabilities.
- Insured women are markets and "billable" resources.
- Our ignorance of how the system works and how technology and drugs are misused can be exploited.
- Our major dependence on government programs means women's services will be the first to be cut or scaled back.

Women, especially women over forty, will have to take the lead in pointing out how these

"REFORMSPEAK": SOME TERMS YOU SHOULD KNOW

Fee for Service. Medical-care providers bill for each medical visit, treatment, service, etc. as a separate item, and, unless restrained, may increase the amount billed from one visit to the next. Conventional insurance companies now handle the majority of health insurance this way under the "indemnity" insurance principle. Most government-sponsored health services are billed and paid this way. Fee for service gives the maximum incentive for medical-care providers to do more and charge more, whether or not services are necessary or beneficial. It maximizes profits for clinics, labs, doctors, hospitals, and insurers but speeds up cost increases for employers, consumers, and taxpayer-supported government programs.

Global Budget. This is the annual, government-established target or spending limit for the country's health expenditures. In its most extreme form, specific limits would be set for each state as well as for the nation.

Health Maintenance Organization (HMO). An HMO is a medical-care-provider corporation organized to deliver both office-based medical care and necessary hospitalization for subscribers who pay one prepaid monthly or annual fee (packages vary). HMOs have their own staff of primary-care doctors and nurses, and expensive visits, procedures, and hospitalization are restrained. Subscribers who seek care outside the HMO will have to pay for bills they incur. HMOs may be for-profit or nonprofit, and can be set up by government, insurance companies, unions, or other groups. HMOs are the oldest type of managed care.

Independent Practice Association (IPA). An IPA contracts with doctors who are in private practice to care also for some patients in different HMOs and other health plans, presumably for less cost.

Managed Care. This is any system that controls costs by monitoring and controlling decisions made by doctors and hospitals under various types of health plans. HMOs and PPOs are two types. Managed care may set up specific guaranteed services of doctors and hospitals to subscribers based on fixed prepaid fees or premiums. A key component of any type of managed-competition plan, managed care is usually profit motivated but may also reduce unnecessary or risky treatments.

Managed Competition. This is an untested theory combining health-care services and financing mechanisms. It is tied to employment and based on the profit-making insurance principle, but with vastly expanded regional markets. A few very large health-insurance plans would be forced to compete for large pools of subscribers in each region. Groups of employers or other subscribers offering benefits, variously called health insurance purchasing cooperatives, or alliances (HIPCs, HIPAs), would "shop" for the best plan. Insurers would be obliged to offer (defined) basic coverage packages to everyone in a prepaid managed- care system with global budgets (package price set in advance) and capitation (a fixed fee to care for each person for a fixed time). Theoretically, the best plan would be the cheapest and would win the competition, keeping prices down and avoiding price control.

PAC Money. Political action committees, special interest groups, give funds to members of Congress to finance their campaigns, securing their loyalty in key legislation battles. (See box page 236.)

Play or Pay. This is a "carrot and stick" approach to employers that would require them to either provide health-insurance coverage for their employees ("play") or else "pay" the federal government, which would provide it through payroll taxes.

Primary Care. Primary care is generally defined by health experts to mean health or medical care given by a *generalist,* someone with broad training who is skilled in recognizing special problems and who will refer a patient to *specialists* if needed. Nurses with additional training, like nurse practitioners, midwives, and physician's assistants, now function as primary-care practitioners in doctors' offices, public health systems, and managed-care programs, as do many physicians, such as family-practice doctors, internists, and geriatricians. The obstetrician-gynecologist, a surgical specialist, is not trained as a primary-care provider and should not be so designated, although many women use them for primary care.

Preferred Provider Organization (PPO). In a PPO, which is one of several managed-care approaches, doctors and hospitals form corporations to give volume discounts to insurance companies to help lower copayments for subscribers who choose from a large list of providers in private practice. PPOs are rarely nonprofit.

Provider. Any health worker or health facility eligible (by license or other mechanism) to receive payment for a medical visit or service, regardless of who pays the bill.

Public Interest. This describes the viewpoint of consumers or citizens, especially to benefit or protect the most vulnerable members of the public, including the poor, the elderly, people with disabilities.

Single Payer. This is a principle similar to public utilities in which one national, centralized nonprofit utility, or a government agency like the Social Security Administration, would be responsible for both collecting and disbursing the money needed to pay medical-care bills. Canada works on this principle and covers everyone for less, with agreed fee schedules for providers and systemwide access for consumers. A single payer would replace the approximately twelve hundred (mostly profit-making) U.S. insurance companies now handling medical claims. Two independent federal agencies agree this saves the most money and is the fairest way to expand coverage. As we go to press, the Health Security Act of 1993 is the most popular single-payer bill before Congress.

Utilization Review. This is the practice of regularly examining all the processes of medical care—tests, treatments, hospitalizations, and other services—so as to limit the unnecessary ones.

assumptions work now, and why they must not be built in to health- and medical-system reform proposals.

Women's Insurance Needs

Millions of women currently lack health insurance, and are the majority of those dependent on government programs for health and medical care.[14] Most uninsured women are women heading families of dependent children or are caring for dependent adults, or both. They are uninsured because they:

- are caring for dependent family members and cannot work outside their homes;
- are working or have worked in small companies that cannot afford to provide health benefits or group coverage;
- work part-time and are not eligible;
- are retired without health benefits; or
- lost whatever benefits they once had as dependents of a working or retired spouse.[15]

Because of changes in the law, employers will be less obliged to provide retirement benefits in the future, so women will be even less likely to have health coverage in retirement.[16]

Too many women are paying a higher and higher percentage of their incomes to buy insurance because they are not part of an employer group.[17] Many women are now "locked in" to jobs they might rather leave, or take jobs they might not like, in order to keep or obtain employer-covered health insurance.

If you are divorced or widowed while part of a group plan, federal legislation may allow you to continue in the plan for a period of time if you can afford the high premiums. Too large a percentage of women still do not have this protection.[18]

Ironically, while most women's health- and medical-care needs, especially at midlife, are often ignored, trivialized, and undertreated, our status as insured women often creates an incentive or "magnet" for unnecessary tests, and surgical or other procedures, resulting in overtreatment.[19]

Women's Reform Proposals

Despite lack of funding to oppose the messages of the special-interest groups and the media, women's health activists and groups are mobilizing to bring the health-reform message to a

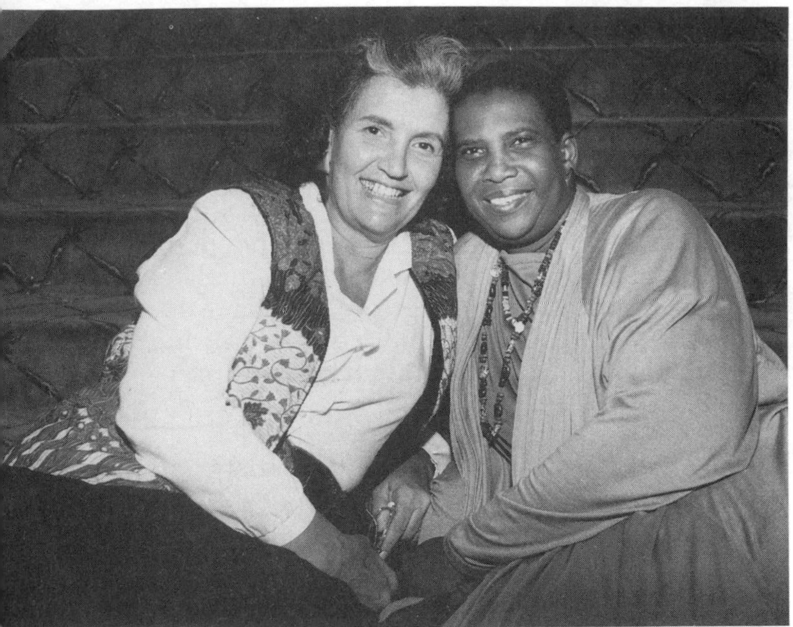

Norma Meras Swenson, Boston Women's Health Book Collective, and Byllye Y. Avery, founder, National Black Women's Health Project *Ellen Shub*

THE MEDIA

Many of us depend on mainstream media like television and daily newspapers for our understanding of both women's health issues and the key points of the health-reform debate. Many conscientious reporters and editors work hard to provide documented facts and thorough analyses; some television producers have also tried to offer discussions that illuminate the nature of the debate. Without them, our understanding of these very complicated issues would be much poorer.

The health industry's special-interest groups have influence in Congress, and influence over the media. We need to know exactly how they are likely to shape decisively any new federal system, if and when it ever becomes law, despite what the people may want. We also need to know that the media are often careless about identifying whether invited spokespeople and "experts" represent special health-industry interests or special political interests rather than the public interest. Reporters sometimes quote study outcomes or results of polls without explaining how these were conducted or who paid for them. Conflicting poll results are sometimes ignored.

Among the media's most pervasive biases, however, has been the failure to question the profit motive in health and medical care at all. They have failed to emphasize sufficiently how the health industries' spectacular rise in PAC (political action committee—see "Reformspeak" box, page 230) donations will

wide diversity of women's groups across the country. They are calling for some basic reforms in women's own health- and medical-care benefits, such as:[20]

- Comprehensive benefits: reproductive/gynecological/childbearing, occupational/environmental, mental, dental, long-term care
- No links to welfare, employment, income, or health status
- Preventive health services, periodic checkups, health promotion for women's health needs—not just treatment
- Access to midlevel practitioners (midwives, nurses) and other health practitioners—not just doctors
- Primary care, especially care designed for women
- Community-based services near home
- Power in the hands of community women
- More training, upgrading, and pay equity for women health workers
- Coverage of services, special treatment needs of HIV-positive and substance-abusing pregnant women

Beyond demands for comprehensive and particular benefits and services for women, many women are also calling for other specific system reforms, such as:

- Recognition of women's unpaid labor as health workers in community, family, and home (income-tax credits or Social Security credits, respite services)
- Better-quality, unbiased women's health information
- Recognition of patients' and consumers' rights and roles, especially women's, in system planning and decision making
- Specific mechanisms of accountability of the system to its users at all levels
- Redress when the system fails or damages us

Women's groups are not simply looking out for their own health in any reform proposals.

influence key members of Congress in coming debates and votes. Recipients of large PAC donations will be expected to favor these industries' preferences and work against progressive legislation. (See PAC box, page 236.)

In addition, the media do not advocate for the public and consumers to have a large and important decision-making and oversight role in such a massive change as national health reform. Media focus on the malpractice issue tends to be dominated by the viewpoint of physician groups, and distorted by a few reports of large jury awards. The media have also virtually ignored women's central and unique place in the entire health- and medical-care system, women's long history of activism and analysis in health reform, and their key stake in progressive change.[1]

The single-payer option (see "Reformspeak" box, page 231) for health reform is rarely mentioned in the news except as something we will not get, even though the government's own fiscal management and budget experts have made it very clear that this system would save the most money for the urgent task of increasing access.[2] Articles critical of the Canadian and other government-sponsored systems abound.[3] Well-packaged, well-placed materials from the special-interest groups are always available for reporters. Often media researchers don't take time to follow up on the viewpoints of reform-movement groups working for the public interest. To learn about other views, the public has to consult public television and radio, and be on the lookout for literature other than daily newspapers and weekly news magazines.

Partly as a result of the media's focus, many Americans have been persuaded to fear progressive reforms, believing they will lose access to "the best" of care.[4] Hostility toward the older generation's entitlement "privileges" and cost of care is also beginning to rise.[5] Few even question why we cannot provide benefits for all ages, as other countries manage to do for so much less cost. We must challenge these assumptions. (See "What One Woman Can Do About Health and Medical Reform," pages 243–47.)

1. An extensive search of both the scientific and "lay" literature in mid-1992 revealed almost no material connecting the idea "Women" with the idea "Health Reform." Search conducted by librarian at the request of the author, Norma M. Swenson, at the Countway Medical Library in Boston, and by the same author at the Newton Public Library, spring 1992.

2. Robert Reischauer, testimony before the Committee on Ways and Means, U.S. House of Representatives, October 11, 1991. Also, the Office of Management and Budget (OMB) produced similar estimates of savings.

3. Jennifer Brundin, "How the U.S. Press Covers the Canadian Health Care System." *International Journal of Health Services,* Vol. 23, No. 2 (1993), pp. 275–77.

4. Erik Eckholm, "Those Who Pay Health Costs Think About Drawing Lines." *The New York Times,* Mar. 28, 1993, pp. 1, 3.

5. Robert P. Hey, "Entitlements Under Fire, but No Big Changes Now." *AARP Bulletin,* Vol. 33, No. 11 (December 1992), pp. 1, 5.

They are interested not only in issues of *cost* and financing mechanisms, *access* and insurance coverage, *quality* of care and services, and *women's health research.* Women are also concerned about many other needs for change in the whole system. These include:

- Universal access and equity
- Elimination of all existing insurance discrimination against women
- Choice of providers
- A single-payer system
- Global budgeting
- Rigorous elimination of waste, fraud, and excess administrative activity
- Fiscal control if a fee-for-service system is continued
- The training and retraining of health professionals in the economic/cultural/psychological and race/gender/age determinants of health
- Better technology assessment and feedback of results
- More investment in evaluation research
- A health-planning system (such as existed in the 1970s)
- Clinical practice standards, reviewed by consumers
- Controls on the drug industry
- More community settings and community-based services

- Improved investment in and recognition of our public health system of services (not only for poor people);[21] better monitoring of health status
- An independent ombudsprogram to guarantee fair adjudication of complaints and claims (see page 252)
- Recognition of violence against women and elder abuse as public health issues (not only as family/mental health/social service concerns)
- Long-term care, rehabilitation and disability services
- Coverage of necessary drugs
- Research on appropriate elements of primary care for women
- Home-care services, including birthing and hospice

NATIONAL HEALTH REFORM

THE CRISIS: COST, ACCESS, AND QUALITY

The "crisis" in the American health- and medical-care system has been regularly announced since the early sixties. Today reform of the system comes near the top of the country's urgent political agenda for many reasons:

1. **Cost.** The costs to government, the economy, individuals, and families have become excessive and are rapidly spiraling out of control. Industry and business claim they are unable to compete because health benefits increasingly erode profits. Some charge that one sector of the economy—manufacturing—is actually subsidizing another—the health industries—through what they pay for employees' health insurance.[22] In fact, paying for health care now consumes so much of our GDP (Gross Domestic Product), currently approaching 15 percent and projected to go up to 20 percent if nothing changes,[23] that health-care costs are themselves a threat to the nation's whole economy and economic survival.[24]

   The President and members of Congress claim that the economy and the deficit problem cannot be addressed successfully without controlling health-care costs, especially those of government programs like Medicaid and Medicare.[25] Too much of what we spend does not even go for medical care. Administrative costs, waste, and fraud are estimated to account for a third of our costs. The more slowly our economy grows, the more costly the whole system becomes, resulting in fewer and fewer people who can afford to pay for health or medical care and must depend on government programs.
2. **Access.** Close to 40 million Americans lack health insurance and are without *access* to health care, and the number is rising.[26] Another large segment of the population is underinsured. As it is, only about half of those living below the poverty line receive health benefits through a public program; Medicaid reaches less than half of those eligible.[27]
3. **Quality.** Not only are we spending too much, but the more we spend the poorer our health becomes. We are not getting our money's worth.[28] Even though the quality of care for everyone has become increasingly poor and uneven, quality issues have a sorry third place in debates over the present crisis.

   Higher-quality care is presented as more costly, because it assumes quality equals expanded access to high-priced specialists and high-technology medicine. Lower quality is feared because it suggests that people who cannot afford to pay will endure "rationing" of needed services. We already ration care in grossly unfair ways that are also ultimately more costly. The idea of appropriate technology in health care has been slow in gaining acceptance. Yet many other medical experts have assured us that simply by eliminating waste and excessive medical treatments we could all be cared for right now.

   Financing, payment mechanisms, and access are very important, but debating them has the effect of keeping our attention focused on them and away from other serious problems with health and medical care like the following:
4. **Accountability.** There are few mechanisms of accountability beyond lawsuits that are available to patients. Most genuine malpractice never becomes a suit. Of the suits, patients win only a tiny fraction, even if a few awards have become larger.[29] Yet reform proposals suggest that patients will have even less access to redress than we do now. We need to fight for our right to create new mechanisms for making medical-care providers accountable, as well as to retain the only recourse we now have.
5. **Equity.** Comprehensive care that is the same for all eliminates the stigma of second-class

status and changes relationships with employers, the welfare system, and providers of care. Tying coverage to employment penalizes women more than men, since women's employment is more marginal, more frequently part-time, and in the smallest companies. It also creates a permanent two-class system within health services. If we completely cover and support the most vulnerable in society, especially women and their children, the whole society will gradually get healthier. Punishing them, denying them care, becomes maximally costly and eventually damages the health and well-being of the whole society.

Two-tier systems do not work, as our own presently existing programs make very clear. The most vulnerable, poorest, and sickest, who are also those with least access to adequate care, are also those most likely to be jettisoned or underserved due to local, state, and federal budget cuts or political considerations. Ironically, the present obsession with cost control often leads to higher costs. People denied preventive and comprehensive care must receive expensive emergency care when in crisis and may even be overtreated as well because of the uncontrolled fee-for-service system. Emergency and crisis care in a two-class system are inevitably the most costly to taxpayers, who support public systems.

Sadly, too few people are willing to demand an equitable system based on American ideals of fairness and social justice. Many Americans today appear willing to tolerate a different and discriminatory quality of health- and medical-care services based on income and social class, or even race and age. Fighting for equity is crucial to the survival and dignity of elders, most of whom will always be women.

6. **Women.** System reforms that do not recognize women's unique relationship to the system as well as their own health needs will not work, any more than ignoring economic conditions, race, and ethnicity can result in a system that meets people's needs.[30]

What Other Industrialized Countries Do

Other industrialized countries, especially in Europe and Japan, are doing much better, spending about half as much as we do and getting much better results for what they pay for health- and medical-care services.[31] For example, Canada, the United Kingdom, and most others provide universal care for less than 10 percent of their GDP.[32] They do this through many different mechanisms, but most include:

- National planning
- Global budgeting and caps on charges
- Universal coverage, comprehensive benefits
- Price controls on the drug industry
- Technology assessment and uniform practice guidelines
- Controlling supplies of expensive equipment
- Emphasizing primary care and limiting the use of specialists

Other countries that manage their health- and medical-care systems better and get more favorable health results from spending less accomplish it by developing a national policy. In 1991, Canada, Germany, and Japan spent 72 percent of their total health expenditures on public health. These countries have better overall health statistics than the United States, which spent more per capita on health but spent only 44 percent of the total on public health.[33] Governments make sure that investments in education, jobs, housing, and preventive public-health programs are more evenly balanced with what is spent on crisis medical care.[34] To be fair, some countries exploit their female labor in the health- and medical-care system, and many of them have devised employer-dependent systems that are in trouble as the world economy continues to contract. But system costs are still nowhere near so out of control as ours, and most of their people are healthier, as shown by their lower infant mortality and higher life expectancy when compared with the United States' population.

National Proposals for a U.S. Health System

The Clinton administration and Congress are offering various proposals both to save government money and to provide basic health-care access for more people—hopefully everybody.

Special Interests

As we go to press, most legislation now being proposed by Congress and the Clinton administration puts profit and control by the major special-interest groups of the health-care industry, especially the insurance industry, ahead of consumer and patients' interests. (See PAC box, see below.)

- **Insurance.** The role of the large, profit-making insurance companies and their increasing involvement in medical-care decision making seems guaranteed.
- **Doctors.** While capping doctors' incomes is discussed, their need to make very high and ever-increasing incomes is not really questioned.
- **Pharmaceutical Industry.** Drug companies' privilege to increase their charges at three times or more than the rate of inflation, far ahead of any country in Europe, without any price controls is criticized but not ended.[35] This crisis impacts on women and seniors the most.[36]
- **Hospital Associations.** Hospitals (whether nonprofit or for-profit) are increasing their expansion, their accumulation of resources, and the development of their profit-making services at public expense.[37]

THE CLINTONS' PROPOSAL

The Clintons are supporting reform with managed competition as its cornerstone. This concept was based originally on some of the ideas of the "Jackson Hole" group, a Wyoming-based organization of leaders in insurance, medicine, pharmaceuticals, hospitals, and other special

PAC (POLITICAL ACTION COMMITTEE) CONTRIBUTIONS AND WOMEN

Lobbying groups, creating PACs as their funding mechanisms for specific political agendas, make donations to candidates through the PAC because federal election laws make it illegal to do so directly. PAC contributions, not strictly illegal but a source of influence over many in Congress, have been a controversial feature of Washington politics for many years, distorting the political process. Because better mechanisms for campaign financing have yet to be devised, the practice will likely continue.

The health industry—insurance, doctors' guilds, the pharmaceutical industry, and hospital associations—has been contributing heavily through PACs to members of Congress, mostly to those powerful on health-care committees, to influence them on health-reform legislation. Not a new practice, PAC donations to the 1990 national election increased nearly 20 percent to a total close to $20 million.[1] More than $2.6 million came from the American Medical Association alone. The insurance industry gave more than $10 million, ahead of almost all other congressional contributors, including banks, real estate, defense contractors, and even the oil lobby.[2]

Lists of the top ten congresspersons receiving the most PAC money from the health industries in both the House and Senate, Democrats and Republicans, include some of the most prominent names in the health-reform debate.[3] In the spring of 1993, when the question of PAC influence was again raised, HEALTHLINE (electronic information on health reform funded by the Robert Wood Johnson Foundation) reported that Congress, with flagrant disregard for its responsibility to protect the public's interest in health reform, voted itself the privilege of being able to continue to accept PAC money for as long as the health-care reform debate lasted, however long that would be.

The issue of PAC contributions and campaign reform aside, however, the sheer scale of the profits that have been made by these industries from the daily labor and savings of everyday Americans is mind-boggling, especially when we realize what a high proportion of women's meager earnings go toward these industries' profits. Huge sums are then available to influence the health-reform process against our needs and all people's needs. We may not be able to stop the health industry PAC contributions, but we can watch who accepts them, and we can make a campaign issue of how they behaved when the health-reform legislation was voted on.

1. Robert Pear, "Whose New Health Plan Is This Anyway?" *The New York Times*, Nov. 15, 1992.
2. Larry Makinson, "Political Contributions from the Health and Insurance Industries." *Health Affairs*, Winter 1992, pp. 119–34.
3. "The Road to Health Care Reform." *The Washington Post*, Jan. 26, 1993.

interests.[38] Though undergoing continual modification, the plan includes an employer-mandated system. Very large, regional health-insurance-purchasing cooperatives or alliances are proposed, at least one per state. These would be made up of large employers or nonprofit corporations or agencies of state government seeking health-insurance coverage for groups of employees or others. These regional alliances would negotiate with competing insurers for the benefit packages for enrollees and must offer a fee-for-service option. Those who do not fit into this system as employees could have their premiums supplemented by the government. States would charter and establish the alliances under federal rules and would monitor the management of the system. "Managed care" (prepaid plans) with fixed annual budgets would also become essential features. Other reform features such as taxes on health benefits are unlikely, and proposals of income caps on doctors or price controls on the drug industry wax and wane.

In sum, this version of the managed-competition plan essentially preserves the insurance industry, and bypasses the employee and consumer as a force in shaping any further changes to the system. To a large extent it even bypasses the providers. Government's role would be relatively weak. Medicaid would be folded into the alliance program. When people turn sixty-five, they would have the option to stay in the alliance or receive Medicare.[39]

Many critics, even within government, say managed competition cannot control costs, as single-payer plans could do. They also claim this system cannot work as proposed in more than one third of the United States, mainly rural areas where competition is not possible. As unemployment continues to rise, tying health care to employment seems increasingly problematic. For some small companies, such a requirement could spell disaster. For women, who work in or own small businesses, work part-time or seasonally, or are often out of the work force for long periods, this type of plan appears least helpful when compared with others.

Bills in Congress

The many and constantly changing bills in Congress include the National Health Service Act (Dellums), which would put government in charge of health-service delivery and build in consumer and citizen control; the Health Security Act of 1993, sponsored by Wellstone, McDermott, and Conyers, the ideal single-payer bill at this writing;[40] and a variety of other proposals from moderates and conservatives.

Basics

Most bills assume some kind of reform of the existing insurance system, some mechanism to produce more primary-care doctors while shrinking the number of specialists, and comprehensive coverage for everyone, however minimal. Managed care will likely continue to grow as a feature of many plans simply because the administration and insurance companies are now interested in it for its reported cost-savings potential. As an alternative to the fee-for-service indemnity system of the past it would appear to slow cost rises and make them more predictable.

Medicare Reform

While Medicare will probably remain part of any new government program, better-off elders will likely be taxed for benefits they could afford to pay themselves. This is fairer and cheaper than means-test programs that require people to prove their financial need. The trend to bring those on Medicare into HMOs or other managed-care plans will probably accelerate, and a slowdown in overall Medicare budget increases is part of deficit reduction in an overall economic plan.

Health Insurance Systems Today

How Health Insurance Works

Insurance is the word used to mean any system that provides benefits, that is, protection against or coverage of costs, in full or in part, for specific named events. Protection is purchased by subscribers or employers in exchange for annual fees or premiums. Health insurance offers benefits that cover part or all of the costs of some health- and medical-care procedures and some services, regardless of whether you, your employer, the federal government, or your state actually pays the premiums designed to cover these services.

Individuals and employers are purchasers of insurance premiums. Insurers and governments are "third-party payers" (neither patient nor medical-care provider). Whether or not some insuring agencies are defined as nonprofit, all insurance systems work on the profit motive, that is, they are designed to make money above the cost of paying the medical bills.

The majority of health-insurance coverage available today is based on the indemnity principle, which means protection is not comprehensive and covers only certain portions of fees for specified procedures or services. These are fee-for-service plans. Many plans will exclude you altogether for "preexisting conditions"—illnesses or injuries you had before joining a plan—that will cost above average to treat. Usually hospitalization or hospital-based services and procedures are included up to a certain limit, but little or no office-based care is included. Premiums paid for benefits received can go up anytime, and benefits may change. Usually, deductibles of a certain amount must be paid by you before payments by the insurance company begin. Coinsurance means that even then the insurer will only pay part of the cost, for example, 80 percent.[41] You must pay the rest. Very few insurance plans pay 100 percent.

THE HEALTH INSURANCE INDUSTRY

There are about fifteen hundred large and small private insurance companies in the United States. About twelve hundred of them sell health insurance, all with different programs and benefit packages, operating primarily under each state's insurance laws. The majority of these plans work on the fee-for-service *indemnity* principle (described above). Plans pay for part of hospitalization costs and sometimes office visits. Often, policies are hard to read and failure to understand their terms can mean very painful surprises if the policyholder must pay for substantial portions of hospital bills, tests, drugs, or follow-up visits.[42]

Fee for Service

The health-insurance industry has become extremely profitable partly because until recently it has supported the traditional fee-for-service system also favored by the medical profession, the hospital associations, the drug industry, and related industries. As the third-party payer, the insurance company continues to sign what are, in principle, virtual "blank checks." The checks are written by providers in the form of bills and invoices for higher and higher charges and fees for each single procedure, visit, or day of stay. In response to these rising charges, the insurance company raises its premiums to subscribers. Providers do more of the most expensive tasks and keep raising the fee.

The effect has been to increase costs with no limits. Companies trying to provide health benefits for their employees and government programs trying to keep costs down have each faced massive, rising drains on their profits or resources. Group indemnity plans make insurance somewhat more affordable for the consumer but do not solve the fee-for-service cost-escalation problem. Most analysts now agree that if costs are to be controlled the indemnity principle and the fee-for-service system must go.

New Approaches

Increasingly, all insurance companies, including nonprofit Blue Cross/Blue Shield and profit-making insurance companies, are moving more rapidly into the business of setting up their own prepaid managed-care health-insurance plans to better control costs and guarantee profits. Built on HMO principles, they may contract or hire their own health professionals and establish their own management system, setting prepaid annual premiums for subscribers who will receive somewhat more comprehensive benefits than under traditional plans. That way, revenues for the insurance companies will be better guaranteed now and in the future, whichever type of insurance plan employers and consumers may choose, and regardless of how the reform proposals finally come out.[43] The companies will also be in a better position to offer a whole series of packages, just as they do now, that would cost progressively more as extras beyond basic care are covered.

Utilization Review

Large insurance companies today are also more involved in monitoring medical care, its costs, and its effectiveness. They have set up utilization-review divisions to monitor diagnostic and treatment decisions refusing to pay for what they deem unnecessary. Physicians and surgeons are becoming resentful that their own judgments and their ability to act are being "second-guessed" by evaluators (some of them nurses) hired by the management companies. That intrusiveness promises to increase further as more insurance companies move into plans with fixed annual fees.

In some cases the insurance companies may be calling into question a doctor's poor or inadequately informed judgment. Medical managers look at outcome studies and other kinds of information that seem to show that certain procedures will not necessarily be in the patient's interest. Given that the profit motive must remain the insurance companies' primary incentive, however, it is impossible to be sure what each decision means. They are not accountable to either the patient or the provider for their decisions. If subscribers are unhappy enough they might switch to another company offering another plan and hope for more satisfaction in the future. Providers have even fewer options, since often they must negotiate decisions with many different insurers.

Health Maintenance Organizations (HMOs) and Other Prepaid Plans

For a flat annual fee these plans offer health-insurance coverage that includes both hospitalization and outpatient care (usually for a small fee each visit). Depending on the premium, HMOs may or may not cover drugs, and some services may not be covered at all. Usually HMOs are set up by an independent, sometimes nonprofit corporation that hires the doctors and other personnel.

Differences in the quality of care between these plans and regular insurance programs may be disappearing. Some say that prepaid plans are better; they have received government support and recognition for their cost savings. Although a different kind of insurance, these programs are nevertheless based on a profit principle, even if some of them are "nonprofit." They too raise their premiums regularly. Physicians are on salary but they have considerable power in negotiating salaries and bonuses. Much of the cost savings in HMOs is achieved through the routine use of nurse-practitioners and other "midlevel practitioners." Most of the rest comes from keeping people out of the hospital and away from expensive procedures.

Preferred provider organizations (PPOs) operate on a similar prepaid principle but generally don't hire their physicians outright and may give subscribers a somewhat wider choice of providers. They are also more likely to be profit-making.

While the standard type of insurance puts you at risk of overtreatment, prepaid plans may be more likely to undertreat you in order to save money. It may be easy to file a complaint in an HMO, but your ability to sue an HMO for malpractice or get your complaints addressed successfully are likely to be much more limited.[44]

Government Insurance (Medicare/Medicaid): "Entitlement" Programs

Medicaid, The State/Federal Program: Poverty and Medical Need

If you meet the standards of *poverty or medical need established by your state, at any age,* you may be eligible for certain benefits under Medicaid. These benefits are decided on, and paid for, jointly by the federal government and your state, if you can find a provider or a facility that will accept the level of reimbursement the state program offers. (Medicaid programs rarely reimburse at 100 percent of the rate most providers and facilities usually charge.) Many services are not office-based, especially the preventive services and screening tests most needed by older women, and may not be covered under Medicaid.[45] Increasingly, many specialists are scaling back the services offered under Medicaid,[46] and indigent women generally have little access to full-fledged specialists.[47]

If you are in an acute medical crisis, you may become temporarily eligible for Medicaid because of medical need, and will become ineligible again as soon as the crisis passes. In many cases you must have proof in writing that you have exhausted most of your financial resources and all of your assets before you can become eligible permanently (even for needed nursing-home care), a process called "spending down" or pauperization. Despite recent efforts to develop plans for advance government financing of nursing-home care for elders, the practice of pauperization continues in most places.[48] Women go through this process most frequently.

Medicare, The Federal Program: Age

If you are *over sixty-five or permanently disabled, regardless of where you live and no matter what your income,* you are probably eligible for Medicare, the federal program that was designed to provide medical care for the elderly. You pay

Medicare (insurance) premiums, which usually appear as deductions from your Social Security check, and Medicare only covers about 40 percent of your costs. Some providers do not even accept Medicare patients because the rate of reimbursement is too low, and many services are not covered anyway. *This means that at sixty-five you will still have to find a way to pay for almost half of your medical care.* Because of deductibles and copayments you either pay out of pocket each time for the difference between what Medicare pays and the billed fees, or if you can afford it you can purchase a private insurance policy to cover part of this difference, sometimes called "Medigap" insurance. (See chart below.) **Warning: While some states allow so-called "long-term care" insurance to be sold, it is usually very expensive and inadequate.** Efforts to regulate long-term insurance have been uneven and largely unsuccessful.[49] Beware of TV ads.

WHAT'S THE DIFFERENCE*

Medicaid	Medicare
Poor people, old or young, on welfare/public assistance or in medical need; mainly children	Older and certain disabled people, rich or poor, on Social Security, Railroad Retirement, or self-pay
States decide eligibility (criteria vary; you prove poverty, citizenship, etc.)	Federal criteria determine eligibility no matter where you live
Benefits vary in each state after basics, always changing	Benefits same in all states, but changed periodically
State money plus federal money	Federal money only, but administered by private contractors/insurers
Office visits/outpatient care usually free: Once pauperized, you usually pay nothing for services covered, drugs, etc. Some states charge some small fees	Office/outpatient never free: Part B premiums deducted from Social Security checks; you pay all drug charges, more than half all provider costs
Home care, hospice care† partly covered if available	Home care, hospice care† partly covered if available
Hospitalization is free but only at certain hospitals; more days covered than Medicare	Hospitalization partly covered: Part A premiums deducted; most hospitals accept Medicare but days limited; you will be asked to pay part; if poor, sick enough, state may help temporarily (known as "medically needy" under Medicaid)
Not all doctors, facilities accept Medicaid patients; few choices	Not all doctors accept Medicare patients or Medicare rates. Facilities' and doctors' rates vary; you pay differences or buy extra insurance if you can afford‡
Nursing-home care covered indefinitely once you get in	Limited days free skilled nursing-home care in lifetime

*This is the way these programs still look as we go to press.
†See Dying and Death chapter.
‡Medigap insurance, supplementary insurance that you must pay for, is designed to help cover the difference between what Medicare will reimburse and what doctors and hospitals charge. It is expensive and may not even cover your needs.

THINGS YOU CAN DO NOW TO GET HEALTH AND MEDICAL CARE

GOVERNMENT PROGRAMS

Many eligible people are not enrolled in government programs of health and medical care and are not receiving what they are entitled to. If you have become disabled due to mental or physical illness or an accident you may be eligible for Social Security benefits.

If your income is low or you are having special medical problems, you may be eligible for Medicaid coverage and not realize it. Ask to speak to a senior services social worker in your community or at the hospital or health center where you receive care. You must visit your state welfare office to determine for sure whether or not you or your family members are eligible to receive Medicaid coverage for medical care. The welfare office can tell you what you must do in order to become eligible. Come prepared to take notes on what you are told; many states will not give out any of their policies in writing because of frequent changes.

If you are nearing Social Security eligibility age, be sure to go to your nearest Social Security office soon to obtain *Your Medicare Handbook* as well as Social Security information and any other available publications that discuss current benefits, advise about purchasing Medigap insurance, or explain health benefits for working retirees. **Don't wait! Premiums will rise if you delay.** If you are disabled, your Social Security office also arranges benefits.

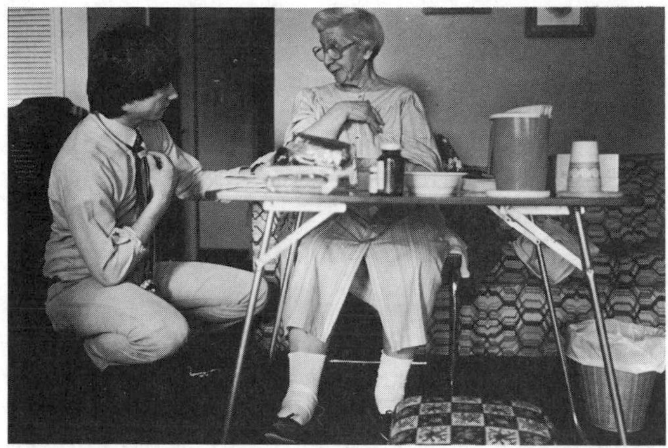

Marianne Gontarz

Both individual states and the federal government are focusing increasingly on Medicaid and Medicare programs as places to make cuts, to increase taxes, and to make other big changes. Because costs of these publicly funded programs are the fastest-rising in the whole health- and medical-care system, we can be sure that something will be done about them. In some states Medicare and Medicaid have already contracted with HMOs and other prepaid group plans to care for the elderly or poor for a flat annual rate. These rates are roughly equivalent to Medicare premiums or a negotiated annual Medicaid fee. Meanwhile, Medicaid costs continue to rise, so cuts and program changes will continue in most states.

You can keep up with proposed changes through the media and join consumer organizations concerned with women's health, the elderly, and other relevant issues. Attend meetings that explain these programs and the proposed changes, and call your state and federal representatives. These are some of the ways we have to keep track and try to make changes that will be fair to the poorest and most vulnerable of us. The time is now!

Working Women's Options: Not Poor Enough, Not Old Enough

If you do not fit into any government categories of poverty or medical need or age, and are working, you have several options:

- If you are a widow or a divorcée of a man who had insurance you may continue your benefits for a limited period, if you can afford to pay the premiums.
- If you work part-time you may be eligible for coverage; some states do require employers to provide health-insurance coverage for part-time workers; be sure to ask.
- If your partner or husband is employed and has health insurance you may be covered through that plan as a dependent.
- You may be insured as part of an employee group (prepaid or indemnity plan) through an employee benefit that pays the premiums for you. Most group coverage is for full-time workers.
- If you do not work full-time or are self-employed, you might get group insurance rates by becoming a member of a professional organization that offers group insurance.
- You may purchase individual private insurance through paying your own insurance premiums under an individual indemnity plan or prepaid HMO.
- You may pay as you go for medical care out of pocket.

Be sure to check all policies carefully; they may not cover your needs. Premiums for individuals in any of these systems are now exorbitant, and are still rising rapidly. Becoming part of a group is the only way most single working women not poor enough or old enough for a government program can afford health insurance. Prepaid plans like health maintenance organizations (HMOs) and preferred provider organizations (PPOs) are the only other alternatives to conventional health insurance but these are only cheaper when employer-based groups subscribe. Some states require employers providing health benefits to offer a choice between prepaid group plans and conventional indemnity coverage. These are just some of the reasons why commercial health insurance and reform systems tied to employment are not good for women.

Reforming Health-Insurance Practices

Women need reform of the insurance system whether or not national reform ever happens.

State-Level Insurance Practices

Many state insurance commissioners have little power and work mostly for the benefit of the insurance industry. But this can be changed through citizen action. Several states have occasionally appointed commissioners who make sure the industry best serves the needs of its citizens. But even when the commissioner is weak, legislators can be prodded into proposing changes to benefit consumers. For example:

Community Rating Versus Experience Rating

By now all of us have heard painful accounts of people who paid out thousands of dollars in insurance premiums over the years only to have their premiums raised exorbitantly or their benefits canceled altogether the moment they used their insurance for illness. Only a few states forbid this practice. This is called "experience rating." Some states require insurance companies to spread these costs among all their subscribers, called "community rating," thus resulting in better coverage for everyone, but somewhat lower profits for the industry. (New York State is implementing such a law in 1993.)

Basic Coverage

States can require that certain basic benefits be covered in any insurance policy sold, such as prescription drugs and mental-health services. Some states, on the other hand, have allowed

OUR RIGHTS AS PATIENTS*

You have the right to control what happens to your body. This includes the right of *informed consent,* which means that before you permit anyone in a medical or mental-health setting to do anything to you, they must first inform you fully as to:

1. What is being planned;
2. The risks and potential benefits of that treatment plan;
3. The alternative forms of treatment, including the option of no treatment at all.

For consent to be truly informed, you must also understand all that is being explained. It is not enough for a provider to simply catalog the risks and benefits in a quick or complicated manner, to do so when you are under the effects of medication, or in English if it is not your first language. You should ask as many questions as you have and wait until they are answered to your satisfaction before proceeding. You might ask for a written statement of the treatment plan in order to monitor your care or in case you choose to seek a second opinion later. Where no medical emergency exists, take as much time as you need to think about your decision. You can make a decision and later change your mind, since informed consent includes the right to refuse *during* as well as before any treatment. And you must agree *voluntarily,* without coercion or pressure applied by physician, family members, or others.

It is essential to read any consent form very carefully and to inquire about any vague or technical terms before signing, since your signature suggests—often incorrectly—that you *were* informed. You may cross out, reword, or otherwise amend a prepared form before signing. Be sure to ask for a copy of any form you sign.

The laws in our country do not recognize an affirmative right *to* treatment, except in the case of medical emergencies seen in a hospital emergency room. *If either transfer or discharge will threaten or adversely affect a patient's condition, then emergency treatment must first be rendered, regardless of ability to pay.*

Ask to see the patient's bill of rights at your hospital. Many hospitals have patient advocates who will help you whenever you have questions or concerns about your rights and about your satisfactions and problems while you are in the hospital. In about a third of the states, patients have a legal right to see, obtain, or have access to their hospital records. Federally qualified HMOs must make records available. Physicians' records, on the other hand, are the doctors' property, though states vary in requiring physicians to make them available to patients. Your local branch of the American Civil Liberties Union can tell you of specific rulings in your state about all aspects of patients' rights.

*Adapted from the Boston Women's Health Book Collective, *The New Our Bodies, Ourselves.* New York: Simon & Schuster, 1992, p. 682.

expensive infertility technology and organ transplants to be covered, even though this means higher premiums for everyone, yet permit policies to be sold that don't cover basic primary care or preventive services.

Drug Costs

For the elderly, but increasingly for everyone, drugs are frequently unaffordable, as prices continue to rise at three and four times the rate of inflation. Drug companies' profits are completely unregulated, triple those of the nearest most profitable industry. State legislatures can also require that drug benefits, for example, be included in insurance policies sold in their state.

HMO Reforms

Only about 15 percent of Americans are now enrolled in HMOs.[50] You deserve the choice of an HMO or other prepaid plan, and some states have been slow to permit them. You can help make sure your state does allow them, and also that some of the recommended federal guidelines are followed, for example, requiring that the board of directors consist of up to one-third consumers/users. Other proposed HMO reforms might include that:

- All HMOs must be nonprofit;
- Medicare patients are welcome (at no increased cost of coverage beyond the federal rate);
- Equitable long-term care is included;
- Strong independent mechanisms are in place that are accountable to subscribers and enrollees in cases of malfeasance and malpractice.

Changes Under Way

Today many states are moving fast on insurance reform and health-system reform, stimulated by their own rising costs and the increasing number of underinsured citizens. States watch national-level debates and see the likelihood that state plans, once implemented, will remain in place. The same health-industry special-interest groups fighting for control of the national reform program are active at the state level.[51] In Hawaii the indemnity plan is mandated as the insurance method guaranteeing universal coverage but resulting in higher rates of surgery and other invasive procedures. Oregon is now trying to set new Medicaid service priorities so as to extend coverage to more eligible people, by eliminating too-expensive procedures or those of doubtful value. New York is now one of thirteen states where experiments with managed care for Medicaid patients are under way.[52] Many other states are working on old or new legislation to change health-insurance coverage or benefits, including setting up one single entity that would receive all medical funds from all sources to pay all bills.

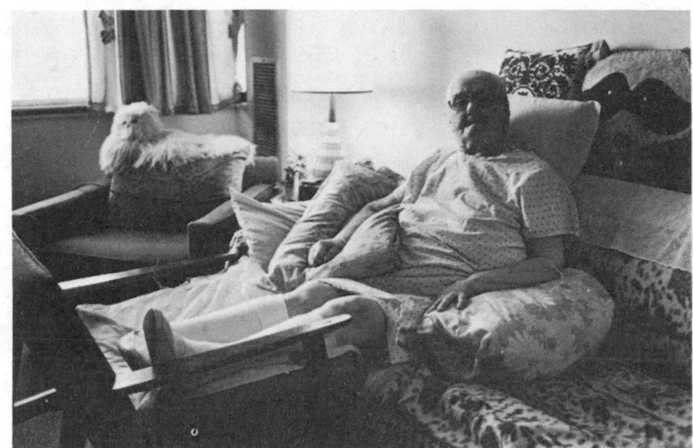
Marianne Gontarz

As national health-system reform appears to move closer, prepaid plans or managed-care plans are certain to be an important feature of any state reforms. Without specific safeguards at the state level, however, patients' rights and consumers' needs might get even less attention than presently. We cannot count on national reform alone.

WHAT ONE WOMAN CAN DO ABOUT HEALTH AND MEDICAL REFORM

National-Level Action

If you are not in regular touch with your congressional delegation about health and medical care reform, call or write the local office of the League of Women Voters to find out who your representatives and senators are. Find out whether or not your representatives and senators have taken PAC (political action committee) money, how much, and from which of the health special interests.

If you belong to a women's group or organization, find out if they are active on this issue and urge them to join one of the large national coalitions of women's organizations that have organized around health-system reform. "Health Care: We Gotta Have It," a group including the

Coalition of Labor Union Women (CLUW) and Church Women United (an ecumenical group), is working to bring grass-roots women's support to health reform. The "Campaign for Women's Health," a coalition of national women's groups spearheaded by the Older Women's League, is another group working to build consensus on what women's health benefits in any plan should be. Look at their evaluations of different proposals coming from the administration and from Congress, how they compare in benefits and costs for women and families, and what proposed structure changes and delivery systems would mean for you and your family. Get their literature, and learn about women's challenges to the reforms. If you haven't been active on women's health issues, this is an excellent time to join or support a national group, or at least to

HOW TO BEGIN TO GET BETTER MEDICAL CARE*

Before Your Visit

Talk to many other women about individual doctors and clinics. In choosing a doctor consider also the hospital at which the doctor practices. Contact women's groups or consumer groups to get more information about costs, attitudes, and medical competence of a number of practitioners and clinics. See *The Directory of Medical Specialists* in your local library or at your local medical society for the doctor's training history and qualifications. Check the medical society or the state board that licenses physicians for complaints against the doctor you are considering. Review your rights as a patient.

During Your Visit

Know your own and your family's medical history. If possible, bring a written record of your own. If you have a problem, write down when it began, symptoms, etc. Write down any questions that you want to ask.

Bring a friend with you.

Firmly ask the practitioner to explain your problem, tests, treatment, and drugs in a clear and understandable fashion.

Take notes or ask your friend to do so. (A tape recorder, if you have or can borrow one, will help in case of long, complicated explanations.) Such record keeping can be invaluable, so try to be assertive even if your doctor reacts defensively.

Ask the doctor to prescribe drugs by their generic rather than brand names (for example, aspirin, not Bayer). This will save you money.

Talk to nurses and assistants. They are often sources of valuable information and support and may explain things better than the doctor.

Ask for a written summary of your visit and any lab tests and X rays.

Remember, you have a right to a second opinion. If a series of expensive tests or surgery is recommended, you can tell the doctor to wait until you consult another doctor. This may prevent unnecessary procedures and treatment.

Don't forget—it's your body and your life. You have a right to make decisions about tests, drugs, and treatments. The questions on page 355 can be modified to apply to other conditions and recommendations to help you make your decisions.

After Your Visit

After the visit, write down an accurate account of what happened. Be sure you know the name of the doctor and others involved, the date, the place, etc. Discuss your options with someone close to you.

"Shop" drugstores, too. Drugstores in poorer neighborhoods may charge more than those in middle-class neighborhoods. Ask to see the pharmacist's package inserts listing medical indications and contraindications. Some drugstores will keep track of all your prescriptions and will check for harmful drug interactions.

Have the name of the drug and clear instructions written on the label, because of the risk to others who may take it in error, and also because when traveling abroad you may be challenged for possession of pills.

If you get poor treatment, if you are given the wrong drugs, if you are not listened to, it subscribe to national newsletters that deal exclusively with women's health issues and that monitor federal agencies and congressional legislation, such as *Network News* of the National Women's Health Network. (See Resources pages 441–44, 482–85.)

Long-term care proposals are growing in number, but are not currently built in to most mainstream reform proposals. These affect midlife and older women the most. Some build in the insurance principle. Many plans provide a continuum of care that allows the frail elderly to remain at home. Some emphasize home- and community-based care recognizing women's unpaid labor caring for vulnerable family members at home. Other proposals clearly plan to exploit that labor. Many plans retain or even expand existing profit-making institutional care. Everyone needs to take a more active role to find support for families and to provide for the long-term-care needs of elders.

We must question how many special interests are protected or even strengthened under the different plans, and where the money comes from to keep paying them. Consider the single-payer option (like Canada's) and then find out who is and is not supporting it in Congress, and why.

From the time I was a young child, I knew how seriously flawed our health-care system was. Starting with the early death of my mother from complications of my brother's birth when she was twenty-seven years old, through the neglect of my sister's deteriorating health because we couldn't afford insurance, and as a young married adult with four children of my own, having to manage without insurance because the only provider we could afford dropped us, my family had suffered everything that could go wrong.

With the Clintons in office I felt someone might listen. So I was one of almost one million people to write to the White House on health reform. I wrote in March 1993 and every letter must have been read, because in October I was asked to testify before the Senate Committee on Health Care Reform. I shared my letter and the senators were very attentive. In my small way I feel I gave life to my mother and my sister, who are remembered through how I live my life today. Don't be complacent. You don't have to be an expert. You can be heard. [a fifty-year-old woman]

State-Level Action

Changes and proposed changes in state-level programs of financing and delivering health and medical care are under way in many states. These changes will surely affect you since they are designed to either reduce costs, increase coverage, regulate the insurance industry, ration care, or change the rules that determine who is eligible for what kinds of state-supported care.

It is likely that any state that has already enacted a state-level plan in anticipation of a national program will be allowed to keep most of

---

is important for your own care and that of other women that you *protest*. Then write a letter describing the incident to one or several of the following:

- the doctor involved
- the doctor who referred you
- the administrator or director of the clinic or hospital
- the director of community relations of the clinic or hospital
- the local medical society
- the state board that licenses physicians
- the organization that will pay for your visit or treatment (for example, your union, your insurance plan, or Medicare)
- community agencies, councils, or boards
- the local health department
- local women's groups, women's centers, newspapers

To complain about a hospital or other health-care facility, contact one of the following:

- Joint Commission on Accreditation of Health Care Organizations, One Renaissance Boulevard, Oakbrook, IL 60181
- American Hospital Association, 840 N. Lake Shore Drive, Chicago, IL 60611

It is hard for one woman to work alone; however, health-care consumers can work together to get the treatment and services they need.

*Adapted from the Boston Women's Health Book Collective, *The New Our Bodies, Ourselves*. New York: Simon & Schuster, 1992, pp. 678–79, based on material originally from HealthRight, Inc.

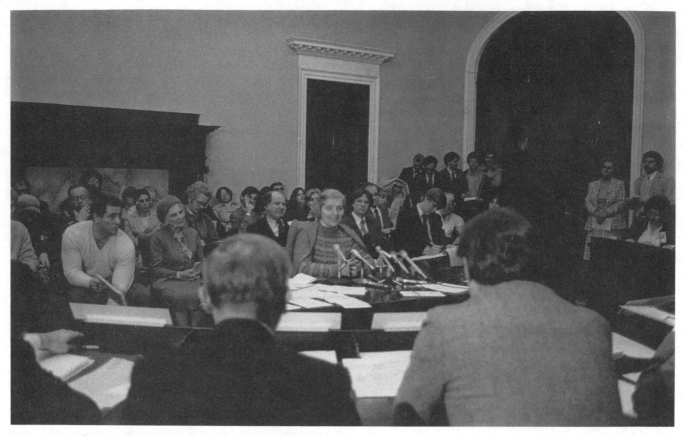

Woman testifying at legislative hearing. Ellen Shub

that plan. As a result, the same special interests trying to prevent serious change in Congress are working at the state level as well. Several states have already begun moving to a managed-competition-type model of care in anticipation of the federal program. Insurance reforms are badly needed in most states, as we describe elsewhere. Medicaid's rising costs stimulate cuts that hurt poor women of all ages and children. These cuts should be opposed. Other states are trying to install managed-care programs for all citizens not covered by private insurance, or play-or-pay models to establish employer responsibility. (See "Reformspeak" box, pages 230–31.)

If you belong to a women's organization, urge them to study these issues in your state, and join with other statewide women's groups to get involved in assessing what your state's legislators are doing about changes in the present health-care system. You can get in touch directly and personally with your representatives in the state legislature, asking what position they plan to take, what bills they are supporting, and why. *Tell them what position you favor, and why.*

Your local group can invite legislators to speak in the community, to explain how they plan to support needed changes that will affect women, especially older women. Help the Older Women's League or League of Women Voters plan a session in your region where all state representatives will be asked to come and explain the basic health-system changes they are proposing or supporting in the different bills—changes in insurance reform, Medicaid benefits affecting the poor elderly, caps in earnings, long-term care, or any other alterations to the existing state system. **Your calls and letters do matter!**

Many women have felt shut out of the legislative and governmental processes in our state and our nation. Many of us have felt alienated and disempowered by our experiences in the health- and medical-care system too. Sometimes we have been treated as if we do not deserve more, and may be given the feeling that we should be grateful for what we have received. Feeling this way alone can be a devastating experience, but knowing you are not alone is one of the most exhilarating experiences women can have. Working with other women to make our vision real is as important as winning. Whether the changes coming will be big or small, women must be part of them, trying to make them happen—for ourselves, our children, our parents, and all those we care for. We hope you will want to work with us for these changes.

NOTES

1. Naomi Maierman, with Dianna Porter and Lisa Lederer, "Critical Condition: Midlife and Older Women in America's Health Care System." Older Women's League Report, May 1992.

2. The Boston Women's Health Book Collective, *The New Our Bodies, Ourselves.* New York: Simon & Schuster, 1992, p. 652.

3. "Healthy People 2000: National Health Promotion and Disease Prevention Objectives." Department of Health and Human Services, DHS-91-50212, 1990.

4. "Women's Health Research: Prescription for Change." Annual Report of The Society for the Advancement of Women's Health Research, Washington, DC, 1991.

5. Testimony by Lynn Rosenberg, Boston University School of Public Health, on The Women's Health Initiative, October 1991.

6. E. Rassell, J. Bernstein, and K. Tang. *The Impact of Health Care Financing on Family Budgets.* Washington, DC: Economic Policy Institute, 1993. (As cited in *Healthcare Trends Report,* Vol. 7, No. 7 [July 1993], p. 5). The 28-page report is available from Public Interest Publications (800) 537-9359 for $5 plus shipping.

7. "One-third of Women Do Not Receive Basic Health Service, U.S. Study Finds." *The Boston Globe,* July 15, 1993; Judy Norsigian, "Women and National Health Care Reform: A Progressive Feminist Agenda." *Journal of Women's Health,* Vol. 2, No. 1 (1993), pp. 91–94; Carolyn M. Clancy and Charlea T. Masson, "American Women's Health Care." *Journal of the American Medical Association,* Vol. 268, No. 14 (Oct. 14, 1992), pp. 1918–20.

8. "Less Access to Care if Family Headed by Woman." *Ob-Gyn News,* Vol. 18, No. 13 (July 1–14, 1993). Article announced publication of "A Growing Crisis: Disadvantaged Women and Their Children" by the U.S. Commission on Civil Rights.

9. "The Menopause, Hormone Therapy and Women's Health," Background Paper for the Office of Technology Assessment, May 1992, p. 101; "Report Finds Health Information Not Easily Available to Women." *Update,* Aug. 12, 1992, p. 19.

10. Doug Podolsky and Joanne Silberner, "How Medicine Mistreats the Elderly." *US News & World Report,* Jan. 18, 1993, pp. 75–79.

11. The Boston Women's Health Book Collective, op. cit., pp. 651–98.

12. "Women's Health Research: Prescription for Change," op. cit.

13. George Annas, et al., "Legal and Ethical Issues, Tort Reform, and Consumer Protection and Participation Working Group Consensus Report." Report to Senator Edward Kennedy, Chair, Committee on Labor and Human Resources, April 9, 1993.

14. "Women Without Health Insurance." National Women's Law Center Report, Washington, DC, April 1993.

15. Older Women's League Report, op. cit.

16. Lawrence O. Gostin and Alan Widiss, "What's Wrong with the ERISA Vacuum?" *Journal of the American Medical Association,* Vol. 269, No. 19 (May 19, 1993), pp. 2524, 2527, 2544.

17. Older Women's League Report, op. cit.

18. National Women's Law Center Report, op. cit.

19. Judy Norsigian, op. cit.

20. "Model Benefits Package for Women," Campaign for Women's Health, c/o OWL, 666 Eleventh St., NW, Suite 700, Washington, DC 20001. Tel. (202) 783-6686. Also write to the Boston Women's Health Book Collective, P.O. Box 192, Somerville, MA 02144, for a copy of the "Statement of the Boston Women's Health Care Coalition, October 1993." See also Vernice Miller, "A Woman's Call to Action." *New Directions for Women,* July/August 1993, p. 4.

21. Helen Rodriguez-Trias and Bertram Yaffe, Presidents, American Public Health Association and Massachusetts Public Health Association, Draft Letter to Hillary Rodham Clinton on Key Points in National Health Reform, March 1993.

22. Vice President Maher, the Chrysler Corporation, talk at a Health Insights meeting, Edgartown, MA, September 1992.

23. *HMQ (Health Management Quarterly),* First Quarter, 1992.

24. Milt Freudenheim, "Study Sees Rise in Medical Costs." *The New York Times,* Mar. 2, 1993, pp. D1, D20.

25. Rep. George Mitchell on *This Week with David Brinkley,* August 1, 1993.

26. *HMQ,* op. cit.

27. National Women's Law Center Report, op. cit.

28. Marcia Angell, "How Much Will Health Care Reform Cost?" *The New England Journal of Medicine,* Vol. 328, No. 24 (June 17, 1993), pp.1778–79; and Lester C. Thurow, "Reality and U.S. Health Care." *The Boston Globe,* Mar. 23, 1993, p. 40.

29. Michael J. Saks, "Malpractice Roulette." *The New York Times,* July 3, 1993.

30. Malcolm Gladwell, "Public Health Experts Turn to Economic Ills." *The Washington Post,* Nov. 26, 1990.

31. Philip R. Lee and Richard D. Lamm, "Europe's Medical Model." *The New York Times,* Mar. 1, 1993, p.A15. William A. Glaser, "The United States Needs a Health System Like Other Countries." *Journal of the American Medical Association,* Vol. 270, No. 8 (Aug. 25, 1993), pp. 980–84; and "National Health Insurance Programs in Different Countries." *The Washington Post,* Apr. 26, 1988.

32. Victor W. Sidel and Ruth Sidel, *A Healthy State: An International Perspective on the Crisis in United States Medical Care.* New York: Pantheon, 1977.

33. G. J. Scheiber, et al., "Health Spending, Delivery and Outcomes in OECD Countries." *Health Affairs,* Summer 1993.

34. Lee and Lamm, op. cit. For a list of books on health reform, see Joseph P. Newhouse, "Health Care Reform: A Reader's Guide." *The New York Times Book Review,* Sept. 12, 1993, pp. 32–33; and Milton Terris, "Lessons from Canada's Health Program." *Technology Review,* February/March 1990, pp. 27–33.

35. Constance Sommer, "Drug Firms Profits Exceed Other Industries, Report Says." *The Boston Globe,* Feb. 26, 1993, p. 57; and "Prescription Costs: America's Other Drug Crisis." *Advocates Senior Alert Process (A.S.A.P.),* September 1992.

36. Special Committee on Aging, United States Senate, "The Drug Manufacturing Industry: A Prescription for Profits," Serial 102-F, Washington, DC: U.S. Government Printing Office, September 1991.

37. Richard A. Knox, "Hospitals' Riches: Excess or Necessity?" *The Boston Globe*, May 9, 1993, pp. 1, 10; "Gap Between Downtown Hospitals, Neighborhood Care Centers Widens." *The Boston Globe*, May 10, 1993, pp. 1, 19.

38. Robert Toner, "Hillary Clinton's Potent Brain Trust on Health Reform." *The New York Times*, Feb. 28, 1993, p. 1, 8.

39. *Implementation Aspects of National Health Care Reform: Reflections on Implementing Medicare*. Washington, DC: National Academy of Social Insurance, 1993. Available free from the Academy at 1776 Massachusetts Ave., NW, Suite 615, Washington, DC 20036.

40. Speech by Rep. McDermott at The Women's Convergence for National Health Care, Cleveland, Ohio, April 30–May 1, 1993.

41. Massachusetts is the only state that forbids insurers from billing for the difference between what the insurer will cover and what the providers might charge. Federal rules limit the percentage above the coverage that can be billed to the recipient.

42. Agency for Health Care Policy and Research, *Checkup on Health Insurance Policies*, U.S. Department of Health and Human Services, Washington, DC: U.S. Government Printing Office, September 1992.

43. Peter Kerr, "Betting the Farm on Managed Competition." *The New York Times*, June 27, 1993, pp. 1, 6.

44. Personal communication, Professor Leonard Glantz, Boston University School of Law, July 30, 1993.

45. Older Women's League Report, op. cit.

46. National Women's Law Center Report, op. cit.

47. Committee on Health Care for Underserved Women, "Ob-Gyn Services for Indigent Women: Issues Raised by an ACOG Survey." The American College of Obstetricians and Gynecologists (n.d.).

48. "Proposed Public Coverage of Nursing Home Care Examined." *Research Activities*, Washington, DC, August/September 1992, reporting on Pamela Farley Short, et al., "Public and Private Responsibility for Financing Nursing Home Care: The Effect of Medicaid Asset Spend-down." *Milbank Quarterly*, Vol. 70, No. 2 (1992), pp. 277–98.

49. "Committee Examines Regulation of Long-Term Care Insurance." *Update*, Aug. 12, 1992.

50. Marcia Angell, op. cit.

51. George J. Church, "Way Ahead of Bill." *Time*, June 28, 1993, pp. 30–33.

52. "States With Managed Care Programs." *The New York Times*, Feb. 1, 1993, p. B1.

17

NURSING HOMES

✦

BY SUSAN LANSPERY

1994 UPDATE BY SUSAN LANSPERY WITH SPECIAL THANKS TO ELMA HOLDER AND BARBARA FRANK OF THE NATIONAL CITIZENS' COALITION FOR NURSING HOME REFORM (NCCNHR) AND LORI ROSENQUIST

RESOURCES FOR THIS CHAPTER ON PAGES 487–89

This chapter assumes that dignity, quality health care, and control over one's own life are basic human rights. This chapter also assumes that a nursing home can be a good choice for some individuals and their caregivers. One's own or a family member's home can sometimes be more isolating than a nursing home.

That night I tossed and turned and I couldn't sleep. I felt so bad that my daughter couldn't go out with her husband because they didn't want to leave me alone. So I made up my mind that I would go into a home. And they tried to talk me out of it, but I said, "In a home I'll be with people my own age and we'll have things to talk about together." So, I've been here almost four years and I haven't been sorry. [a woman in her nineties]

My mother benefited from the mental stimulation of being surrounded by a lot of different people and activities which could never have been achieved in her own home. She was able to make new friends she never would have met had she lived alone in her apartment with a series of hired caregivers. I am sure the quality of her life during those years, although by no means ideal, was much better than it had been in those lonely and sick years before her collapse.[1]

After my husband had a devastating stroke, everything in my life other than that stopped. He was in hospitals, then in nursing homes, and then I took him home against everybody's advice. I felt like I was retired from life. It seemed as though the world deserted us. I used to say, "I'll never put my husband in an institution again. Home is the best place for him." But I was wrong. I really was wrong because there was very little contact with others and no diversions for him at home. [a woman in her sixties]

One reason so many of us react negatively to nursing homes is that serious problems *do* exist in many nursing homes. Even "better" nursing

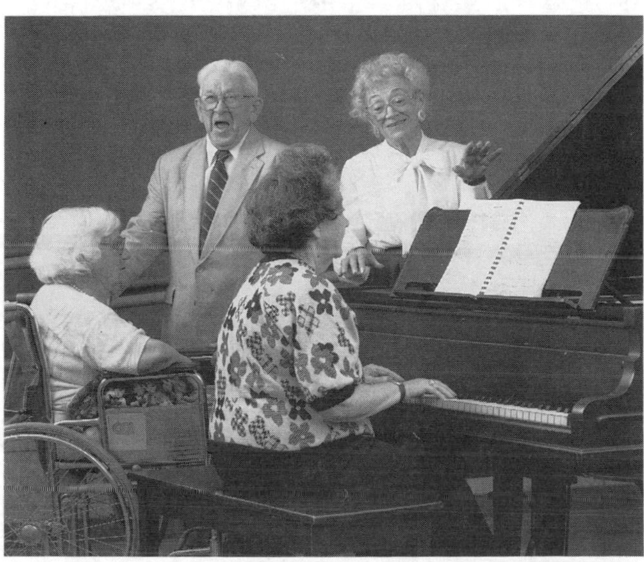

Peter Jones/Hebrew Rehabilitation Center for Aged

homes that provide a clean, safe environment and competent basic medical service may infantilize and dehumanize residents, ignoring their needs, desires, and rights for choice, control, privacy, and meaningful lives. All of these problems are part of our society's tendency to write off older people and people with disabilities, wherever they reside.

The solution to these problems lies in action. Successful nursing-home placement, care, and reform require information, planning, and maximum consumer/family involvement; in other words, a sense of control.

It's never too late—or too early—to start learning about nursing homes. Although less than 5 percent of people over sixty-five are in institutions at a given time, up to 43 percent of people over sixty-five may spend at least some time in one.[2] We must all recognize the need for alternatives to family-based care. While many such alternatives are evolving (see Housing Alternatives and Living Arrangements chapter), nursing homes remain necessary for a small percentage of the population. Education and a positive attitude will enhance our success whichever we choose.

It is particularly important for women to understand as much as possible about nursing homes. Women outnumber men as nursing-home residents, as primary caregivers who may help others to make nursing-home decisions and adjustments, and as workers in nursing homes. Most (75 percent) nursing-home residents are women, and percentages increase dramatically by age group.[3]

Furthermore, the number of poor older women is growing rapidly. Their poverty (often a lifetime's worth) increases their chances of poor health and of a need for long-term care. We must extend the feminist ideals of empowerment, action, hope, cooperation, and respect to them—to us.

DIFFERENCES AMONG NURSING HOMES

One way that nursing homes vary is in type of ownership.

- *Proprietary nursing homes* are profit-making. Most nursing homes are proprietary. Since the 1970s, the trend toward proprietary chains, in which one corporation owns many individual homes, has been increasing.
- *Nonprofit nursing homes* are operated by such organizations as religious groups, service clubs, and labor unions. Some have endowments and receive private contributions. They may also provide volunteers from their membership.
- *Public nursing homes,* also nonprofit, are generally supported by city, town, county, or state funds.

Nursing homes vary in the extent to which they meet government standards, whatever their type of ownership. There are excellent proprietaries and inferior nonprofits, although proprietaries (perhaps unfairly) tend to have the lesser reputation.

Even nursing homes that meet basic standards, however, vary in atmosphere, physical design, services offered, and areas of specialization. Some meet one individual's needs better than another's. Tips on choosing a facility appear later in this chapter.

Nursing homes once varied markedly by state and by level of care provided. This began to change when Congress enacted the December 1987 Nursing Home Reform Amendments as part of PL 100-203, the Omnibus Budget Reconciliation Act. The new law, often called "OBRA '87," grew out of years of consumer advocacy, a 1982 Reagan administration attempt to shift nursing-home regulation to states, and the recommendations of the landmark 1987 report of the Institute of Medicine (see Resources for this chapter). OBRA '87 directs the U.S. Department of Health and Human Services to incorporate residents' rights into regulations that every nursing home must meet in order to participate in Medicare or Medicaid. It places new emphasis on nursing-home residents' dignity, choice, quality of life, and self-determination. OBRA '87 also includes provisions for nurse-aide training, testing, and registration; increased nurse staffing; comprehensive resident assessments; and prescreening of residents for mental illness and mental retardation (see box, page 260).

PAYMENT

Rates for nursing homes vary greatly around the country according to type of facility, location, services offered, size of room, number of roommates, etc. Like other medical costs, nursing-home rates have risen faster than the overall rate of inflation. They are generally higher than people expect.

Almost all nursing-home residents pay for their care with private funds, Medicaid, or Medicare. Though virtually all homes accept private funds, most homes also participate in the Medicaid program, and could not survive without it: well over half of nursing-home income is derived from Medicaid funds. Medicaid is for people who cannot afford the health care they need. Most residents either are Medicaid-eligible upon admission or become eligible after they exhaust their assets by paying for care themselves. If your income is not enough to cover what you are charged, if your assets are below the limit for Medicaid set by your state, and if you need nursing-home care, Medicaid will generally pick up the difference.[4] A home that does not accept Medicaid can legally evict residents when their funds run out. Thus you should make sure that the facility you choose accepts Medicaid. Protect yourself to some degree by getting assurances concerning Medicaid—and anything else related to finances—in writing. Don't be afraid to consult a lawyer before signing anything. Medicaid-eligible nursing-home residents are permitted a personal-needs allowance; that is, they can retain a portion of their income for personal expenses.

The following example shows roughly how Medicaid reimbursement works with respect to the personal-needs allowance. Say Medicaid reimburses XYZ Nursing Home $40 per day for a bed in a three-bed room, or $1,200 per month in a thirty-day month. Resident A, who receives Medicaid, lives in a three-bed room. Her monthly income is $535—$335 from Social Security and $200 from a pension. The personal-needs allowance in her state is $35 per month.[5] She or her designee pays the nursing home $500, keeps $35, and the nursing home then bills Medicaid for the remaining $700.

Many older people expect that Medicare will pay for nursing-home care, but it rarely does. Medicare is *short-term* health insurance and pays only 2 percent nationally of costs for skilled nursing-home care.

THE SYSTEM AND ITS PROBLEMS

Discrimination against Medicaid recipients in the admissions process is only one of many problems in the nursing-home system. Because Medicaid generally pays nursing homes less than the homes would be able to charge private-pay residents, many are reluctant to admit Medicaid-eligible residents. In most communities it is widely accepted that only people with private funds are likely to find nursing-home placement.

My mother was on Medicaid and languishing in a hospital, waiting to be more settled in a nursing home. Every local facility had a one- to two-year waiting list for Medicaid or private pay. But we were sure these mainly applied to people on Medicaid. Finally my husband and I took out a second mortgage to pay for at least a few months of care. Shortly after we called around again, one facility notified us that a bed had "just" opened up. [a woman in her fifties]

Assistance from an advocate may expedite Medicaid admissions.

The home my father and I wanted for him kept telling us to wait. I contacted an agency to set up all the in-home services I could. The woman I spoke to felt that my father did need nursing-home care, and she called the home we wanted. A place became available for him soon after. [a forty-eight-year-old woman]

Elder advocates argue that nursing-home admission should be based on need, not ability to pay. Nursing-home owners argue that they have to make enough money to run their businesses, and that no one is served when proprietary nursing homes close due to unprofitability.

Prospective residents and their families should be aware that federal law prohibits nursing homes participating in Medicaid from seeking or accepting funds or gifts over and above Medicaid reimbursement. You should seek assistance (see Resources for this chapter) if such requests are made of you. Advocates argue that this provision applies to various common practices such as requiring, upon admission, a guarantee of funds sufficient to pay privately for a specified amount of time even if the prospective resident is Medicaid-eligible, or restricting admission to private payers.

Complex issues arise from the tension between private enterprise and public welfare, public financing, and public health oversight. Some believe that a free-market approach would result in lower costs and care of a reasonable quality. Others believe that quality care will never be achieved through a private system. In the words of Elma Holder, Executive Director of the National Citizens' Coalition for Nursing Home Reform (NCCNHR): "Care that is driven solely by the profit motive is unconscionable. A system that largely puts mammon* first, and workers and residents last, is contrary to the maintenance of quality care." NCCNHR, a group of advocates, professionals, and residents, is the leading source of information, analysis, and advocacy at the federal level. NCCNHR was founded in 1975, its goal to present a united consumer voice to the nursing-home industry and government. They were joined in their work by ombudspersons† and others (see Resources for this chapter).

This continuing debate does not solve the admission problem faced by Medicaid recipients. Some states have attempted to address the problem through specific laws. For example, Ohio nursing homes participating in Medicaid cannot have more than a fixed percentage of private-pay residents; in Minnesota, participating facilities' private rates cannot be higher than Medicaid rates. Another proposed solution is higher Medicaid reimbursement rates.

A related type of discrimination concerns evictions and transfers that occur when a resident can no longer afford to pay privately.

Discrimination also exists against "heavy-care" people, especially those on Medicaid. Because heavy care costs the facility more and is more troublesome, nursing homes sometimes narrowly interpret or limit the services they provide, or exaggerate the length of their waiting list.

The first nursing home said they couldn't handle a catheter—but we knew of a wealthy resident there who had one. The second place said they didn't take alcoholics—but my father's main problem was a stroke. His minor liver problem did result from alcohol abuse, but he hasn't had a drink in twenty years. The third home, after saying they had a long waiting list, said they'd like to "take the liberty of suggesting" that we should consider a chronic-care hospital instead of a nursing home. [a woman in her fifties]

People of color and people from various ethnic or religious backgrounds may also face discrimination. Admission may be denied outright; hostile insinuations may be made, such as "We don't feel she'd be comfortable here—the other residents are prejudiced." Subtler problems arise in the lack of attention to traditional foods and customs, such as religious services, and language barriers. Nursing homes that offer alternatives to white middle-class food, language, and activities are usually sponsored by or affiliated with ethnic or religious organizations.

My mother was much better able to cope with Western food when she could look forward to occasional Eastern meals at the nursing home's new "international nights." Her health and attitude improved and she began talking to other residents and staff about her native Korean recipes.

In November 1985, the South Cove Manor Nursing Home opened to accommodate Chinese-speaking residents in Boston. The staff observed a dramatic improvement, noting in

TRANSFER AND DISCHARGE RIGHTS

Only facilities that do not accept Medicaid can evict residents when they can no longer pay privately. A nursing home must maintain identical policies and practices regarding transfer, discharge, and the provision of services required under Medicaid for all individuals. Generally, a transfer or discharge is allowed only if:

- It is required for the resident's welfare;
- The resident's health has improved and she or he no longer needs nursing-home care;
- The health or safety of other residents is endangered;
- The resident has failed, after reasonable notice, to pay an allowable facility charge for an item or service that the resident requested.

Facilities may move a resident from a "private-pay" to a "Medicaid" bed under some circumstances, but both residents and their representatives should be given advance notice and the reason for transfer. You should seek recourse if you feel that these rights have been violated or you or a loved one has been harmed.

*A biblical reference to pursuit of riches.

†The nursing home ombudsprogram is federally mandated to investigate and resolve or refer concerns related to resident care and residents' rights. It is officially known as the nursing-home or long-term-care ombudsman program. "Ombudsman" is from a Swedish word for a government official who investigates citizens' grievances against the government. This chapter uses "ombudsprogram" and "ombudsperson."

particular a 104-year-old woman who had been erroneously diagnosed as demented because no one understood her at the old nursing home.[6]

Deinstitutionalization of people with psychiatric illnesses presents a different kind of problem. It has resulted in the transfer of many to nursing homes, where other residents may fear or snub them. The nursing-home staff often doesn't know how to deal with former psychiatric patients' special medication and communication needs. The result is a lower quality of care for all residents. Many of these individuals may fare better in noninstitutional settings; others continue to need residential psychiatric care.

Systemic problems also arise from government policies. For example, currently popular cost-containment measures encourage hospitals to discharge patients as soon as possible. Thus, people entering nursing homes or receiving home care upon a hospital discharge may need more services than if they had been kept in the hospital longer. In addition, if a person is Medicaid-eligible, the state can decide whether she needs nursing-home care and, if so, at what level. This may not be good for that person, since the state can underestimate her need for care just to save money.

Other problems relate to the fact that all nursing homes that accept Medicaid and/or Medicare are expected to meet stringent federal and state regulations, including regular inspections. Those few nursing homes that accept only private payment must meet only state regulations. The regulations—both state and federal—cover licensing, safety, cleanliness, staffing, food, programs, and medical care, among other things. Some are too vague; some are too weak. Some reinforce resident dependence. Others overemphasize details and foster compliance with the letter, not the spirit, of the law. The 1987 National Nursing Home Reform Act (see page 250 and box, page 260) strengthens regulations across states and places new emphasis on spirit or outcome (what actually happens) rather than on letter or process (what could happen based on "paper compliance").

But perfect regulations perfectly enforced are only part of the story. A nursing home that is "in compliance" may not be homey, or loving, or fun.

At one facility, I saw residents who were very active despite numerous disabilities. Staff attitudes were excellent, and the atmosphere was cheery and warm. The stairwell walls boasted a brightly colored mural which residents had helped to paint. The mural extended to, but clearly outlined, the fire exit. The administrator said the home had received a deficiency on its last survey because this unorthodox mural supposedly obscured the exit. [a nursing-home ombudsprogram volunteer][7]

DIFFICULT CONDITIONS IN NURSING HOMES

"Medicalization" is an unfortunate fact of life in nursing homes. As in hospitals—although they are called "homes"—nursing homes' medical orientation encourages a narrow approach to residents' well-being. Loneliness, confusion, depression, and behavior problems resulting from a lack of freedom and meaningful activity are addressed medically (if at all). Drugs or other restraints are too often the first choice, rather than the last resort, in dealing with what are often sane reactions to an impossible situation. The medical model requires efficiency and hierarchy. Because it cannot incorporate the chaos of individuality and assertiveness, it treats residents as patients or cases instead of as people and rewards those who conform.

LOSS OF AUTONOMY

The medical, institutional approach fosters regimentation and loss of privacy and autonomy. Most residents must share rooms, follow schedules, and accept a preplanned menu. Activities offered are often limited to the large-group, lowest-common-denominator type. Negative attitudes among staff and a lack of resources rarely allow for excitement or choice. Also, because passivity is built into the medical approach, even kind and caring staff members tend to overprotect. Too much help takes away a resident's right to risk, experience, and learn.

Three groups from the same home were asked to complete a puzzle. One group was assisted by staff members. A second group was left to itself. A third received less help than the first group, more than the second. Result: those who received the most help thought the puzzle most difficult. The less help received, the easier the puzzle seemed.[8]

Lack of control over daily life has serious consequences for residents' well-being, contributing to a vicious cycle of increasing dependence.[9] Residents themselves identified choice and control as key components of quality care in a national research project.[10]

I make my own bed. It's a small thing but it's important. I've seen those people who think they can't do anything. Sometimes their families or the staff don't take the time to encourage them or teach them. Soon they can't do anything for themselves. Any little thing you can do for yourself helps keep you going. [a seventy-year-old woman]

Sometimes, nursing homes can rise above their limitations and rescue residents from a medically dictated oblivion.

When [my mother] collapsed, her doctor advised me to find a nursing home "for her to die in."... As soon as she arrived at the nursing home, their doctor stopped all treatment: the tranquilizers, IVs, catheters. The dentist replaced her dentures.... The physical therapist had her up in a wheelchair and doing exercises, and the attendants and I started feeding her. Within two months, she was walking and talking. She lived for another four years as an active, loving, thinking, feeling individual, not the "vegetable" her doctor had predicted she would be.[11]

Abuse

A tragic problem inside and outside nursing homes is elder abuse and neglect. Within an institution, staff members are usually the guilty parties. Outside, family members are most often involved. The problem often stems from a history of abuse, including alcohol or drug abuse—for example, parents who abused their children may later find themselves victims; a nurse's aide who abuses alcohol or takes drugs may find it hard to maintain caring behavior.

In addition, both family caregivers and nursing-home staff often feel frustrated, isolated, and under stress. In a home caregiving situation, a single caregiver may be responsible twenty-four hours a day. Nursing-home staff are often underpaid, overworked, and inadequately trained and supervised. These conditions increase the likelihood of abuse.

Symptoms of abuse and neglect range from bruises, burns, other wounds, bedsores, malnutrition, and infections to social withdrawal, weight loss, and dehydration. Such symptoms can arise from disease, but none should be ignored.

Less Obvious Problems

Other common problems in nursing homes are less dramatic but no less damaging. They are difficult to detect, and prejudiced attitudes toward older people with disabilities may blind us to their seriousness. For example:

- *Overmedication,* or inappropriate medication, may be intentional, an attempt to control a resident's behavior. It may be the result of ignorance about the effects of medication on older people. Or it may occur because the nursing-home's drug-monitoring systems are inadequate. In any case, this is very dangerous.
- *Physical restraints* are a problem in some facilities. While OBRA '87 (see page 250 and box, page 260) does not require a totally restraint-free environment, it mandates that facilities minimize use of restraints. It has fostered alternatives to restraints that include treatment of underlying problems such as pain or constipation, behavioral management strategies, more appropriate activities, and emotional support. Under OBRA '87, residents have the right to: (1) be free from physical or mental abuse, corporal punishment, involuntary seclusion, or disciplinary use of restraints; and (2) be free of restraints used or psychoactive drugs administered for staff convenience rather than residents' well-being and not required by a physician's written order to treat medical symptoms.
- *Verbal indignities* can be harmful even when not extreme. A statement that doesn't sound threatening to a visitor may terrify a resident. A patronizing tone and low expectations may create or reinforce confusion, depression, and dependence.

I encouraged the residents to talk, but no one spoke. To get the discussion started, I asked one interested-looking resident to read a proclamation of independence written by another group of residents. The activities director quickly said, "Oh, she can't read." But the resident took the paper and read it to the group. [a nursing-home ombudsprogram volunteer][12]

- *Subtle, daily neglect* gradually wears residents down and may lead to withdrawal or apathy.

No one was cruel, but I just wasn't very happy. Then, after the new administrator started, little things started going right again and so did my spirit. Hot coffee, crisp toast, medication that comes at about the same time each day, and fewer clothes lost in the laundry—it made all the difference. [a woman in her eighties]

- *Financial exploitation* can take many forms. Family members, acquaintances, or nursing-home staff or administrators may steal cash, property, or other assets outright. They may pressure the older person for gifts. Or they may deprive the older person of control over her or his resources.

- *Inadequate rewards and training* affect all staff, even the most caring and competent, and reflect the low status of nursing-home residents. High turnover and unprofessional behavior are too often the result.

Another area of concern is the potential for easy spreading of infectious diseases, such as tuberculosis[13] or influenza. Some facilities don't take appropriate precautions. Others are so overcautious that residents lose access to visitors and activities both inside and outside the home in return for only a marginal improvement in safety.

NURSING-HOME PLACEMENT

This section mainly addresses long-term rather than short-term placements. However, it is worthwhile to resist the impulse to assume that a stay will be long-term and to try to keep your options open. (See Housing Alternatives and Living Arrangements chapter.)

THE DECISION

Many, if not most, nursing-home decisions are made in the midst of a crisis. But prospective residents and caregivers who prepare in advance retain more control of the process and cope better with the strong feelings evoked by such a major transition. The likelihood of a waiting list adds to the importance of advance planning. All of us, even those who are healthy, should make our wishes known to loved ones in advance. Or, as caregivers, we can sensitively approach the subject before our loved one becomes incapacitated or we become exhausted.

My brother can't seem to handle what he calls the "sin" of abandoning Ma to strangers, but he lives 600 miles away. I'm the one who has to deal with the day-to-day problems, and I've run out of patience, energy, and understanding. My health, my job, and my other relationships have all been affected. I've just about lost my sense of humor, which always got me through the roughest days. [a woman in her sixties]

Decision making should involve the prospective resident to the greatest degree possible. Even confused people can respond to caregivers' attempts to communicate lovingly the realities of a difficult situation. Avoiding the topic or misleading the prospective resident—even if intended as kindness—can have a devastating effect on morale.

How is it? Don't even ask. I was living by myself in Florida. My husband died many years ago. Four months ago my son came down to visit me and said, "Ma, I'm taking you home with me." He did take me to his home for one night, but the next day he brought me here and

QUESTIONS TO KEEP IN MIND AS YOU DETERMINE WHETHER YOU—OR A FAMILY MEMBER OR FRIEND—NEED A NURSING HOME:

What kinds of services are needed and how many are available in your community? Home health care, homemaker assistance, personal care, visiting nurses, Meals on Wheels, congregate meals, shopping and chore services, and respite care are some of the services to look for. However, it is usually difficult to find quality in-home assistance, especially for evenings, nights, and weekends. Most workers do their best, but their salaries, benefits, professional prestige, training, and supervision are often inadequate. Consider what you would do if helpers quit, arrived late, got sick, or went on vacation.

What can you afford? Will Medicare, other insurance, or Medicaid pay for the home care you need? Are there other financial-assistance programs in your community or are services available on a sliding-fee scale?

What financial or other assistance can your family, friends, and neighbors realistically provide? The answer should be fair to both caregivers and the people they're helping. An exhausted caregiver helps no one.

What is your housing situation? If you are living in a high-crime area, or if your home needs numerous or extensive repairs, or if you simply feel isolated, a move of some sort may be wise. Again, a nursing home is only one option to consider if you decide you should change your living situation. It's hard to move from a home you love; but the further in advance you can plan for it, the better you will be able to cope.

dropped me off. I've only seen him once since then. [a ninety-year-old woman]

Involvement in the decision, on the other hand, can have quite the opposite effect.

My mother was lonely and miserable, but would not even talk about moving. As her health deteriorated, my sister and I knew we had to look at facilities that would accept her. The dishonesty of a companion/aide finally shook her sufficiently, and I'm sure made her feel so helpless that she was willing to look at the places we had screened. Our preference was a small place, but she chose a larger one, hoping to have a greater selection of bridge partners! She selected her clothes and those few belongings one is allowed to take. It seemed a pathetic end. Yet this was not the end. She is now in many respects more alert and interested and in constant contact with people. [a fifty-six-year-old woman]

Remember that a nursing home is only one of many options. Sometimes it is the right choice; sometimes it isn't. The more you plan for the *possibility* of living in a nursing home, the better you will be able to control the move if you need to make it.

The Search

In many communities, you can find nursing-home directories, information on how to select a home, and information about residents' rights. Such information can come from the nursing-home ombudsprogram, a nursing-home licensing agency, the area agency on aging or other elder service organizations, advocacy groups, or your state's nursing-home association (see Resources for this chapter). If you are in the hospital, the discharge planner or continuing-care coordinator should help you. Word of mouth is another good source of information, although opinions may be colored by emotions, stereotypical attitudes toward nursing homes and residents, and conclusions drawn from an unrepresentative incident.

The following general suggestions should be helpful in a search.

- *Be organized.* Make a checklist so that you can compare and contrast facilities. Make notes about items of importance.
- *Check into the track record of facilities you're interested in.* Your licensing agency (see Resources for this chapter) conducts regular inspection surveys, the results of which are matters of public record. You should be able to call the agency with specific questions. Survey reports are supposed to be available from the agency and at your local Social Security office. Information on the home's financial status is also important. Financial troubles or negative survey reports can be precursors of a home's closing. (Homes close for other reasons too, such as an owner's desire for high profits from a condominium conversion.) For some residents, especially for those who are very frail, the stress of having to move from a facility can be fatal.
- *Set your priorities.* Do you prefer a large or small home? Where should it be located? (The choice of location should take into account both your preferences and the distance from family and friends.) What services do you need? What level of care do you need? Do you want a facility where you can move from more to less dependence or vice versa? Do you prefer an ethnically and religiously homogeneous or diverse community? You'll probably have to compromise, but first set your priorities.
- *Visit homes that meet your criteria.* There is no substitute for a personal visit. This visit will not only help you evaluate the facility, it will help you adjust to it when and if you move in. It is worth some inconvenience. If the prospective resident definitely cannot make the trip, a trusted friend or relative should be dispatched instead. (In some communities, professionals will evaluate homes for you for a fee.) The person who visits should keep the prospective resident's needs and desires in mind. If any kind of visit is impossible, a phone conversation with residents and staff might be useful.

During your visit, ask questions, participate, and talk to as many people as possible—especially residents. Look for positive staff attitudes and resident independence. You should look for evidence of family and community involvement. As one resident put it, "If you know you're having lots of company, you'll keep your house clean."

If possible, visit more than once, and at varying times of the day, week, and month.* Make one visit at a mealtime. Check the activities board. Use all your senses. Be critical, but be balanced: For example, a strong urine smell *probably* indicates a cleanliness problem and/or too little emphasis on progressive ways of manag-

*It is very useful to visit at night and on weekends, since understaffing is especially troublesome at these times.

ing incontinence. However, the odor may result from an unusual series of accidents or a temporary staff shortage, so a second visit may be warranted. Also, a slight odor may be tolerable if the facility suits you well in other ways. (Totally odor-free facilities sometimes achieve that status by discriminating against incontinent and other heavy-care people, or by emphasizing cleanliness to the exclusion of other important qualities, such as resident activity.)

The Transition

Deciding to enter and choosing a nursing home are only the beginning. To make your transition as smooth and easy as you can, you should:

- *Think about your personal belongings.* Most nursing homes allow you to bring a few possessions, and some will store a few valuables. What do you want to have with you? What would you like to give to loved ones? What can you sell? Do you want to keep anything in storage—especially in the event that your nursing-home stay is short?
- *Think ahead about adjustments you will have to make.* You will probably have to get used to one or more roommates, a large group of people in close proximity, a loss of privacy, and having a daily schedule set for you. Many residents do make good adjustments; humor, a spirit of compromise, and self-confidence help. Think about ways to retain as much autonomy as possible.

Once you're in the facility:

- *Get to know the staff and their procedures.* You as well as your family and friends will feel comfortable more quickly, retain more control, and get more satisfaction if you know who handles complaints. For example, do you tell the dietitian, the nurse, the cook, the administrator, or the residents' council if you have a problem with the food?
- *Become involved in the resident assessment and care plan.* Residents, families, and friends must be notified about and have the right to participate in this process, which must occur within fourteen days of entry and include an assessment of functional, medical, and psychological status; the resident's rehabilitation, activities, and discharge potential; and life-long and current habits, interests, strengths, and needs. A multidisciplinary team must devise a specific, personalized care plan based on this joint assessment.
- *Encourage family and friends' visits.* A companion on your first day is especially helpful.

I stayed with my mother for most of her first day. Together we got to know the home, met the staff and learned their names, found out about schedules and procedures, and visited several residents. We set up her room and had lunch together. When I had to leave, we both felt sad, but we had both expected it to be much worse. [a forty-two-year-old woman]

Visits will keep your morale high, provide you with mental stimulation, and ensure better care for you and others. Do your best to make visits pleasant. If family and friends fail to visit, don't blame yourself. Some people feel so distressed by a hospital or nursing home, anticipating physical and emotional discomfort, that they are literally unable to visit.

Family and friends who don't know how to create an enjoyable visit, especially if their loved

Nursing-Home Residents: The Experts on Quality Care

In *A Consumer Perspective on Quality Care: The Residents' Point of View,* published by the National Citizens' Coalition for Nursing Home Reform (see Resources for this chapter), nursing-home residents around the United States were asked to describe the elements of quality care. The 457 participants named choices in and control over their lives as the most important. They also recommend:

- Active, caring, informed management and staff
- Decent wages and other rewards for staff
- A wide variety of activities
- Food that is fresh, tasty, and varied to reflect cultural and individual diversity
- Explicit, workable, and sensitive channels for problem resolution
- Safety of the environment
- Maximum autonomy for residents
- Strong, enforced regulations
- Resident participation in facility and public policymaking and quality control
- Community involvement

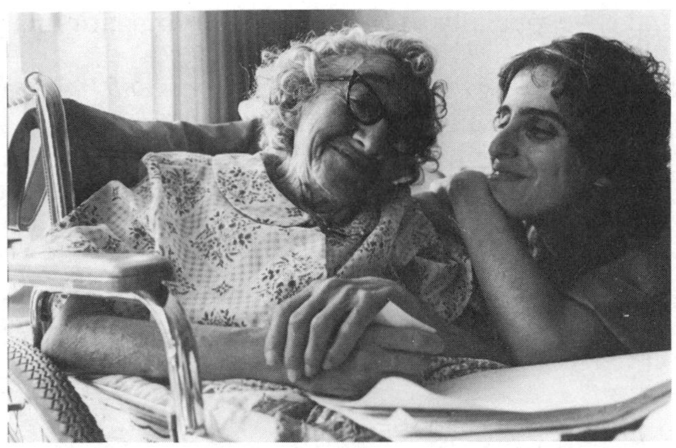

Marianne Gontarz

one finds communication difficult, should ask for help. Nursing-home staff or other experienced people may have suggestions. Many people have solved difficult communication problems in spite of overwhelming odds against them.

Mama awakened, and I put her hand on my head, our code for showing her it was I. She is completely deaf and almost blind. "Oh, dear child!" she said with a delighted smile of recognition. "It's my youngest!" I took her hand and moved it up and down in a vertical signal to "nod" yes, and gave her a big hug and kiss. Her fragile warm hands took one of my big strong cold hands and rubbed it lovingly. I thought to myself, "How lucky I am to be receiving all this caring love!" [a sixty-three-year-old woman]

If you are a family member who feels guilty about placing your loved one in a nursing home—and most do—try not to withdraw from the situation. Keep visiting as often as you can. Nursing-home staff who advise you to stay away because the resident "gets too upset" are looking for a short-term solution or trying to save themselves work. In the long run, visiting almost always pays off and makes both families and residents feel better.

Talking with others in similar situations can also help. Some nursing homes and communities sponsor family-support groups. If none exists, consider starting one. Nursing-home staff or self-help groups may be able to make specific suggestions for dealing both with your emotions and with any anger a resident may feel. Above all, remember that you are a human being too, with legitimate time, financial, and other constraints. Self-sacrifice almost always leads to resentment and that helps no one, least of all the person for whom the sacrifice is made.

FIGHTING FOR RIGHTS AND CHANGES

The key to reform of the nursing-home system is the concerted effort of residents and their allies—families, friends, community groups, and professionals. All must cooperate to improve both the present situation and the future of long-term care.

Numerous coalitions of such interested parties have developed since the early 1970s. Many of them work together through the National Citizens' Coalition for Nursing Home Reform, which can refer you to other groups in your area.

Resident involvement is an increasingly important part of reform. A major "discovery" resulting from this trend is that even frail residents are more able and willing to get involved than most people would expect. Their involvement lends legitimacy to reform movements—who knows more about nursing-home life than the people who live there? It also provides crucial opportunities for residents to exercise control and choice, and counter the negative effects of institutionalization.

We struggle against illness, and the tiredness of our age; against isolation from the larger community. . . . But I am here to tell you that we have a lot to offer and to ask you to listen to us. We need a chance to share our ideas, to speak our mind with nursing-home staff and administrators and with the government people who make the rules and make sure they're enforced. [a nursing-home resident speaking at a press conference of NCCNHR]

As a resident, you can advocate for yourself through a number of channels. Residents do not lose their civil rights, such as the right to vote, when they enter a nursing home (unless they have been declared incompetent in court). They and their families also enjoy other rights, such as the right to full disclosure concerning facility policies and medical treatment, to privacy, to access to the community, and to a maximum amount of independence. This "Bill of Rights" (see box, page 260) should be prominently posted in your facility. You can also obtain a copy from the facility or a nursing-home ombudsperson.

Residents are also protected under their state's consumer-protection laws. Information on these laws should be available from the ombudsprogram, a legal services agency, the state attorney general, or the state consumer-affairs office.

Residents' councils, sometimes formally

elected by the residents, meet regularly in an increasing number of nursing homes. They are important channels for resident involvement. Such councils range from the very effective to the purely symbolic (similar to company unions), which never do more than vote on which film to show next week. Some administrators and staff sabotage councils because they seem threatening (and indeed they can be). Others like the council idea but don't know how to help the residents get started. Still others provide support that empowers and enables residents to play a role in the facility's operation. Residents' councils should meet regularly and privately—ideally, staff and administration should attend by invitation only.

If your residents' council is inactive or ineffective, don't give up. Build from small achievements to larger ones. Choosing and planning activities help build the confidence to discuss and decide bigger issues. Group projects, such as forming an orientation committee for new residents, can provide a real but nonthreatening service while strengthening the council. A group meeting with the administrator to discuss grievances might be a good next step.

If you do have a grievance, as an individual or a group, usually it's best to go to the staff member involved. If you're uncomfortable dealing with that staff member, try her or his immediate supervisor. Be polite, fair, and sensitive, but be firm: don't apologize for wanting a decent life within the limitations of a nursing-home structure. Use your common sense in making suggestions for resolutions. Be as specific as you can in describing the problem and possible solutions. If your complaints are serious and you fear retribution, you should go immediately to the administrator or outside the facility, to families, the ombudsprogram, or the licensing and enforcement agency.

Community-wide residents' organizations are also increasing in number. There are now at least fourteen major residents' organizations nationwide, most of them coalitions of residents' councils. You can get information about them from the National Citizens' Coalition for Nursing Home Reform (see Resources for this chapter). These organizations bring together residents from many facilities and support your involvement in your own facility while giving you opportunities to examine and act on broader policy issues. They can also help you to meet residents from other facilities and become more involved in your community.

One example of such an organization is L.I.F.E. (Living Is for the Elderly), founded in 1972. It has helped thousands of Massachusetts nursing-home residents to become activists. In the words of some L.I.F.E. leaders:

The nursing-home residents band together, go to the State House, and speak before the committees. We get there any way we can, in wheelchairs and using canes. We also write letters to the governor, representatives, and senators. We fight for things we know are right. [a seventy-eight-year-old woman]

I've become educated about the legal process. You have the feeling that you are contributing to the welfare of other people. When you advocate, it helps everyone! [a seventy-year-old woman]

You are not alone—you belong to a group with people you have never met and learn to help yourself and others. [a woman in her eighties]

We are a group of people working to make our lives in nursing homes as close as possible to what life in our own homes has been. [a woman in her seventies]

One of our nurses talked roughly to a patient. I knew that there was a law that said that people can't abuse us, even by yelling. They have the laws posted on the bulletin board, but a lot of residents don't understand them. I spoke to the head nurse and she spoke to the nurse on duty. A representative from L.I.F.E. had educated me to know I could go to someone. I think the solution to abuse is education. Teach us that we do have rights and that we can go to someone if we have a problem. [a woman in her middle seventies]

Family councils and other family groups are important adjuncts to residents' groups. Family (and friend) involvement encourages residents and keeps the nursing home on its toes, greatly improving the quality of care. Some nursing homes have even gone out of their way to encourage family groups—a "we're all in this together" approach.

Like residents' councils, family councils must work toward an effective, not a symbolic, voice in the facility, and may combine forces with the residents' council toward this end. Some family councils consist of only a couple of family members; others are large. Effective ones usually meet regularly and keep in close communication with staff and administrators. Members should be aware of residents' rights and facility policies, and present their concerns and suggestions in the most organized and sensitive way they can. (To put it another way, they should be assertive but not aggressive.) Families must also recognize residents' need for independence. Sometimes family members are guilty (as staff can be) of overprotectiveness, which only encourages dependence and helplessness.

Community involvement can also be instrumental in improving the quality of life within nursing homes. For example, individuals and groups can volunteer at nursing homes, join with resident and family councils and other advocates to improve and reform nursing homes, and encourage nursing homes to make space available for community meetings and caregivers' support groups. Residents who have no family or friends benefit most from community involvement. For those of us who are not residents, vol-

The Nursing-Home Reform Act (OBRA '87)*

Nursing-home residents have the right to:

- Choose their personal physicians.
- Be given full information and participation in planning for their care and treatment.
- Have reasonable accommodation of individual needs and preferences.
- Choose social, religious, and community activities; schedules; and health care consistent with interests, abilities, and needs.
- Voice grievances about care or treatment without fear of discrimination or reprisal, and to receive a prompt response.
- Organize and participate in resident groups in the facility. (Families have the right to organize family groups).
- Have privacy and confidentiality in treatment, accommodations, personal visits, written and telephone communications, meetings, and records.
- Be free from abuse and unnecessary restraints (see page 254).

Nursing homes must:

- Provide residents with facility inspection results and correction plans.
- Notify residents and their families or responsible parties in advance of plans to change their rooms or roommate.
- Inform residents of their rights at admission and, upon request, provide a written copy of those rights.
- Inform residents in writing of services covered by private-pay rates and by Medicaid, and of extra charges for extra services.
- Display and provide clear information about how to apply for and use Medicaid benefits, including, if applicable, how to receive a refund from Medicaid for previous private payments.
- Permit immediate visits by a resident's personal physician, representatives from the health department and ombudsprogram, and relatives (with resident's consent).
- Permit visits "subject to reasonable restriction" for others, including organizations or individuals providing health, social, legal, or other services, subject to a resident's consent.

Other Provisions

Staffing:

- Nurse aides must receive seventy-five hours of training in specified areas, pass an exam, and register with the state. Nursing homes must consult this registry to check potential employees' training, competency, and history concerning resident neglect or abuse or misappropriation of resident property.
- Facilities must usually provide licensed nursing coverage twenty-four hours a day, and a registered nurse eight consecutive hours every day.

Individuals with mental illness or developmental disabilities must be screened to determine appropriate placement. They are eligible for nursing-home placement as long as their primary need is for nursing-home care.

Resident assessments: see page 257.

*Adapted from "Fact Sheet on Nursing Homes," prepared by the National Citizens' Coalition on Nursing Home Reform for the American Association of Retired Persons (see Resources for this chapter).

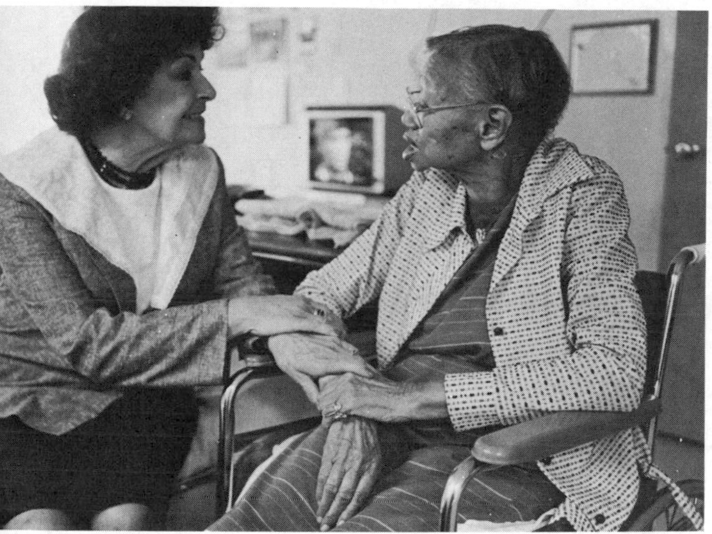

Marianne Gontarz

unteering or just visiting is the ideal way to learn about and confront our feelings about nursing homes.

Why do I devote time to this residents' group? That's simple. I want something like it around if I ever become a nursing-home resident. [a fifty-year-old community volunteer]

The nursing-home ombudsprogram investigates, resolves, or refers concerns related to resident care and residents' rights. The program exists in all states. Some states have only a small ombudsprogram staff, while others offer a large network of local staff and volunteers. Although the program has been criticized for being relatively powerless and overly bureaucratic, ombudspersons around the country have helped residents and families to organize and strengthen councils, intervened with staff and administrators when residents or others felt hesitant to complain, and helped to decertify administrators who have flagrantly violated the law. Ombudsprograms also educate residents and others about residents' rights and other long-term-care issues.

Legal Aid can be a nursing-home resident's best friend. Despite funding cutbacks, you can still find in most communities attorneys providing free nonroutine services to older people who meet low-income guidelines. If you can't find a listing for "legal services" or "legal aid" in your phone book, check with your local agency on aging or with your nursing-home ombudsperson. Legal Aid lawyers have helped countless income-qualifying residents assert their rights; protect their personal funds from unscrupulous families, staff, administrators, and owners; and improve care. In addition, they have helped research and draft legislation beneficial to nursing-home residents.

Nursing homes are part of our lives. The more we learn about them, the better we will understand them. Openness to new possibilities and a positive attitude will help residents, prospective residents, families, and friends face problems and influence the system, and will provide residents with opportunities for choice, control, and more meaningful lives.

In the words of five hundred residents attending a L.I.F.E. conference in Massachusetts, "We have the power to make the changes!"

NOTES

1. Mickey Spencer, "Nursing Homes," *Broomstick: A Bimonthly National Magazine By, For, and About Women Over Forty,* Vol. 8, No. 4 (July–August 1986). (See p. 446 for address.)
2. *Aging America: Trends and Projections.* U.S. Department of Health and Human Services (FCOA) 91-28001. Washington, D.C.: U.S. Government Printing Office, 1991, p. 162.
3. Ibid., p. 163.
4. Medicaid-eligible individuals must be officially screened to establish the level of nursing-home care they need—if any—in some states.
5. The amount of the personal-needs allowance is set by each state, but by federal regulation it must be at least $25.
6. Doris Sue Wong, "Nursing Home Ends a Language Barrier." *The Boston Globe,* Jan. 27, 1986, p. 21.
7. Personal communication, staff member, L.I.F.E. (See Resources for this chapter.)
8. From *Investigative Newsletter Institutions/Alternatives,* Vol. 7, No. 9 (September 1984), p. 12.
9. This point is documented in various articles and books, notably Ellen Langer, *Psychology of Control.* Beverly Hills, CA: Sage Publications, 1983.
10. *A Consumer Perspective on Quality Care: The Residents' Point of View.* National Citizens' Coalition for Nursing Home Reform (NCCNHR), a study of quality care with 457 resident participants.
11. Spencer, op. cit.
12. Personal communication, staff member, L.I.F.E. (See Resources for this chapter.)
13. W. W. Stead, et al., "Tuberculosis as an Endemic and Nosocomial Infection Among the Elderly in Nursing Homes." *The New England Journal of Medicine,* Vol. 312, No. 23 (June 6, 1985), pp. 1483–87.

18

JOINT AND MUSCLE PAIN, ARTHRITIS, AND RHEUMATIC DISORDERS

✦

BY ROBIN H. COHEN

MATERIAL ON TMJ BY MARTHA WOOD AND RENÉE GLASS

SPECIAL THANKS TO JEANNE L. MELVIN

1994 UPDATE BY ROBIN H. COHEN; TMJ BY RENÉE GLASS

RESOURCES FOR THIS CHAPTER ON PAGES 489–90

My left leg hurt all the time, down the outside, across the foot, behind the knee. My hip joint ached mightily. I thought, "What do you expect, over sixty?" But it turned out a nerve in my spine was being pressed—and there were things I could do to hurt less. [a woman in her sixties]

I noticed in exercise class that I had pain when performing certain motions with my arms—my shoulders would not let me do things I had always done before. I wish I had paid attention to the slight signs earlier. Now I've lost quite a lot of shoulder motion. [a sixty-one-year-old woman]

As we grow older, we may experience aches in our joints and muscles. We may fear pain and immobility as a result of these conditions. It is important that neither we nor our health-care providers dismiss pains and aches as inevitable signs of age. We should not assume discomfort is normal and so neglect preventable and correctable conditions.

As we age, our spines may change shape in response to stresses placed on them. Bony growths, called spurs, may limit joint motion. The soft tissues that stabilize the joints can become inflamed by overuse or strain. Arthritis can attack our joints. Muscles may weaken or become tight with disuse, tension, and postural habits, making it hard, for example, to look back when we drive or to hook a bra. What hurts and what shows up on X rays don't always go together. As we understand the environmental and life-style factors that affect our joints, we can find ways to stay limber and comfortable.

A joint is formed where two bones meet. It is surrounded by a capsule of soft tissue lined with a synovial membrane that produces a rich fluid. This fluid lubricates the cartilage-covered bone ends as they move against each other. The cartilage absorbs shocks, protects the ends of the bones, and receives nourishment only through exercise. Ligaments, which attach bone to bone, and tendons, which attach muscle to bone, keep bones stable while permitting them to move. Bursae, small, pillowlike sacs lined with synovial membrane, cushion the movement of muscle over bone, or of one muscle over another.

Inflammation is an indication that the body is attempting to heal and repair injured tissue. Injury can result from many causes, including a blow, strain, overuse, or reactions to foreign substances or anything the body interprets as foreign. The symptoms of inflammation can be local pain, heat, redness, swelling, or general discomfort, including headaches and weakness.

Pain may arise from:

- *Overuse*—stressing joints or soft tissues by repetitive motions, such as hammering
- *Underuse*—not moving enough, resulting in stiffness and limiting mobility of the joint
- *Incorrect use*—habitually moving in ways inappropriate for the way the body is made, such as holding the phone to one ear with a raised shoulder
- *Reactions to stress*—muscle spasm and pain created by habitual tension in the muscles
- *The pain-spasm-pain cycle*—the cycle of pain causing further tightening or spasms in other muscles, creating still more pain
- *Inflammation*—in the joints (arthritis), tendons (tenosynovitis or tendonitis), bursae (bursitis), muscles, or blood vessels
- *Changes in bone shape*—changes that can cause bones to press on nerves, causing other pains

Prevention of Joint Pain

To prevent joint problems and to prevent reinjury or disability from them, you can:

1. Keep muscles strong with exercise and flexible with gentle stretching.
2. Reduce muscle tension. Regularly use relaxation techniques, such as systematically tensing and relaxing groups of muscles from head to toe, meditating, and getting massages.
3. Deal with difficulties in movement as soon as you notice them. Be alert to any difficulty you may have in performing daily activities, to pain where you never had it before, and to changes in the ease and range of your motion. For example, if you have trouble climbing stairs, your knees, hips, or front thigh muscles (quadriceps) may need attention.
4. Try to manage your weight. Being very heavy stresses the joints.
5. Use good body mechanics. This means using the body in ways that minimize joint stress. Use the largest and strongest joint for any given task—for example, push with your hips or thighs instead of with your hands.
6. Wear comfortable shoes. Foot problems can affect the whole body. Wobbling on high or thin heels creates strain on the knees, hips, and back as these joints try to stabilize the body when the feet can't do the job.

Home Care for Sprains, Mild Injuries and Inflammation, and Joint and Muscle Pain

Pain in joints and soft tissues often responds to home care and will heal in two to six weeks given rest, hot or cold compresses, and time. Rest gives the body a chance to make repairs and helps reduce inflammation, but too much bed rest for back pain caused by muscle or ligament strain may result in loss of muscle strength.[1] You may want to immobilize the joint with a sling, splint, or corset. Once or twice a day, move resting joints through their normal range of motion, because inflammation can make tissues stick together and become hard and tight ("frozen"). Heat relaxes muscles, while cold reduces

When to Use Heat and When to Use Ice

If there is swelling and warmth from inflammation in the joint or muscle, ice packs or ice massage (passing ice over the painful area, without pressure, for twenty minutes) is generally more beneficial for reducing swelling, inflammation, and pain.

When the main problem is stiffness and there is no swelling, moist heat—such as a shower or bath, wet compresses, or a wet washcloth placed between the skin and a plastic-covered heating pad—is more effective than dry heat. Guard against scalding or burning.

When an area is sore and painful and an application of heat does not bring relief, it is likely that an ice pack will.

For trauma to a joint, such as twisting an ankle or a knee, the best treatment is ice to decrease swelling and bruising.

If you "pull" your back muscles while exercising, the pain felt afterward is usually caused by a spasm in the muscle. It may be more comforting to apply heat at first. However, if you do not get good relief with heat, ice packs or ice massage can often be beneficial.

The treatment that gives the greatest relief is best for you.

swelling and inflammation, and can ease muscles in spasm.

SIGNS OF FURTHER PROBLEMS

The following symptoms require more complete investigation.[2] **Contact your health-care practitioner if:**

- your temperature is over 100° F
- you feel numbness or tingling
- the pain runs down your leg to your foot or down your arm to your finger
- the pain persists or is very bad
- you can't use the joint
- you have severe pain and swelling in one or more joints
- you have trouble in the same joint on both sides
- you have stiffness that lasts more than one hour after waking up
- you feel weak, fatigued, or generally unwell
- you have lumps under the skin, particularly near the elbow

MANAGING LONG-TERM PAIN

I've really learned to listen to my body. All my life I wasn't listening. My mind was too ambitious. But now, if I don't feel good one day and can't do anything, I say the hell with it and wait. If you say, "I'll do it tomorrow," somehow tomorrow comes. [a seventy-five-year-old woman]

Living with pain is physically and emotionally stressful. Work with a physical therapist may be essential to reduce pain but you may also have to use drugs before you can try the following important self-help program.

Exercise

When in pain we tend to tighten muscles and move less (the pain-spasm-pain cycle), so even a few gently performed small movements can have an astonishing effect and lead to larger pain-free movements. Even those confined to a wheelchair or bed will find exercise helpful. Mobility and strength do not develop in a straight line; remember that you will have bad days as well as good days.

Every morning and before I go to bed I do bicycling on my back, knee-chest stretches, leg lifts, and turn my head. When I rest I practice breathing from my diaphragm instead of my chest. I work on posture and thigh muscles by bending my knees and sliding my back up and down against the wall. [a seventy-five-year-old woman]

Listen to your body. Exercise gently and slowly, with relaxation between repetitions, only as much as is comfortable, up to but not beyond the point of pain. Increase exercise very slowly. One or two rest days a week may help. You may even need to begin exercising in the supportive environment of warmed water.

When my body seemed stiff beyond repair because of the pain-spasm-pain cycle, I used water to support me as I turned my head from side to side or slowly walked back and forth in the pool. Small changes gradually led to larger ones. Now I swim a half-mile. [a sixty-one-year-old woman]

I won a victory over arthritis in my fifties. I was acting in a mime troupe and walking got so painful I was crying as I was walking with the pain in my hip. A surgeon suggested surgery, but I refused. I started using a whirlpool and doing exercises in a swimming pool for a year, three times a day. I was so successful that at fifty-eight I learned to ski. [a fifty-nine-year-old woman]

I'm always stiff when I get up in the morning. Then I stand in a hot shower, and I'm okay for the rest of the day. [an eighty-five-year-old woman]

I don't like to use dishwashers. I like to do dishes by hand in hot water. The water feels so friendly to my hands. [a seventy-eight-year-old woman]

The YWCA, YMCA, or the local chapter of the Arthritis Foundation in your area may offer exercise classes in water for people with joint problems.

The Feldenkrais method and Alexander technique (see Moving for Health chapter) realign our bodies and show people how to move with less effort. Yoga has helped many people with arthritis. Like any other exercise, yoga must be modified to suit you.

I came to yoga in my fifties when my mother was dying. I couldn't sleep because I would see her dying face. All my pains got worse. When I read a book on yoga, I could feel that my body was full of tension. I got a record, took a course, and grew limber. When I saw my osteopath, he was astounded at how flexible I had become.

But my yoga teacher insisted that I could do a shoulder stand, which I knew was not right for me. Against my better judgment I tried it and injured my neck. I had to wear a collar until it healed. [a seventy-five-year-old woman]

Rest and Energy Conservation

Pain is exhausting, and feels worse when you are tired. You need to find the right balance between exercise and rest, and to avoid tiring yourself by learning to conserve energy.

Plan rest times into your day. Plan work spaces so you do not waste steps. Sit to work instead of standing, use gadgets that avoid straining your joints, and plan restful tasks between more energetic ones. Your body will tell you when you've done too much.

I thought I had done everything right in planning a small party. I bought most things, made others on three different days. The day of the party I felt good and ran around a lot instead of resting. The next morning I could not get out of bed. Everything hurt. It took a week to get over it. [a sixty-one-year-old woman]

Only by trial and error can you discover the balance between rest and activity best for you.

I told my physician I had tickets for a show, but I was in such pain how could I go? He asked, "If you stay at home, will the pain go away? So why not go?" And that did a lot for me. I went. I had to stand against the wall from time to time, but I went, and I kept going. Once, when I felt like giving up, the same doctor said, "If you don't keep active, you'll end your days in a wheelchair." That shook me. I put a fancy scarf around my neck collar and I went out. [a seventy-five-year-old woman]

Dealing with Stress

Emotional or physical stress seems to increase pain, perhaps by suppressing endorphins, the body's natural painkillers. Try to limit the effects of stress you cannot avoid. Exercise, relaxation techniques, and daily meditation are all useful methods for increasing endorphins.[3]

Sex

Sex can help to reduce pain. For helpful suggestions on sex when you or your partner has pain or limited mobility, see Sexuality in the Second Half of Life chapter.

Self-Help Groups

Self-help groups make it possible to exchange ideas for managing back and joint pains and rheumatic disorders, to share experiences, and to give and get support. The nearest chapter of your state's Arthritis Foundation, a local hospital, YWCA, or YMCA may know of a group—or you can start one yourself. Managing these disorders requires a lot of support. An important resource in coping with pain is the ability to *ask for help*.

My husband said to me, "Don't be a baby." I was terribly hurt. I was hysterical. He doesn't know how much pain I'm in. But my group knows. [a woman in her sixties]

Exploring What Is Available in Your Community

Physical therapy, occupational therapy, massage, acupuncture, meditation and other relaxation techniques, visualization (making mental images of the way you want to be), and hypnosis have helped many people. Myotherapy (pressing on spots in the body that send pain to other parts) may relieve muscle spasms.[4] Acupressure, a form of massage that includes pressure on acupuncture points, has been a help to many.

During an acupressure massage, the masseuse found a very sore spot on my back. When she pressed it for a while, some of the pain on my right side went away. Now, if my right side pains me when I am walking, I just reach around and press the sore spot and the pain goes away. That's a wonderful trick to know. [a sixty-five-year-old woman]

Drugs

Drugs are often prescribed to break the pain-spasm-pain cycle and to reduce inflammation. Aspirin is useful because it relieves both pain and inflammation. Diazepam (Valium), however, is potentially addictive and is frequently misused and overused. See page 275 for a summary of antiinflammatory and other drugs.

COMMON JOINT PROBLEMS

FOOT PROBLEMS

It is important to take special care of our feet, since the entire body depends on them for mobility and stability. Much foot discomfort comes from the restrictive styles of women's shoes, which are rarely designed for comfort and health. High heels force our weight onto the metatarsal joints in the ball of the foot, distort our walking gait and posture, and strain other joints, including the back and neck. Pointed-toe shoes can push the big toe out of its normal position and place pressure on the joint, causing bunions. Instead of being a modern version of Chinese footbinding, women's shoes should provide the same level of comfort as good men's shoes. Try them sometime. You'll be amazed at the toe room.

A comfortable shoe should outline the shape of the foot—broad in front with rounded toes, heel wide enough to distribute weight, and with room enough for the top of the foot.[5] It should have plenty of room for the toes to wiggle and thick crepe or soft rubber soles and heels. Sandals and properly shaped shoes give the foot room to spread.

I have found a style of flat sandals with built-in supports that keeps me pain-free. I wear them all the time. On the rare occasions, such as a wedding, when I feel I must wear another style of shoe, I change my shoes in the ladies' room so I wear the less comfortable shoes for the shortest time. [a fifty-four-year-old woman]

Check the bottoms of your shoes. If they are worn down unevenly, that can be an early sign of a problem. Repair your shoes frequently, because walking around in unevenly worn shoes can produce strain on your knees and back. If you have pain on top of your feet where laces tie, choose shoes with more than two shoelace holes on each side and loosen the laces over the painful area.

As we grow older, our toenails may be harder to cut. They may become horny, we may have difficulty reaching them, or our hands may not have sufficient strength to work the clippers. Try large clippers with long handles and a spring. Cut nails straight across a little at a time. Ask for help. You might want to exchange pedicures and foot rubs with a friend.

If you need molded shoe inserts (orthotics) but have flexible feet (feet with very loose joints), be sure the orthotics are molded without your weight on them but with your foot supported in the correct position.[6] People with flexible feet are often more comfortable in shoes with very flexible soles.

Flat feet may cause more pain as you get older. Exercise and well-fitting shoes, perhaps with arch supports, will make your feet and legs more comfortable.

If your second toe is longer than your big toe, you have a Venus de Milo foot. This sounds nice, but it may contribute to back pain because the long toe changes the way the foot rolls when walking. Padding under the ball of the foot may help.

Bunions (swelling, tenderness, and redness of the big toe joint) do not usually cause pain if we wear comfortable shoes. A tendency to have them may be inherited, but the shoes we wear may also be at fault. If you see a bunion coming, visit a podiatrist or a physical therapist who specializes in foot problems. An orthotic or new shoes can reduce the stress that produces the bunion.

Morton's neuralgia, a condition in which a tender nerve at the base of the third and fourth toes causes tingling and numbness in the middle toes and pain in the ball of the foot, is common among middle-aged women. It can often be relieved by changing to shoes with wide toe room, support for the metatarsal arch, and low heels.

If your foot joints are affected by rheumatoid arthritis, ask your health-care provider to monitor the circulation in your feet.

BACK PROBLEMS

Almost everyone has a back problem at one time or another. Most back pain comes from muscle or ligament strain, muscle spasm, sacroiliac joint strain, disc problems, excessive curvature of the spine (kyphosis), or arthritis. Once injured, the back can take several weeks or months to heal.

The backbone, or spine, supports us and lets us twist, bend, and turn. It consists of bones (vertebrae) alternating with flexible units (discs) containing a soft center. The nerves of the spinal cord, which connects brain and body, pass through openings in the vertebrae. When viewed from the back, the spine should appear to divide the body in two equal parts. When viewed from the side, the spine has a characteristic S-curve that helps absorb shocks.

Avoiding Back and Neck Problems

Observe the basic rule: Don't do anything that causes pain. If something causes pain, stop doing it, and follow the suggestions for home care beginning on page 263.

The suggestions above for preventing and managing pain apply especially to the two most common causes of back pain—back muscle sprains and sacroiliac joint inflammation. The following suggestions may prevent problems, ease the pain you have, and save you from rein-

VERTEBRAE OF THE SPINE

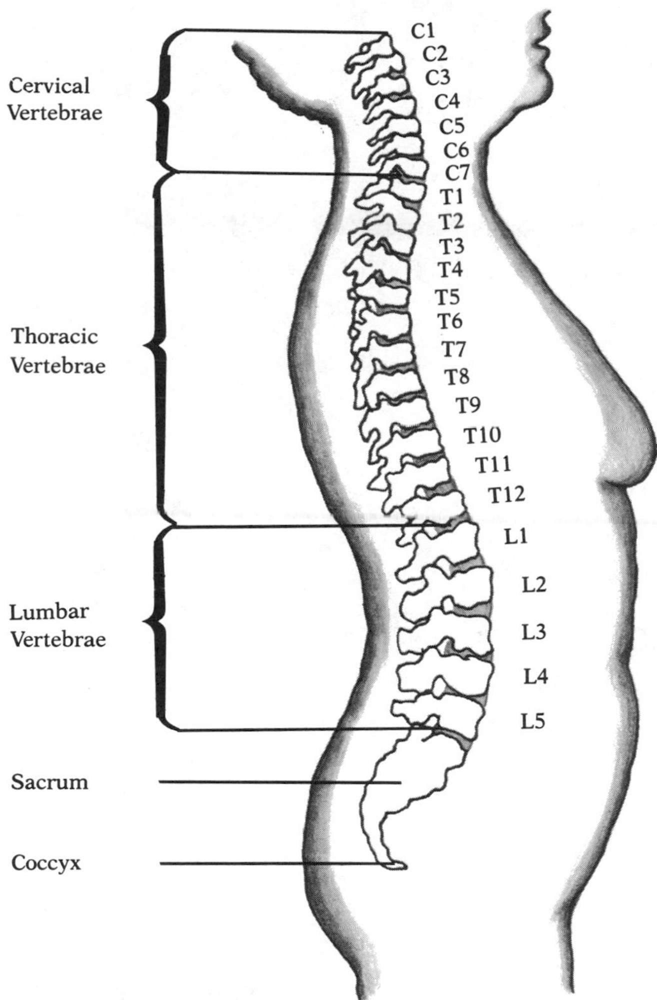

juring or aggravating a bad back or neck.* Suggestions marked with a bullet (•) are particularly useful for disc problems.

1. Strengthen your abdominal and back muscles. (See page 76.) Excessive back sway from weak muscles, a slack or protruding abdomen, and poor posture place severe stress on the muscles and joints of the lower back and can cause pain.

•2. When you sit or stand, try keeping your feet at different levels. Rest one foot on a stool, a book, a bar, or on the floor of the cabinet underneath the sink when washing dishes.

*Some Ys, health centers, HMOs, and hospitals conduct back classes where they teach body mechanics, flexibility exercises, and pain management. They may also include group self-help discussions.

3. If your mattress sags, put a ¾-inch plywood board under it. The best mattress is soft on the top so it contours and supports weight evenly but firm enough so it doesn't sag. However, you need to sleep well, and what is comfortably firm to one person may be a bed of nails to another.

•4. Don't sleep on your stomach. Sleeping on your stomach is especially bad for neck problems. If you can't sleep any other way, place a pillow under your waist to prevent the swayback position. If you sleep on your side, place pillows in front of you to support your top shoulder and top knee.

5. If your days are sedentary, get up often and walk around or lie down. While sitting, periodically round and straighten your back or, holding your elbows in opposite hands, twist gently to the right and left.[7] During car travel, stop and walk around every hour. Move around in a train and airplane as much as possible and exercise in your seat. Two examples of exercises to be done slowly and gently are stretching alternate arms upwards and lifting one knee at a time toward opposite elbows.

•6. Some positions put more pressure on lower-back discs than others. Sitting exerts more pressure than standing, and both more than lying down. When you have to lift an object, don't twist. Lifting and twisting puts four hundred times more pressure on your lumbar spine than lying down.[8] Bending over and lifting can also harm your back. Don't bend at the waist, but instead bend your knees, keep your back straight while lifting, and hold the weight close. If you can't bend your knees that far or need help to get up, support your back by leaning a hand on a nearby solid object, or by resting a forearm on your own thigh. If you need to move furniture with someone, you should be the one in front with your hands behind your back.

7. Change a baby on furniture of comfortable height. Do not bend over. Carry an infant with her back resting on your forearm, and her head cradled in your hand. Don't lift children. Let an older child climb on your lap. Some of us can kneel or sit to let an older child climb on our backs to be carried.

8. Carry all objects close to your body *above* waist level. Use a backpack. If carrying shopping bags, divide the load in two so you are balanced. Lighten the load whenever possible.

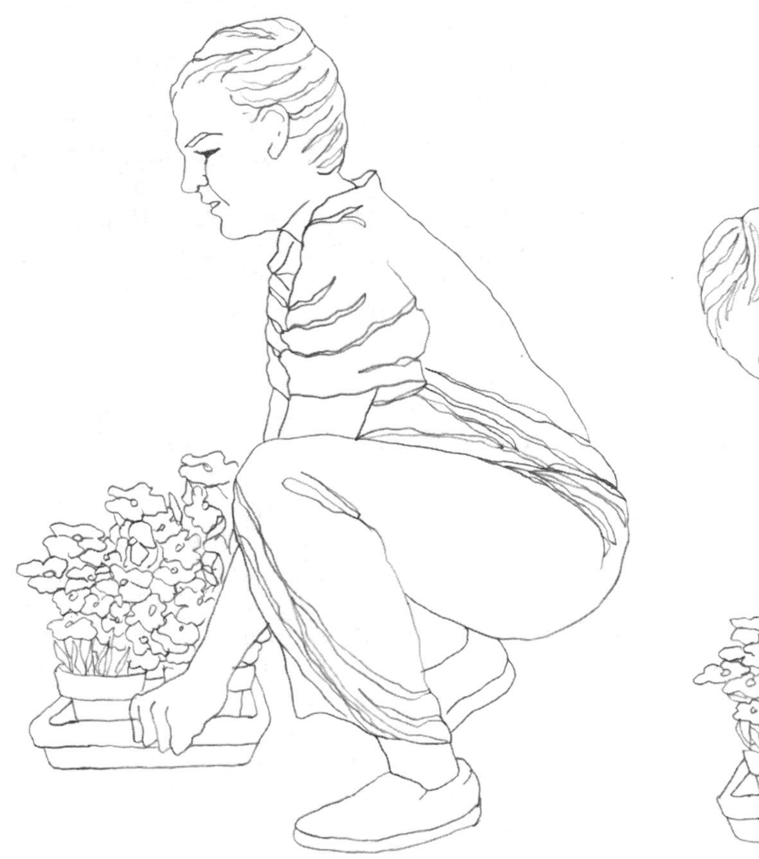
DO THIS

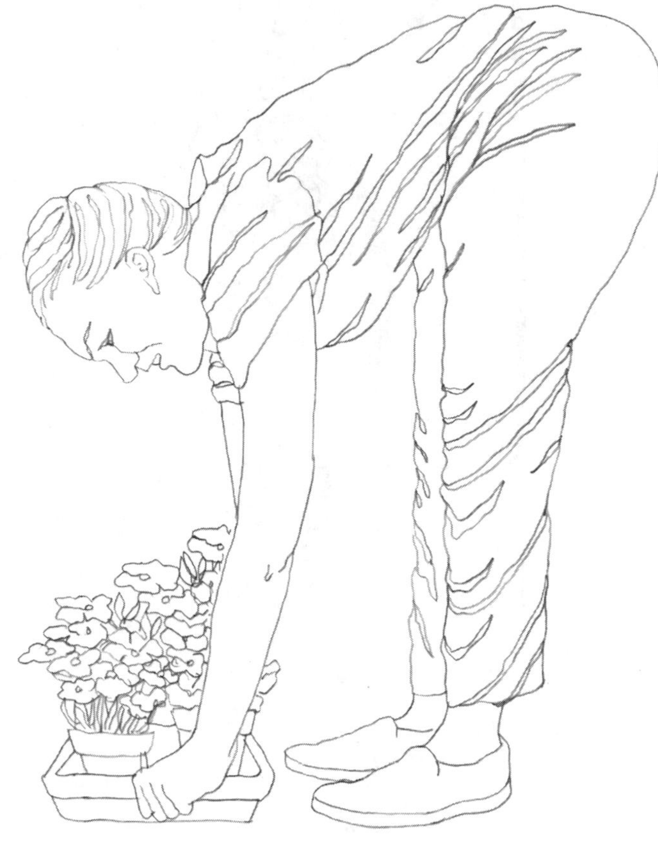
NOT THIS

- •9. Don't reach for or lift an object over your head; stand on a stool so that you can keep your elbows bent.
- 10. Since most chairs do not provide support for the lower back, supply it yourself by folding a towel or sweater 6 to 8 inches wide and about 1½ inches thick in the middle. Put it in the hollow of your back. You can do this at the movies or while riding in a car.
- 11. At work and at home, try to use chairs that are adjustable in height, so your feet can be flat on the floor with your knees bent at 90 degrees. Your chair should have an adjustable backrest placed where the back curves most inward. It should be upholstered in a nonslip material and be soft at the edge of the seat so that circulation in the thighs is not cut off. It should have arms whenever possible.
- •12. Get up from a chair by sliding to the edge so that your weight is directly above your feet. Do not spread the knees wide apart. Don't lean forward, for this increases the pressure on your discs. Use the chair arms to help you, or push with your hands on your thighs to support your back as you straighten up.
- 13. Share helpful hints with others. You may find it easier to lie on your back in bed to put on shoes and socks. If pulling up the emergency brake in a car hurts, it may help to press against the dashboard with the other hand when you do it.[9]
- 14. If your back hurts, relax in the position that is most comfortable for you.

For me the most comfortable position is lying on my back, legs loosely together and raised at right angles at the hips and knees, with my calves and feet on a hassock or chair seat. Sometimes I even put the hassock in bed with me. [a fifty-five-year-old woman]

For most people, specific exercises are essential to help prevent back pain. Exercises that strengthen your back muscles, abdominals, and front thigh muscles (quadriceps) will help protect your spinal discs. Abdominal muscles provide the sole support for the lower lumbar vertebrae and help hold us erect. Women of middle age characteristically have weak abdominals. If your quadriceps are strong, you have less tendency to rely on back muscles to lift you up. If you have repeated bouts of back pain, go to a physical therapist who specializes in back problems for an individualized exercise program.

While exercise is important, choose sports with care. Warm up and gently stretch your back muscles before doing sports or heavy labor. Some sports are harder on your back than others. Walking and swimming are good, but you may need to select and modify your strokes. The breast and back stroke, for example, arch the back and may cause pain.

DISORDERS OF THE SPINE (Front View)

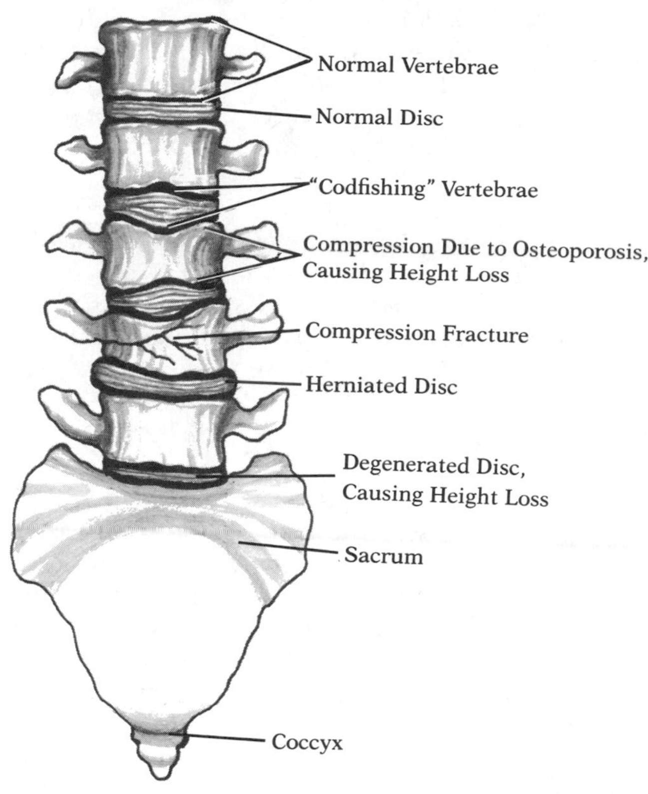

Some Special Back Problems

Only 5 percent of back problems require surgery. A magnetic resonance imaging (MRI) or a CAT (computerized axial tomography) scan may be used for diagnosis. Before MRIs were developed, most doctors performed a myelogram, in which a flow of dye is injected into the space surrounding the spinal cord so that anything that blocks the flow will show up on an X ray.

New techniques have reduced the discomfort of myelograms but 10 percent of those who have one will still suffer severe headaches and backaches; the discomforts are lessened when water-soluble dyes are used. Although the development of MRIs has cut the use of myelograms, for certain problems, as in the neck, a myelogram may reveal more than an MRI. People who wear pacemakers or other metal in their bodies cannot have an MRI.[10]

A **herniated disc** occurs when the soft center inside the disc is forced through the outer casing. This may cause pain when it presses on a nerve. Most likely to herniate are the two lower lumbar discs, which can press on the sciatic nerve. When this happens, the lower back may hurt, followed by pain running down the back or side of the thigh, the outside of the calf, and possibly into the toes. You are most likely to have a herniated disc when you are between thirty and sixty. As we age, our discs dry out, becoming thinner, harder, and less likely to herniate. A sudden severe pain in an older woman is more likely to be a fracture from osteoporosis than a disc problem. The majority of people with disc problems do not require surgery but respond partly or completely to conservative, nonsurgical treatment. The most common treatment used to be bed rest, which is so debilitating for older people that many doctors no longer recommend it.

At one time, chymopapain (the enzyme from papaya used in meat tenderizers) was injected into the herniated disc. Chymopapain is now rarely used in the United States, since it was not effective. It is still in use in other places, so note that the injection is given only in hospitals under anesthesia, and involves risks equal to those of surgery. The doctor should first determine whether you are allergic to the injected material.[11] As with any surgery, always get a second opinion before undergoing the procedure.

Vertebrae tend to develop rims of extra bone, called *spurs,* around their edges and on the projections at their rear. While spurs and/or narrowed spaces between vertebrae may combine to press on a nerve, not everyone who has rims and spurs experiences back pain. Stretching exercises, relaxation techniques, and traction may relieve discomfort.

Spinal stenosis is the name for a narrowing of either the spinal canal or the openings for nerve roots in the vertebrae. Appearing mainly in people over fifty, it is now diagnosed more often than before as a source of pain, numbness, and weakness in the legs because it can be seen with the CAT scan. The pain usually increases gradually over time. Treatment may involve appropriate exercise, antiinflammatory drugs, a corset or brace, steroid injections, and, as a last resort, surgery.

I saw many doctors for my pain. I liked a woman neurologist best because she talked with me for forty-five minutes. I had a CAT scan. It was spinal stenosis. The neurologist said that 80 percent of the people operated on for this problem felt better, but before surgery I would have to have a myelogram. I didn't want to have one. She said there was no hurry to decide. [a woman in her sixties]

Scoliosis is a condition in which the spine curves to one side. Mild scoliosis is common in adolescent women and, as we age, can contribute to tight muscles or limited motion and strain on the back. If you have scoliosis, ask your health-care practitioner about the role it may play in your back pain. Be sure to monitor the degree of curvature, especially after pregnancy, for any change. Chiropractic techniques cannot correct this condition. Deep breathing and exercise can be helpful in counteracting the strain created by scoliosis.

Getting Help with Back Problems

What kind of specialist is most likely to help with back pain? An informal survey of former back patients indicates that they were most satisfied with sports medicine practitioners and physiatrists (physicians specializing in movement). They also had kind words for rheumatologists. The former back patients received temporary relief from osteopaths (physicians who may prescribe medications) and chiropractors (who cannot prescribe medications), both of whom manipulate the spine; but manipulation is not advisable for herniated discs or sciatica. They found yoga teachers who understand back problems helpful. Physical therapists helped with massage and taught useful exercises, and occupational therapists showed how to perform daily tasks comfortably. The study indicates that the greatest long-term help came from life-style changes. A practitioner who, regardless of specialty, understands the interaction of bones and soft tissues in movement and encourages changes in daily habits gives the most help.[12]

OTHER COMMON JOINT PROBLEMS

Knees

Many knee problems really originate in the foot. People who walk are less likely to develop knee problems than joggers or runners. Serious overweight stresses the knees. Keeping your quadricep muscles strong stabilizes the knee. Arthritis and bursitis are also common causes of knee pain.

Meniscus cartilage cushions the bones of the knee joint. Two thirds of the people in whom this cartilage is removed develop arthritis and pain five to twenty years later. Make every effort to retain the cartilage if possible.[13]

Hips

Finding the exact source of pain in the hip is often difficult because the joint is located deep in

STEPPING OUT WITH A CANE

We hurt, we're stiff, we want to get around more in spite of the difficulties—but use a cane? Never! Everyone will think we're old!

But a cane can really help. Problems that severely limit our mobility can often be eased by the proper use of a cane. Like fans, which are so helpful for the hot flashes of menopause, canes used to be more fashionable than they are now. Let's make them so again. We can decorate them to match our outfits or save up for an elegant one with fancy carving. We can use a cane to get a seat on the bus, or stamp the floor with it when we want to emphasize a point. A cane can say "Don't mess with me" if we choose.

Usually, hold a cane in the hand opposite the sore leg. Your elbow will be at a 120-degree angle if the cane is the right height for you. Step out with the cane and the sore leg at the same time. The cane lessens pressure on the sore leg, resting it and giving it time to heal.

Be sure to have the height and your use of a cane (or crutches) checked by an experienced physical therapist or nurse. You can cause damage by incorrect use.

the body. The pain may come not from the hip but from arthritis of the spine. Pain caused by arthritis of the hip is usually felt in the groin, and may radiate to the area above the knee. Pain felt on the outside of the hips (at the widest part) is usually caused by bursitis and is often most painful when we are climbing steps or rising to a standing position.

Shoulders

Pain in a shoulder most often comes from bursitis or tendonitis and is usually the result of repeated motions such as overhead work, throwing, or racquet sports. A progressive loss of motion with some stiffness and pain may be so gradual that we don't notice it until it has become quite serious. "Frozen shoulder" occurs often in women over fifty. If not cared for, this condition can become permanent. Rest, hot packs, ice massage, and ultrasound treatments from a physical therapist can prepare the way for passive exercise (someone moves your arm for you) and regular exercise.[14]

Neck

When you sleep, your neck should be supported so that it is in a straight line with your spine. If you awaken with neck pain, the position you slept in may be the cause. For sleeping, fold a hand towel lengthwise to a width of four inches, wrap it around your neck, and pin it with a safety pin.[15] Or try a cervical pillow shaped to fit under and support the neck. Neck pain may also come from vertebrae or disc problems in the spine.

Jaw

I suddenly awoke about 4 a.m. with a severe earache. Aspirin kept the pain down, but it hurt to chew. A few days later it became painful to talk or even swallow. A friend who is a dental hygienist had told me about TMJ but I hadn't really paid much attention at the time. Then it dawned on me that this might be my problem. It was. My right jaw joint had slipped out of kilter.

The jaw joints—the temporomandibular joints (TMJ)—work twenty-four hours a day when we eat, talk, yawn, drink, and sleep. They must be synchronized to allow four-way movement: up and down, side to side, forward and back, and rotation, gliding simultaneously. When these joints get out of alignment, a wide range of symptoms may occur, among them noisy or jammed jaw joints, headaches, earaches or ringing in the ears, eye pain or redness, dizziness, lower-back pain, neck and shoulder stiffness, numbness in the limbs, and other seemingly unrelated pain or dysfunction.

The causes of TMJ syndrome are diverse and some are not yet known. We do know that poor occlusion, or misalignment of the teeth, and grinding or clenching of teeth under stressful conditions are often causes, as are occupational, sports, and vehicular injuries to the head, whiplash, various types of arthritis, and injuries at birth caused by such practices as forceps delivery. Misalignment can be natural, caused by faulty dental work or orthodontics, or caused by other problems, such as ill-fitting dentures.

For years physicians and dentists dismissed those with TMJ symptoms, especially women, as complainers. It is now known that jaw joint disorders are very common and often overlooked, particularly among older people.

I'd had headaches for years that sometimes were so bad I really couldn't function. When the dentist did a lot of work, including realigning my teeth, my headaches stopped. When I remarked about my headaches stopping, my dentist said it might be TMJ syndrome—something I'd never heard of. He examined me closely and then made a mouthguard for me to wear at night. [a sixty-three-year-old woman]

TMJ problems should not be ignored. When diagnosed and treated early, TMJ can be helped. When ignored, misdiagnosed, or mistreated, it can become intractable, forcing sufferers to stop working and socializing. The keys, therefore, are a careful diagnostic workup done by a physician or dentist who is knowledgeable and sensitive to jaw joint problems, and treatment by an experienced practitioner. Physicians and dentists should recognize TMJ as a legitimate clinical entity and work together to find solutions for each sufferer. TMJ is not just a dental problem.

The treatment of TMJ syndrome is controversial and is almost as varied as the symptoms and causes. Support groups are helpful. Treatment can include a temporary switch to soft foods, behavior modification, stress management, corrective dental work, physical therapy, muscle relaxants, and, in rare cases, surgery. However, always get an independent second opinion—perhaps a third—before taking any strong drugs, having teeth ground down or removed supposedly to balance your bite, or undergoing surgery or any other irreversible treatment.

TMJ sufferers need to band together in self-help groups and as advocates to get better care from dental and medical groups. Insurance companies often define TMJ problems as dental problems and, therefore, deny payment under medical insurance policies that do not include dental payments. We must organize to make sure that reimbursement for needed treatment is included under both medical and dental policies and covered by workmen's compensation.

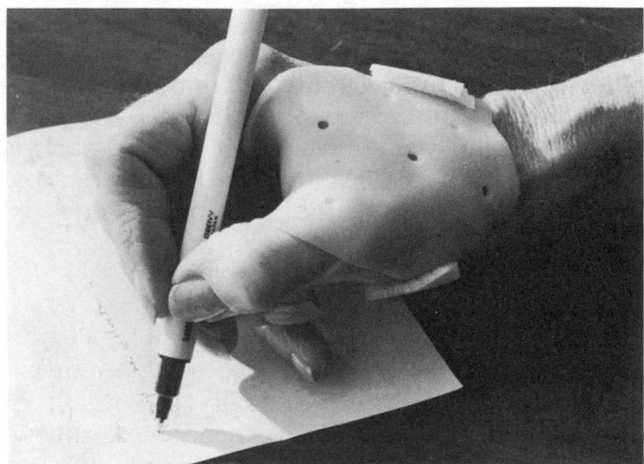

Pam White/Arthritis and Health Resources Centres, Inc.

Elbows

Much used and in a position to be bumped, our elbows are particularly subject to bursitis and tendonitis. Tennis elbow, which can come from any repeated strenuous movement (not just tennis), is a form of tendonitis. A wrist splint made by an occupational therapist to immobilize the wrist muscles that attach at the elbow is more useful than an elbow bandage.[16]

Wrists

Inflamed or swollen tissues in our wrists may squeeze a nerve as it passes through a tunnel on the underside of the wrist, causing pain in the wrist, prickling, numbness (usually in the thumb and first three fingers), and pains shooting up the arm. This syndrome, called *carpal tunnel syndrome,* is common in women who are garment- and electronics-industry workers, food service workers, cashiers and clerical workers,[17] and some musicians. It is increasing among computer users, especially if the chair, desk, and keyboard are not adjusted for your height. Discuss with your health-care provider whether you would benefit from using a wrist splint, available from hospital supply stores. Arthritis in the wrists can make many usual motions painful. The Arthritis Foundation's *The Self-Help Manual for Patients with Arthritis* (see Resources for this chapter) has helpful suggestions.

Hands and Fingers

Arthritis affects our fingers in many different ways. The sign language alphabet is excellent exercise for the fingers. Osteoarthritis may enlarge just the joints nearest the fingernail (these enlargements are called Heberden's nodes). These swellings may be painful, but they do not usually interfere with activity and do not require medical consultation.[18] A tendency to have these seems to run in families. Rheumatoid arthritis can affect all of the joints in the hand and wrist, especially the knuckles and middle joints of the fingers, and warrants immediate medical attention. Splinting, cold or heat, and exercise are necessary to keep the fingers from becoming deformed.

Many women complain of pain and swelling in the lower part of the thumb, near the palm.[19] Ice packs are helpful for this. Pictured is one type of splint that rests the sore joint while still permitting movement in the rest of the thumb.

The base of my thumbs hurt for two years. It got so bad that I couldn't write letters. Medications didn't help. An occupational therapist made a small lightweight plastic splint to support and immobilize the base of my thumb so the joint could rest. In two weeks the inflammation was gone. Now I use the splint during stressful activities such as writing and shopping to prevent pain and irritation. [a fifty-year-old woman]

A sixty-four-year-old woman who spends most of her working day typing ran tape from the back of her hand around the thumb joint to her palm to rest her sore joints in the evening.

ARTHRITIS AND RHEUMATIC DISORDERS

The word *arthritis* describes a condition in which a person has inflamed, painful, stiff, and sometimes swollen joints and muscles. *Rheumatism* is an older word for the same symptoms.

There are many conditions that produce these discomforts, however, so if a health-care provider uses these general terms, ask her or him to be more specific.

By age sixty-five to seventy, about 80 percent of all women have some arthritic complaint.[20] People who have arthritis and the health-care providers who work with them are firm in stating: *All arthritis can be helped.* Although people with arthritic disorders require more rest than most others, millions of people with arthritis are living normal, rich, and fruitful lives. Ninety percent of people with arthritis are employable, although some may need help changing to more appropriate jobs. Only 3 percent of those with arthritis are seriously disabled, and prevention, self-help, early diagnosis, and new methods of treatment are reducing that percentage. Many react with disbelief at the pain and stiffness that may be the first indicator of arthritis.

I refused to consider that anything was wrong with me until I found myself going down the stairs one at a time holding the banister with one hand and the wall with the other. I was only forty-three. [a sixty-one-year-old woman]

GETTING HELP WITH RHEUMATIC DISORDERS

We can find appropriate people to help us when we have arthritis or another rheumatic disorder. We must not assume, as some physicians do, that pain, stiffness, and decreased mobility are inevitable. Treatment *can* be effective in old age. A thorough examination is essential. A physician specializing in internal medicine (an internist) can coordinate the evaluation and the care we may need. You may also want to consult a physician who specializes in joint and tissue diseases (a rheumatologist). A surgeon who specializes in bones (an orthopedist) is useful for an early consultation even if you do not intend to have surgery, but he or she should not be used exclusively. Nurse practitioners are skilled at helping you manage chronic conditions. Podiatrists fit orthotics and help with foot care; occupational therapists help adapt equipment for your use; physical therapists can teach body mechanics and evaluate which exercises are best for you. In addition, many women find relief through the services of acupuncturists and massage therapists.

OSTEOARTHRITIS

The most common form of arthritis is osteoarthritis, called "wear-and-tear arthritis" or degenerative joint disease (DJD) because of the gradual wearing away of joint cartilage. Although almost all adults past forty show signs of osteoarthritis on X rays, only 10 percent of them have any symptoms. So don't worry if an X ray shows some osteoarthritis; just follow the suggestions for prevention of joint pain (page 263).

Osteoarthritis is a localized, mechanical problem rather than an illness involving the whole body. It develops earlier in previously injured or stressed joints. Osteoarthritis also occurs in the spinal joints. As with all osteoarthritis, pain or stiffness in the spinal joints is worst after inactivity and may improve as we move around.

Managing osteoarthritis involves combining rest, exercise, and pain relief (including, if necessary, drugs). Sometimes losing weight relieves the pain. Exercises involving gentle stretching of all muscles two or three times a week are helpful in reducing pain and maintaining mobility. Gently stretch frequently during the day to reduce stiffness. When you feel up to it, *slowly* begin an aerobic activity such as walking, swimming, or bicycle riding (if your knees can take it).

Keep warm—people with arthritis are often sensitive to cold, dampness, and changes in barometric pressure, which change the pressure inside the joint.

You may be tempted to move to a drier climate. This does not always help. Try a visit first. Moving can be one of life's most stressful experiences, and the loss of one's friends and familiar environment may be more painful than bad weather or aching joints.

RHEUMATOID ARTHRITIS

Rheumatoid arthritis (RA) is an inflammatory illness that affects the whole body. It feels, and is, systemic, like flu. While it may affect many organs, it usually causes most problems in the joints. In RA, the lining of the joint capsule (synovial membrane) becomes severely inflamed, producing enzymes that damage cartilage, bone, and soft tissue, in severe cases destroying the joint.[21]

RA affects three times as many women as men. While it first strikes most often between twenty-five and forty-five, half the women who have it are over fifty years of age. What causes the inflammation is not clear but may involve autoimmunity, in which the body attacks its own cells.

Joints, almost always the same ones on both sides of the body, become painful, stiff, swollen, warm, and tender. Early diagnosis and therapy can do much to prevent the disabling aspects of the disease: of those who start treatment *within twelve months* of the early signs of the disease, 75 percent will show substantial improvement. Physical and occupational therapy should start early. Unfortunately, people sometimes wait years before seeking treatment, enduring needless suffering and sometimes causing irreversible damage.

A major U.S. study found some increase in RA at menopause, but found a particularly high instance of it in women who had had both ovaries removed (bilateral oophorectomy). Something other than estrogen may be involved, since neither oral contraceptives nor postmenopausal hormones are effective in preventing or treating RA.[22] For this and other reasons, removal of healthy ovaries should be avoided.

People with arthritis do best when they are active participants in managing their disease. Be sure you understand your illness, with its painful flare-ups alternating with good periods, and your consequent emotional ups and downs. You will be the best monitor of your condition.

The progress of this disease is so individual that it is entirely up to me to determine (by listening very hard to my body) what is appropriate, what is too much, when to rest, when to cut back on activities, when to call it quits. This entails constantly reassessing goals, resetting the "clock" back to zero when I overextend. It is very frustrating but even more so when friends and family pressure me, however subtly. A close friend said to me that the five-hour train trip to visit her is easy. "After all, you're sitting down all the way." It gets so hard to always have to explain. [a thirty-eight-year-old woman]

LUPUS

Systemic lupus erythematosus (SLE), like rheumatoid arthritis, is an autoimmune disease—that is, a disease in which substances produced by our bodies attack our own cells or tissues. The inflammatory processes of lupus can attack connective tissue in any organ system, making the disease difficult to diagnose. It was not even recognized as a disease until 1946. Of the 500,000 to 1,000,000 people in the United States who have lupus today, 90 percent are women; lupus is more frequent among black and Hispanic women. About half of the people with lupus will have symptoms similar to the symptoms of rheumatoid arthritis.

Early diagnosis is important to protect the kidneys; checking kidney function is part of living with the disease. Before the use of corticosteroids, lupus was often fatal within three years. Now 90 percent of people with lupus survive at least fifteen years.[23] Since corticosteroids tend to drain the body of calcium, people with lupus should pay particular attention to calcium intake. They require even more rest than those with other rheumatic disorders. Some drugs may cause lupuslike symptoms, which cease when the drugs are stopped. Lupus may get worse after a viral infection, ultraviolet light exposure, surgery, stress, or ingestion of alfalfa sprouts.[24]

OTHER RHEUMATIC DISORDERS

Inflammation that attacks the connective tissues of the body can cause other rheumatic disorders. Three of these disorders are relatively common:

Fibrositis is often called fibromyalgia or myofascial pain syndrome. Symptoms, including aching, pain, stiffness that has persisted for at least three months, sore spots that radiate pain elsewhere when pressed, fatigue, and sleep disorders, may continue for months or years and then taper off. A long-lasting remission is possible. Antiinflammatory drugs, minute doses of an antidepressant to relax muscles, therapeutic exercise, relaxation techniques, stress management, and the attention of a physical therapist can make an enormous difference in the quality of life.

For some months I had been feeling sore, stiff, and tired. All my joints hurt. Then my cheekbones began to hurt (no joints there!) and pain in my shins kept me awake. My physician told me the sheaths of my muscles were inflamed. He prescribed an antiinflammatory drug and physical therapy. I was astonished at how limited my movements had become. I began a slow program of specific exercises, working up to walking and swimming. After ten months I feel much better. The main limitation is that I must avoid fatigue or choose to pay the price in pain. [a sixty-one-year-old woman]

Polymyalgia rheumatica, an inflammation of the small blood vessels that supply the muscles, has been recognized as a disease only since 1969. It appears often in women over fifty; the average age of onset is seventy. One woman in several hundred experiences this increasingly recognized condition, which causes stiffness and aches. The symptoms of inflammation in the temporal arteries may include headaches on the side of the forehead and sudden severe stiffness in the shoulders and neck, on one side or both. **Inflammation in the arteries in the temple (temporal arteries) must be treated immediately with corticosteroids to prevent blindness.**[25]

Sjögren's syndrome involves inflammation of the excretory glands, such as those that produce tears, saliva, and moisture in the vagina. Ninety percent of people with this syndrome are women, many but not all of whom already have some form of arthritis. Dry eyes may cause ulceration of the cornea; dry mouth may encourage tooth decay and cause hoarseness, chronic cough, and difficulty in chewing and swallowing; a dry vagina may make intercourse painful. Artificial tears and frequent sips of water help the eyes and mouth; lubricants or corticosteroid creams help the vagina. Your primary-care provider should also be alert for damage to the internal organs and the increased likelihood of developing lymphoma, and should work with other specialists such as a dentist, ophthalmologist, and rheumatologist.[26]

Drugs for Rheumatic Disorders

Control of inflammation and pain is essential for the management of rheumatic disorders. Inflammation can be so damaging to the body that even those who dislike taking medication may decide to do so. When necessary, medication can enable us to lead normal lives or can even save our lives. (See OTC and Prescription Drugs, pages 31–33.) Several groups of antiinflammatory drugs are described below. All of them must be carefully monitored because people react to them in individual ways. What works for one person may not work for another. If one prescribed drug does not agree with or help you, talk with your physician about others. Patience is necessary to find the drug that works best for you.

Research indicates that very high levels of fish oils may have an antiinflammatory effect. It is not clear, however, that the expensive omega-3 fatty acid supplements now sold by several drug companies contain the effective ingredient. Moreover, high doses, especially if combined with other drugs that retard clotting, such as aspirin, may result in excessive bleeding.[27] Instead of taking expensive unproven supplements, make fish a regular part of your diet. It is high in protein and vitamin D, low in fat and cholesterol, and may possibly have an antiinflammatory effect.

Antiinflammatory nonsteroidal drugs reduce inflammation and pain. Among these drugs are aspirin, ibuprofen, sulindac, and many others. Acetaminophen is a painkiller with a slight antiinflammatory effect. All these drugs tend to irritate the stomach, so are best taken after food. Aspirin, the standard against which the other drugs are measured, is the cheapest. When prescribed to control inflammation, it is used in high doses over long periods of time. For some, the amount of aspirin necessary to control inflammation may cause ringing in the ears or other undesirable effects, or may not work at all.

One antiinflammatory drug, piroxicam (Feldene), which can cause gastrointestinal ulcers and bleeding, was in several countries labeled harmful to people over sixty but was marketed in the United States for several years before a warning label was finally added.[28]

Serious undesirable effects accompany two other nonsteroidal drugs, phenylbutazone (Butazolidin) and oxyphenbutazone (Tandearil). These two drugs are dangerous, because on rare occasions they can kill most of the white or red blood cells.[29] Older people cannot replenish these cells as quickly as young people. These drugs also cause fluid retention, which can lead to heart failure in older people.

Some people with rheumatoid arthritis respond well to antimalarial drugs: chloroquine (Aralen) and hydroxychloroquine (Plaquenil). Because these can cause damage to the retina, possibly resulting in blindness, eye examinations every six months are necessary.

For many of those who have severe rheumatoid arthritis, gold salts or penicillamine can bring dramatic relief. These drugs may actually halt the progression of the disease. However, both treatments also have rare but severe and sometimes fatal effects.

Corticosteroids (hormones obtained from the adrenal gland, most commonly cortisone and prednisone) are appropriate, even lifesaving, treatments for some rheumatic disorders. They have severe effects, among them masking symptoms of acute infection, raised blood pressure, slowed healing of injuries, osteoporosis, cataracts, diabetes, water retention, and increased appetite. They can cause fat deposits on the face, shoulders, and abdomen. Never take corticosteroids without supervision; carry a warning card if you do take them. Don't decide on your own to stop or reduce the amount of corticosteroids you are taking even if you feel well.[30] **Stopping steroids suddenly or failing to taper off slowly can cause serious problems, even death.** Advise any new health-care practitioner if you have been under corticosteroid treatment within the past two years.

Cortisone given by injection into a joint affects that joint but not the entire body. Its use should be limited to no more than three injections in the same joint in a year.

The anticancer drug methotrexate has been helpful even for very old people but must be monitored carefully and should not be taken with aspirin.[31]

Surgery for Rheumatic Disorders

Long-endured pain makes us vulnerable to the hope that surgery may solve the problem. Since speed is rarely a factor in surgery for arthritis, we have time to get other opinions. When joints are so seriously affected that the results are disabling, surgery may be helpful. Arthritis surgery requires special skills and should not be performed by a surgeon who does such operations only occasionally.

For example, surgery can reposition tendons in the hands and feet moved by the bone changes of rheumatoid arthritis, thereby restoring some function in these joints. A synovectomy—removing the inflamed lining of a joint—can provide dramatic pain relief for some years, but the painful symptoms usually return.

You may choose to have a hip or knee replacement if you have severe and worsening pain even when at rest, have great difficulty walking or performing movements such as putting on or removing shoes and stockings, and if other methods have not helped. Over 120,000 hips and knees are replaced each year and the number is rising. The main complications of these procedures are blood clots and infections (but a good facility for hip replacement will have an infection rate of only 0.5 percent to 1 percent—ask). Hip replacements are more successful than knee replacements, but both can improve the quality of life. Take time to consider; waiting will not affect the results. Be aware, though, that limping because of hip pain can increase pain and arthritis in the opposite hip.

A hip replacement is a temporary solution to a serious problem. The replacement will wear out in ten to fifteen years, but those years may be more mobile and pain-free than without the operation. No one is too old for a hip replacement, but those unable to take anesthesia or who are very heavy may not qualify. Replacements wear out faster under the impact of heavy weight.

A hip replacement has two parts. One, a polished metal ball and stem, attaches to the leg bone nearest the hip (the femur—see illustration). The other attaches to the hipbone and is a socket into which the metal ball fits and moves. A glue or cement similar to Lucite holds these parts onto the bones.

I had both hips replaced in separate operations. I learned bed exercises from a physical therapist, what positions to avoid, how to use the toilet, get into the tub, and manage stairs. I was on crutches for three months, then one crutch, then a cane. At first, I needed help getting dressed. I exercised on the floor, but now I swim and walk every day. The hips are not like my own when they were healthy, but they don't hold me back from anything like when my own were bad. If I knew someone who needed a hip replacement, I'd say, "Go ahead and do it!" [a seventy-two-year-old woman]

I had problems with my hip for over two years and wanted to avoid surgery partly because of the discussion in your first edition. I want you to know that I'm now home from a total hip replacement. I stood on the floor the second day after the operation, used a walker on the third day and a cane on the seventh day. Now after two and a half weeks I can walk with hardly any pressure on the cane. I have been on a bus and can climb stairs with no difficulty. I am allowed to drive. [a sixty-eight-year-old woman]

Knee-joint replacements wear out faster, and have more complications and a slightly higher infection rate than hip-joint replacements. Restriction on weight is important; regular physical-therapy exercises are essential for a satisfactory outcome after the operation. Knee replacements have limited motion, but you should be able to get up from a chair, go up and down stairs, and walk without pain.

I had two hips replaced eight years ago because of osteoarthritis. They've been fine. But my knees also had

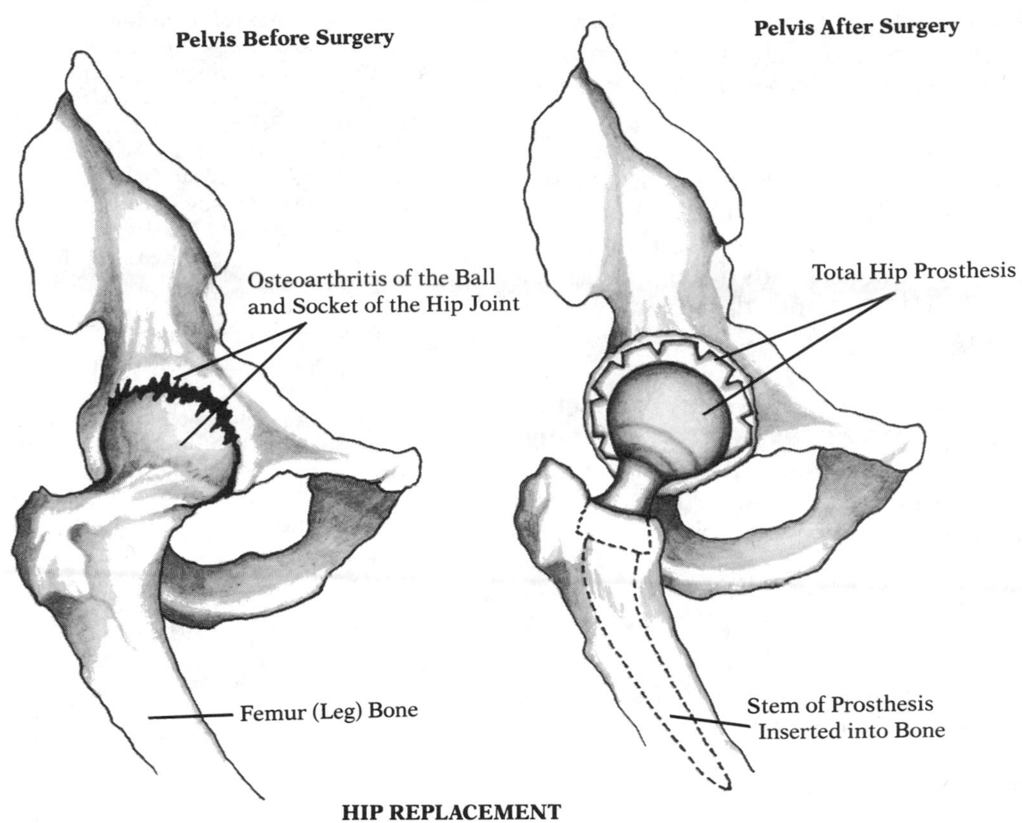

HIP REPLACEMENT

osteoarthritis, and when I could no longer take walks with my husband, which I like to do, I had them both replaced. I worked hard at exercising in the hospital. I'm losing weight now. I take exercise classes and swim. I have a little limitation of motion in my hips and I can't cross my legs any more. But I can walk and do most of the things I want to do. [a sixty-two-year-old woman]

Two years ago after a very brief examination, an orthopedic surgeon advised a knee replacement. I sought a second opinion from an arthritis clinic in a teaching hospital. They examined and questioned me for an hour and said I did not need an operation. One corticosteroid shot and their suggestions helped the problem and it hasn't returned. [a seventy-six-year-old woman]

Unproven Remedies

One characteristic of rheumatic disorders is that periods of pain alternate with periods of relief (spontaneous remission). People who experience this may be convinced that whatever they did just before the relief caused the relief, and therefore may easily adopt unproven remedies, thinking they are miracle cures. Many people make money promoting such cures. *Consumer Reports* estimated in 1979 that for every dollar spent for research in arthritis, $25 was spent on useless or, in some cases, dangerous treatments—more than $1 billion a year of wasted money.[32] Except for the value of eating fish for their fatty acids, research has not yet confirmed claims that vitamin therapy or dietary changes can help arthritis. Eating well will improve your general health whether or not it has a direct effect on your arthritis.

New developments must be watched for their long-term effectiveness and safety. Chicken type II collagen[33] and gammalinolenic acid[34] (GLA from plant seeds such as borage and in oil of evening primrose) are the latest to warrant further research.

Some unproven cures may be relatively harmless, such as wearing copper bracelets or observing dietary restrictions that do not interfere with good nutrition. Some, like DMSO (a chemical that can carry medication through the skin), not only have no value for arthritis but may cause other problems.[35] Many people take medications that indeed make them feel better, only to pay a terrible price in unhealthful effects later, if they have been unknowingly taking corticosteroids or hormones without supervision and necessary testing. Never take drugs if you don't know what they are, especially if they are provided by someone who does not oversee their use.

If you seek help from an arthritis center, look for one that has individually designed programs, including physical therapy, occupational therapy, counseling, nutritional advice, and exercise. The federal government funds fifteen arthritis centers at hospitals around the country (see Resources for this chapter).

Protecting joints, exercising daily, balancing activity and rest, learning to ask for help, trying different techniques to relieve pain—these add up to changes (often modest, sometimes sweeping) that can help us enjoy life in spite of arthritis and joint pain.

I used to do ceramics, painting, leatherwork. The first time the doctor said "Stop before the pain starts," I said, "You must be crazy. I'm involved in creative work. I have to finish it!" It took years before I learned. Later I discovered that flower arranging did not drain my strength and gave me pleasure. It became a new creative outlet for me. I joined a garden club and won several ribbons. [a seventy-five-year-old woman]

NOTES

1. Richard A. Deyo, et al., "How Many Days of Bed Rest for Acute Lower Back Pain? A Randomized Clinical Trial." *The New England Journal of Medicine,* Vol. 315, No. 17 (Oct. 23, 1986), pp. 1064–70; and Nortin M. Hadler, "Editorial: Regional Back Pain." *The New England Journal of Medicine,* Vol. 315, No. 17 (Oct. 23, 1986), pp. 1090–92.

2. Adapted from James F. Fries, *Arthritis: A Comprehensive Guide to Understanding Your Arthritis,* rev. ed. Reading, MA: Addison-Wesley, 1986, p. 6.

3. John Hoffman, et al., "Reduced Sympathetic Nervous System Responsivity Associated with the Relaxation Response." *Science,* Vol. 229 (Jan. 8, 1982), pp. 190–92.

4. Bonnie Prudden, *Myotherapy: Bonnie Prudden's Complete Guide to Pain-Free Living.* Garden City, NY: Doubleday, 1984.

5. René Cailliet, *Foot and Ankle Pain,* 2d ed., Philadelphia, PA: F. A. Davis Co., 1983, p. 115.

6. Personal communication from Bruce Woods, M.D.

7. Suggested by Connie Slater, physical therapist.

8. Personal communication from Alf Nachemson, M.D.

9. Jack R. Tessman, *My Back Doesn't Hurt Anymore.* New York: Quick Fox, 1980, pp. 59–60.

10. Interview with Daniel Swerdlow, M.D.

11. G. Timothy Johnson and Stephen E. Goldfinger, *The Harvard Medical School Health Letter Book.* Cambridge, MA: Harvard University Press, 1981, pp. 135–38.

12. Arthur C. Klein and Dava Sobel, *Backache Relief.* New York: Times Books, 1985, pp. 13–54.

13. Elisabeth Rosenthal, "Mending or Replacing Torn Cartilage in the Knee." *New York Times,* Nov. 11, 1992.

14. For exercise suggestions, see Kate Lorig and James F. Fries, *The Arthritis Helpbook: What You Can Do for Your Arthritis,* rev. ed. Reading, MA: Addison-Wesley, 1992.

15. Fries, op. cit., pp. 192–93.

16. Personal communication from Jeanne L. Melvin.

17. "Women's Health." Report of the PHS Task Force on Women's Health Issues, Vol. I. *Public Health Reports,* Vol. 100, No. 1 (January–February 1985), p. 92.

18. Personal communication from William P. Docken, M.D.

19. Letters to *Broomstick,* Vol. IV, No. 4 (July–August 1982), p. 29, and Vol. VI, No. 6 (November–December 1984), p. 36.

20. Jane Porcino, *Growing Older, Getting Better: A Handbook for Women in the Second Half of Life.* New York: Crossroad Continuum, 1991, p. 248.

21. Fred G. Kantrowitz, "Rheumatoid Arthritis." *Medical Times,* Vol. 110, No. 2 (February 1982), p. 73.

22. Preliminary Results from the Nurses' Health Study, Harvard School of Public Health. *Menopausal Status, Estrogen Use, and Incidence of Rheumatoid Arthritis,* abstract presented at the 110th Annual Meeting of the American Public Health Association, 1982.

23. John J. Condemi, "The Autoimmune Diseases." *Journal of the American Medical Association,* Vol. 268, No. 20 (Nov. 25, 1992), pp. 2882–92.

24. Ibid., p. 2884.

25. Fries, op. cit., p. 63.

26. Condemi, op. cit., pp. 2888–89.

27. "Should You Begin Taking Fish Oil Supplements?" *Tufts University Diet and Nutrition Letter,* Vol. 4, No. 11 (January 1987), pp. 1–2.

28. "Feldene: Canada and Germany Protect Older People Better." *Health Letter,* Public Citizens Health Research Group, Vol. 2, No. 4 (September/October 1986), pp. 14–15; "Feldene." *Health Letter,* Vol. 3, No. 1 (January 1987), p. 18.

29. Fries, op. cit., pp. 106–7.

30. Lorig and Fries, op. cit., p. 218.

31. *The Merck Manual of Geriatrics.* Rahway, NJ: Merck & Co., 1990, p. 696.

32. Fred Kantrowitz, *Taking Control of Arthritis.* New York: HarperCollins, 1990, p. 170.

33. David E. Trentham, et al., "Effects of Oral Administration of Type II Collagen on Rheumatoid Arthritis." *Science,* Vol. 261 (Sept. 24, 1993), pp. 1727–30.

34. Lawrence J. Leventhal, et al., "Treatment of Rheumatoid Arthritis with Gammalinolenic Acid." *Annals of Internal Medicine,* Vol. 119, No. 9 (Nov. 1, 1993), pp. 867–73.

35. Annabel Hecht, "Hocus Pocus as Applied to Arthritis." *FDA Consumer,* U.S. Department of Health and Human Services, September 1980, HHS Pub. No. (FDA) 81-1080.

19

OSTEOPOROSIS AND FRACTURE PREVENTION

✦

BY KATHLEEN I. MACPHERSON

1994 UPDATE BY DIANA LASKIN SIEGAL WITH HELP FROM NORMA MERAS SWENSON AND KATHLEEN I. MACPHERSON AND WITH SPECIAL THANKS TO DONALD J. DERASKA

RESOURCES FOR THIS CHAPTER ON PAGES 490–91

Lately, osteoporosis is mentioned everywhere we turn—in newspapers, women's magazines, and television talk shows. An illustration of a woman with a "dowager's hump" is used repeatedly, implying that such a fate is inevitable if we do not take hormones. This media blitz has resulted, as a recent survey of women showed, in high recognition of the word *osteoporosis,* but confusion about what it is and how it affects women[1] and men.

In this chapter we will explain osteoporosis but will also include the real public health question: How can we prevent fractures? In the United States, people suffer 1.5 million fractures annually, including more than 275,000 hip fractures, 500,000 vertebral fractures, and 200,000 wrist fractures. In 1987, the cost of care and lost earnings due to fractures was estimated at $10 billion.[2] Fractures are often devastating to old people, many of whom succumb to complications caused by the same underlying diseases or disabilities that contributed to their fall.[3]

While osteoporosis is a cause of fractures, it is only one cause among many. Fractures are also the result of environmental hazards found everywhere, including our homes; the prescribing of sleeping pills, tranquilizers, and other medications that cause unsteadiness; and cultural customs such as a sedentary life-style, the pressure to be as thin as possible, and wearing high-heeled shoes. Osteoporosis, as we will explain, results from much more than our bodies' natural decline in estrogen as we age.[4]

We need to reduce the many causes of fractures. Do not be lulled into a false sense of security encouraged by drug-company advertising and those doctors who imply that we are safe as long as we take hormones.

UNDERSTANDING OSTEOPOROSIS

Our bones are made up of living cells in a state of constant breakdown and repair. Except for the skin, no other substance in the body has such excellent regenerative powers as bone. As new bone is produced, it is actually laid down on the solid outer shell (cortical bone). Old bone disappears from the softer, less dense substance inside (trabecular bone) where calcium can enter and leave. Normally, our body balances the two processes of building new bone and removing old bone so that our bones remain strong. This continuous building process is called remodeling. When new bone formation no longer keeps up with bone loss, bones begin to thin and weaken.

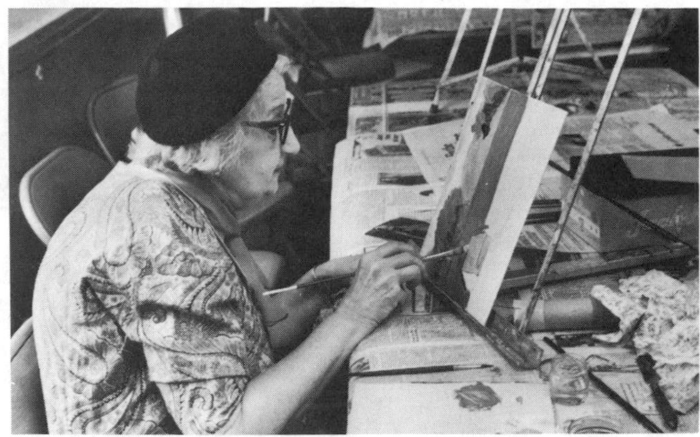
Norma Holt

We lose a certain amount of lean muscle tissue and some bone cells as a natural result of the aging process, although most of us will not develop osteoporosis. Bone loss starts in women a few years after bone density peaks at about age thirty-five. The loss increases slightly in the four to five years following menopause.[5] There are large differences in the rate and amount of thinning among individuals.[6]

Through an intricate process, the level of calcium in the blood is kept within a very precise, narrow range necessary for muscle contractions, transmission of nerve impulses, and blood clotting. If the level of calcium in the blood is higher than necessary, the body excretes whatever cannot be absorbed. Calcium can be leached out of the bones if the level of calcium in the blood drops below normal.

Osteoporosis is a complex condition that usually takes years to advance to the stage where it can be detected. Many interrelated factors affect the exchange of calcium between the blood and bones. These factors include the amount of calcium in the diet, how efficiently our bodies absorb it, hormonal balance, and our level of physical activity. Decreased ovarian estrogen after menopause is only one factor—often overemphasized in the mass media and medical literature—that contributes to the development of osteoporosis. We can understand these factors and make changes that will slow bone loss and improve bone remodeling.

For example, when we are young, diet is our chief source of calcium. Vitamin D is added to milk because it helps the body absorb calcium from the small intestine and also promotes the transportation of calcium into bone. The level of calcium in the blood, in turn, controls the amount of hormone secreted by the parathyroid gland (parathyroid hormone, or PTH). If the level of calcium in the blood decreases, more PTH, which triggers leaching of calcium from the bones, will be produced to correct the deficit in the blood. Other hormones also play a role—normal estrogen levels protect women from producing too much PTH; steroid hormones (such as hydrocortisone, cortisone, and prednisone) have several effects that cause osteoporosis.

It is also important to understand how activity, or the lack of it, affects bone strength. Bone mass will increase or decrease according to the demand placed on it. The total amount of calcium in the body increases with exercise, but muscle strength, bone-mineral content, and specific bone mass will vary depending on activity patterns. For example, tennis players have thicker bones in their dominant arms. Demand in an active part of the body will pull bone mineral away from inactive parts. In one study, women aged thirty-five to sixty-five in an aerobic-movement program showed loss of mineral in upper-body bone, which was regained when upper-body resistance exercises were added.[7] (See Moving for Health chapter for a balanced exercise regimen.)

Many factors—reduced activity, reduced calcium absorption in our intestines, and reduced levels of estrogen to counteract the effects of PTH—result in increased calcium loss as we age.

A GLOSSARY OF BONE CONDITIONS

Osteopenia: a general term for decreased bone density. Osteopenia refers to all forms of bone weakness, including osteoporosis and osteomalacia.

Osteoporosis: from "osteo," referring to bones, and "porosis," full of holes. In this condition, the actual bone is normal—there is just not enough of it. When osteoporosis exists, certain bones become thin and more likely to fracture or become compressed as a result of even a minor fall, making a bed, or opening a door.

Osteomalacia: the adult form of rickets, a softening and weakening of bones due to the lack of vitamin D, the inability of the body to use vitamin D, or other causes. In this condition, bone cells are abnormal and the bones may actually change shape.

Risk Factors

Biological Risk Factors

Sorting out age, sex, and race risk factors is not simple. It is generally stated that women are at greater risk of osteoporosis than men because men have 30 percent more bone mass at age thirty-five than women, and they lose bone more slowly as they age. If you are black, the chances of your developing osteoporosis are rare. Black women have 10 percent more bone mass than white women, and may have more calcitonin, the hormone that strengthens bones.[8] But the consequences of fracture are greater for blacks possibly because of the effects of poverty, inadequate health care, and the greater likelihood of having other underlying diseases. Asians are considered, like whites, at risk, but one study showed that Japanese women continue to gain bone mass until thirty-five to thirty-nine years of age[9] and another study showed a lower rate of hip fractures in Hong Kong than in the white U.S. population. Indeed, over the age of eighty, males in the United States had higher rates of hip fractures than women in Hong Kong.[10] If you are of Hispanic, Mediterranean, or Jewish ancestry, the risk seems to fall between the low risk for blacks and the high risk for Northern European white women and Asian women. The fairer your complexion, the greater your risk.

A person's risk of hip fracture doubles approximately every six to seven years, regardless of sex or race. At any age, the risk for white women is approximately double that for black women. The unusual susceptibility of white women is, thus, not simply due either to sex or race, since there is no clear gender correlation among blacks and no clear race correlation among men. This suggests that there is a similar underlying process that increases fracture risk in all groups as they age, but that this process either begins earlier or presents symptoms earlier in white women.[11] Although you cannot change your biological factors, you can make a special effort to prevent osteoporosis by eating a calcium-rich diet and exercising.

In addition, talk to your mother, aunts, and grandmothers to find out whether any of your close relatives have had a dowager's hump, many fractures, or a diagnosis of osteoporosis. You need to take special precautions if your relatives have had this condition, although it is not known if the tendency is inherited or comes from a shared environment or diet.

Women who have never had a child or breastfed an infant have missed out on the temporary surges of estrogen that accompany pregnancy and follow breastfeeding and help protect us against osteoporosis in later life. Although estrogen levels temporarily drop during lacta-

Factors That Increase Your Risk of Osteoporosis

Life-Style Factors

- Lack of exercise
- Excessive exercise
- Smoking
- High alcohol intake
- Low-calcium diet
- Vitamin D deficiency
- Prolonged dieting or fasting
- High caffeine intake (over two cups a day)
- High salt intake

Environmental Factors

- Inadequate fluoride level in the water supply
- Living in a northern climate
- Being confined indoors

Medical Factors

- Oophorectomy (removal of ovaries)
- Use of certain prescription and over-the-counter drugs
- Extended bed rest or immobilization
- Surgical removal of part of the stomach or small intestine
- Anorexia
- Celiac disease
- Chronic diarrhea
- Diabetes
- Kidney or liver disease

Biological Factors

- Being female
- Having a family history of osteoporosis
- Having Northern European ancestry
- Being thin and short
- Having fair skin and freckles
- Having blond or reddish-colored hair
- Early natural menopause
- Childlessness
- Lactose intolerance
- Teenage pregnancy
- Scoliosis

tion and calcium leaves bones to go into milk formation, as soon as you stop breastfeeding your estrogen level rises again. This helps strengthen the bones in preparation for another pregnancy.

A nutritious diet during pregnancy will help bones get stronger. If you are not on a nutritious diet, pregnancy and breastfeeding can actually draw calcium out of the bones—hence the adage about losing a tooth for each child. When the mother's own bones are not fully formed, adequate calcium is especially necessary. The adolescent mother can suffer as much as a 10 percent loss in bone content after four months of breastfeeding.[12] We can't change our own childbearing history, but we hope this information will influence young women to delay pregnancy until their own growth is complete, or, if they become pregnant and breastfeed, to eat wisely. Recommended dietary allowances for pregnant teenagers include a 2,500-calorie diet daily, including 76 grams of protein and 2,000 milligrams of calcium.[13] We believe this intake of calcium, 2,000 mg during pregnancy and 2,200 mg while breastfeeding, is best for women of any age.

Medical research in this country reports that women experience increased bone loss for three to six years following the onset of menopause.[14] After that, with adequate calcium and vitamin D, the amount of loss levels off. If you have an early natural menopause, before age forty, you are at risk of osteoporosis because the cessation of menstruation causes estrogen levels to drop.

If you experience diarrhea, cramps, and gas after drinking milk or eating milk products you may be lactose intolerant—without enough lactase, the enzyme that helps us digest milk properly. If you are lactose intolerant, see the Eating Well chapter for dealing with this condition and for good alternative sources of calcium. About 70 percent of blacks and Asians are lactose intolerant, compared with 15 percent of the general population. Sixty percent of women with osteoporosis are lactose intolerant, compared with 15 percent of the general population.[15] Note, however, that blacks have a low rate of osteoporosis despite their high rate of lactose intolerance, which shows that other factors are involved.

Medical Risk Factors

Certain diseases or chronic conditions can make us vulnerable to excessive bone loss. Women with anorexia, for example, may develop osteoporosis as early as age twenty-five—even to the point of having spinal crush fractures, which are usually seen only in elderly women.[16] Extremely strenuous exercise, as a result of which the percentage of body fat drops so low that menstruation stops, can also lead to osteoporosis.

Celiac disease in childhood (malabsorption of food usually caused by sensitivity to the gluten in wheat) is never completely outgrown, and even if controlled may recur in adults when irritating food is eaten. Chronic diarrhea caused by ulcerative colitis or Crohn's disease (chronic inflammation or tuberculosis of the small intestine) also prevents the calcium in food from being absorbed.[17] Production or ingestion of excessive thyroid hormone weakens bones.

If you have diabetes, you have to contend with frequent urination, which causes excessive loss of calcium, and high blood acidity, which interferes with the absorption of vitamin D. If you have kidney or liver problems, the calcium in your food is not efficiently absorbed; kidney dialysis adds to calcium deficiency.

Certain surgery can also put you at risk for osteoporosis. Surgical removal of the ovaries, especially before, but even at the time of, menopause, reduces estrogen production more rapidly and for a longer period of time than a normal menopause. If you undergo this surgery, you need to take special care to maintain an adequate calcium intake and exercise program. Many researchers report a high rate of osteoporosis if hormone-replacement therapy isn't started soon after removal of premenopausal ovaries.[18]

Stomach surgery (a gastric bypass for weight reduction or ulcer removal) and intestinal surgery can also place you at risk for osteoporosis; stomach surgery can lead to insufficient hydrochloric acid, which is necessary for the proper digestion of food before it passes into the small intestine.[19] Calcium can get into the bloodstream only through the small intestines or bones. If there are problems with intestinal absorption, your bones pay the price.

It's also necessary to consider medications often taken for chronic health problems, such as cortisone for severe arthritis, phenobarbitol or phenytoin (Dilantin) for seizures, and aluminum-containing antacids for ulcers or heartburn. Excessive dosage of thyroid hormone can also accelerate bone loss. Exercise and a nutritious diet are a must if you take these drugs, because they all interfere with the body's ability to absorb calcium from food and calcium supplements.

Life-Style Risk Factors

Avoiding osteoporosis isn't as complicated as we are led to believe. Most of us can take immediate steps at any age to improve bone strength by changing our daily habits.

Nutrition, for example, plays a major role in preventing and treating osteoporosis. (See the Eating Well chapter for a full discussion of the role of calcium in a balanced diet.).

Vitamin D is a vital factor in the body's use of calcium. In order for vitamin D to aid in calcium absorption, it has to be converted into a hormone in the liver and in the kidneys. Osteoporosis may occur when the conversion is not taking place, and hence may be a symptom of liver and/or kidney disease. In addition, vitamin D can't be converted to its active hormone form when the blood is too acid due to stress, diabetes, or fasting, or if you have a magnesium deficiency. Certain medications such as anticonvulsants, laxatives, cortisone, and mineral oil can also interfere with the absorption of vitamin D.

A summer holiday in the sun allows us to store vitamin D for prolonged periods of time. Half an hour in the sun with 30 percent of the body exposed several times a week is sufficient. This is especially important if we live in the North, in overcast areas, or are confined indoors. Walk in the morning and be sure to avoid excessive exposure to the sun.

Foods rich in vitamin D are egg yolk (if hens are allowed outside), certain fish, fish liver, and butter. Vitamin D is added to milk—8 ounces of milk contain 100 IUs—but is not added to other dairy products. We need 400 IUs daily. Over the age of sixty-five we need 600 to 800 IUs daily because our bodies have a decreased capacity to absorb and convert vitamin D as we get older, which may be a significant factor in osteoporosis. You can take a supplement if you don't drink milk. Supplementary amounts over 1,000 IUs a day interfere with calcium absorption and, because vitamin D is stored in the body for long periods of time, higher amounts can be toxic.*

The amount of phosphorus (which aids in the development and maturation of bones)[20] we consume should be equal to the amount of calcium we consume. Most of us, however, probably take in too much phosphorus from eating red meat, processed cheese, baked goods that contain phosphate baking powder, cola and other soft drinks, instant soups and puddings, bread, and phosphate food additives. Dried skim milk is very high in phosphorus—each 100 grams of milk contains 950 mg of phosphorus[21]—so if you add powdered milk to soups or casseroles for extra calcium, take care to cut out other unnecessary sources of phosphorus. Excessive phosphorus causes bone loss.

We also need magnesium for strong teeth and bones. The amount of magnesium we consume should be at least half the amount of calcium we consume—perhaps equal to it.[22] If magnesium intake is too low, the body is not able to utilize calcium or vitamin D, even if a sufficient amount of those substances is available. There is a rich supply of magnesium in nuts, whole grains, sprouts, beans, fresh vegetables, and fruit.

It's also important that we get enough zinc and manganese, because calcium added to the diet decreases their absorption. Zinc is found in whole-grain breads and cereals, nuts, and seeds. Manganese is found in sunflower seeds, nuts, rice, barley, oats, and blueberries.

Prolonged dieting and fasting are common in our society because of the obsession with slenderness. If you habitually eat little, your daily requirements for calcium and related nutrients are not met, so that calcium has to be taken from your bones. Adequate weight and fat tissue offer protection from osteoporosis. The weight on the bones makes them work to produce new bone tissue, and the fat tissue helps to maintain some estrogen in the body after menopause. Some women with low bone density do not fracture. One reason can be that they have more fat on the hip that absorbs the impact of the fall. After trying to be as thin as possible for fashion, we can now buy hip padding to add the protection that we have dieted away. Encouraging residents to wear hip protectors has been tried in several nursing homes and has significantly reduced the incidence of hip fractures.[23]

Other life-style factors, such as alcohol and caffeine use, can also contribute to bone loss. Both caffeine and alcohol act as diuretics that can cause loss of calcium and zinc in the urine. Alcohol damages the liver, interfering with vitamin D metabolism. However, one or two cups of coffee or four cups of tea,[24] a beer or a glass of wine, or 1½ ounces of hard liquor daily probably do no harm.

Smoking is a known risk factor in osteoporo-

*Prudent advice to most postmenopausal women is to have 1,000 to 1,500 mg of calcium and 400 to 800 IUs of vitamin D daily. Robert P. Heaney, "Thinking Straight About Calcium." *The New England Journal of Medicine*, Vol. 328, No. 7 (Feb. 18, 1993), pp. 503–5.

sis. It is directly toxic to the ovaries. Women who smoke often experience menopause up to five years earlier than nonsmokers. Smoking may also interfere with the body's metabolism of estrogen, and may affect bone remodeling in other ways.[25] Smoking often accompanies high alcohol or caffeine use.

Lack of exercise is another major risk factor that you can control. Part of the geographical and racial differences among women relative to the incidence of osteoporosis may be due to differences in physical activity.[26] In the past, women generally didn't exercise vigorously. To sweat was unfeminine, and our society equated femininity with a small frame, low weight, and a passive attitude toward life; certainly there was no approval of a female "jock" type. Fortunately that is changing and it's never too late for us to start exercising. Weight-bearing exercises such as walking, jogging, jumping rope, and dancing all make our bones work harder and strengthen the muscles and ligaments supporting the skeleton. One researcher reported that weight-bearing exercise that excluded upper-body activity resulted in a 3.5 percent increase in spinal bone during an eighteen-month period, but a 3.6 percent decrease in wrist bone.[27] It is important to make our arms work also, by swimming, wearing weights on them as we walk, doing push-ups, or other arm exercises.

A study of bones from two centuries ago showed fewer hip fractures and more bone density at all ages, including after menopause, compared with women today.[28] The reasons for these differences are unclear but one factor may be the lower amount of steady daily physical activity in present-day women. Adding exercise clearly shows benefits in improved bone density, decreased bone mass loss as we age, and improved muscle strength, which supports bones and improves our vigor and steadiness.

Environmental Risk Factors

Fluoridation of drinking water has been successful in the prevention of tooth decay—and it may also prevent bone fragility and osteoporosis.[29] Studies of the relationship between levels of fluoridation and the rates of hip fractures (commonly used as the measure of the amount of osteoporosis) have shown mixed results. A recent NIH workshop concluded that further research was needed.[30] Levels as low as one part fluoride to 1 million parts water are reported to reduce hip fractures by up to 40 percent.[31] You may wish to check the fluoride level of your public or bottled water supply. People now ingest fluoride through the use of toothpastes and mouthwashes as well as food and beverages manufactured in communities with fluoridated water. Individual fluoride supplementation may not be needed.

Three quarters of hip fractures occur indoors and environmental hazards contribute to two thirds of them.[32] Look around your home to eliminate hazards likely to cause falls, such as slippery surfaces, loose rugs, and electric wires on the floor. Install rubber mats and grab bars in showers and tubs and near toilets, and lights and railings in all stairways. Wear shoes and slippers with low heels and nonslip soles. If you are unsteady on your feet, use a cane or a walker. If you need glasses, wear them, but never walk around with glasses that are meant just for reading.

Make sure your house temperature is at least 65 degrees at night. Cold temperatures can lead to dizziness and falling. Dizziness can also be caused by low blood pressure, by certain medications, or by getting up too quickly after eating, lying down, or resting. Always use special caution when walking outdoors on wet and icy pavements.[33] Speak up for better snow and ice removal and sanding.

Among women in Japan, wearing broad, flat-heeled shoes rather than high heels, sleeping on futons or low beds rather than in high beds, years of squatting and kneeling resulting in greater strength of the thigh muscles, and their lower use of tranquilizers and alcohol protect them from falls and fractures and are strategies we could adopt.

When We Need Professional Help

If you have several of the above risk factors, or just feel you want further information, you can seek out a health provider who is knowledgeable about osteoporosis. Nutritionists can be extremely helpful in planning a preventive diet to your liking; exercise instructors can tailor a regimen that will strengthen the muscles and ligaments supporting your bones; nurses and nurse practitioners can help you establish osteoporosis-prevention habits and understand the politics of the current osteoporosis controversy;[34] physicians can order screening tests and medication for osteoporosis.

If you choose to visit a physician, ask other women to recommend one who treats each woman as an individual, who has an understanding of the complex factors that cause osteoporosis and doesn't give simplistic answers—for example, one who doesn't suggest hormone therapy for all postmenopausal women. If you live in an urban area, you may be near a metabolic bone disease or osteoporosis clinic that offers screening and treatment. If you have doubts about a medical recommendation, get a second opinion.

In the past, most physicians have concentrated on treatment of existing osteoporosis at the expense of early prevention. They have often prescribed, after a fracture has occurred, the very procedures that might have prevented osteoporosis from developing in the first place—replacement calcium, vitamin D supplements, and exercise. Some physicians are very "promedication"; others warn of its dangers and encourage exercise and dietary modifications instead.[35]

Warning Signs of Bone Loss

Several years ago, I developed a pain up under my right breast and I couldn't imagine what it was. It hurt to move and it hurt to breathe and I ignored it for a little while. Finally it got so bad that I went to the doctor and he ordered X rays of my back and rib cage. He said, "Oh, my, your bones are so thin I'm amazed you haven't broken everything you've got." The vertebrae had thinned and compressed—one was pressing on a nerve which caused the pain in my chest. [a fifty-nine-year-old woman]

Early warning signs of osteoporosis include wrist fracture following a simple fall or blow, and muscle spasms or pain in the neck while at rest or while doing routine daily work such as making a bed or picking up an object from the floor. This pain comes on suddenly; most women can recall the exact moment it began. It is often caused by the spontaneous collapsing (a spinal crush fracture) of small sections of the spine that have been severely thinned or weakened. These compression fractures can lead to "dowager's hump," which shortens the chest area and makes digesting food more difficult. Because compression fractures do not always cause prolonged, severe pain or disability, some women are not aware that they have this condition, although 20 percent of women do by age seventy.

Loss of height is another early sign of spinal crush fractures and osteoporosis. It would be wise to measure your height routinely. In extreme cases, women can lose as much as eight inches of height, all from the upper half of the body.[36]

Screening and Diagnosis

Because the loss of bone cells leading to osteoporosis is so gradual, we need to be very alert to early signs. Screening and diagnosis of this condition can be difficult since low bone density alone does not necessarily indicate osteoporosis. There is substantial similarity in the bone density of women with and without fractures.[37] As yet there are no criteria for the diagnosis of osteoporosis on the basis of any tests. So always ask how the results are obtained and on what the interpretation is based. You may find that the test indicates only how your bones compare to other women your age, so you'll then need to ask on what group of women the scores were developed. Other factors, such as the strength of the muscles and ligaments supporting the bones, also affect susceptibility of bones to fractures.

Loss of teeth during midlife and thinning of the bones supporting the teeth are warning signals. This bone thinning may be detected by dental X rays. A recent study reports that loss of teeth at midlife occurs more often in women than in men, and in white women much more often than in black women. Women who lost their teeth early and smoked developed osteoporosis three times as frequently as women who did not smoke.[38] However, we women will have to question and convey information between our physicians and dentists, since they so rarely communicate with each other.

Ordinary X rays don't clearly detect osteoporosis until at least 30 percent of bone density is lost, and are not suitable for screening purposes. One screening tool is a bone-density scanner, of which there are several types: single- and dual-photon absorptiometry, dual X-ray absorptiometry, and quantitative CT (computered tomography). This is another name for a CAT scan (computerized axial tomography).

Single-photon absorptiometry (SPA) scans are most common and least expensive—they take less than fifteen minutes and usually cost less than $100. Radioactive iodine is directed at the patient's arm, which is submerged in water or placed in a rubber collar, and a detector counts how much radiation passes through the bone, thereby gauging bone density. The amount of radiation received from this procedure is less than 1 percent of that received from an X ray.[39] However, though SPA is a relatively simple and accurate measure of bone density in the hand and arm, it doesn't predict bone density in the hip and the spine. The risk of *nonspine* fractures with decreased bone density, however, was predicted equally well by bone-density measurement of the hip or spine by dual X-ray absorptiometry (DXA) and of the wrist by SPA.[40] Some centers, however, use SPA as a screening technique for detecting osteoporosis.

Dual-photon absorptiometry (DPA) can be used to scan the whole body, including the spine and hip. This method is also low in radiation but is expensive. It is becoming less popular than DXA because its radioactive source must be replaced periodically and the accuracy of its measurements changes over time. DXA is similar to DPA but uses X rays. It can measure bone density of any area in a reliable manner with a low radiation dose. Quantitative CT scanning (qCT), which is a special type of CT scan, is the most accurate method of detecting osteoporosis anywhere in the body. However, it is expensive, involves exposure to more radiation than the SPA or the DPA, and is not useful for comparing tests over time.

In order to be certain that osteoporosis is the major problem, and not the result or symptom of another disease, other tests, possibly even a bone biopsy, are needed. A bone biopsy to test for osteoporosis is usually taken from a hipbone.

Most doctors outside of large research centers will probably continue, at least in the near future, to conclude that osteoporosis is the culprit whenever a female patient over fifty fractures a bone. The well-to-do can afford to be monitored and tested early if they wish, but poorer women generally do not have this option. If screening can predict osteoporosis before a fracture occurs, then it should be available to all middle-aged women.

Such early detection is meaningless, however, unless it is accompanied by incentives for women to make the changes in diet and life-style that will strengthen bone mass or at least slow down its loss. Understanding the risk factors described in this chapter may go a long way toward achieving that end. The screening methods can then be used by those with high risk factors.

THE USE OF HORMONES

Many physicians are likely to prescribe hormone therapy for osteoporosis even though low hormone levels have not been proven to be the direct cause of this condition. Until 1973, physicians in the United States who viewed menopause as a "deficiency disease" rather than as a natural event usually prescribed estrogen alone. Use declined after estrogen was linked to an increased rate of endometrial cancer. They then added progestogen. This combination "imitates" the hormones of our menstrual cycle. Estrogen (usually 0.625 mg daily for 25 days) and progestogen (commonly medroxyprogesterone in a dose of 10 mg daily on days 16 through 25 of a 28-day cycle), in combination, are supposed to prevent the lining of the uterus from building up to a dangerous precancerous level. Now the emphasis is on the use of these hormones for osteoporosis. Research is under way to determine if doses small enough not to cause periods are still effective in preventing osteoporosis. But some physicians don't prescribe this combination of hormones because:

- Research on the long-term effects is not yet available;
- Progestogens in the birth-control pill increase the risk of high blood pressure, strokes, and breast cancer; some researchers claim that medroxyprogesterone (Provera), the progestin most commonly prescribed for postmenopausal women, has a weaker adverse effect than the form used in birth-control pills or "the shot";
- This combination of hormones causes menstrual-type bleeding;
- Extra medical examinations—such as regular Pap smears, pelvic and breast exams, blood-pressure monitoring, and endometrial biopsies—are necessary to monitor the effects of these drugs.

Prevention or Treatment?

There is a fundamental confusion in the medical literature and in the popular media between recommending hormone therapy to *treat* osteoporosis and recommending it to *prevent* osteoporosis. In April 1984, a National Institutes of Health Consensus Development Conference recommended the use of estrogen for Caucasian women to prevent osteoporosis, despite the known risks.[41] Now many physicians are indiscriminately prescribing hormone therapy for prevention.

To recommend widespread use of hormones to prevent osteoporosis without assessing the needs of each individual woman is the same as recommending that everyone take antihypertension drugs to prevent high blood pressure. Rarely is anything as dangerous as hormones recommended for prevention. Considering the serious risks of taking hormones, each woman for whom hormones is recommended, as either prevention or treatment, must balance the risks of using hormones against the degree of osteoporosis and other risks for fractures.

One researcher recommends estrogen therapy both for what he calls Type I osteoporosis—which occurs in women within ten to fifteen years after menopause, resulting in spinal crush fractures and dowager's hump—and for Type II osteoporosis—which affects elderly women and men and is caused by inefficient calcium absorption.[42] Estrogen therapy does appear to offer some protection against bone loss for three to five years. We must remember, however, that both these types of osteoporosis can be affected by the life-style factors discussed previously, and that if we start hormone therapy and then stop we will lose just as much bone as if we never started.[43] Along with postponing the bone loss may come some reduction in fractures. Some physicians recommend, therefore, that hormone therapy be continued indefinitely. Others limit its use to high-risk women for a short period of time, while helping the women make dietary and exercise changes.

Physicians Disagree

Among physicians, we find a wide range of opinions on hormone therapy as a preventive measure. Some advocate it for all postmenopausal women,[44] some promote it for women at high risk for osteoporosis, while others are against mass campaigns that recommend hormones for prevention.[45]

Generally, practicing physicians, in contrast to medical researchers, are more likely to use hormone therapy both to prevent and to treat osteoporosis. These physicians have direct contact with women and are thus forced to come to some decision regarding the prescribing of hormones. Women themselves may ask for hormones. The physician should explain the risks and possible benefits so that an informed decision can be made by the women themselves. Some physicians worry about the possibility of a lawsuit if they do not prescribe hormone therapy for a woman who later develops osteoporosis. The lawsuit could be based on the contention that the physician was unaware of "prevailing use" or "common medical practice"; after all, there has been a deluge of articles, advertisements, and public-relations campaigns on osteoporosis. But many medical researchers, on the other hand, are concerned with the possible dangers of hormone therapy (especially cancer and gallbladder conditions).[46]

Lowered estrogen levels after menopause are only one of several factors involved in osteoporosis. Almost all studies of bone loss in aging women show that the process begins before age forty in the bones of the hands, spine, hip, and wrist. The loss accelerates for a few years after menopause and then returns to the gradual premenopausal rate of loss.[47] Furthermore, researchers have shown that while the age at which menopause occurs is relatively constant, enormous geographic and racial differences exist in the incidence of fractures related to osteoporosis.[48] Differences in fracture rates may be due to differences in nutrition and physical activity as well as to genetic factors.

Most of us who don't take hormones won't develop osteoporosis severely enough to cause fractures, and many women treated with hormones still experience fractures. There can be a similar amount of bone mass for women with and without osteoporosis, so that selecting appropriate subjects for preventive hormone therapy remains beyond the ability of medicine at this time.

Hormones as Treatment

Doctors do not agree on the advisability of *treating* osteoporosis with hormones, either. Some believe that since hormones cannot reverse the course of osteoporosis, they only expose women to unnecessary cancer risks without any obvious benefit. Moreover, there are now other treatment options available.

Both doctors I consulted advised me that the history of cancer in my family was so strong—breast cancer particularly—that it was better not to take estrogen for my osteoporosis. They said it was better to leave it alone, so I did. [a fifty-three-year-old woman]

One woman with osteoporosis decided reluctantly to take hormones:

I've had a bad back for a long time—I walk stooped over and I can't stand up straight . . . it's gotten worse, especially the pain. After I was advised by three doctors to take hormones I started on estrogen and progesterone to prevent further development of osteoporosis. Does it help the pain in my back? No. The disadvantage is that I got my periods again and that feels just awful. It isn't natural for an older woman like me to be having periods. I was really against taking hormones, but when the three doctors told me to I didn't give up on my skepticism, but I did stop resisting. [a seventy-six-year-old woman]

Hormones did not help her pain, but physical therapy might.

Another woman decided to participate in an experiment:

I'm short, slim, and light-skinned and worried because my mother developed osteoporosis. I'm willing to be part of a research project in which I'm taking calcium plus estrogen and progestin in such low doses that I do not have periods. [a fifty-five-year-old woman]

One physician warns that decisions about whether, when, and how much of what hormone to prescribe should be based on individual evaluations after a diagnosis of osteoporosis has been confirmed.[49] When we have osteoporosis, the most hormones can do is to help prevent further bone loss and keep our bones at the level they were when treatment started.

Women who should not take estrogens include those with a history of some kinds of cancer and breast cysts; high blood pressure; blood clots; atherosclerosis; strokes; kidney, liver, gallbladder, or heart disease; sickle-cell anemia or trait; asthma; epilepsy; uterine fibroids; endometriosis; adenomyosis; and vaginal bleeding that has not been diagnosed as due to a benign condition; and women who took DES during pregnancy. Though women who smoke are at high risk for osteoporosis, their use of estrogen further increases their risk of blood clots, heart disease, and stroke.

Women who have not had a hysterectomy and who take estrogens are advised to take progesterones to reduce the risk of endometrial cancer. **Be aware that the effects of long-term use of progesterone are not known.** Progestin can cause changes similar to those of diabetes, can unfavorably alter blood fats and so may increase the risk of heart disease and strokes, and may stimulate the growth of breast-cancer cells, which are more frequent in older women. Some brands of estrogens also include tranquilizers or testosterone. Some women taking hormone therapy experience nausea, water retention, weight gain, breast enlargement and tenderness, or depression.

If you have been on hormone therapy and decide to stop, consult your health-care provider on how to taper off. A sudden drop in hormones can cause hot flashes and other discomforts; a gradual drop may be more comfortable.

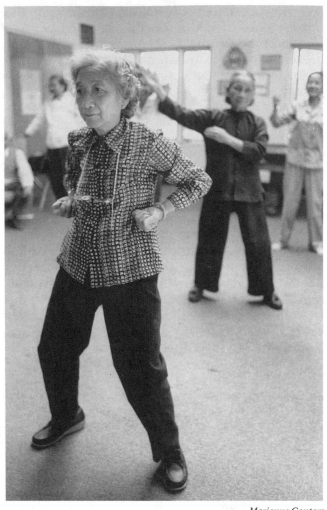

Marianne Gontarz

The Hormone Industry

When a condition has received as much publicity as osteoporosis has recently, there are enormous profits to be made by drug companies. Hormones are particularly profitable, and manufacturers are constantly seeking new markets. Wyeth-Ayerst Laboratories (now a subsidiary of American Home Products), manufacturer of the most commonly used estrogen (Premarin), aggressively advertises in magazines and medical journals and hired a public-relations firm in 1982 to run a massive public education campaign on osteoporosis.[50] This campaign has been very successful in making osteoporosis a popular subject for TV talk shows and magazine articles and has culminated in the passage of federal legislation for an annual Osteoporosis Awareness

Week. A carefully orchestrated campaign by the pharmaceutical industry presents hormones as the best defense against osteoporosis. Pharmaceutical companies and some physicians are advocating a return to an "estrogen forever" approach. This idea, however, is not supported by all members of the medical community.

By the year 2000 there will be 20 million of us over the age of sixty-five—a potentially lucrative market for hormones if we and our physicians can be convinced of the simplistic point of view that hormones are the best means for preventing and treating osteoporosis. It seems advisable, in light of the lack of information about the long-term effects of progestogen and the DES tragedy,* to look at these claims with a healthy degree of skepticism. We must strengthen our resistance to the promotion of hormones as a universal way to avoid or treat osteoporosis, yet at the same time be able to recognize when their benefits outweigh their known dangers. We can always change our nutritional and exercise patterns first before opting for chemical solutions.

The present debate over whether to prescribe hormones to prevent or treat osteoporosis will continue. We believe that it is unethical and medically unsound to prescribe hormones for all menopausal women. Instead, we support a public health campaign to prevent fractures by focusing on injury prevention, on osteoporosis prevention by reducing the number of unnecessary oophorectomies, by increasing women's knowledge of the risk factors, and by encouraging exercise, good nutrition, and avoiding or ending the habits of smoking and drinking excessive alcohol.

*DES (diethylstilbestrol), a synthetic form of estrogen, was prescribed for millions of women in the United States between 1941 and 1971 for many uses, including prevention of miscarriage. It was marketed under more than two hundred brand names in pills, injections, and suppositories. Although studies as early as the 1930s showed estrogen to be carcinogenic in laboratory animals and as early as 1953 showed that DES was ineffective in preventing miscarriage, the FDA did not warn against its use in pregnancy until 1971, after its link to cancer was established. It is still prescribed for other uses.

Women who took DES thought they were taking a wonder drug but are now, many years later, showing an increased incidence of cancers of the breast, uterus, cervix, and ovaries, and noncancerous tumors of the uterus. The daughters and sons of women who were given DES during pregnancy have suffered abnormal structural development in their uteruses and testes, abnormal and cancerous cells, and other problems, including fertility problems. By questioning the indiscriminate use of drugs and hormones, we can prevent similar medical mistakes from happening again. (See Cancer resources if you or your mother took or might have taken DES.)

Sodium Fluoride

Besides the small amounts of fluoride being added to the water supply, fluoride is also being used in higher doses experimentally to increase bone mass and lessen the chance of new fractures. One study found that a fluoride-calcium-vitamin D regimen helped hip-fracture patients prevent future fractures.[51] Other recent studies using fluorides showed increases in spinal bone density but decreases in forearm bone density and increases in nonspinal fractures.[52]

Fluoride is not approved as treatment by the FDA and should only be used to treat severe osteoporosis under careful supervision and be accompanied by a good nutrition and exercise program. Sensitivity to fluorides varies; some people experience nausea and vomiting, inflamed joints, and gastric pain and should not take them.

Bisphosphonates

Currently etidronate (Didronel) is the only bisphosphonate approved by the FDA for use in this country. Experience with it comes from its use in Paget's disease (the skeletal disease, not the breast cancer). It is absorbed into bone and prevents bone breakdown. But if given long enough or in high enough doses, it weakens bones, causing osteomalacia. To avoid this, it is given once daily by mouth for two weeks every three months. It seems to increase spinal bone density. It must be taken on an empty stomach, and very rarely causes stomach upset or diarrhea, which disappears when the drug is stopped.[53]

Calcitonin

Calcitonin is a hormone made by the thyroid gland that seems to block the bone breakdown that releases calcium into the blood and so increases the total body calcium content. Calcitonin is available as synthetic preparations of salmon and human forms. Both are expensive but the salmon form is more potent and less expensive. It is used unless someone has an intolerance or develops antibodies to it. In this country calcitonin is given as a daily or every-other-day injection under the skin. The nasal spray form used in Europe is not yet approved by the FDA and can only be used in a research project. Some people develop flushing, nausea, urinary urgency, and dizziness but these symptoms are minimized by starting with a low dose and increasing gradually. Usually the symptoms go away with continued use.[54]

NEW RESEARCH

Several new drugs are currently being studied for their effectiveness against osteoporosis. These include calcitriol (the body's working form of vitamin D), a synthetic parathyroid hormone, androgenic anabolic steroids (steroids that increase bone mass but cause masculinization and adverse effects on blood lipids), thiazides (diuretics that reduce the amount of calcium lost in the urine), more potent bisphosphonates, "ADFR" (a complex system of several drugs), and various drug combinations. Calcitriol and calcium (with or without calcitonin) show promise in slowing down corticosteroid-induced bone loss in the lumbar spine.[55] If your doctor offers you these drugs, you should know that their efficacy and safety have not yet been established. We urge an emphasis on life-style modifications to prevent bone loss and careful consideration of the judicious use of medications by an individual to prevent bone loss only if the benefits outweigh the risks associated with the use of that drug. We also stress the need for adequate long-term testing for safety and efficacy of any drugs before they are marketed.

LIVING WITH OSTEOPOROSIS

After I was told that I had osteoporosis, I slowly got my act together and began to realize that I, too, must help. I started reading about vitamins and calcium and had long talks with people who had gone the health-food route. I changed my diet. This, with walking up to one hour per day, gradually brought my health up to par. [a sixty-seven-year-old woman]

Many of the same steps that help us live with osteoporosis can help us prevent it. An exercise program as short as six months can reduce the risk of bone fractures. When we have osteoporosis, exercise must be vigorous enough to strengthen but not fracture the bones. Some exercise programs offer muscle-strengthening regimens and physical therapy in a swimming pool.[56]

Lifting can be hazardous and should be done with care. See page 268 for correct methods. For fractures of the spine that can cause a "dowager's hump," a back brace or support is sometimes fitted. It helps you to avoid strenuous bending, provides pain relief by supporting the spine, and reduces the degree of curvature. Long-term use, however, can weaken the very muscles that need strengthening. Exercises to strengthen the back muscles, increase flexibility, and encourage straighter posture are important. A firm mattress is helpful. Place plywood under a soft one, and put a foam pad or old soft quilt on top of a firm one for comfort.[57]

Now the osteoporosis means little to me. My doctor told me not to worry about it. He said, "You're going to have aches and pains as this thing progresses. Be careful but don't let it ruin your life." So I didn't. When I asked him about cross-country skiing and the awful falls I take, he asked, "Do you enjoy it?" And I said, "Yes, I do!" He said, "Then do anything you enjoy, and when it hurts, stop." I believe that I shouldn't let it interfere with my life-style. The only concession I made was when I decided to wait to do cross-country skiing until after my daughter's wedding. I want to be on both feet for the ceremony. [a sixty-year-old woman]

When I was eighty-two I fell down a flight of stairs and injured a vertebra and my hip, and I have pain in one leg. The doctor told me I had osteoporosis, which I had never heard of before. He gave me a lot of information about it. I developed it after being on thyroid medication for ten years. My doctor said there was no cure but we could arrest it. We had a long session about the alternatives. I decided to use exercise and nutrition. I walk at least three to four blocks a day. If the weather is bad I walk up and down the corridors of the apartment building. I use a set of exercises I learned at a course on aging and I do them every day. I have lost only a little height, am still very flexible and can touch my fingers to the floor. I drink four glasses of skim milk a day. I used to have a lot of salt but now I reduce it. I have red meat only one or two times a week. I'm a Southerner so I like to have collard greens and other vegetables. I'm still very active and belong to many organizations. [an eighty-six-year-old woman]

One of the best things you can do if you have osteoporosis is join an existing self-help group or start one with other middle-aged and older women. It is especially important to have a place to discuss what we read and hear about osteoporosis and the pros and cons of hormone therapy—outside the medical arena. As we tell each other about our experiences and feelings about living with osteoporosis, about ways to cope, treatments by physicians and/or self-help ideas, we start to feel less alone and we can help each other make desirable life-style changes.

Notes

1. Katie Maslow, "Concerns About the Availability of Accurate Public Information About Post-Menopausal Osteoporosis." U.S. Congress, Office of Technology Assessment. Prepared for the NIH Workshop on Menopause, March 22–24, 1993.
2. "Fast Facts on Osteoporosis." National Osteoporosis Foundation. Also the figure according to the American Academy of Orthopaedic Surgeons quoted by Judy Foreman, "Inroads Being Made Against Osteoporosis." *The Boston Globe*, Apr. 5, 1993, pp. 29, 32–33.
3. Julie E. Dunn, et al. "Mortality, Disability, and Falls in Older Persons: The Role of Underlying Disease and Disability." *American Journal of Public Health*, Vol. 82, No. 3 (March 1992), pp. 395–400.
4. Kathleen I. MacPherson, "Osteoporosis: The New Flaw in Woman or in Science?" *Health Values*, Vol. II, No. 4 (July/August 1987), pp. 57–62.
5. Diane M. Raab and Everett L. Smith, "Exercise and Aging Effects on Bone." *Topics in Geriatric Rehabilitation*, Vol. 1, No. 1 (October 1985), pp. 31–39.
6. A. Michael Parfit, "Definition of Osteoporosis: Age-Related Loss of Bone and Its Relationship to Increased Fracture Risk." Paper presented at the National Institutes of Health Consensus Development Conference on Osteoporosis, April 2–4, 1984. National Institutes of Health, Bethesda, MD.
7. Raab and Smith, op cit., p. 37.
8. Morris Notelovitz and Marsha Ware, *Stand Tall! The Informed Woman's Guide to Preventing Osteoporosis.* Gainesville, FL: Triad Publishing Co., 1982.
9. H. Okano, et al., "Effect of Menopause on Bone Loss in Japanese Women." Presented at the NIH Workshop on Menopause, March 22–24, 1993.
10. Suzanne C. Ho, et al., "Hip Fracture Rates in Hong Kong and the United States, 1988 Through 1989." *American Journal of Public Health*, Vol. 83, No. 5 (May 1993), pp. 694–97.
11. Mary E. Farmer, et al., "Race and Sex Differences in Hip Fracture Incidence." *American Journal of Public Health*, Vol. 74 (December 1984), pp. 1374–79.
12. Gary M. Chan, et al., "Decreased Bone Mineral Status in Lactating Adolescent Mothers." *The Journal of Pediatrics*, Vol. 101 (November 1982), pp. 767–70.
13. NIH recommendation quoted in American Academy of Orthopaedic Surgeons, *Calcium*, no date.
14. B. Lawrence Riggs and L. Joseph Melton, "The Prevention and Treatment of Osteoporosis." *The New England Journal of Medicine*, Vol. 327, No. 9 (Aug. 27, 1992), pp. 620–27; and "Letters to the Editor." Vol. 328, No. 1 (Jan. 7, 1993), pp. 65–66.
15. Notelovitz and Ware, op. cit., p. 93.
16. Judy Foreman, "Study, Anorectic Women May Have Osteoporosis." *The Boston Globe*, Dec. 20, 1984.
17. Betty Kamen and Si Kamen, *Osteoporosis: What It Is, How to Prevent It, How to Stop It.* New York: Pinnacle Books, 1984.
18. J. M. Aitken, et al., "Oestrogen Replacement Therapy for Prevention of Osteoporosis After Oophorectomy." *British Medical Journal*, Vol. 3 (1973), pp. 515+.
19. Notelovitz and Ware, op. cit., pp. 58, 73.
20. L. G. Raisy and B. E. Kream, "Regulation of Bone Formation, Part II." *The New England Journal of Medicine*, Vol. 309 (1983), pp. 83–89.
21. Kamen and Kamen, op. cit., p. 157.
22. Jane Porcino, *Growing Older, Getting Better: A Handbook for Women in the Second Half of Life.* New York: Crossroad Continuum, 1991, p. 233.
23. J. B. Lauritzen, M. M. Petersen, and B. Lund, "Effect of External Hip Protectors on Hip Fractures." *Lancet*, Vol. 341 (Jan. 2, 1993), pp. 11–13.
24. Douglas P. Kiel, et al., "Caffeine and the Risk of Hip Fracture: The Framingham Study." *American Journal of Epidemiology*, Vol. 132, No. 4 (1990), pp. 675–84.
25. John A. Baron, "Smoking and Estrogen-Related Disease." *American Journal of Epidemiology*, Vol. 119, No. 1 (1984), pp. 9–22.
26. J. Chalmers and K. C. Ho, "Geographical Variations in Senile Osteoporosis: The Association with Physical Activity." *Journal of Bone and Joint Surgery*, Vol. 52B (1970), pp. 667–78.
27. Fran Pollner, "Osteoporosis: Looking at the Whole Picture." *Medical World News*, Vol. 14 (January 1985), pp. 38–58.
28. Belinda Lees, et al. "Differences in Proximal Femur Bone Density Over Two Centuries." *Lancet*, Vol. 341, No. 8846 (March 13, 1993), pp. 673–75.
29. D. S. Bernstein, N. Sadowsky, D. M. Hegsted, et al., "Prevalence of Osteoporosis in High and Low Fluoride Areas in North Dakota." *Journal of the American Medical Association*, Vol. 196 (1966), pp. 85–90; O. Laitinen and O. Simonen, "Does Fluoridation of Drinking Water Prevent Bone Fragility and Osteoporosis?" *Lancet*, Vol. II, No. 8452 (Aug. 24, 1985), pp. 432–34.
30. S. L. Gordon and S. B. Corbin, "Summary of Workshop on Drinking Water Fluoride Influence on Hip Fracture on Bone Health." *Osteoporosis International*, Vol. 2 (1992), pp. 109–17.
31. *Fluoridation, Nature's Tooth Protector.* Division of Dental Health, Massachusetts Department of Public Health, January 1986.
32. Lauritzen, Petersen, and Lund, op. cit., p. 13.
33. National Institute on Aging, *Age Page: Preventing Falls and Fractures*, 1992.
34. Kathleen I. MacPherson, "Osteoporosis and Menopause: A Feminist Analysis of the Social Construction of a Syndrome." *Advances in Nursing Science*, Vol. 7 (July 1985), pp. 11–22.
35. Sydney Wolfe, E. Borgmann, C. Lacheen, et al., Statement of Public Citizens Health Research Group. Read before the National Institutes of Health Consensus Development Conference on Osteoporosis, Bethesda, MD, April 2–4, 1984.
36. Notelovitz and Ware, op. cit., p. 32.
37. Pollner, op. cit.
38. Harry W. Daniel, "Post-menopausal Tooth Loss: Contributions to Edentulism by Osteoporosis and Cigarette Smoking." *Archives of Internal Medicine*, Vol. 143 (September 1983), pp. 1678–82.
39. Product Reports, "Osteoporosis Diagnostic Centers Multiplying Rapidly." *Hospitals*, Vol. 59 (May 1985), p. 126.
40. D. M. Black, et al., "Axial and Appendicular Bone

Density Predict Fractures in Older Women." *Journal of Bone and Mineral Research*, Vol. 7 (1992), pp. 633–68.

41. National Institutes of Health, *Osteoporosis Consensus Development Conference Statement*, Vol. 5, No. 3. Washington, D.C.: U.S. Department of Health and Human Services, Office of Medical Applications of Research, 1984.

42. Pollner, op. cit.

43. Robert Lindsay, et al., "Bone Response to Termination of Oestrogen Treatment." *Lancet*, Vol. 1 (1978), pp. 1325+.

44. One physician advises others not to "get bogged down with fancy tests, most of which aren't sensitive enough anyway," and just to increase the quality of life for midlife women by prescribing hormones. Pollner, op. cit.

45. Wolfe, et al., op. cit.

46. Patricia Kaufert and Sonja McKinlay, "Estrogen Replacement Therapy: The Production of Medical Knowledge and the Emergence of Policy." In Ellen Lewin and Virginia Olesen, eds., *Women, Health and Healing*. New York: Tavistock Publications, 1985, pp. 113–38.

47. Robert Lindsay, et. al., "Long-term Prevention of Post-menopausal Osteoporosis by Estrogen," *Lancet*, Vol. 1, No. 7968 (May 15, 1976), pp. 1038+; and S. Meema et. al., "Preventive Effect of Estrogen on Post-menopausal Bone Loss." *Annals of Internal Medicine*, Vol. 135 (1976), pp. 1436–40.

48. Chalmers and Ho, op. cit., pp. 667–75.

49. Herta Spencer, "Osteoporosis: Goals of Therapy." *Hospital Practice*, Vol. 17, No. 3 (March 1982), pp. 132–51.

50. Tacie Dejanikus, "Major Drug Manufacturer Funds Osteoporosis Public Education Campaign." *The Network News* (Publication of the National Women's Health Network), May/June 1985, p. 1.

51. Pollner, op. cit.

52. B. L. Riggs, et al., "Effect of Fluoride Treatment on the Fracture Rate in Postmenopausal Women with Osteoporosis." *The New England Journal of Medicine*, Vol. 2 (1992), pp. 109–17.

53. T. Storm, et al., "Long-term Treatment with Intermittent Cyclical Etidronate: Effect on Bone Mass and Fracture Rate"; and C. H. Chestnut, III, et al., "Etidronate Cyclical Therapy for Treatment of Postmenopausal Osteoporosis: 4 Year Experience," *Journal of Bone and Mineral Research*, Vol. 7 Suppl. (1991), pp. S117, S143.

54. K. Overgaard, et al., "Effect of Calcitonin Given Intranasally on Bone Mass and Fracture Rates in Established Osteoporosis: A Dose-Response Study." *British Medical Journal*, Vol. 305 (1992), pp. 556–61.

55. Philip Sambrook, et al., "Prevention of Corticosteroid Osteoporosis: A Comparison of Calcium, Calcitriol, and Calcitonin." *The New England Journal of Medicine*, Vol. 328, No. 24 (June 17, 1993), pp. 1747–52; and "Is Steroid-Induced Osteoporosis Preventable?," pp. 1781–82.

56. Joseph Lane, "Postmenopausal Osteoporosis: The Orthopedic Approach." *The Female Patient*, Vol. 6 (November 1981), pp. 43–45, 49–50, 54.

57. Suggestions taken from "Strategies for Persons with Osteoporosis: After the Vertebral Fracture." *The Osteoporosis Report*, Vol. 9, No. 1 (Spring 1993), pp. 8–10.

20

DENTAL HEALTH

✦

BY MARTHA C. WOOD

1994 UPDATE BY MARTHA C. WOOD

RESOURCES FOR THIS CHAPTER ON PAGES 491–92

Dental health is important not only in itself but also for total health and well-being. Yet, although we are among the wealthiest nations in the world, 98 percent of American adults have caries (dental decay or cavities) and periodontal (gum and bone) disease.[1] One fourth of all Americans over age forty-five and 41 percent over the age of sixty-five are missing all their natural teeth.[2] Many people believe that tooth loss is a natural part of aging, but this is not the case.

Prevention of dental disease involves self-care and regular visits to a dentist or dental clinic. Having good dental health can help prevent a whole range of potentially debilitating and isolating conditions among older people. Continual tooth pain saps our energy and can distract us for days and weeks at a time. Tooth loss can prevent us from eating well if we don't learn to substitute nutritious soft foods for those we can no longer chew. If we are embarrassed about our appearance, we may avoid going out. We may avoid smiling and speaking, and we may feel awkward.

FOUR IMPORTANT RULES FOR GOOD ORAL HEALTH ARE:

- Brush your teeth after you eat anything and floss daily.
- Eat well and drink fluoridated water when possible.
- Schedule regular visits to a dental office for cleaning and checkups (even if you have dentures).
- Keep your natural teeth—avoid dentists who are quick to extract teeth (get a second opinion).

Many people, especially older people, never get the dental care they need because it is expensive. Despite the fact that chronic dental problems increase with age, more than half the U.S. population over sixty-five has not been to a dentist in at least five years or has never been to one.[3] Most of us expect that once we are over sixty-five, Medicare will cover all of our health-care needs, but we learn that quite a number of things aren't covered, among them dental-care problems.

Medical insurance should include dental coverage. We need a Medicare program and a national health-insurance program that recognizes the importance of and provides for dental care. Dental care should not be a commodity available only to those who can afford to pay for it. For some of us, raising the money to pay for needed dental care can be a major triumph.

Yesterday I got three brand new teeth—a permanent bridge; and I am as excited as when I awaited the tooth fairy at age five. They are crafted to match my original long, strong, yellow teeth, and since they hit my bottom teeth I can chew even better than with the originals.

They embody my new dedication to taking care of myself. I made the decision to save the surrounding teeth. And I alone paid for those three expensive additions to my upper right jaw.

What seems to make them most special is the fact that I am the only person who can see them. They are the three last teeth on the upper right; I can admire them in the mirror only when I pull my cheek back. They are my own special gift to me. [a fifty-seven-year-old woman][4]

Special Dental Problems of Older Women

The risk of losing teeth increases as we age, and women have higher rates of tooth loss than men.[5] Older white women have a higher rate of tooth loss than white men or black women of the same age. Yet white women practice more careful dental hygiene than white men and have lower rates of periodontal disease than black women. For these reasons, some researchers have begun to suspect that postmenopausal bone loss may be a factor in tooth loss for older white women.[6] Paying attention to prevention of osteoporosis, especially by not smoking and by getting enough calcium and fluoride, may have the added benefit of protecting us against losing teeth in our older years. Also, there are more than four hundred common medications that have effects on dental health.

Home Care for Teeth and Gums

Many of us were not taught as children to take proper care of our teeth and gums. The idea of preventive dental care dates back only to the 1950s in the United States. A seventy-eight-year-old woman remembered her father calling tooth brushing a thing "only sissies do."

Many dentists believe that an individual's careful attention to diet and self-care will do more to prevent tooth problems than the best professional care.[7] Proper tooth brushing and flossing are essential parts of this. Ideally, brushing should be done after every meal but not less than twice a day and flossing at least once a day, preferably at night. A machine that directs a stream of water to the gumline can be a helpful adjunct but does not replace brushing and flossing.

Tooth-brushing guidelines have changed over the years. Now the preferred method is to use a brush with soft, rounded nylon bristles. (Natural bristles act as a bacteria reservoir because they take too long to dry.) Hold the brush alongside the teeth at about a forty-five-degree angle against the gumline, wiggle it in a circular motion and then brush away from the gum.[8] Move the brush back and forth several times, using a gentle scrubbing motion. On the biting surfaces of the teeth, again use a back-and-forth motion. If you can't grasp a toothbrush easily, try wrapping it with adhesive tape or something like a sponge hair curler to enlarge the handle. If you have shoulder problems that make it hard to brush, try an electric toothbrush or extend the length of your toothbrush by gluing a strip of wood or plastic to the handle. Replace your toothbrush when it wears out (after about six months or sooner if bristles begin to spread) and after each time you have a cold or flu.

A mild, only slightly abrasive commercial toothpaste with fluoride is best for the teeth. Baking soda can be used, but don't brush with salt because salt damages the surface enamel of the teeth. Brush your tongue and the roof of your mouth, too. Bacteria collect on the tongue and then spread to the teeth. Plaque—the sticky, colorless layer of bacteria that forms around the teeth and along the gumline—often forms more quickly and in larger amounts because of reduced saliva flow as we age. (Saliva production is part of the mouth's cleaning process.) After brushing, rinse your mouth with warm water.

Floss between all teeth. Start with an 18-inch piece of floss. Wrap the ends of the floss around the third finger of each hand. Use your thumbs and forefingers to guide about 1 inch of floss at a time between the teeth. Holding the floss tightly, gently insert it to the gumline. Curve the floss against one tooth in a C-shape and gently rub up and down the whole height of the tooth side. Repeat on each adjacent tooth. In case you have trouble holding the floss, dental-floss holders are available at most drugstores. Or you might try cutting a 12-inch length and tying the ends together to form a circle. You can have someone prepare these for you if you have trouble tying the knots. If you haven't been flossing regularly, your gums will probably bleed when you start but will stop bleeding after a few days.

I hate to floss, but I've had a lot of gum problems and the dentist says I must floss. I've found it's more pleasant to do in the tub. [a fifty-four-year-old woman]

Dentures

If you have dentures, you should brush them with a soft brush. Soaking dentures, even in a denture cleanser, is never enough. Dentures must be brushed with a commercial denture powder or paste, hand soap, or baking soda. Never use scouring powders, as they damage the denture. Fill a sink about one third full of water and place a washcloth on the bottom to prevent damage in case you drop the denture. Hold the denture over the water while brushing and brush thoroughly both inside and out. Rinse with cool water (never hot) before putting the dentures back in your mouth. Dentures should never become dry, because they may crack or warp. When they're not in your mouth, immerse them in water. To remove stains from full dentures, soak them overnight in a commercial denture cleanser or a combination of bleach and water (1 teaspoon chlorine bleach to 8 ounces warm water). Never use bleach alone, as it can change the color of the pink base of the denture, and never use bleach at all on a partial denture, as it may harm the metal clasp. To remove stains from partial dentures, soak them in white vinegar or a commercial denture cleanser.

Dentures should be relined when they start to slip. The reason for the slippage can then be determined and the soft tissue checked for damage. Relining and other denture adjustments or repairs may be cheaper at a dental school than by your regular dentist. Denture adhesives are not very effective and should be used for a limited time only. The denture will still wiggle, and this cuts the inside of the mouth and interferes with chewing. Overusing adhesive powders can irritate the gums and soft tissue in the roof of the mouth.

It is important to wear dentures regularly. If you don't wear them for a few weeks, the shape of your mouth will start to change and the dentures won't fit. The tissues will then have a hard time readjusting to the old set of dentures. And if you don't wear your dentures, you are less likely to eat a nutritionally balanced diet, since you won't be able to chew properly. Make sure you massage and brush your gums and the roof of your mouth daily with a soft toothbrush or washcloth.

Denture problems may be caused by poorly made or poorly fitting dentures, not enough mouth tissue to cushion the fit, or even emotional upsets—or a combination of these factors.

I've had false teeth for over twenty years—a full upper plate and a partial on the bottom. I still see my dentist three times a year, since I have periodontal problems with my few remaining teeth and want to keep them at all costs. I have my dentures adjusted almost every time I see my dentist because my mouth tissue keeps changing. No one told me about bone reabsorption when I got my dentures. I've had three dentures made over time and both of the first two relined. Your jawbone just naturally gets narrower and shorter as you get older, though I think having your teeth pulled makes it happen more so. My current dentist is terrific and I can eat raw carrots, apples, and anything I want. But I expect to live another thirty-five years and I worry about whether I'll have enough bone left for my teeth.

My dentist says I should leave my dentures out at night to give my mouth tissue a rest. He may be right, but I don't feel self-confident—and certainly not sexy—without my teeth.

There are times I can't wear my partial for days due to soreness on my gums, not just from cuts but from when I have the flu or am under stress at work. My gums react and are extremely painful. [a fifty-one-year-old woman]

If you leave your dentures in while you sleep, be sure to remove them for some time each day to let the tissues in your mouth repair. Partial dentures increase plaque formation, so remove partial dentures each day and thoroughly clean the remaining teeth.

Dental Implants

The use of dental implants increased 73 percent between 1986 and 1990.[9] These implants are attached to the tissues or bone and once in place "you don't think about their not being real," one woman noted. The dentist must follow the implant closely for several months. A failed implant may be painful, may have to be replaced, and may lead to infection. Choose a dentist who has completed at least 300 hours of training in implantology. Implants are more costly than dentures and are not covered by insurance, although insurance should pay for extracting the teeth and for the required bridges.

Mouthwashes

Mouthwashes, lozenges, and toothpaste can't cure bad breath. They only cover it up for a brief period of time. Warm, salty water is the best mouthwash. Persistent bad breath may be a sign of a medical or dental problem that needs attention, such as postnasal drip, digestive problems, diabetes, gum disease, or badly decayed teeth. It may also be caused by medicines or smoking.

Dry Mouth

If your mouth feels dry, you should discuss the problem with a doctor. A slight decrease in saliva may occur as we grow older, but frequently dry mouth (xerostomia) is caused by prescription or over-the-counter drugs. More than two hundred medications, including antihistamines, decongestants, diuretics, and some drugs used to treat Parkinson's disease, ulcers, and cancer can cause dry mouth. In addition, smoking dries and irritates the mouth. Caffeine and alcohol both have dehydrating effects. Thus, the proper treatment may be as simple as rinsing with a saltwater solution several times a day or avoiding very spicy foods. In some cases an artificial saliva may be prescribed. Dry mouth can also be caused by a blocked saliva gland. Because saliva is essential for a healthy mouth, not taking care of dry mouth can lead to tissue breakdown, tooth decay, gum disease, and ill-fitting dentures.

Nutrition

Good nutrition is an important factor in keeping teeth and gums healthy. Here are some pointers to keep in mind:

- Among the many good reasons to eat protein are that it doesn't form plaque and that it builds and repairs mouth tissue.
- Eating fiber helps to remove food particles trapped between the teeth (chewing gum won't do this).
- Sugar plays a major role in causing cavities so keep the use of table sugar low, and watch for hidden sugars in such things as ketchup and lunch meats.
- If you do eat sweets, eat them with meals rather than in between. Acid produced from the bacteria formed by food particles eats into tooth enamel. The more often you eat decay-promoting foods, the more "acid attacks" the teeth suffer.
- The longer sugar is in the mouth the more chance the bacteria have to produce destructive acid, so avoid hard candy, cough drops, or anything else that is high in sugar and is sucked or chewed for a while. Foods like raisins and honey stick to the teeth and so remain in the mouth a long time.
- As we grow older we need more vitamins C, A, and B complex, as well as calcium. Vitamin C helps with healthy gums and tissue repair. Vitamin A keeps tissue soft. Vitamin B complex prevents tissues in the corner of the mouth from breaking down and also prevents sore tongue and other mouth sores.[10] Calcium strengthens the bones that support the structure of the mouth. Try to get these vitamins and calcium by eating healthful foods.

Dental Checkups

It's important to have regular dental checkups that include a thorough cleaning. Someone with severe gum disease or diabetes should have a cleaning every three months. For most of us, twice a year is best. Only a dentist or hygienist, using special instruments, can remove hardened plaque, also called *calculus* or *tartar*, from the teeth. It is also important to have your gums examined regularly. You need regular dental checkups even if you have full dentures.

If you don't have a dentist, ask a friend, call a dental school, or ask your physician for a referral. (Dental societies or associations merely recommend from a list with no preference to quality.) If you can't afford a private dentist, ask your community health department about dental clinics in your area. These may be affiliated with a dental school, a dental hygienist school, or a low-cost medical clinic.

A dentist should take a thorough medical and dental history. Make sure she or he offers emergency care. Avoid dentists who won't talk to you about fees, give estimates, itemize bills, or discuss a payment plan. (However, prompt payment keeps fees down, since billing costs money.) Beware of exceptionally low fees, as they may indicate a dentist who cuts corners on laboratory costs. Compare your dentist's fees with those of your friends' dentists. Interview a prospective dentist to make sure she or he is someone with whom you can feel comfortable.

Avoid dentists who want to extract teeth without discussing alternatives. There is almost always some way to save a tooth, and it is almost always to your advantage to do so. Saving a tooth or teeth is usually the healthiest and most economical thing to do in the long run. Six million teeth are removed unnecessarily each year. False teeth just can't do what natural teeth can. Some people are unable to wear dentures comfortably because of the shape of their mouths—a sad fact often not discovered until it is too late. Be sure to get a second opinion, not only about the need for extraction but about your ability to wear dentures. Sometimes pulling a tooth is necessary, but if that is the case a space saver must be fitted permanently into its place so the entire jaw structure doesn't shift.

Don't allow any dental work to be done without getting a full explanation of what it is, the amount of discomfort likely, other possible treatments, the consequences of postponing treatment a few weeks or months, and potential complications. Get a written cost estimate, and never be embarrassed to obtain a second opinion.

Because of a severe toothache I sought a dentist in the state where I spend half the year. He said an artificial tooth on a bridge had to be taken out, extensive gum surgery was needed, and then a replacement would have to be fitted. The estimated cost was very high. I took my X rays with me to seek another opinion. Meanwhile, the tooth holding the artificial tooth broke and fell out with the bridge.

I went to the dentist I have used for many years in the state where I spend the other half a year. He explained how he would grind down the broken tooth and fit in two artificial teeth, and drew a picture for me. He recommended that I have my teeth cleaned twice a year instead of once a year and that I floss regularly. He did not think I needed gum surgery. He encouraged me to check his price, saying that I would find some prices higher than his and some lower. I checked with a dental school and another clinic for their prices and for the way he was proposing to do the work. The estimated price was lower if students did the work or if other materials were used. I decided to have him do the work because he has treated me well through the years and explains everything clearly. The total cost will be much less than that quoted by the first dentist. Now I floss every night while I watch TV. [a seventy-six-year-old woman]

X Rays

X rays are used to detect abscesses or underlying decay, broken tooth roots, bone loss from periodontal disease, and ill-fitting dental restorations. Full-mouth X rays as part of a regular checkup aren't necessary more often than every three to five years. Bite-wing X rays, taken with the film holder held between the teeth, may be taken yearly—a clinical exam will not always find cavities between the back teeth and under fillings. X rays are usually necessary when a problem is suspected. While X rays are being done, your neck and body should be covered with a lead apron. Legally your X rays belong to you, not to the dentist. Take them with you if you change dentists so you don't have to have them done again unnecessarily.

Dental Decay

Cavities (caries) can form at any age. As we age we are more susceptible to root caries (60 percent of persons sixty-five and older have root caries). Drinking fluoridated water reduces cavities in adults by 50 percent and contributes to stronger bones, thus reducing the possibility of fractures from osteoporosis.[11] Some evidence is emerging that very small cavities can actually be remineralized—that is, the tooth can rebuild itself—if we drink fluoridated water.[12]

Having work done on a root canal is one way to save a tooth when the nerve of the tooth is infected. In a root-canal procedure, the nerve within the tooth is removed, and the nerve canal is cleaned and filled. The tooth can remain healthy and structurally sound. There is an alternative to root-canal work, which can be used if decay has reached but not infected the tooth's nerve. In this option, a lining is placed over the nerve before the tooth is filled.

A crown is a cap or jacket over the stump of a tooth. It is used to support a badly decayed tooth, for cosmetic purposes, or to anchor a fixed bridge. The dentist grinds the natural tooth to a stump, caps it with pure gold or gold mixed with other metals, and sometimes covers it with porcelain. (The all-gold is the most expensive but less durable than other materials.) If your dentist suggests crowning a decayed tooth and you can't afford it, ask about having a filling with reinforcing pins, which should cost much less.

Periodontal Disease

Periodontal disease is actually a group of diseases involving the gums and the supporting bones under the teeth in an infective process. Older people have more periodontal disease than previously reported. A recent study showed that 56 percent of people over age seventy had severe periodontal disease—more than twice the amount previously reported.[13] Gingivitis (surface inflammation of the gums caused by irritants) is a risk factor but does not always develop into periodontitis (inflammation or infection of the bone).[14]

Plaque is the most common cause of periodontal disease. Other causes include grinding or clenching teeth, a bite that doesn't fit together (malocclusion), or an irregular jaw configuration. In addition, hereditary predisposition, hormonal imbalances, diabetes, and thyroid problems may worsen gum problems, since they impair the body's defense against disease.

The symptoms of periodontal disease include red gums, swollen gums, bleeding, loose teeth, and drifting teeth. It may be painless and often involves no bleeding. Only a dentist or hygienist can detect it in its early stages. Prevention of the disease begins with proper brushing and flossing. If it is caught early enough, treatment involves root planing or smoothing, scraping under the gum, and, if needed, prescription antibacterial mouthwash. In more advanced cases, where the disease has caused deep pocketing, treatment becomes more complex. Most surgical procedures are done in a dental office or, depending on the extent, in a hospital. A local anesthetic is used and a medical dressing is placed over the wounded area for a week or so while it heals.

I had gum surgery around two teeth and then two other surgeons recommended more gum surgery. Instead I've followed my dentist's suggestion to brush with a soft brush or ADA-approved electric brush, floss, use a fluoride rinse, and have my teeth cleaned, including minimal scaling, three times a year instead of the usual two. My gums are fine. [a sixty-one-year-old woman]

Since the late 1970s a nonsurgical treatment, the Keyes technique, has been used by some periodontists. This technique combines deep scaling and antibacterial agents applied by the dentist plus a special paste treatment used at home daily. Baking soda and peroxide toothpastes are a commercial variation of the special paste. The technique is a respected conservative treatment that does not replace surgery but can be tried first. (See Resources for this chapter.)

SMOKING

Smoking and using snuff or chewing tobacco can damage the tissues of the mouth, increase the risk of oral or nasal cancer, stain the teeth, and cause bad breath. Anyone who uses a tobacco product should see a dentist or hygienist frequently—at the very least once a year but twice a year is best. Smoking can also cause dryness in the mouth, resulting in chewing and swallowing problems as well as tissue damage and tooth decay.

DENTAL CARE IN NURSING HOMES AND HOSPITALS

People in nursing homes have special dental-care concerns. Although they need regular dental exams, their dental care is often neglected. Even in states that require nursing homes to have a dental consultant, the homes may have difficulty finding dentists who accept Medicaid, who have portable equipment, and who have offices accessible to people who can't climb stairs.

A frequent problem in hospitals and nursing homes is loss of dentures. A few states have passed legislation requiring that all false teeth be marked with the owner's name when they are made or relined. There are also other ways of marking dentures, even in a nursing home, ranging from etching to simply writing the name in ink and covering it with a clear acrylic finish. Dentures should be identified with the wearer's name (not a number or code) so they can be returned to the correct person quickly.

NOTES

1. "Teeth." *Health Facts*, Vol. II, No. 10 (July–August 1978).
2. Marvin Glasser, Keynote: Proceedings from National Consortium meeting, January 7–9, 1992.
3. Jane Porcino, *Growing Older, Getting Better.* New York: Crossroad Continuum, 1991, p. 312.
4. Excerpted from an unpublished manuscript by Carolyn Ruth Swift.
5. Ronald J. Hunt, et al., "Edentulism and Oral Health Problems Among Elderly Rural Iowans: The Iowa 65+ Rural Health Study." *American Journal of Public Health*, Vol. 75, No. 10 (1985), pp. 1177–82.
6. Harry W. Daniell, "Postmenopausal Tooth Loss: Contributions to Edentulism by Osteoporosis and Cigarette Smoking." *Archives of General Medicine*, Vol. 143 (September 1983), pp. 1678–82.
7. *Health Facts*, p. 4.
8. Ibid.
9. Naomi Stillman and Chester W. Douglass, "The

Developing Market for Dental Implants." *Journal of the American Dental Association,* Vol. 124, (April 1993), pp. 51–56.

10. Maury Massler, "Oral Aspects of Aging." *Postgraduate Medicine,* Vol. 49 (January 1971), pp. 179–83.

11. O. Simonen and O. Laitinen, "Does Fluoridation of Drinking Water Prevent Bone Fragility and Osteoporosis?" *Lancet,* Vol. II, No. 8452 (Aug. 24, 1985), pp. 432–34.

12. National Institutes of Health, *Challenges for the Eighties.* National Institute of Dental Research Long-Range Research Plan 1985–89. U.S. Department of Health and Human Services, Public Health Service, December 1983, NIH Publication No. 85-860, pp. 2, 19.

13. Chester W. Douglass et al., "Oral Health Status of the Elderly in New England." *Journal of Gerontology,* Vol. 48, No. 2 (1993), pp. M39–M46.

14. Steven Shepherd, "Brushing Up on Gum Disease." *FDA Consumer,* Vol. 24, No. 4 (May 1990), pp. 9–10.

21

URINARY INCONTINENCE

✦

BY NORMA MERAS SWENSON AND DIANA LASKIN SIEGAL

SPECIAL THANKS TO GRACE Q. VICARY AND MARY D. FILLMORE

1994 UPDATE BY DIANA LASKIN SIEGAL WITH SPECIAL THANKS TO CATHERINE DUBEAU

RESOURCES FOR THIS CHAPTER ON PAGES 492–93

Urinary incontinence, the involuntary loss of urine, is a common problem among women, and yet we are ashamed to talk about it. The barrier to discussion is only one of the obstacles to finding satisfactory solutions. We also have to deal with professionals who do not keep current with new advances and with the myth that only surgery helps. Many of us have arrived at adulthood and even old age without ever receiving adequate, accurate information about our bodies and how they work.

Bladder-control problems should not be looked upon either as an inevitable part of aging or as a disease, but rather as a problem that can be managed and possibly corrected if you are determined to do so. Shame, guilt, anxiety, fear, embarrassment, loss of self-esteem, and depression are common, understandable accompaniments to this problem but only make matters worse if they contribute to inaction. Finding the courage to take action is an important step in regaining self-confidence. Realize that you are not alone, and that many other women are finding ways to escape the prison that incontinence problems impose. Be aware that about 30 percent of incontinence is temporary.

Current figures show that up to 30 percent of women sixty-five years of age and older living in the community report bladder-control problems. Over 50 percent of all those in long-term-care institutions, mainly nursing homes, have urinary incontinence problems.[1] These problems may have contributed to the reasons for their admission to the nursing home. Cost estimates for dealing with this problem in nursing homes are $3.3 billion annually, more than half of which comes from public funds.[2] The cost for the care of the incontinent elderly in all institutions is estimated at over $8 billion per year.[3] Many of these people could be helped through timely evaluations and care if more staff were hired and trained in behavior modification, medication, surgical treatment, or some combination of these techniques. Since women compose the majority of the elderly and the overwhelming majority of the nursing-home population, bladder-control problems are a major public health issue for women.

Only about 15 percent of all the incontinent elderly are institutionalized.[4] More elderly incontinent men are cared for outside of institutions, with the direct, unpaid burden of caring for them falling, in the majority of the cases, on female caregivers in the home. In other words, whether we have the problem or whether we care for those who have it, incontinence is overwhelmingly a women's problem. The good news is that increasing attention, more accurate diagnosis, and more appropriate treatment are resulting in complete cure or great improvement in about two thirds of those with the problem.[5]

Women apparently suffer from bladder-control difficulties far more than men, both in number (approximately two to one) and in degree of severity, and the difficulties increase with each decade of age. These facts tend to reinforce the belief that incontinence is an inevitable accompaniment of female aging, yet fail to explain why some elderly women have the problem and others don't. The problem is underreported. Many women are too embarrassed to speak about the problem, especially to a male physician; others don't speak about it because they believe nothing can be done. Most physicians never ask about bladder control. Sadly, many women who have had the courage to bring it up have found their doctors uninformed, unsympathetic, and often embarrassed themselves.

We hope this chapter will help you know more about how your body functions, what the different types of incontinence are, what you can do about bladder-control problems for yourself or for others, and how to find competent help. Fortunately, new materials are available to help us deal with these problems and to educate health providers to assist us better (see Resources for this chapter).

CONTROL OF OUR SOCIAL LIVES

One of the very first ways we learn as little girls that we are different from boys is that if we can't "go" in some places, we can't "go" at all. Girls may be restricted from certain places or events because there are no toilets. It's usually okay for little boys to simply turn around, discreetly or otherwise, and pee if there isn't a toilet nearby, but it isn't always okay for little girls.

At a festival by the river in Cambridge, the nearest public toilets are several blocks away. I overheard a little girl about five years old say she needed to "go." She was then scolded by the man who appeared to be her grandfather. "Didn't you go before you left the house?" and all that. Because I have incontinence problems, I stepped in and asked whether he would just take a little boy over to the bushes. When he responded, "Yes, of course," I suggested he take the little girl there also. He was embarrassed but then the girl's grandmother, who had been sitting nearby, offered to take her. [a woman in her sixties]

Bladder control can be difficult for young girls to learn, and for women to maintain, because while we are being taught to control our bladders and anal sphincters we are also being taught that "nice" girls do *not* feel or experiment with anything "down there," especially with the nearby sensations coming from our clitorises, vulvas, and vaginas.

When we are aware of our bladder sensations we are often required to ignore them. Many of us remember when times to go to the bathroom were strictly regulated in schools. Adult women are also restricted in where they can urinate. There are usually few public toilets in shopping malls, none in grocery stores and subways, and not enough in sports arenas and theaters, forcing women to brave bars and other places they may not want to enter just to find a toilet. Public toilets are often so filthy and unsafe that women can't use them.

At the Montreal Olympics I passed the time while waiting in the long lines for the ladies' room by counting the number of men and women leaving the toilets. I observed that the men's line moved four times faster than the women's line. Architects should take that into consideration when designing rest rooms. [a woman in her fifties]

Many workplaces still have inadequate toilet facilities for female employees. In rural areas where migrant workers are employed, often there are no toilet facilities whatsoever, and women sometimes feel they have to wait until dark to pee, trying to "hold it" hour after hour.

Even where toilets are available, women may have to sit hour after hour doing clerical work, with little chance to walk around or get other exercise. When there is a chance to take a break, that, too, is often spent sitting. Sitting is very destructive to the abdominal, pelvic, and back muscles. All of these situations can contribute to bladder problems by forcing women to hold urine, which overstretches the bladder, and by weakening muscles. These conditions may in turn lead to chronic infections, cystitis, and bladder-control problems.

Our ability to manage our urine actually controls our social life far more than we realize. Finding a bathroom is a constant worry for many women, young and old. To lose urine, to wet one's pants visibly, or to smell of urine is simply unacceptable. Not only would we give offense, but we might be thought of as not fully adult—childish, regressed, or even "senile." We all try to learn how to "hold it," often longer than we should, without realizing that doing so may contribute to infections from urine retention. If the anxiety about making it to a toilet in time is too distracting, we may decide not to attempt errands and trips, or only do so after we know exactly where the bathroom is and are sure we can be near it. We may resort to pads, or "adult diapers," now widely advertised, rather than tell anybody. In many cases of incontinence, women feel obliged to withdraw from social life altogether, not going out and often not having people in, either. Use pads and other aids temporarily, if necessary, rather than avoiding people and activities, but do not assume that nothing can be done about incontinence.

An older person's inability to control urine is often the last straw for an overstressed caregiver, and institutionalization often becomes the solution. Pads are often used in place of adequate evaluation and treatment, especially in nursing homes with overworked and undertrained staff. What is labeled incontinence is often ignoring a patient's request for a bedpan or toilet until she has no choice except to wet herself.

HOW BLADDER CONTROL WORKS

As shocking as it is, even experts know little about the basic anatomy and physiology of the female genitourinary system, as the female genitals and urinary tract together are called. The classic text, *Gray's Anatomy,* devotes several pages to the male genitals and urinary tract but only one sketch to the female urinary system. Most doctors see the female urinary system as an inadequate or defective variation on the male system, rather than as a complex system in its own right. Following is a summary of what experts believe about how the female genitourinary system works.

Urine comes down two tubes called ureters (one from each kidney) to fill the bladder. The bladder and the urethra (the tube opening from the bladder to the outside) constitute a unit for the purpose of storing and emptying urine. Normally, the bladder relaxes while it is filling with urine and the urethra tightens along its whole length from where it joins the bladder neck down to the outside opening, in order to hold urine in. When it is time to pee, the urethra opens along its entire length, and the top of the bladder (the fundus) contracts, expelling the urine. The urethra then closes along its entire length and the whole bladder again relaxes.

The anus has a true sphincter musculature that is capable of closing off completely in response to a conscious act of will. The vagina never closes off completely. The neck of the bladder and the area near the opening of the urethra have some muscle tissue, but not like the anal sphincter. The urinary structure is capable of perfect control by the following mechanisms. Normally, the urethra will not open until we decide it should. At a certain point we become aware of the sensation that the bladder needs emptying, but we postpone it rather than wetting ourselves. This is the first stage of control. Though it feels automatic, this postponement until we can get to the right place is a discipline we learned years ago during toilet training.

As the pressure builds up, we deliberately control the muscle surrounding both the urinary and vaginal openings, called the pubococcygeal or levator ani muscle. This muscle is part of a group of muscles woven like a large sling or hammock under the bladder and uterus and around the delicate tubes of the vagina, urethra, and anus. The entire area controlled by this muscle, from the clitoris at the front to the anus at the back, is called the pelvic muscle (see diagrams, page 75 and page 304). Using this muscle is the second stage of control.

Anxiety about promptly getting to a place where they are comfortable urinating plays a role in incontinence for many women, especially if they know from experience that they may not make it. But even for a woman without special anxieties, after postponement has gone beyond a certain point, pain may set in and it will take squeezing her legs together and even holding her hands against her labia to keep urine from escaping before she gets somewhere to pee. This is the third stage of control.

Once at an acceptable place, we have to deliberately decide to release the urine, an act of relaxation, which may be quick or take some time, depending on how distracted we are, how anxious we feel, and how long we have been postponing release. Sometimes sexual arousal may either stimulate or delay the release of urine.

It is also not clear how we know when we are really finished urinating, because we can voluntarily stop and start again. We think we're finished when no more urine comes out and the initial sensation of pressure is gone. Yet some women retain small or large amounts of urine in their bladders even after the sensations cease and the urethra recloses.

In fact, bladder functioning is one of the most

complicated, sophisticated mechanisms of the female body. As many as thirty different reflexes may be involved in the retention and voiding of urine. Incontinence in women involves a complex interaction of anatomical, medical and neurological, functional, environmental, social, and psychological factors.[6] Be sure your practitioner considers all these factors in your evaluation for treatment.

TYPES OF INCONTINENCE

Experts do not agree on how to describe the various types of incontinence. Since many women have a combination of types, individualized assessment and treatment are needed. We are naming the categories we will discuss as follows:

1. "Transient" incontinence
2. Stress incontinence
3. Urge incontinence
4. Overflow incontinence

"Transient" incontinence may last a short or a long time but is due to other conditions. When the other conditions are cleared up, further treatment of the incontinence may not be needed. Examples of causes of transient incontinence include the use of certain medications, symptomatic urinary-tract infection, delirium or confusion caused by a disease, restricted mobility, such as a flare-up of arthritis that slows down a person's ability to rise and move to the bathroom, excess urine production caused by drinking too much fluid or having an underlying disease that causes storage or loss of too much fluid, and stool impaction.

Stress incontinence is a condition in which there is a loss of urine at times when sudden activity increases the pressure in the abdomen and bladder, such as when you cough, sneeze, laugh, lift, swing a club or racket, or run. This type of incontinence is very common even in younger women. Often stress incontinence is combined with one or more other types of incontinence. Current theory suggests that urine loss results when the urethra is increasingly unable to maintain control along its entire length against the ever-filling bladder, changing the balance of pressure between the two systems. The bladder neck has probably widened, often in response to relaxation of muscles (against pressure of the bladder); the urethra may be stretched wider and wider at the top, and shortened, much the way a nylon stocking is when you take it off, compared with how it was when you took it out of the package. The only remaining control mechanisms then are a very short area of the urethra near the outlet and the pubococcygeal muscle. Even when weak, the pubococcygeal muscle can usually permit normal functioning, but is unable to handle the "stress" of the laugh, cough, sneeze, or bearing-down pressure.*

Urge incontinence refers to a sudden urge to urinate that is unexpected and so powerful that it is not always possible to make it to the bathroom. The feeling may or may not be uncomfortable or painful. The key aspect is the suddenness and strength of the urge, which may occur even shortly after urinating. Most gerontologists and urologists believe that urge incontinence is most common among women over the age of sixty-five.

What gets me is that often I'll be fine all day out shopping—no trouble at all. Then just as I get home and start to put the key in the door, I'll suddenly have to go so bad that I can hardly stand it. Sometimes I just make it to the bathroom, but sometimes I lose it right there at the front door.

Overflow incontinence is the problem in a smaller percentage of cases. Usually, it comes on with no warning—no sensation or signal at all—and urine unexpectedly "overflows" after a woman changes position, such as standing up after sitting, or sitting up after lying down. We may lose a relatively small amount—a few drops—or enough to require a pad.† Often there is a desire to urinate again a few minutes later, but very little urine emerges, a sign that the bladder is not emptying completely. The risk of bladder infection is high with this problem, which often happens because we have been sedentary or have learned to hold our urine too long. It also may happen after bladder suspension surgery or other pelvic surgery.

*A few women who have this type of relaxation of the pelvic floor are apparently perfectly continent, and others with stress problems do not seem to have any noticeable relaxation of the pelvic floor, but this is not the general rule.

†Rarely, an abnormal passage (a fistula) may have occurred as a result of a difficult childbirth, radiation treatments, or surgery, and not been detected. This often results in a more or less continuous drip from a break between the vaginal wall and the bladder or urethra. Most fistulas can be repaired surgically.

Causes of Bladder-Control Problems

Aging Is Not *a Cause*

Aging does not by itself cause female incontinence, even if the chances of being incontinent do tend to increase as women age. This is probably the single most important fact to get across to the medical profession and to the general public.

Weak Muscles

Our whole way of life in this culture has traditionally worked against women's maintaining good muscle tone. Many generations of women were brought up to think of exercise as something for men only. In these generations it was poor women who often had adequate muscle tone because of the physical work they did. A general fitness campaign directed at adult women as well as men, and also including the elderly, has only recently been started, and this is too often directed only to the affluent.

After midlife, the muscle tone that we tended to take for granted as younger women slowly decreases. Keeping in shape may take much more effort than previously. This partly depends on how active you have been throughout life. Without a fairly systematic and vigorous program, already weak muscles may deteriorate more rapidly. Even women who were active previously, however, will lose muscle tone and may gain weight through inactivity. "Use it or lose it" is as true for the pelvic muscles as it is for any others. The good news is that we can improve muscle strength at any age.

There is solid evidence that weak pelvic and abdominal muscles contribute to stress incontinence, and perhaps to other incontinence problems. Severe and prolonged immobility can contribute to incontinence problems such as "overflow." Exercise such as running, aerobic dancing, even walking may aggravate bladder

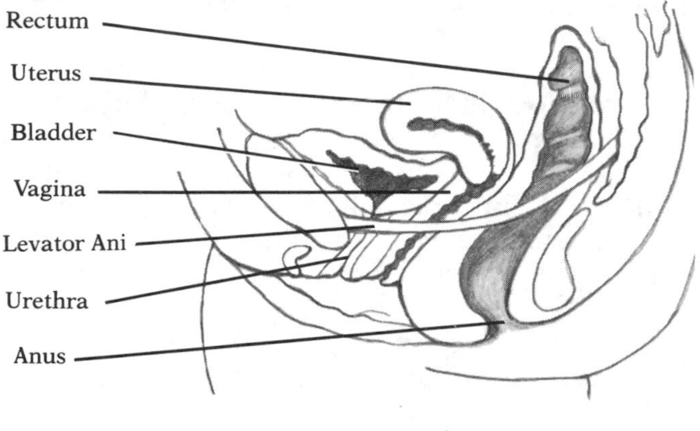

Normal

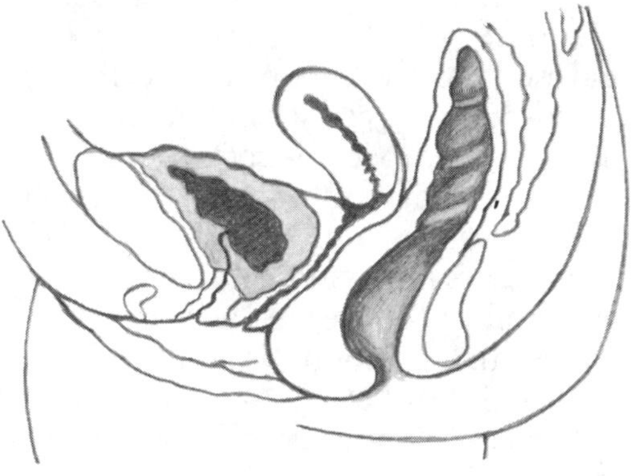

Cystocele: Bladder protrudes into vaginal canal

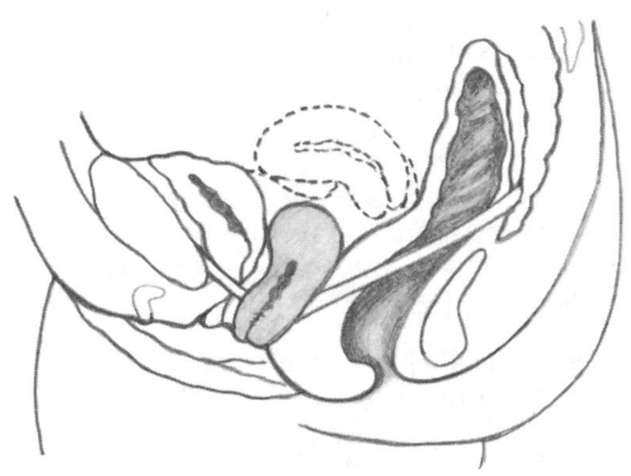

Prolapse of the uterus: Uterus descends into vaginal canal

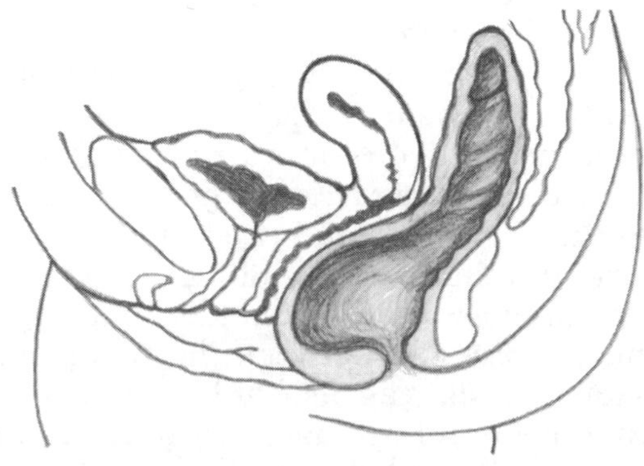

Rectocele: Rectal wall protrudes into vaginal canal

problems because of the jarring and gravitational pull on the genital and urinary organs. Yoga and swimming strengthen without jarring. Breaking the cycle begins with Kegel exercises for getting control of that key set of pelvic muscles.

The Kegel exercises can be done conveniently and invisibly, whether sitting, standing, lying down, or during sex, and can, when done consistently, bring improvement and even cure stress incontinence and improve other kinds.[7] Women frequently report a noticeable improvement in sexual response as well as urinary control when Kegel exercises are practiced regularly (see Moving for Health, pages 75–77).

Reproductive Events and Hormonal Changes

Reproductive events may contribute to a woman's bladder-control problems or create problems where none existed before. For example, slight bladder-control problems, which may be temporary or permanent, are often associated with childbirth. While childbirth itself is often blamed for these problems, the actual cause may be damage caused by obstetric practices, such as the use of forceps, episiotomy, the lying-down position in which most women have been required to labor, and pushing uphill to give birth, often with a partially full bladder.[8]

The reduction of ovarian estrogen production around the time of menopause, which may bring some degree of thinning, drying, or shrinking of vaginal tissues, often affects the nearby urethra as well. Some women may for the first time experience some type of incontinence, which may be temporary and disappear once the body has adjusted to its different production of estrogen (less from the ovaries but some from the adrenal glands and fat tissue) or may persist.

Nutrition and Water

The role of nutrition in incontinence is somewhat controversial, but it is clear that diet inadequate in basic nutrients can contribute to repeated bladder infections and poor muscle tone. Inadequate water intake can lead to bladder infections and to constipation, which can cause urinary incontinence.

Magnesium deficiencies have been reported to contribute to bladder instability, but there is no solid evidence for this. However, magnesium (available in fruits and vegetables) is an important mineral for bone strength in elderly women, and should accompany calcium, which is also important for muscle fitness.

Drinking too much water, coffee, tea, alcoholic beverages, sodas, and other liquids can also contribute to incontinence. Some women report that the artificial sweetener aspartame (NutraSweet and Equal) seems to contribute to their problems.[9]

Infections and Inflammation

One cause of some urinary-control problems is a long-term pattern of chronic bladder and urethral infections. A vicious cycle is often involved in incomplete emptying of the bladder. Infection builds up in the stagnant urine, which may inflame the lining of the bladder and infect the urethra itself. One result may be intermittent, temporary, or permanent urge incontinence. Many women have low-grade infections of this type almost constantly, without even being aware of them until they flare up and overwhelm the system.

Interstitial cystitis also causes frequent urination and pain similar to the symptoms of bladder infection. Urine tests are negative, however, because the symptoms are caused by chronic inflammation and scarring of the bladder lining, which may bleed, rather than by bacterial infection.[10]

Medications and Drugs

Several specific prescription drugs for hypertension, heart disease, and fluid buildup (diuretics), as well as some sedatives, hypnotics, tranquilizers, and antidepressants, may provoke temporary incontinence. Many types of drugs (including many over-the-counter antihistamines and nonsteroidal antiinflammatories) can cause the bladder to retain urine and lead to overflow incontinence. Always bring to your health-care practitioner for review a list of all the prescribed and over-the-counter medicines you use.

Trauma and Medical Treatment

Violent sexual penetration, gynecological surgery—especially hysterectomy and other procedures carried out via the vagina—as well as radiation treatments for cancer all may contribute to problems with urinary control. In the case of hysterectomy, the cause may be physical—the loss of support that the uterus provides for the bladder and urethra[11] or damage to the urinary structures or nerves during surgery—or it may be hormonal. For many women, hysterectomy causes a drop in estrogen levels, even when the ovaries have been retained. This drop can, in turn, affect the urinary structures. In some cases, repair of a uterine prolapse or cystocele may remove the blockage that was actually helping to control the urinary flow.[12]

Specific Diseases

Other causes of urinary-control problems include diabetes, congestive heart failure, and progressive degenerative diseases involving the brain or spinal cord such as Alzheimer's disease, multiple sclerosis, brain or spinal-cord tumors, and Parkinson's disease. Other specific physical causes include spinal-cord injuries, stones in the urinary system, obstructive tumors, bladder cancer, strokes, or TIAs (transient ischemic attacks). Before diagnosing incontinence, a competent physician should rule out each of these conditions, and, if any are present, plan a treatment program that includes treating the incontinence as well.

Emotional Problems

Finally, there are bladder problems that result primarily from stress, anxiety, and depression. Since emotional factors are rarely the sole cause of the problem, it is vital to rule out physical causes first, while recognizing that the state of our emotions may aggravate any bladder-control problem we may have.

I started to wake up at night to urinate—sometimes once or twice, but sometimes every two hours. A gynecologist put me on estrogen cream that caused bleeding, so then he wanted to do a D&C. I said goodbye to the cream and to him and also to the leading urologist, who wanted to put me on antidepressants. He had said after observing me—and I was tearful—"The sorrow that has no tears to cry makes the body weep." I realized I had this dependency on "Doctor, doctor, make it better!" The only initiative I was showing was going to doctors. Then I decided to do as much as I could for myself. So I changed my whole pattern of eating to vegetarian (macrobiotic) foods, started swimming and doing Kegels regularly. I try to understand what is happening. Now I see that my waking up is related to stress and anxiety. I still expect to wake up once most nights, but when I have had a massage, I usually sleep through the whole night. [a fifty-five-year-old woman]

GENERAL SELF-HELP

Before seeking any type of medical solution to an incontinence problem in the absence of other symptoms, we encourage you to observe and record your problems and take some simple steps to try to help yourself. The first step is to review your diet, hygiene, and exercise habits.

Are you drinking enough or too much water and other liquids? Many women avoid drinking in order to avoid accidents. The result is more likely to be urinary-tract infections and dehydration, which can actually trigger accidents and may even become life-threatening. Try cutting down drastically on caffeine, alcohol, and soft drinks (including "diet" sodas) and substitute water and clear unsweetened fruit juices such as apple juice. Drink six to eight glasses of water (64 ounces) throughout the day, most of them before your last meal. Some women develop problems because they are drinking too much water.

To empty the bladder more completely, stand up when you think you've finished, wait a few seconds, then sit down and try again. Another way is to lean forward or press on the abdomen while seated.

Toilet hygiene tends to become more important as we age. Some women were never taught that it is important to wipe from front to back to avoid fecal contamination. Some may find that moist wipes do a better job now than conventional dry toilet paper. If you can get access to a bidet or a "telephone" shower (shower-head extension with a flexible hose) for post-toilet cleansing, or switch from tub baths to showers, you may have fewer urinary infections.

A diet high in whole grains, fruits, and vegetables, including some fish, and low in white flour, sugar, fats, and meats, can help keep the acid balanced in the urinary and vaginal systems to discourage infections and also improve overall digestion, muscle tone, and urinary output. Vitamin C, including bioflavonoids, is sometimes helpful. Many women find that unsweetened cranberry juice prevents or fights infections. Some women discover that spicy foods aggravate their problems.

Are you getting enough general exercise, at least walking regularly every day? Decide now that you are not going to stay home or avoid exercise for fear of having an accident, but will find whatever kinds of protective devices and clothing you need in order to have brief walking trips, preferably every day (see Resources for this chapter). Wear comfortable shoes when walking, and pay attention to posture to correct the alignment of the entire pelvis.

Next, check your overall weight and health. Many women find that losing weight through a nutritious diet and exercise improves their continence noticeably, though it isn't always clear why. It may be a combination of improved diet and increased exercise, removal of the drag of heavy fat across the abdomen, plus the improvement in self-esteem.

If you hold your urine for several hours and then have urge problems, make an effort to identify earlier the feeling of needing to urinate, which you may be ignoring. Go to the toilet regularly, either at the very earliest sign of fullness or at scheduled intervals regardless of sensation. If feelings of urgency are *very* frequent, allowing the bladder to fill up more may help. This is called "bladder retraining." Breathe deeply and relax and the urge may pass. Urinate five minutes later. Gradually increase the time between the urge and urination.

If you have never done Kegel exercises, start today. While exercising this important set

Keeping Records

While you are taking the initial steps in the self-help process, you may also want to keep a careful watch on your symptoms, both for your own use and to help any professional you decide to consult. A competent doctor or nurse will ask you many specific questions as one part of a thorough history and evaluation. Keeping this record will help you to be ready with answers. For example, many doctors ask, "How many pads do you use in a day?"

Begin by making a note of *every* time you urinate. Mark if it was on purpose or an "accident"—exactly when it happened, what you were doing, where you were, how much urine you lost in ounces (approximately), and what you did about the loss. Try to remember when you first began to have a problem. How did it begin? Does it seem to be getting worse? Did it begin suddenly? Did it start for the first time after an operation or childbirth, after you started taking some new prescription drugs, after an accident, after a time of stress, or after some episode of illness? Is it worse during the day or during the night? How long can you hold your urine after you sense a need to go? Do you feel your bladder completely empty? Do you strain to empty? Do you regularly wear pads to catch escaping urine? In some cases, simply keeping a record like this can improve bladder control by helping you pay attention to your patterns.

One of the things you need to establish is whether your condition is temporary or chronic. Try to distinguish between different types of episodes. Do you ever experience pain with an accident? What kind of pain (sharp, dull)? Is there itching, burning, or a feeling of pressure? Is it something that happens only when you laugh, sneeze, cough, run, jump, or lift something? Does it happen when you stand up quickly from a sitting position, turn suddenly, or stoop down? All the time or only sometimes? Have you gained weight recently? Do you (or did you) ever wet the bed at night while you are asleep? Do you drink caffeine or alcohol regularly? What does your usual diet consist of (include all liquids and snacks between meals, as well as meals)? Do you sometimes lose urine without any urge or warning? Do you experience sudden, overwhelming urges to urinate that you cannot control? Does the sound of running water cause you to start urinating? Do you have a history of chronic infections of the bladder or urinary tract? What is your menopausal status?

If you answer these questions carefully and keep records for several weeks, you should be able to get a rough idea of whether or not you fall into one of the major categories of urinary incontinence or whether you seem to have signs of more than one type. Mixed problems will call for several types of treatment, but many women will discover that they fall mainly into one category or another, which clearly calls for a specific set of medical or surgical options, and for which other approaches will probably not be as useful. When you have assembled this information, you will be better prepared to work with your health-care practitioner to develop an effective treatment plan.

of muscles may not prevent or solve all problems of urinary control, it almost always brings some improvement (see Moving for Health chapter, pages 75–77).

In my early forties I had some stress incontinence which I stopped by doing Kegel exercises. In my early fifties I started waking several times a night and, once awake, needed to urinate. When I went on a camping trip for several months I didn't like getting out of the sleeping bag and tent so many times at night. At first I kept a plastic container in the tent to pee in but then I decided to ignore the feeling and go back to sleep. By the end of the trip I was sleeping through the night. For a few years after that I was awakened several times at night because of hot flashes but never had to urinate more than once a night. Now that my hot flashes have subsided I am again sleeping through the night. [a fifty-five-year-old woman]

Next, review all your prescription and over-the-counter drugs (see pages 31–32). Your pharmacist can tell you whether any of these drugs or combination of drugs actually aggravate bladder-control problems, as well as whether certain foods or drinks taken at the same time may make a drug's effects even stronger.

As you try all of these approaches, a self-help group can be extremely useful. Composed of other women like you, groups offer an invaluable opportunity to realize that you are not alone, and to hear what others with the same problems have found helpful. Other women are the major source of information on this subject. You may learn from one another who and where the really helpful professional people are and how to avoid inappropriate care. If you attend a group sponsored by "experts," be sure you evaluate their biases. You may have to start your own group.

SEEKING COMPETENT MEDICAL CARE

One of the most serious barriers to a better understanding of the connections between the reproductive and the urinary system is their traditional separation into two different areas of specialization: gynecology and urology. The two physical systems, in fact, are subject to the same hormonal influences and are separated only by a thin layer of tissue. The whole unit is anchored together on the bladder side to the abdominal cavity.

Obstetrician-gynecologists generally have little training in urology—the study and treatment of the urinary system.[13] Some gynecologists are so eager to treat any incontinence with standard surgery that they may fail to ask even the most basic questions before proceeding. This often results either in failure to notice an underlying disease or in misdiagnosis of the specific type of incontinence. The urologists, meanwhile, know little more than the basics about female reproductive organs. Few doctors in either specialty are trained to treat middle-aged and older women. At least there is now a set of clinical practice guidelines with a commonly agreed-upon terminology.[14]

Whom should you see? As women, we tend to refer ourselves to gynecologists for most problems, without always realizing that they are surgeons, trained primarily to offer a surgical solution to many problems that might be better treated in other ways. Sometimes a medical or surgical approach (or combination thereof) is warranted. However, many women continue to suffer from bladder-control problems as a direct *result* of surgical or medical treatment (a phenomenon known as iatrogenesis, or illness caused by medical treatment). In some cases, the doctor did not diagnose the bladder problem correctly, or prescribed treatment such as gynecological surgery or certain drugs that caused bladder-control problems for the first time. Yet if surgery is appropriate, all of us want to be sure we are in the hands of the most skilled and knowledgeable people. Since so few surgeons have adequate training for successful treatment of female urinary-control problems, you may have to make considerable effort to locate satisfactory care.

Using the new Agency for Health Care Policy and Research (AHCPR) guidelines, primary-care physicians (internists, geriatricians, family-medicine practitioners, general practitioners, nurse practitioners) are able to take care of many of the urinary incontinence problems affecting women. They can refer, if needed, to a specialist for additional evaluation, development of a treatment plan, and further treatment. If surgery is recommended, request that the physician or nurse continue to work together with you and the surgeon to help define the right approach to your treatment. You should decide about surgery in the context of your total health and life situation. Do not be rushed into agreeing to surgery.

"Continence clinics" are now available in most major cities. Look for one that will work with your primary-care practitioner and that has an interdisciplinary staff, including educators and physical therapists.

A new medical specialty is developing called "urogynecology." Physicians in this field are surgeons who specialize in female urinary problems. Their numbers are growing but they are still rare.*

MEDICAL DIAGNOSIS

A diagnosis involves many different processes, and you are an important part of all of them. How you feel and what you experience and remember definitely help the health-care practitioner identify the cause of your problem. If you feel you are not being listened to or are contradicted, or if a detailed history and questionnaire about your bladder functioning are not taken before tests are done, you may want to consult another practitioner.[15] The one you choose should make a diagnosis based on an extensive history, your observation of your own symptoms, clinical examination, and, where appropriate, diagnostic tests. A combination of different diagnostic tests and treatment options may be indicated for women who have an overlap between stress and urge incontinence, for example.

Diagnostic Tests

Tests alone, as important as they can be, cannot substitute for clinical judgment, and vice versa. *Most experts now agree that a test for stress incontinence performed with the surgeon's fingers alone, while the patient is lying down or standing, is an inadequate basis for planning surgery.*

Standard Tests

A urinalysis and a urine culture should be done first, in order to rule out infection as a temporary or chronic cause of bladder or kidney problems. Some doctors say only a clean specimen taken by catheter is adequate. Part of the urinalysis should also include screening for excess sugar, since some bladder problems (like too frequent urination) may actually be an early sign of diabetic or prediabetic conditions. In old women, incontinence with swollen ankles may be a sign of heart failure, which requires treatment. The physical examination should include two pelvic (internal gynecological) exams, one while the woman is standing and the other while she is lying down, to check that the position of the internal organs is not a problem. Basic neurological testing should rule out damage to the brain, spinal cord, or peripheral nerves. If physical causes are ruled out, a thorough practitioner usually looks for depression or other psychological causes of the symptoms.

Trial Use of a Pessary

One intermediate approach to testing whether or not you are an appropriate candidate for stress-incontinence surgery is the use of a pessary. A pessary is a silicone or rubber device varying in size and shape that fits into the top of the vagina, somewhat like a diaphragm, except that it is a little larger and less flexible. Many women used pessaries for uterine prolapse in the days when surgery was not as safe or available (or insured) as it is today. One effect of the pessary is to raise the neck of the bladder to a position more nearly normal, thus reducing the tendency to stress incontinence. Today, the pessary is becoming more popular again as a diagnostic test and as a solution.

If there is significant reduction of stress incontinence when the pessary is in place, then the chances are improved that surgery (properly performed, of course) will be successful.[16] For some elderly women who are not good candidates for surgery because of other physical problems (heart condition, etc.) or for any woman who wishes to avoid surgery, the pessary may also prove to be a valuable permanent alternative to surgery, as it sometimes was in the days of our grandmothers. It requires considerable manual dexterity (the kind necessary to use cervical caps, for example) for a woman to remove and clean the pessary herself, but many do. Otherwise, a health-care practitioner will have to do this regularly for you.

I've had the pessary for about a year and a half. Before that everything was sliding down—there was a big "thing" [the prolapsed uterus] in my body and I had to pee every half hour or so. Once in a while the urine would leak out but mostly I got to the bathroom in time. Now I don't leak urine.

I think in the beginning the pessary was too small and it came out. Then they put in a bigger one. It was uncomfortable for about a month but then it was all

*As of July 1993, there were 556 members of the American Urogynecologic Society, of which at least 15 percent were women. Membership is open to researchers and clinicians. Call (312) 644-6610 for referrals.

right. About every two or three months they take it out and wash it and put it back again. It hurts when they are putting it in but once in it stops hurting. [a ninety-one-year-old woman in a nursing home]

Neurological Tests

Clinicians should test to see whether incontinence could be caused by damage to the nervous system itself. If this type of testing is to be done, however, consider having a separate examination by a neurologist/psychologist team experienced in identifying TIAs (small strokes), Alzheimer's disease, or other neurological problems. Distinguishing among these conditions is difficult but crucial for planning treatment.

Urodynamic Studies

These tests, also called urodynamic pressure profiles, evaluate how well the bladder, urethra, and anal sphincter function. A catheter is inserted in the bladder, filled to capacity, and various measurements are taken while the patient is lying down, standing, and urinating.[17] While they provide a more complete evaluation, they may be stressful and unnecessary for elderly women.[18] Bladder training programs often bring improvement without such detailed testing.

Tests in Preparation for Surgery

Today there are multiple diagnostic tests available to surgeons planning specific types of surgery, usually for stress incontinence.

Other common tests include cystoscopy and urethroscopy, a direct look inside to check the condition of the bladder and urethra. Bladder and kidney X rays, using fluorescent dyes, also help visualize the shape and position of both the urethra and the bladder. Some tests have the purpose of determining the precise angle of the urethra, but the importance of correcting this angle is under debate. Some doctors rely on physical examination for this, while others insert a beaded chain into the urethra, take an X ray, and then remove the chain.

I went to a urologist who insisted on doing a cystoscopy in his office. He was aware of my great reluctance because an earlier cystoscopy was very painful, even under anesthesia, but he said he could not determine what he wanted to know when the patient was asleep. He was very reassuring and so was the nurse. He was so gentle and the procedure was so painless that I would not hesitate to recommend having this done in a doctor's office, if done by a doctor of this caliber. After doing the cystoscopy the doctor said he did not find anything wrong except a prolapsed bladder. He said he did not recommend an operation. This doctor said that stretching the urethra, which other doctors recommended, is a very outdated urological technique and he does not do it. [a woman in her sixties]

If your surgeon recommends a test, ask exactly which test it is, how it will be done, what it will show, and how that information will be used in planning the surgery, if necessary. If you do have the test(s) done, ask to see the results yourself and have them explained to you. Together with diagrams of the surgery being proposed, this should enable you to participate more meaningfully in the final treatment decisions.

MEDICAL AND SURGICAL TREATMENTS

Drug and Behavioral Treatments

Drugs are sometimes prescribed to treat incontinence. They can be used with the self-help strategies and Kegel exercises discussed earlier and with behavioral techniques such as timed voiding and bladder retraining.

Drugs are used to help regulate the bladder or urethra during the filling or the emptying phases. Certain drugs reduce the tendency for the "irritable" bladder to contract. Others may improve the tone of muscles at the bladder opening. However, most drugs to treat incontinence also produce unpleasant effects, such as dry mouth or irritability, and should not be used without consideration of your total health condition and the other medications you take. Be sure to check all drugs with your doctor and pharmacist for the availability of newer formulations, and for possible undesirable effects. Behavioral techniques have no adverse effects.

Treatments of Mild Stress Incontinence and/or Vaginal Dryness

Many doctors routinely recommend synthetic estrogen drugs either for complaints of vaginal dryness or urinary-control difficulties around the time of menopause. A condition mild enough to respond to estrogen treatment might respond to less risky nonhormonal moisturizers, and dietary and exercise changes as well. On the other hand, if these other approaches have been tried and a thorough medical history and evaluation do not reveal any significant anatomical problems with the bladder or urethra (and estrogen is not contraindicated), estrogen is an option some women have found helpful. It may be that a low-dose estrogen cream for a short time is all that is needed for some mild problems (see page 90).

Treatments for Severe Stress Incontinence

SURGERY

After the less drastic approaches mentioned above have been tried, you and your surgeon may conclude that surgery is the only way to correct a dropped bladder or the overstretched muscles and/or ligaments in the pelvic area that contribute to stress incontinence.

For example, a woman with fairly severe stress incontinence may feel that the exercise/weight-loss approach, including Kegel exercises, is too slow (sometimes it takes several months), or she may have already tried it and found the amount of improvement unsatisfactory. Sometimes she has already had surgery that failed and wants to try again.

The major goal of most surgery for stress incontinence is to restore the bladder neck to its normal position slightly above and behind the major bones that come together at the front of the pelvis (beneath the mons). Ideally, the dynamics of the normal pressure between bladder and urethra will thus be restored. Once raised, the bladder neck is "tacked" into its new position by attaching it to the bones or ligaments of the pelvis.

We do not have space here to describe all the possible surgical procedures for stress incontinence. Techniques for repositioning the bladder—specifically, the bladder neck—vary from suspensions such as tacks inside the vagina alongside both sides of the urethra (much like creating a short tunnel for a drawstring) or tacking the bladder neck to an abdominal ligament, to more complex sling devices, some made from a woman's own muscle tissue, others from a synthetic substance like Dacron.

While all of these surgical procedures for stress incontinence *may* result in improvement, some of them do so by permanently altering the relationship of the internal organs to one another—actually cutting the bladder away from its natural attachment to the vagina or anterior abdominal wall. None actually alters the primary cause of the dislocation of the bladder, the stretched or weak levator ani or pubococcygeal muscles of the pelvic floor. Every woman considering surgery should obtain full information on the risks, benefits, complications, and alternatives before giving her consent.

After many years of bladder problems and avoiding a gynecological examination or evaluation, my mother finally had to submit to a vaginal hysterectomy because of a seriously prolapsed uterus. She was seventy-nine. At the same time, her doctor performed urethrovesical suspension surgery (she called it "tucking her up"), which has been totally successful. My mother has been liberated from the constant anxiety of having to be near a bathroom at all times. She only regrets not having done it much sooner.

SLINGS

Many surgeons believe women with stress incontinence need some type of sling that can help support the bladder in a new position. It may be appropriate for very severe stress incontinence that has not responded to other treatment. However, this operation may offer only limited benefit if the urethra has become shortened, scarred, and rigid due to repeated infections or surgeries.

DILATION

Some doctors, including respected urologists, still practice a surgical procedure called dilation or dilatation, the insertion of a tube or a scalpel-like coring mechanism into the urethra to break up scar tissue. Today most specialists say this only further damages tissue already scarred from repeated infections, almost never yields permanent results, and frequently makes the condition worse.

Treatments for Urge Incontinence

Women need to be wary of snap diagnoses offered without thorough evaluations. Newer approaches to bladder-control problems of the urge type are emerging that involve combinations of nonsurgical techniques such as biofeedback, exercise, drugs, bladder retraining, and going to the toilet at timed intervals.[19] Most women need to urinate every three to four hours. If you feel the need to urinate in less than two hours and you do not have a bladder infection, you might want to try some bladder retraining to overcome the urge. When you feel an urge, take two or three deep breaths and use any kind of relaxation method that you have learned. (See Aging and Well-Being chaper.) You may find the urge goes away. Then wait five minutes and void. Gradually try to extend the time between feeling the urge and voiding. You may be able to retrain yourself to a three- to four-hour schedule.

Women may also be helped by certain antispasmodic drugs. Whenever a doctor recommends drug treatment, however, it is crucial to investigate exactly what is being recommended and why, as well as to make sure that other drugs already prescribed for you are being taken into account. In most cases, all these approaches involve long-term monitoring and follow-up. Any treatment you try should include competent and committed supervision. Such programs may use catheters or other devices to measure how much bladder control a woman is able to exert, and how that control is improving over time.

Most experts believe that urge incontinence must result from some type of neurological impairment. Unfortunately, the classification "neurological" means different things to different doctors. Some perceive it as a damage or a defect in the central nervous system's ability to transmit messages, perhaps because of a stroke or because of some other disease. Other doctors interpret "neurological" to mean "psychiatric," concluding that the problem behind urge incontinence is somehow "emotional" or "psychological" in origin, or represents evidence of senility. As a result, they conclude that nothing can be done about it. Most doctors are taught in medical school that complaints without any verifiable anatomical cause are "functional," implying, in psychiatric language, that, although the symptoms may be real enough, the patient's complaint probably serves some other purpose in her life or relationship with her doctor, such as attracting attention.

Many older women with urge incontinence have actually suffered unknowingly from some type of neurological problem. Testing for various neurological abnormalities can't hurt and may yield benefits. If, for example, a small stroke is discovered, it is possible to commence both rehabilitation therapy and preventive therapy for future strokes at the same time that the incontinence is being treated.

However, it is entirely possible that no neurological cause will be found, even on the most searching examination. An "unstable bladder" (detrusor instability[20]) is the name given bladder contractions for which no neurological cause can be found. As a result, the term *unstable bladder* has become a wastebasket category for many, often unrelated, conditions. In some cases of incontinence, women are given tranquilizers, which can make the problem worse, or are referred to psychiatrists instead of receiving the examinations they need. Many psychiatrists are also unaware that the complaint of incontinence may require physical and neurological evaluation.

Nevertheless, there may be some psychological aspects to the origin of urge incontinence. Also, the loss of bladder control in and of itself is capable of *causing* depression. This reaction is well within the range of what is normal, given our culture and given the social loss that this crucial malfunction represents. In fact, most incontinent people report their first reaction to this problem was one of depression. Many women have experienced noticeable improvement when antidepressant drugs are given for incontinence, even in the absence of a diagnosis of depression.[21] It is now known that some antidepressant drugs reduce bladder contractions and increase sphincter resistance. It may also be that some forms of depression actually bring on incontinence difficulties.

Treatments for Overflow Incontinence

In cases of overflow incontinence, a program of regular, frequent, timed trips to the toilet is effective. Such a program helps reestablish normal signals to prevent overflow and infection. For urine retention, self-administered catheterization or clean intermittent catheterization (CIC) may be desirable. Indwelling catheters are more controversial, and are rejected for overflow incontinence by many doctors because of the high risk of infection, even though they offer improved control. For certain conditions they may be necessary temporarily.[22]

ISSUES TO CONSIDER REGARDING SURGERY

What factors should you consider in evaluating surgery as an option? First, there is a high failure rate—up to 50 percent and a 20 to 30 percent rate of complications. Many surgeons dismiss these figures, saying that of the patients who come to them as "failures" from previous surgery, a significant percentage show that the original diagnosis was wrong or that the correct procedure was not performed in the first place.[23] However, it is also true that even many successful procedures become failures after several months or a year or two. Most procedures require general anesthesia, with its known risks. There are also risks of damage to nearby organs. Such damage may not be classified as a failure by the surgeon, but for the woman it most certainly is one.

If something goes wrong after surgery, we need to ask not only "Was the correct diagnosis made?" but also "Was the appropriate procedure performed?" The best approach is to take our postsurgery symptoms and complaints seriously and seek a second opinion for verification.

You might consult one of the major centers for the evaluation and treatment of incontinence that exist in the United States and Canada, usually in teaching hospitals or geriatric centers, especially if you have already undergone unsuccessful surgery. You might also call the nearest center for a referral to someone knowledgeable in your community. While we do not have many firsthand accounts of women's experiences with such centers, we believe that, because of their interdisciplinary approach, you should receive a more thorough evaluation and a wider range of options for treatment of incontinence. This way you will be more likely to avoid unnecessary surgery than when you seek care directly from a gynecologist or urologist. However, you must always keep your critical awareness active in any medical setting.

A major issue when considering surgery for incontinence problems is whether to have a procedure done "from below"—that is, entirely through the vagina—or whether to undergo an abdominal, or "suprapubic," procedure. As with hysterectomy, there are advantages and disadvantages to both, and disagreement among experts. Many gynecologists have preferred vaginal techniques because the invasion of the body cavity, which is always risky, may lead later to adhesions (scar tissue) on the surrounding organs and recuperation takes longer. Many women prefer vaginal surgery just to avoid a scar; even the so-called "bikini cut" (near the top line of the pubic hair) may show, especially on older women with less pubic hair. Nevertheless, the complication/infection rate in the case of hysterectomy, for example, is significantly higher with vaginal surgery than with abdominal surgery. There is also the risk of damage by gynecologists to the urethra and ureters during vaginal surgery (and during both abdominal and vaginal hysterectomy), which may actually cause incontinence. Many expert urological surgeons do perform corrective procedures through the vagina.[24] A painful bone condition called osteitis pubis, a slow disintegration of the pubic bone, is another complication frequently resulting from surgery that attaches stitches to the bony structure rather than to one of the ligaments. You will have to discuss the choices of techniques, consider your surgeon's experience, and compare your preference with your surgeon's preference.

When we realize how little scientific knowledge is available on this subject, and how poorly prepared most medical professionals are to help us, it is easy to feel depressed about incontinence. On the other hand, progress has been made since our first edition, encouraging us to continue to break through the barrier of silence surrounding this condition.

NOTES

1. Neil M. Resnick and Subbarao V. Yalla, "Current Concepts: Management of Urinary Incontinence in the Elderly." *The New England Journal of Medicine,* Vol. 313, No. 13 (Sept. 26, 1985), pp. 800–805.
2. T. W. Hu, "Impact of Urinary Incontinence on Health Care Costs." *Journal of the American Geriatrics Society,* Vol. 38, No. 3 (1990), pp. 292–95.
3. Resnick and Yalla, op. cit., p. 800.
4. Ibid.
5. Ibid., p. 803.
6. "Structural, Neurological, Psychological Factors in Female Incontinence." *Ob. Gyn. News,* Vol. 17, No. 12 (June 15–30, 1982).
7. Patricia A. Burns, et al., "A Comparison of Effectiveness of Biofeedback and Pelvic Muscle Exercise Treatment of Stress Incontinence in Older Community-Dwelling Women." *Journal of Gerontology,* Vol. 48, No. 4 (1993), pp. M167–M174.
8. Sally Inch, *Birthrights.* New York: Pantheon Books, 1984.
9. Joan K. Glickstein, ed., *Focus on Geriatric Care & Rehabilitation,* Vol. 3, No. 10 (April 1990), p. 4.
10. Adriane Fugh-Berman, "Standard Bladder Infection Treatment May Bring on Interstitial Cystitis." *The Network News,* Vol. 10, No. 3 (May/June 1985), pp. 4–5; The Boston Women's Health Book Collective, *The New Our Bodies, Ourselves.* New York: Simon and Schuster, 1992, pp. 595–96; Rebecca Chalker and Kristine E. Whitmore, *Overcoming Bladder Disorders.* New York: HarperCollins, 1991, pp. 133–79.
11. Joanne West, "Urinary Problems Resulting from Hysterectomy." *HERS Newsletter,* April 1983, pp. 3–4.
12. David A. Richardson, et al., "The Effect of Uterovaginal Prolapse on Urethrovesical Pressure Dynamics." *American Journal of Obstetrics and Gynecology,* Vol. 146, No. 8 (Aug. 15, 1983), pp. 901–5; and Emil A. Tanagho, "The Effect of Hysterectomy and Periurethral Surgery on Urethrovesical Function." In Donald R. Ostergard, *Gyne-*

cologic Urology and Urodynamics. Baltimore, MD: Williams & Wilkins Co., 1980, pp. 293–300.

13. "Women Need Same Services That Urologists Provide for Men." *Ob. Gyn. News,* Vol. 18, No. 21 (Nov. 1–15, 1983), pp. 1–14.

14. Agency for Health Care Policy and Research (AHCPR), *Clinical Practice Guidelines: Urinary Incontinence in Adults: Clinical Practice Guidelines.* AHCPR Pub. No. 92-0038. Rockville, MD: Agency for Health Care Policy and Research, Public Health Service, U.S. Department of Health and Human Services. March 1992. (See p. 482.)

15. "Chart for Urodynamics and Gynecological Urology History." In Ostergard, op. cit. (Chart is copyright 1978 by Donald R. Ostergard.); and AHCPR *Guidelines,* op. cit.

16. N. N. Bahtia and A. Gergman, "Urinary Incontinence: Pessary Test Predicts Surgical Outcome." *Modern Medicine,* September 1985. Taken from article in *Obstetrics & Gynecology,* Vol. 65 (February 1985), pp. 220–26.

17. Kathleen Poole, "A Useful Way to Diagnose Bladder Disorders." *RN,* Vol. 47, No. 8 (August 1984), pp. 51–52.

18. J. A. Fantl, et al., "Efficacy of Bladder Training in Older Women with Urinary Incontinence." *Journal of the American Medical Association,* Vol. 265, No. 5 (1991), pp. 609–13.

19. William Frewen, "Role of Bladder Training in the Treatment of Unstable Bladder in the Female." *Urologic Clinics of North America,* Vol. 6, No. 1 (February 1979), pp. 273–77; Evan C. Hadley, "Bladder Training and Related Therapies for Urinary Incontinence in Older People." *Journal of the American Medical Association,* Vol. 256, No. 3 (July 18, 1986), pp. 372–79; Kathleen A. McCormick and Kathryn L. Burgio, "Incontinence: An Update on Nursing Care Measures." *Journal of Gerontological Nursing,* Vol. 10, No. 10 (1984), pp. 16–23; and AHCPR *Guidelines,* op. cit.

20. "Detrusor Dyssynergia: A Rare Cause of Urinary Incontinence in Women. Questions and Answers." *Journal of the American Medical Association,* Vol. 241, No. 12 (June 1985), pp. 15–30; and Neil M. Resnick and S. V. Yalla, "Detrusor Hyperactivity with Impaired Contractile Function: An Unrecognized but Common Cause of Incontinence in Elderly Patients." *Journal of the American Medical Association,* Vol. 257, No. 22 (1987), pp. 3076–81.

21. Alan J. Wein, "Pharmacology of the Bladder and Urethra." In Stuart L. Stanton and Emil A. Tanagho, eds., *Surgery of Female Incontinence.* New York: Springer-Verlag, 1980, pp. 195–96.

22. Diane K. Newman, Diane A. Smith, and Gail Goetz, "Neurogenic Bladder Dysfunction Causing Urinary Retention." *Journal of Home Health Care Practice,* Vol. 4, No. 4 (1992), pp. 45–60.

23. Stanton and Tanagho, op. cit.

24. Shlomo Raz, ed., "Vagina Surgery." *Seminars in Urology,* Vol. 4, No. 1 (February 1986), pp. 1–61.

22

HYSTERECTOMY AND OOPHORECTOMY

✦

BY DOROTHY KRASNOFF REIDER

SPECIAL THANKS TO GENEVIEVE CARMINATI

1994 UPDATE BY DOROTHY KRASNOFF REIDER

RESOURCES FOR THIS CHAPTER ON PAGES 493–94

Our reproductive organs, like most other parts of our bodies, have multiple functions. We are only beginning to identify and do not yet fully understand the many ways these organs affect our health and our sexuality. Therefore, our bodily integrity should never be tampered with unless absolutely necessary. Yet for well over a century in the United States, women's uteruses and ovaries have been subjected to routine medical abuse. Although the extent of unnecessary removal of the uterus and ovaries has been exposed, the rates are still too high. Anyone considering either of these procedures needs to be aware of *all* the possible consequences. Hysterectomy (removal of the uterus) and oophorectomy or ovariectomy (removal of the ovaries) can be lifesaving procedures, but before undergoing them every woman must be sure that they are truly necessary and understand the possible consequences.

UNNECESSARY HYSTERECTOMIES AND OOPHORECTOMIES

Hysterectomy and oophorectomy have their place in sound medical practice, mainly as treatment for confirmed cancer. As women get older the risks of uterine and ovarian cancer increase, so regular gynecological checkups including Pap smears are advisable.

In 1991, 546,000 hysterectomies and 458,000 oophorectomies were performed on women in the United States.[1] Women are surprised to learn that only a small proportion of hysterectomies—8 percent to 12 percent—are performed to treat cancer and other life-threatening diseases.[2] Most hysterectomies are elective, that is, not clearly necessary. Almost every woman has a need to believe that her hysterectomy was necessary. However, studies challenge her belief. The number of hysterectomies thought to be unnecessary is estimated at 10 percent to 90 percent, depending on the source.[3] And many surgeons unnecessarily remove healthy ovaries while performing a hysterectomy. Ironically, a large percentage of hysterectomies are performed on women just before menopause, even though menopause itself often resolves some of the problems for which the hysterectomies are recommended.

Some of the reasons for the high rates of hysterectomy may be economic. Obstetricians-gynecologists can make money faster by performing a hysterectomy than they can with "watch and wait" approaches, office treatments, checkups, follow-up visits, or lesser surgery. Doctors do them for training and status in teaching hospitals and perform them for population control on poor and minority women who were not fully informed about what was being done.[4] Hysterectomies have been done for birth control in place of simpler tubal ligations. Hysterectomies also provide income to compensate for the declining birth rate and resulting loss of hospital and obstetrical fees. The tendency to recommend unnecessary surgery, including hysterectomies, is greater where there is an overabundance of surgeons and hospital beds.

In the United States, hysterectomies are far more frequent among women who have "fee for service" medical care, covered by insurance, than among women who belong to health maintenance organizations. However, a study of seven managed-care organizations (see Chapter 16) in which the incentives are to perform less surgery still reported 10 to 27 percent unnecessary hysterectomies.[5] Insured women, both rich and poor, have much higher rates of surgery than the uninsured. Under national health plans, the rate of hysterectomies in England is half, and the rate in Norway and Sweden is one third that of the United States, without any evidence that women are suffering poorer health.[6]

Hysterectomy rates vary dramatically from one region of the country to another. One study shows, for example, that 70 percent of women in one Maine city had had hysterectomies by the age of seventy, while in another Maine city the figure was 20 percent.[7] These wide variations among similar groups of women indicate that the practices of physicians should be closely examined.

Although most hospitals have committees to monitor surgeons' performances and ethics, they examine cases *after* surgery has been performed, and the findings are kept confidential. Presumably, surgeons who perform too many questionable hysterectomies are sometimes told to restrain themselves, but surgical-review committees are not designed to protect patients.[8] The time for us to review a recommendation for surgery is *before,* rather than after, the surgery occurs. Part of the problem is that: (1) physicians believe that hysterectomies are good for women who are having problems and are past childbearing age (even female gynecologists may urge hysterectomy too casually); (2) women are uninformed about less drastic alternatives to hysterectomy; and (3) the permanent adverse effects of a hysterectomy have not been well publicized.

The good news is that there has been a steady decline in the number of hysterectomies since 1975.[9] This may be because of the rise of consumer-advocate groups and other critics of excessive hysterectomies and oophorectomies, the use of less invasive technologies, more openness among women about the negative aftereffects, the policy of Medicaid and some other insurance plans requiring a second opinion before a hysterectomy is performed, and the recent appearance of informative literature written by concerned gynecologists.

But women need even more information. If all women knew in advance the many risks of a hysterectomy, the rate could be greatly lowered.

Pressures to Have a Hysterectomy and Oophorectomy

Women in their forties and fifties who have gynecological problems face pressure to have hysterectomies and oophorectomies. They are encouraged to do so by medical authorities, many of whom believe older women have little to lose, since in their view the uterus and ovaries have outlived their usefulness and merely provide a potential site for cancer. They also believe, incorrectly, that artificial hormones can safely make up for whatever may be lost in surgery. Alternatives to hysterectomy are usually suggested only if the woman still wants children or if she is under forty.[10]

Some psychoanalysts have suggested that women's problems after hysterectomy are caused by emotional problems rather than by surgery. Women have been told over and over that removing the uterus and ovaries only improves the quality of life, as long as we have the "proper" attitude. Being "too attached" to the uterus is considered "infantile," a sign that a woman's sexuality is inappropriately confused with her ability to reproduce. Most gynecologists and some psychiatrists still believe this. The few studies that did document problems were generally ignored.[11]

Older women were not generally raised to love and appreciate their bodies and their bodies' functions, such as menstruation and sexuality. Some may view menstruation as a "curse" rather than as a part of nature's ingenious design. Many of us grew up in a time when the public's awareness of cancer increased and when surgery was the primary method used to treat cancer. Fearing cancer, we may be vulnerable to the medical profession's cavalier attitude—take it out! To compound the problem, most of us have been brought up to follow physicians' recommendations without question.

Moreover, as we approach menopause, our bodies are changing. The unpredictable nature of menstrual periods before menopause can be nerve-racking if we do not understand what to expect. Women who do not realize that gushes and clots of blood are common at this time of life may be terrified and look for quick solutions. Fear of accidental pregnancy later in life, coupled with fewer safe contraceptives available for older women, may make the idea of removing the uterus seem appealing. In addition, the vast number of women who have had hysterectomies gives us a false sense of confidence in the procedure. Is it any wonder that so many women accept, and some even request, a hysterectomy?

Reader: Be Wary

Most books and articles over the last two decades, even those written by women, stressed the benefits of hysterectomies, rarely mentioned the drawbacks, or else blamed women themselves for any adverse results. Though out of date, these misleading books are still in libraries. For example, one book written in 1976 blatantly states:

Far too many women remain convinced that the removal of the uterus will result in (1) a change in physical appearance, (2) a radical shift in weight, (3) a deterioration of sexual performance. Although these possibilities are at best remote, and have no medical basis at all, any woman can bring them about merely by believing strongly enough that they are inevitable.[1]

Another book falsely states:

The uterus has nothing whatsoever to do with a woman's libido or capacity to enjoy sex. It is simply an organ for childbearing.[2]

Most books disregard reports from women who have had hysterectomies or discredit them as "old wives' tales."

No expert is more dogmatic than the woman who has had a hysterectomy and is suddenly the center of attention at bridge parties and coffee breaks, who determinedly hangs on to this attention by reciting all the horrible "changes" in her life that she attributes to a hysterectomy.[3]

1. Nancy Nugent, *Hysterectomy.* New York: Doubleday & Co., 1976, p. 85.
2. Harry Huneycutt and Judith L. Davis, *All About Hysterectomy.* New York: Reader's Digest Press, 1977, p. 257.
3. Ibid., p. xi.

Possible Aftereffects of Hysterectomy and Oophorectomy*

Each woman is different, and it is impossible to tell in advance how a hysterectomy will affect her. Neither age, marital status, work, sexual preference, severity of symptoms before surgery, nor the number of children she has had will indicate how a woman will feel after a hysterectomy. Many women report a variety of adverse physical and emotional effects of hysterectomy, many of which are permanent and irreversible.

Both the ovaries and the uterus have important functions in the body long after the reproductive years are over. A study that tested ovarian function in 2,132 women whose uteruses were removed found that many ovaries continued to function for up to twenty-five years after the operation.[12] In fact, hot flashes can appear when a woman's ovaries are removed years after her menopause occurred.[13]

Healthy ovaries should not be removed. Removal of the ovaries from premenopausal women causes an immediate "surgical menopause" that is often more severe than normal menopause and may make more likely the recommendation to use hormone replacement therapy, at least up to the average age of menopause. Removal of ovaries creates many problems and dilemmas for a woman. Some women find that they cannot tolerate the effects of hormones or they are allergic to them. Additionally, estrogen is contraindicated for those women who have past or present thromboembolic events (strokes, phlebitis, pulmonary embolus, or heart attack), endometriosis, breast or endometrial or any other estrogen-stimulating cancer, severe liver

*We wish to be clear throughout this chapter about whether we are discussing hysterectomy, oophorectomy, or both. We will try to avoid the inaccurate, but common, error of referring to the removal of any part of the uterus or ovaries as a hysterectomy.

disease or chronic impairment of liver function, or gallbladder disease. Consider avoiding estrogen use if you smoke or have hypertension, migraine headaches, seizure disorders, or heart disease or kidney disease associated with fluid retention.[14] On the other hand, since premature menopause raises the risk for osteoporosis, bone and joint pain, vaginal dryness or shrinkage, and atherosclerosis, most experts recommend estrogen for women whose ovaries are removed before they reach age forty-five.

The relationship between hormones and osteoporosis is discussed in the Osteoporosis and Fracture Prevention chapter on page 286. In addition to knowing what is stated there, women should be aware that hormone therapy, either estrogen or the estrogen-progestin combination, does *not* replace the androgens secreted by functioning ovaries. Androgens contribute to the libido (sexual desire).* And the hormonelike substances called *prostacyclins* that circulate in the uterus and help keep arteries open, keep blood platelets from excessive clotting, and help to prevent heart attacks are not replaced through hormone therapy.[15]

Even when the ovaries are left in place, a hysterectomy can cause a significant drop in hormone levels. The uterus is a living, functioning organ that secretes hormones and responds to ovarian hormones for many years after menopause. It is more than just a "baby carriage." When the uterus is amputated, a delicately balanced system (which includes ovaries, fallopian tubes, cervix, vagina, and clitoris and their blood and nerve supplies) is disrupted. Major blood vessels, nerves, and connective tissues are cut, leaving raw edges to heal and scar, which may permanently alter sensation. In addition, if the cervix is cut out, the top of the vagina must be sewn shut, resulting in a shortened vagina and a loss of elasticity.[16]

More than two hundred women who contacted a support group in New York reported varying degrees of fatigue, memory loss, and loss of sexual feeling following a hysterectomy. *None of the women had been forewarned by their doctors about any possible aftereffects.* Those who retained their ovaries had hot flashes for several weeks after surgery, but then the flashes disappeared if the women were premenopausal. Also reported were breast pain, breast enlargement and engorgement, cystic breasts, and feelings of lactation and oily skin. Those who had their ovaries removed reported severe hot flashes, bone and joint pain, and dry skin. Many of the women did not realize that their problems might be linked to their surgery until they talked with other women who had suffered similar problems following hysterectomy.

Other consequences reported by women after hysterectomy with or without oophorectomy are: depression, loss of sexual sensation in the breasts and other parts of the body, lessened sexual desire, weaker orgasms, insomnia, vaginal dryness and shrinkage, loss of firm body tone, hair loss, premature graying, weight gain (despite dieting and exercise), unpleasant vaginal odor, protruding abdomen, constipation, bloating, recurrent vaginal yeast infections, urinary incontinence (see Chapter 21), dry eye syndrome, lower resistance to colds and infections, and less intense emotions.

Hysterectomy means the loss of uterine contractions during orgasm, which for many women reduces sexual pleasure. Many women report the loss of pleasure from penetration, fewer sexual fantasies, slower arousal, lack of interest in seeking lovers or a mate, loss of desire to masturbate, and sometimes even an aversion to being touched.

My hysterectomy had a result that I was most unprepared for. With breast stimulation, intercourse, and orgasm, there was a definite loss of a sensation which I can only describe as uterine. Having had a number of losses and having helped others through the losses that seem to come to us throughout life, I felt prepared for anything that life had to offer . . . meaning anything that I could conceive of. This was one thing that I had never conceived of. My greatest need at the time was simply to talk with someone who knew what I was talking about. I received a lot of unhelpful responses. The most insensitive came from female sex therapists. [a forty-one-year-old nurse]

One study reports that 33 percent to 46 percent of women experience varying degrees of diminished libido and diminished physical sexual responses after hysterectomy.[17] Estrogen therapy is of no benefit in this regard.[18]

The worst thing since my hysterectomy is the lack of desire. No more delicious cravings and wonderful radiating feelings of exciting anticipation. I always felt that my desire and enjoyment of sex was a special gift, my own

*Testosterone (one of the androgens) has been used to enhance libido but also results in "masculinizing" effects such as facial hair, acne, and permanently lowered voice. (See The Boston Women's Health Book Collective, *The New Our Bodies, Ourselves,* New York: Simon and Schuster, 1992, pp. 228–29, 601.)

private joy that could never be taken away from me even if I lost material things in life. If something turned me on, whether it was a love scene in a movie, a touch, or a thought, my body would feel all tingly and flushed. Even if I didn't get sex right away, I could luxuriate in thinking about it—how I would do it, where, and when.

Now there is just emptiness inside. I feel I could go one hundred years without sex and I'm aware of the enormous void. To me it is tantamount to death. I was so overcome by the loss that I cried to everyone about it. [a fifty-year-old woman]

For other women, loss of the cervix may prevent orgasm if they were dependent upon cervical stimulation. Some women also report loss of nipple and clitoral sensation; this may be the result of severed nerves and ligaments and loss of blood flow to the pelvic area. Changes in vaginal structure, loss of cervical mucus, and the loss of the copious discharge resulting from monthly ovulation and hormonal changes also contribute to the sexual deficits created by this surgery.

Depression is a common aftermath of hysterectomy. One physician who had a hysterectomy described her feeling as that of "chronic sorrow." One study found that 70 percent of women suffered depression after hysterectomy, which was double the rate of other postoperative depressions.[19] Depressions usually occur within three to six months after surgery and can be severe. The causes of posthysterectomy depression have not been researched thoroughly enough. One theory is that removal of the uterus lowers the estrogen level by altering the blood supply to the ovaries, and lowered estrogen level is associated with a lowered blood level of *tryptophan,* an amino acid that may prevent depression.[20] Recent attention has focused on beta endorphins, substances circulating in the blood that contribute to feelings of well-being. One researcher has linked posthysterectomy depression to a sudden drop in beta endorphins, which occurs in women within six months after oophorectomy and in the 50 percent of women whose ovaries stop cycling after their uteruses are removed.[21] Other possible reasons for posthysterectomy depression may be the rage resulting from loss of sexual feeling or from concluding that one's surgery was unnecessary.

The removal of the uterus sometimes results in a surprising feeling of devastation over the loss of fertility.

After my hysterectomy, I grieved over the end of my childbearing potential, although I was fifty-five. Before I left the hospital, my concentration on babies became pronounced. I watched a TV program on adoption and fantasized about a foster child or about becoming a Big Sister or a Foster Grandparent. The woman across the hall told me that she found she could not look at new babies because she was grieving over having had her hysterectomy and never having had children. She was surprised at her grief at being childless because she had, she thought, long ago chosen to be a lesbian and to have no children. Now, she was once again having to reinforce that choice. [a fifty-seven-year-old woman]*

Some women also regret other changes in their bodies.

I miss my periods so much. I think there's something barbaric about cutting off a woman's periods before her time. Two months after my hysterectomy I developed a raw spot in my internal scar that had to be cauterized. The procedure made me stain for a few days. I tried to pretend that the blood on my pad was a period. But I knew it wasn't and I felt sad. [a fifty-year-old woman]

Not everyone reacts negatively to having a hysterectomy. Some women are pleased with the outcome.

From the moment I woke up from the surgery I was optimistic. The recovery was smooth and swift. About three months later I began having hot flashes. (My ovaries had also been removed, at my wish.) I began a regimen of estrogen and later a progestin was added. From the recovery on, I have not had a bad day. It is a joy not to be bleeding either regularly or irregularly and to be interested in sexual activity any day of the month. The sense of security and comfort of not having periods is great. If I knew it would be so easy after the operation I would have had it at thirty-nine, when my heavy bleeding started. My youngest child was then seven and I knew that I wanted no more. [a fifty-three-year-old woman]

The important point is that women should be made aware of all possible reactions to and consequences of hysterectomy before surgery is undertaken.

When the doctor recommended a hysterectomy for a fibroid, I tried desperately to get information from at least ten women who had the operation. Each one willingly told me about her hospital, her doctor, and the anesthesia

*From an unpublished manuscript by Carolyn Ruth Swift. The writer has since become a substitute grandmother for a lesbian couple raising a child and a biological grandmother to another.

she had. Not one of these women told me how she really felt afterwards, or mentioned a single word about aftereffects. Some of them encouraged me to have the surgery. From all this I naïvely concluded that a hysterectomy is not too bad.

When the shock of the sudden, unwelcome changes from my hysterectomy hit me with its full impact, I became overwhelmed with anger and hurt at these women for not telling me anything. I felt betrayed. Why didn't anyone warn me? Could they have all been so satisfied with their results? Could they have been too embarrassed to talk about sexual changes? If I had known more truths I would have tried harder to avoid the surgery!

Could they have simply not wanted to scare me or to assume too much responsibility in case my operation was really necessary? Or is there a baser emotion, a certain reluctance in some people to spare another person from making the same mistake they made—something like "misery loves company"? When anyone comes to me asking, "What is a hysterectomy like?" I tell them everything I've experienced and let them take it from there. [a forty-nine-year-old woman]

When Hysterectomy Is Necessary

There are times when a hysterectomy is life-saving; each case must be evaluated individually. Some conditions that may require surgery are:

1. Invasive cancer of the uterus (endometrium), ovaries, cervix, or fallopian tubes. This operation should be planned in consultation with both a gynecologist and an oncologist (cancer specialist) to review all the treatment options.
2. Hemorrhaging (severe uncontrollable bleeding) combined with anemia that has not responded to medical treatments—such as a D and C (dilation and curettage, or scraping, of the uterus), hormone therapy, or laser technology—or to nonmedical treatments.
3. Fibroid tumors (common, noncancerous growths) that obstruct bowel or urinary function (a rare occurrence) and that are too large to remove by myomectomy (removal of the tumor alone). Frequent urination is usually not a sufficient reason for a hysterectomy.
4. Advanced pelvic inflammatory disease (PID), in which infection spreads to the peritoneal cavity (membrane that lines the walls of the abdomen). Sometimes a bad infection can be fought successfully with massive combinations of antibiotics (administered intravenously) and complete bed rest.
5. Severe uterine prolapse, in which the uterus descends completely through the vagina.
6. Severe endometriosis (the presence of tissue of the uterine lining elsewhere in the abdominal cavity), if it is untreatable by hormones or other drugs, or if it recurs with severe pain and bleeding after minor surgery.
7. Certain other obstetrical catastrophes and very rare cases of tuberculosis of the uterus.

Some Common Problems and Alternatives to Hysterectomy

The following conditions will often correct themselves with the coming of menopause. They rarely require hysterectomies and never require oophorectomies.

Fibroid Tumors

Fibroid tumors (myomas or leiomyomas) are the most common reason for hysterectomy in women between thirty-five and fifty. Fibroids are knobs of muscle tissue in or attached to the uterus. Do not automatically think of cancer when you hear the word *tumors;* 99.7 percent of all fibroids are benign (noncancerous).[22] Nearly 40 percent of white women over thirty-five have fibroids, and the incidence is even greater in black women. The growth of fibroids is stimulated by estrogen, so if you know you have fibroids you should avoid birth-control pills and estrogen therapy. Fibroids may stay the same size or grow in spurts, plateau, and shrink many times during a woman's reproductive years, often peaking just before menopause. Usually they recede slowly after menopause as estrogen levels drop. A uterus can accommodate a surprisingly large number of sizable fibroids without showing any symptoms. The uterus can retain a normal pregnancy and birth (although sometimes premature) despite the presence of a large fibroid.[23] The presence of large fibroids, and even feelings of heaviness and mild pressure, are not necessarily reasons for a hysterectomy.

The three most common types of fibroids, named according to their location in the uterus, are:

- *Subserous*—Located outside the uterus. These usually do not interfere with uterine function,

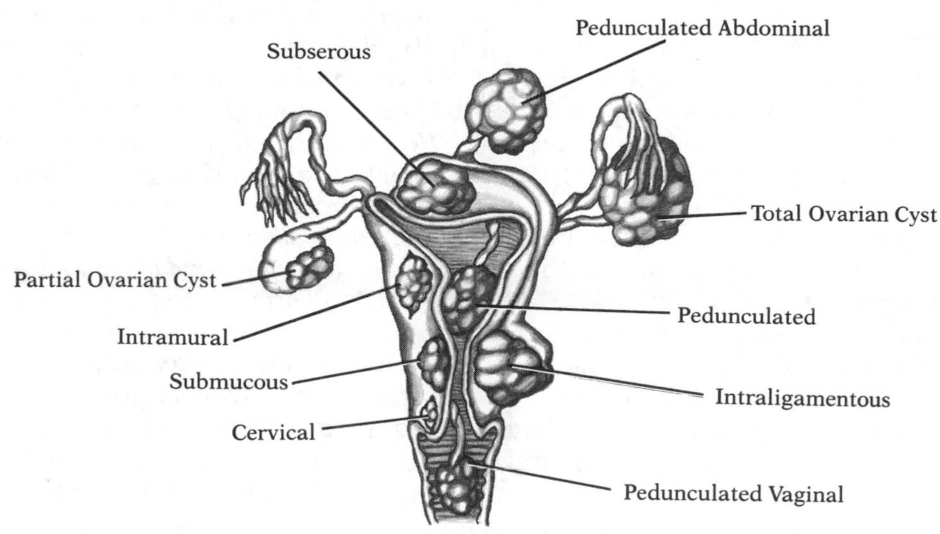

FIBROIDS (MYOMAS) OF THE UTERUS

This is a composite drawing. No one has all these fibroids.

even if they are large (though very large ones may eventually disturb other organs).

- *Intramural*—Located outside the muscle wall of the uterus. May cause pain and bleeding (not true hemorrhaging) at menstruation.
- *Submucous*—Located just under the surface of the uterine lining and jutting out into the uterine cavity; this type of fibroid sometimes causes serious bleeding. Fortunately, this is the least common of the three.

Sometimes a fibroid is attached to the uterus with a *pedicle* or *peduncle,* a narrow-based stalk, which may twist and cause pain. The pedunculated fibroid is the easiest to remove regardless of its size. The size and location of fibroids are determined by uterine X ray, ultrasound test (sonogram), D and C, the new vaginal ultrasound, and, sometimes, magnetic resonance imaging (MRI).

We may be alarmed when doctors tell us we have "large" fibroids. How large is a "large" fibroid? Hospitals approve surgical removal of a fibroid that grows beyond a twelve-week-pregnancy size, or is larger than four to five inches (the size of a grapefruit) when palpable from the abdomen. Some gynecologists consider a uterus massively enlarged if it is the size of a fourteen- to eighteen-week pregnancy. Unfortunately, many surgeons perform hysterectomies for much smaller fibroids. Sometimes nothing more than a surgeon's clinical judgment is used to measure these growths. A slight increase in size can make a fibroid seem enormous to the touch, and a gynecologist might rush a woman into a hysterectomy, telling her that fibroids are overtaking her uterus. In the operating room these "enormous" tumors often turn out to be much smaller than originally perceived.

Some women become alarmed because they think the rapid growth of a fibroid may be a sign of malignancy, although this is extremely rare. How does a woman know how rapid is "rapid"? Ultrasound tests can be repeated at three-month intervals in order to compare sizes. A fibroid that increases by one third its size in three months might be considered to show rapid growth, although most fibroids that grow rapidly are benign.

Fibroids may have to be removed if they cause extreme bleeding or pain, if they degenerate because they have outgrown their blood supply, or if they become infected. But in such cases the operation of choice is usually a myomectomy, *not* a hysterectomy.

If you are approaching menopause and have bothersome fibroids, you may choose to wait until menopause, when fibroids usually recede, before making a decision about surgery. Try the following suggestions in the meantime. Patience is advisable in this situation, because fibroid shrinkage may be very gradual, over a period of months or even years after the last menstrual period.

Self-Help for Women with Fibroids

1. Do not take estrogen.
2. Do not take steroids, unless needed for a life-threatening illness. (Steroids stimulate the adrenal glands, which also produce estrogen and so may enlarge fibroids.)
3. Try to keep your percentage of body fat down by exercising. Estrogen is produced in the fat cells of the body.
4. Reduce the total percentage of fat in the diet. Cut out or cut down on sugar. Increase vegetables and whole grains. Cut out alcohol.
5. Try to manage and reduce stress. Many women recall that their fibroids enlarged after a particularly stressful time. Reactions to stress can stimulate the adrenal glands to produce hormones.
6. Try alternative healing techniques. Some women report help from acupuncture and from visualizing a uterus free of fibroids.
7. Find or form a network of other women who are living with troublesome fibroids and who are trying to wait them out.

Myomectomy for Fibroids

Myomectomy, or surgical removal of fibroids without removing the uterus, was rarely done in the past and was reserved for younger women who wished to have children. However, with new awareness of the value of retaining organs, an increasing number of skilled surgeons are performing myomectomies on older women who do not intend to have children but who wish to preserve their uteruses. In 1990, thirty-eight thousand myomectomies were performed in the United States.[24]

During a myomectomy the surgeon will make an incision into the abdomen and examine the uterus. Fibroids on the outside of the uterus (subserous) can be removed. If the fibroids are inside the uterus, the surgeon will cut into the uterine cavity and remove the fibroids, which peel out like oranges peel from their skins. She or he will then repair and close the uterus. Uterine tissue heals easily.

Myomectomies are now covered by insurance companies to the same extent as hysterectomies.

I just had my second myomectomy in sixteen years because of extensive periods. Before the myomectomy, I had periods that were two weeks long, I looked five or six months pregnant, had to pee frequently because the fibroids were pressing on the bladder, and experienced discomfort during sex because of the fibroid in the cervix. The surgeon compared the sizes of the fibroids to fruits. He said he removed one grapefruit, one orange, several lemons, and a bunch of grapes. I had problems with my insurance policy because the bill was much higher than the usual allowance for a myomectomy. This was because of the time and the two units of blood needed to do such extensive surgery. [a forty-one-year-old woman]

Though not necessarily more difficult to perform than a hysterectomy, myomectomy does require a surgeon experienced in that technique. Such surgeons are more apt to be found in teaching hospitals and fertility clinics.

Every effort must be made to remove even the smallest fibroid during a myomectomy, since regrowth can occur in 10 percent to 25 percent of cases. An older woman is less likely than a younger woman to have fibroids regrow to a size that requires a second myomectomy. Fifteen, thirty, and even more fibroids have been successfully removed without damaging the uterus.

New methods of myomectomy with laser beams now exist, which cause less bleeding and require a much shorter recuperation time than conventional surgery.[25] Laser surgery through a hysteroscope (a device that allows the surgeon to see into the cavity of the uterus) can destroy submucous fibroids. Long-term advantages of this technique over a standard myomectomy are being studied.

Unfortunately, gynecologists who are unfamiliar with or unskilled in performing myomectomies may discourage a woman from having one by telling her that it is dangerous, that it might require a second operation, that it is silly at her age, or that she should accept a hysterectomy instead.

My periods had increased in length to two weeks or more, and were accompanied by cramps, extreme weakness, and sometimes fever. Most of the rest of the month I suffered from PMS [premenstrual syndrome] and back pain. A doctor told me I had to have a hysterectomy. He said my uterus was the size of a four- to five-month pregnancy due to fibroids. While he mentioned myomectomy, he said it was a much more dangerous operation and I shouldn't think about it unless I felt strongly about having a child. I was not planning to have a child. He called the uterus a "baby-carrying sac" with no other purpose. A second doctor had the same opinion. A third doctor, more thorough, gave me a sonogram, which showed my en-

larged uterus pressuring my kidneys and rectum. While he did not push hysterectomy over myomectomy, he also felt that the basis of my decision should be whether I wanted a child.

A diagnostic D and C reduced the length of my periods but the other problems remained. I wanted more information. At a hysterectomy support group I learned of a wide range of side effects of a hysterectomy, which none of the doctors had told me about. I arranged for a myomectomy with the third doctor, who had solid experience doing them and was up on the latest methods. I felt compelled to tell him, however, that the basis for my decision was that I wanted a child. I had six fibroids removed. One was the size of a small grapefruit, and three others were the size of tennis balls.

Now, a year later, my period is two and a half days long with little pain. I have PMS just two or three days before my period. For me, myomectomy was the best choice. [a forty-year-old woman]

Since the growth of fibroids is stimulated by estrogen (fibroids are never found before puberty and only rarely after menopause in women who are not taking estrogens), drugs that suppress estrogen are being increasingly used. These drugs induce a reversible menopause that shrinks fibroids to an average of 50 percent of their original size. The various formulations—danazol, and synthetic variations of the hormone that inhibits each new menstrual cycle (called GnRH analogs) such as leuprolide or nafarelin—are expensive and must be considered with caution. They can cause hot flashes, vaginal dryness, and (except danazol) may reduce HDL ("good" cholesterol) levels and cause bone-mass loss. Danazol, a derivative of the male hormone testosterone, is not without its own potential additional effects—namely, depression, liver damage, weight gain, loss of libido, and masculinizing reactions such as growth of facial hair and deepening of the voice. Also, the fibroids may grow again when the drug is stopped. Studies are under way to see if small doses of hormones can be administered along with these drugs to reduce the harmful effects yet still shrink fibroids.[26] The treatment may be used by itself as a way to "buy time" until menopause, or may be used to shrink fibroids before a surgical myomectomy is performed. It is important to note that some surgeons prefer to do a myomectomy on fibroids that have not been so treated because they feel untreated fibroids are better delineated.

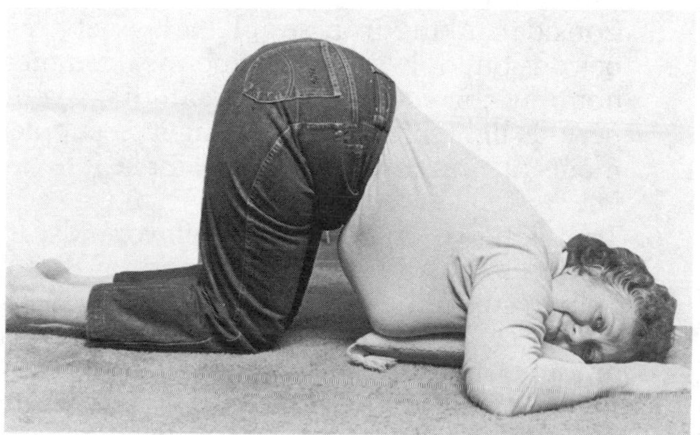

Knee-chest position Pam White

Pain During or Between Periods

Do not have a hysterectomy just because you have pain in the lower abdomen during or between periods. Pelvic pain can arise from a variety of causes, including endometriosis, fibroids, ovarian cysts, and infection or scar tissue from previous pelvic surgery. All possible sources for the pain, including childhood physical and sexual abuse and psychogenic causes, should be professionally investigated and treated before resorting to surgery.[27] A thorough diagnostic workup should be done to discover whether the cause of the pain might be from the digestive system, the urinary tract, the bones, or the joints. Do not automatically assume that the pain is gynecological.

Visualization, relaxation training, and hypnosis for pain control are often helpful. Pain can sometimes be caused by *premenstrual syndrome,* which sometimes increases in duration and severity in women nearing menopause[28] and then subsides after menopause.

If self-help techniques are not effective, prescription drugs may be necessary. A group of antiarthritic drugs (generic names: ibuprofen, naproxen, and mefenomic acid; trade names: Motrin, Anaprox, Ponstel) may relieve menstrual cramps and pain from fibroids. These drugs contain prostaglandin-blocking substances that often lessen excessive menstrual flow as well.[29] One drug may work better for one woman than another. Take these drugs with milk, as they can cause stomach upset.

To relieve the pain caused by a fibroid in a tipped-back uterus that is pressing on the rectum, try the knee-chest position several times a day. This position will help straighten the uterus, thus lessening pressure on the rectum.

HEAVY OR PROLONGED MENSTRUAL BLEEDING (MENORRHAGIA)

Even though women are used to menstrual bleeding on a regular basis, unexpected and unpredictable bleeding can be frightening. We need to know that irregular or heavy menstrual flow is very common in women approaching menopause. Heavy or irregular bleeding can also occur from the use of an IUD (even after it is removed), polyps, fibroids, ovarian cysts, infections of the cervix, or shifting hormone balances. Discuss prolonged heavy bleeding with your health-care provider. Also, **any bleeding in a woman well past menopause should be checked.**

A hysterectomy should not be done merely to stop heavy bleeding, at least until the reason for the bleeding is determined and all other efforts to control it have failed. Many hysterectomies performed because of bleeding are done without a preliminary D and C, hysteroscopy and suction curettage, or endometrial biopsy. In a letter to a medical journal, an indignant physician wrote, "Generally, menorrhagia seems to be diagnosed on the basis of a woman's description of her menstrual loss and is rarely confirmed by the methods available. I am unaware of any other important organ that is electively removed without first assessing its degree of malfunction."[30]

Be sure that you do not overestimate the amount of blood lost during a period. We suggest women keep menstrual charts, recording the number of days from the beginning of one period to the beginning of the next period, the number of days bleeding lasts, how many napkins or tampons used, whether there are clots (red or brown), and any other details that seem relevant. You may be able to establish some pattern to the bleeding to discuss with your physician.

In addition, heavy loss of blood may lead to anemia, which causes fatigue, paleness, and heart palpitations. A blood test for anemia should always be given to a woman who is bleeding heavily. Normal hemoglobin values range from 12 to 16 grams per 100 milliliters; normal hematocrit values (the ratio of red blood cells to the volume of whole blood) range from 33 percent to 46 percent. A mild anemia can often be improved by eating more iron-rich foods and taking iron supplements after you eat. Foods rich in vitamin C eaten at the same meal as iron-rich foods help increase the absorption of iron.

I'm forty-two years old and walking around with a twenty-weeks-pregnant-size uterus from fibroids. Several years ago, my uterus was eight- to ten-weeks size. I was told then to have a hysterectomy. My periods were heavy, on and off. Once I was so frightened that I took a cab to a hospital emergency room, but the bleeding subsided by the time I got there. I was told I was anemic. Two years ago I started taking iron pills. My red blood cells [hematocrit] went from twenty-nine in February to thirty-five in June and thirty-eight in October. The iron upset my system only slightly and cost $2 per 100 tablets. For the first five months my bleeding decreased significantly. But two months ago the doctor said my uterus is still twenty-weeks size, and he seems thoroughly disgusted with me that I haven't had a hysterectomy. I'm really in a quandary, with probably another six years to go before menopause.

In the absence of any diagnosed pathology, you can try these self-care and alternative treatments for heavy bleeding:

1. Try to remain calm. Anxiety can increase blood flow by raising your blood pressure and making the heart pump faster. Don't panic.
2. Stay off your feet, with your legs elevated, if "flooding" occurs. An ice pack applied to the abdomen for an hour or two (fifteen minutes on, fifteen minutes off) can stop or reduce bleeding. Also, try applying cold to the lower back with a towel that has been dampened and chilled in the freezer.
3. Avoid heating pads, hot showers, or baths on heavy-flow days. Heat increases blood flow.
4. Avoid aspirin products, garlic, and mint. They increase bleeding.
5. Consider taking iron supplements between periods but only if you are anemic. Iron pills not only correct anemia but can make your periods lighter. *Caution:* Taking iron supplements during your period may make it heavier.[31]
6. Try taking vitamin C with bioflavonoids. In amounts under 1 to 2 grams per day, these help to strengthen the walls of blood vessels and may reduce bleeding. Above this amount, vitamin C is sometimes toxic, and may actually increase bleeding. The white part of citrus fruits contains bioflavonoids.
7. Try taking 10,000 IUs of vitamin A twice a

day.[32] Amounts in excess of 25,000 IUs per day can be toxic. One carrot contains about 8,000 IUs.

8. Calcium, vitamin D, and magnesium encourage blood clotting and blood vessel contractions.
9. Acupuncture and other alternative healing methods have helped some women.
10. Try over-the-counter antihistamines the first day or two of the period.[33]

If self-help approaches do not work, some doctors may prescribe progestins. For women approaching menopause, the most common reason for heavy bleeding is that they are not ovulating. If your production of progesterone is not sufficient to balance estrogen's buildup of the uterine lining, you may want to work with your physician to find the right dosage and duration of progestin before resorting to a hysterectomy. *Caution:* Do not use progestins if you have had phlebitis, emboli episodes, cerebral hemorrhage, or breast cancer, or if you might be pregnant or having a miscarriage.[34]

A D and C is a diagnostic procedure that can also remove polyps (strawberrylike benign growths) and hyperplasia (the overgrowth of normal uterine tissue) that may be causing bleeding. For routine diagnosis, an aspiration-suction curettage done in the doctor's office costs less and is safer than a D and C. It involves neither the risk of damaging the delicate lining of the uterus nor the risk of anesthesia.

Laser ablation surgery is now used experimentally for uterine conditions, especially to treat heavy bleeding. The surgeon needs special training to use a flexible glass rod with a laser beam tip to burn away (cauterize) the uterine lining. The resulting scar tissue will not bleed. The surgeon is able to view the inside of the uterus through a hysteroscope inserted through the vagina and cervix. Being able to see the lining this way may have advantages over a D and C, which is performed blindly. The newer Nd:YAG laser beam can be focused more precisely than a CO_2 laser. Danazol is given for three weeks before the surgery to thin the endometrium. This procedure is not recommended for women with any signs of cancer or active pelvic inflammatory disease. *This procedure causes sterilization* but seems to preserve other uterine functions. It carries the risks of anesthesia and perforation but the heat created and lack of incision minimize infection. Moreover, it can usually be done on an outpatient basis with immediate resumption of normal activities. Few surgeons are skilled in the technique and it has not been in use long enough to evaluate long-term effects.

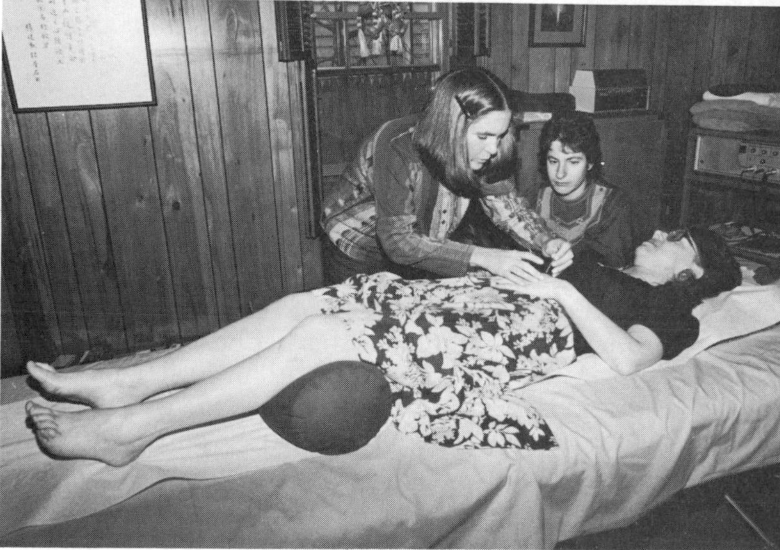

Acupuncture treatment for heavy bleeding. Betsy Shapiro

UTERINE PROLAPSE (DROPPED WOMB)

About 35 percent of hysterectomies in older women are done for uterine prolapse, or dropped womb. In general, prolapse results from stretching of the ligaments that support the uterus and/or weakness of the pubococcygeal muscle, which supports the pelvic floor. See drawing on page 304. There are three stages of uterine prolapse:

- *First degree*—The uterus has descended into the vaginal canal, but not yet into the vaginal opening.
- *Second degree*—The cervix actually appears outside the vaginal opening, in whole or in part.
- *Third degree* (called complete prolapse)—The entire uterus descends to the point that it shows outside the vagina entirely. This type is most common in women over seventy.

To prevent uterine prolapse and to improve your pelvic muscle support system, no matter how slight or severe your prolapse, do Kegel exercises regularly (see Moving for Health chapter, page 75). Symptoms usually do not occur with first-degree prolapse, except for occasional bearing-down discomfort. *If you cannot tell you have a prolapse, then surgery is not necessary*.

Some women can avoid surgery by use of a pessary, a plastic or rubber device that helps hold the uterus in place. Pessaries come in various sizes and shapes and must be fitted and inserted by a physician experienced in their use. They must be removed periodically for cleaning. Any woman who wishes to avoid surgery or is a poor risk for surgery because of age or vulnerability to anesthesia might find this her best choice.

A less drastic surgery than hysterectomy to correct prolapse is uterine suspension surgery (sometimes called by women a "plastic"). This is abdominal surgery that lifts the uterus into its correct position by shortening the ligaments that hold the uterus in place. Unfortunately, some surgeons prefer to remove the uterus rather than repair it, based on their own value judgment that losing her uterus does not matter to a woman beyond a certain age.

Endometriosis

Endometriosis is a condition in which tissue of the uterine lining is found outside the uterus. This tissue thickens and bleeds with the menstrual cycle each month, forming cysts. The main symptoms of endometriosis are pain during menstruation or intercourse and heavy bleeding. The symptoms tend to get worse as the endometriosis spreads and grows. Endometriosis is often a cause of infertility.

Doctors sometimes diagnose endometriosis when they find tender, nodular growths behind the uterus during a manual pelvic exam, but a laparoscopy (examination of the pelvic organs with a lighted, periscope-type instrument through a half-inch incision in the navel) provides the most definite diagnosis.

Endometriosis is often treated with birth-control pills or other hormones that bring on a state of pseudopregnancy. This can dry up the growths completely and is effective in about 50 percent of cases. However, relief is temporary, since the tissue can regrow, and the hormones have certain unpleasant and/or dangerous effects. Birth-control pills are very dangerous for women over the age of thirty-five who smoke and women over forty with a second risk factor for heart disease such as diabetes or hypertension (see page 103). Danazol (previously discussed on page 323) is reported to be effective in the treatment of endometriosis. Instead of, or in addition to, danazol, you may choose to undergo conservative surgery, in which an abdominal incision is made and the endometrial implants removed, either by laser beams or by electric cauterization. Recently, GnRH analogs are also being used to shrink endometrial implants prior to laparoscopic surgery.

Hysterectomy is usually a last resort for endometriosis, especially in near-menopausal women whose symptoms will probably recede after menopause. Since endometriosis, like fibroids, is estrogen dependent, you can follow some of the same self-help tips for it as you do for fibroids (see page 322).

Adenomyosis

Adenomyosis is a condition in which endometrial tissue that lines the inside of the uterus (and which is shed each month during the period) becomes embedded in the walls of the uterus. Previously the condition was called internal endometriosis, since both involved endometrial tissue in unusual places. Adenomyosis, however, is usually found in women in their forties and fifties who have borne children, while endometriosis is most commonly found in younger women who have not borne children. One theory is that the tissue becomes trapped as the uterus shrinks to normal size after pregnancy. Some degree of adenomyosis is so common that it is found in up to 60 percent of women whose uteruses are removed and examined for some other reason. With adenomyosis, the examining physician may find that the uterus is firm and diffusely enlarged, but only 20 percent of these women may experience heavy or prolonged periods and menstrual pain. A D and C will not help adenomyosis because the tissue is embedded in the wall of the uterus. Since the tissue swells with the increase of estrogen each month but is trapped in the uterine wall, use of estrogen or progesterone will only make it worse. See cautions (above) on the use of danazol. Try the self-help suggestions for heavy bleeding, pain, and fibroids. Menopause, with its drop in estrogen, brings relief.[35]

Precancerous Conditions

Many women have hysterectomies because of supposed "precancerous" conditions. Always question a doctor's suggestion that an area of tissue is precancerous. It is not clear whether precancerous means the tissue will almost certainly become cancerous or whether it means the condition can revert to normal, become cancerous, or stay the same. Sometimes what is called a precancerous condition may disappear without treatment or can be treated with medication, self-help techniques, or less drastic surgery. If your doctor tells you that you have a precancerous condition, ask for a copy of your pathology report and get another pathologist to review your slides.

Be sure to have a second, or even third, Pap test several weeks or even a month after the earlier one before agreeing to surgery or any other treatment to destroy questionable cells. If the results of the Pap tests warrant further investigation, the physician should view the cervix with a colposcope. Areas of the cervix can be removed for study by a *punch biopsy* (removal of a small plug of cells for examination). Suspicious cervical cells have sometimes returned to normal when women had their male sexual partners use condoms to keep sperm from contact with the cervix. Then cauterization (with heat, electricity, or chemicals), cryosurgery (freezing the cells), or laser surgery can destroy small patches of malignant cells. *Cone biopsy,* or *conization* (removal of a ring of the cervix around the opening to the uterus), may also be recommended. These procedures can remove small amounts of tissue, reduce the spread of cervical cancer, and prevent hysterectomies.

The cells of the lining of the uterus (endometrium) can also undergo changes, many of which are not serious enough to justify hysterectomy. One such change, *hyperplasia* (an increase in the number of normal cells), is not cancer, rarely becomes cancer, and can be treated with medication or a D and C. A hysterectomy is not necessary to diagnose uterine or ovarian cancer. An endometrial biopsy performed in a physician's office or a D and C can diagnose cancer of the uterus with reasonable accuracy. A laparoscopy (described earlier in this chapter) can provide a view of the ovaries and even take samples of tissue or fluid for examination. This procedure requires general anesthesia. Even if the diagnosis of ovarian cancer is found, you do not always have to be "cleaned out." Cancer specialists are finding that many women treated by having only the diseased ovary removed do just as well as those in whom everything is taken out as long as the surgeon does a thorough search for tumor spread.[36]

TYPES OF HYSTERECTOMY

There are three different types of hysterectomy:

- *Total hysterectomy,* sometimes referred to as *simple hysterectomy*—Removal of the uterus and cervix (mouth of the womb) but not the ovaries and fallopian tubes. A woman continues to produce hormones from her ovaries, but not at her optimum output, and the regular cyclical pattern of ovulation may be interrupted. Sometimes the ovaries are irreparably "shocked" and never resume functioning after the uterus is cut away.[37]
- *Total hysterectomy with bilateral salpingo-oophorectomy*—Removal of the uterus and cervix as well as both tubes and ovaries. Ovarian hormone production ceases abruptly.
- *Subtotal hysterectomy*—Only the body of the uterus is removed. The cervix is left in, with the surrounding stump of uterus. The tubes and ovaries remain.

Physicians rarely did a subtotal hysterectomy, on the theory that the cervix may develop cancer later. Many women and some physicians are now questioning whether a healthy cervix should be removed. The rate of cervical cancer is no higher after a subtotal hysterectomy than it is in women whose organs are intact.[38] Researchers do not yet know whether the remaining cervix and piece of uterus will provide the body with beneficial hormones as a piece of ovary will. Also, leaving the cervix in when a hysterectomy is performed avoids the necessity of cutting the bladder completely away from the uterus, as the surgeon does in a total hysterectomy. The advantage of letting the bladder remain with the cervix is that it may prevent the prolapse of the vault of the vagina, as sometimes occurs after a total hysterectomy.[39] Leaving the cervix in may prevent the loss of sexual response among women who depend on cervical stimulation for orgasm.

If the cervix is left, then be sure to continue to have regular Pap tests.

HYSTERECTOMY: THE OPERATION

As with all surgery, hysterectomy presents hazards. The death rate is one to two per thousand women—approximately eight hundred women die each year from a hysterectomy. Most of these deaths are anesthesia-related. As many as half of

FEMALE PELVIC ORGANS

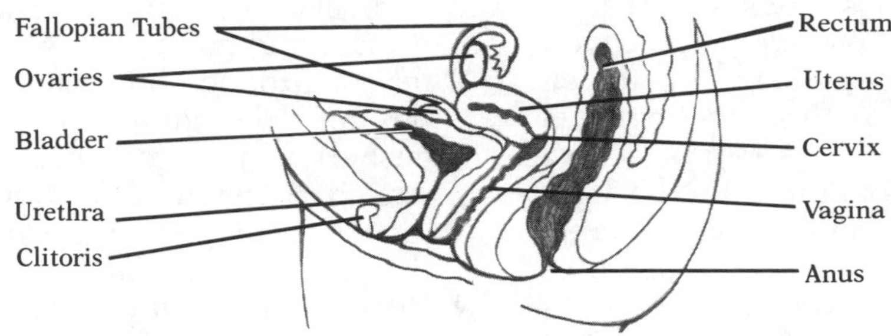

TYPES OF HYSTERECTOMY

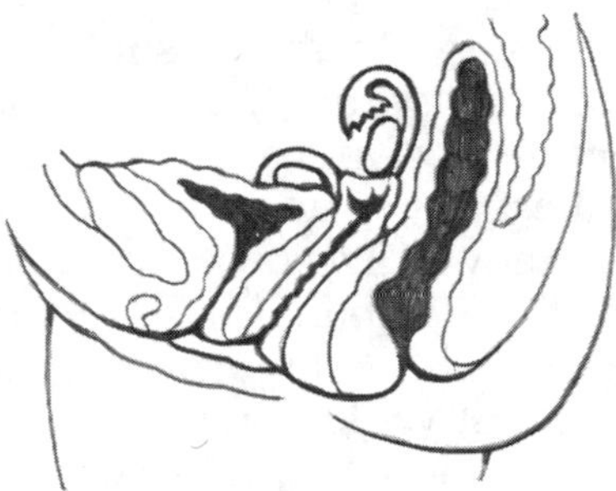

Subtotal or Supracervical:
Removal of uterus leaving cervix, fallopian tubes, and ovaries

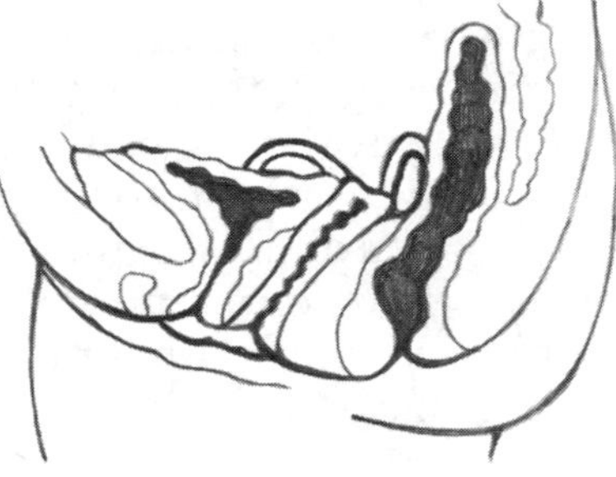

Total or Complete:
Removal of uterus and cervix, leaving ovaries and fallopian tubes

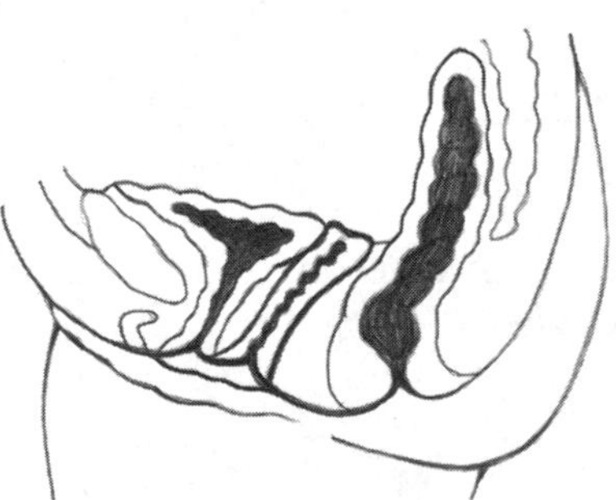

Total with Bilateral Salpingo-Oophorectomy:
Removal of uterus, ovaries, and fallopian tubes

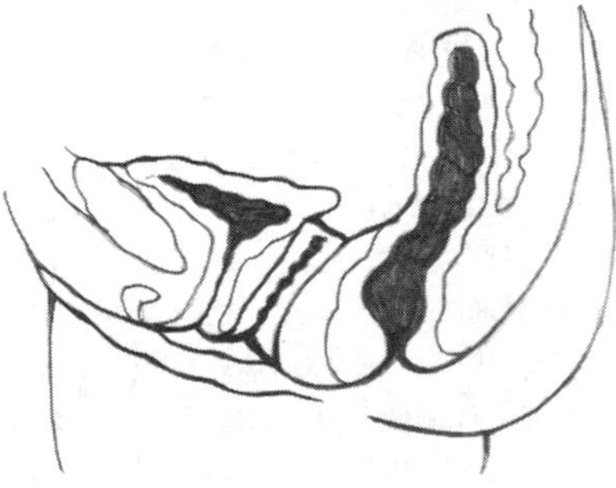

Radical:
Removal of uterus, ovaries, fallopian tubes and top of vagina

all patients experience some operative complications, including adverse reactions to anesthesia, hemorrhaging that requires transfusion (one in ten women),[40] infections, abdominal adhesions, injury to the bladder, bowel, or rectum, and postoperative blood clots. Long-term effects include ovarian failure and urinary and constipation problems.

The surgery commonly involves five to seven days in the hospital and four to six weeks of recovery at home. As with any surgical procedure requiring general anesthesia and involving opening the abdominal cavity, strenuous activity is usually curtailed for several months. Some women experience prolonged fatigue and loss of energy for six months to a year after surgery.

The operation may be done from inside the vagina (leaving no visible scar) or through an abdominal incision. Vaginal hysterectomies seem to involve a shorter recovery period and faster healing. However, many urologists and gynecologists specializing in the treatment of incontinence believe that the vaginal approach carries too much risk of damage to the urinary system, and that the abdominal approach is preferable for that reason. (See Urinary Incontinence chapter.) Don't lose sight of the major question, "Is it necessary to remove an important organ?" The cheery tone of the term *bikini cut* trivializes the seriousness of a hysterectomy.

Ovaries In or Out Over Forty?

The threat of ovarian cancer does not justify routine removal of healthy ovaries. Ovarian cancer, while a serious disease, is relatively rare, occurring in less than 1 percent of all women. While the risk increases in postmenopausal women, it should be noted that the average age of diagnosis of ovarian cancer is sixty-one, and this does not justify routine removal of healthy ovaries from women in their forties or fifties. In the United States a woman has a 1.3 percent chance of developing ovarian cancer by her seventy-fourth year.[41] One source estimated that seventy-five hundred healthy ovaries would have to be removed to prevent a single cancer death.[42] The risk of ovarian cancer is no higher in hysterectomized women who keep their ovaries than in women who do not undergo a hysterectomy. Furthermore, because ovarian tissue can occur elsewhere in the abdominal cavity, removal of the ovaries does not absolutely guarantee that ovarian cancer will never occur.[43]

During a hysterectomy, the ovaries should be examined for abnormalities. In *advance* of surgery, a woman should discuss with her doctor the conditions under which she consents to the removal of her ovaries. Often a gynecologist will say, "If the ovaries are unhealthy we'll take them out," without specifying what is meant by "unhealthy." A cyst, for example, can be cut out from an ovary without removal of the entire ovary. Most ovarian cysts in menstruating women are harmless and disappear after several cycles. Sometimes cysts collect fluid or blood and can be drained (aspirated).[44] There is no evidence to date showing that the presence of cysts means an increased risk of ovarian cancer at any age.

If the ovaries are retained after a hysterectomy, regular ovarian checkups are advised just as if you never had a hysterectomy. The ovaries are actually easier to examine once the uterus is out of the way, and any question as to their size or consistency can be checked by vaginal ultrasound or other scans.

Do's and Don'ts for Women Contemplating Elective Hysterectomy

A woman who has been advised to have a hysterectomy is often not at her best physically and emotionally. She may feel weak or sick and be under too much stress to be an assertive, active information seeker. The pressures are often strong to "get it over with." But it is important to persist, for a thorough knowledge of your condition is your best assurance of making the right decision.

- *Do* have someone with you when you see your health-care provider. Bring a person who will help you ask questions, assess the answers, and support you so you will not feel intimidated into making a quick decision.
- *Do* seek other opinions if surgery is recommended. In a medical system as geared to hysterectomy as ours, a second opinion may not be enough. Many insurance programs today will pay for second or even third opinions. *Don't* feel that you must agree if the second doctor also recommends hysterectomy.
- *Do* talk with other women. *Do* try to find a hysterectomy or a menopause support group in your community and attend a meeting. The women there cannot make your decision for you, but they will give you information

unavailable elsewhere and, possibly, a physician-referral list. Some groups have a twenty-four-hour hot line. Other women's honest assessments are one of your best tools.

- *Don't* have a hysterectomy for sterilization purposes. (See Birth Control for Women at Midlife chapter.) This practice is not permitted by the American College of Gynecologists.
- *Don't* have a hysterectomy because that was the medical practice popular in your mother's and aunts' era.
- *Do* search out the most current information. Check copyright dates: books written even five or six years ago do not have the newest information about alternatives to and aftereffects of hysterectomy. Women's health centers and hospital medical libraries may help you find the newest information. Technical language may be difficult at first, but conquering the jargon is well worth the effort. *Do* check the source of all information read. A pamphlet produced by a drug company, for example, may subtly encourage surgery that would necessitate taking their drug.
- *Do* use an internist, family practitioner, or general practitioner as your primary physician. She or he is more apt to see you as a total person, rather than just a set of gynecological organs. This primary physician can recommend nonsurgical treatments and can refer you to a gynecologist or an endocrinologist (a specialist in glands and hormones) if necessary. *Caution:* Many physicians have been trained to regard hysterectomies as routine procedures.
- *Do* try to find a physician who is treating someone else's gynecological problem conservatively without a hysterectomy.
- *Do* try to be optimistic. This is very difficult when physicians take a somber, pessimistic approach to your condition. In an effort to manipulate you into a hysterectomy, some doctors may accentuate the negative.
- *Do* try to reduce stress by every means possible. Stress exacerbates all gynecological problems.
- *Don't* automatically reject proposed treatments because you do not want to take drugs regularly. Some drugs may be far less risky than a hysterectomy, which involves anesthesia, prophylactic antibiotics, and possibly long-term hormone-replacement therapy, not to mention the potential irreversible aftereffects of the surgery.
- *Do* realize that you have a right to refuse or withdraw from any treatment or surgery at any time, even *after* you have entered the hospital.

IF YOU HAVE ALREADY HAD A HYSTERECTOMY

Although no treatment, drug, or regimen can replace or restore what was lost, women have found some ways to feel better.

- Give yourself time to grieve your loss. If yours was an unnecessary hysterectomy, your feelings of rage are normal and understandable. Having an unnecessary hysterectomy or being denied full disclosure, like being raped or abused, is a violation that requires time for recovery. Make every effort to seek support. Keep a journal, join or form a hysterectomy support group, talk with sympathetic friends and family, or become an advocate of women's health issues. Use your anger to help other women.[45]
- Make sure you know exactly what was removed during the procedure. Many women do not know that they have had one or both ovaries removed. Ask for a copy of your medical record. Gather all the facts. This might help you to cope more effectively.[46]
- If you want to be sexually active, make extra efforts to promote sexual desire. This may be difficult if your interest in sex is low, but just thinking about sex as well as engaging in it increases hormone production in the ovaries and/or adrenal glands and contributes to health and well-being. Sometimes vaginal moisture helps to boost sexual desire as well as make sex more comfortable. Practice Kegels (see pages 75–77) and see suggestions on pages 89–91.
- Pay special attention to your diet. Avoid caffeine, sugars, salt, alcohol, and red meats. Hysterectomies often produce hormone imbalances that can lead to low blood sugar (hypoglycemia). Try to eat small meals high in protein or complex carbohydrates (see Eating Well chapter) every two to three hours. Vitamin supplements, especially B complex and vitamin E, may help deficiencies caused by hormone loss.
- Exercise helps to lessen depression and builds stronger bones, helping to prevent osteoporosis. Some women find that yoga, swimming, dancing, and walking are especially helpful after a hysterectomy. Exercise helps firm mus-

cles and increase muscle and tendon strength, which is helpful in preventing urinary problems and osteoporosis.

- If you undergo an oophorectomy before menopause, you may wish to consider estrogen or estrogen-progestin replacement therapy only until the time when menopause would be expected, tapering down gradually to imitate a natural menopause. If you are undergoing menopausal changes or if you are postmenopausal already, you may prefer not to add hormones when your system has already decreased its production.

Seeking Legal Recourse for Hysterectomy Abuse

If you feel you have been wronged by your surgeon, you should not delay too long before contacting a lawyer, since the statute of limitations (the definite time within which you may initiate a lawsuit) varies from state to state (Pennsylvania's is only two years). Some women's health groups keep a list of health-law specialists. In several recent court cases, women have successfully used the right of informed consent to fight hysterectomy abuse. *Informed consent* (see page 242) means that a woman must have the opportunity to refuse a diagnostic procedure, treatment, or any type of medical care if she decides the contemplated procedure involves unacceptable consequences. Women have won court cases because of doctors' failure to inform patients of possible consequences before getting their consent.[47]

New state legislation in California (1988) and New York (1991) requires doctors who recommend a hysterectomy to a woman to provide her with information detailing the surgical operation and its consequences and to explain alternative procedures. Ask your state representative or senator to work with you, your support group, and other women's health activists to pass a hysterectomy law in your state.

The "good patient" attitudes that were held in high esteem in our growing-up years cause us to be brave and all-accepting in the face of medical adversity. Sometimes the "good patient" attitude works to our disadvantage and makes the older woman an easy target for medical abuse. As we learn more about pelvic cancer, we can become more courageous about questioning or refusing treatments that may risk our good health to save us from a disease we are not likely to contract.

NOTES

1. Estimated figures from the National Center for Health Statistics.
2. The Boston Women's Health Book Collective, *The New Our Bodies, Ourselves*. New York: Simon and Schuster, 1992, p. 599.
3. The 10 percent figure is from one HMO cited in Steven J. Bernstein, et al., "The Appropriateness of Hysterectomy: A Comparison of Seven Health Plans." *Journal of the American Medical Association*, Vol. 269, No. 18 (May 12, 1993), pp. 2398–2402. The 90 percent figure is in Herbert A. Goldfarb with Judith Grief, *The No Hysterectomy Option*. New York: John Wiley & Sons, Inc., 1990, p. 202.
4. Claudia Dreifus, ed., *Seizing Our Bodies*. New York: Vintage Books, 1978.
5. Bernstein, op. cit.
6. Kristen Kjerulff, et. al., "The Socioeconomic Correlates of Hysterectomies in the United States." *American Journal of Public Health*, Vol. 83, No. 1 (January 1993), pp. 106–8
7. John E. Wennberg, "Dealing with Medical Practice Variations: A Proposal for Action." *Health Affairs*, Vol. 3, No. 2 (Summer 1984), pp. 6–32.
8. See Marcia Millman, *The Unkindest Cut: Life in the Backrooms of Medicine*. New York: William Morrow and Co., 1977.
9. National Center for Health Statistics. By age sixty, however, over one third of U.S. women have had a hysterectomy. "Hysterectomy—the second most common major surgery." AHCPR *Research Activities*, No. 167 (August 1993), p. 9.
10. The use of myomectomy to remove just a uterine fibroid rather than removing the entire uterus is increasing. Karen J. Carlson, et al., "Indications for Hysterectomy." *The New England Journal of Medicine*, Vol. 328, No. 12 (Mar. 25, 1993), pp. 856–60.
11. Katherine Dalton, "Discussion on the Aftermath of Hysterectomy and Oophorectomy." *Proceedings of the Royal Society of Medicine*, Vol. 50 (1957), pp. 415–18. Surveyed women for ten years after surgery.
12. Brooks Ranney and S. Abu-Ghazaleh, "The Future Function and Fortune of Ovarian Tissue Which Is Retained in Vivo During Hysterectomy." *American Journal of Obstetrics and Gynecology*, Vol. 128, No. 6 (July 15, 1977), pp. 626–34.
13. Sherwin A. Kaufman, *The Ageless Woman*. New York: Prentice-Hall, 1967, p. 127.
14. National Women's Health Network, *Taking Hormones and Women's Health: Choices, Risks and Benefits*. Washington, D.C., 1993.
15. James D. Shelton, "Prostacyclin from the Uterus and Woman's Cardiovascular Advantage." *Prostaglandins, Leukotrienes and Medicine*, Vol. 8, No. 5 (May 1982), pp. 459–66.
16. Vicki Hufnagel, *No More Hysterectomies*. New York: New American Library, 1988, pp. 42–44; *H.E.R.S. Newsletter*, Vol. V, No. II (1993), p. 3.
17. L. Zussman, Shirley Zussman, R. Sunley, and Edith Bjorson, "Sexual Responses After Hysterectomy/Oophorectomy: Recent Studies and Reconsideration of Psychogenesis." *American Journal of Obstetrics and Gynecology*, Vol. 140, No. 7 (Aug. 1, 1981), pp. 725–29.

18. Wulf H. Utian, "Effect of Hysterectomy, Oophorectomy and Estrogen Therapy on Libido." *International Journal of Gynaecology and Obstetrics,* Vol. 13, No. 3 (1975), pp. 97–100.

19. J. Anath, "Hysterectomy and Depression." *Obstetrics and Gynecology,* Vol. 52, No. 6 (December 1978), p. 729.

20. D. H. Richards, "A Post-Hysterectomy Syndrome." *Lancet,* Oct. 26, 1974, pp. 983–85.

21. Winnifred Berg Cutler, *Hysterectomy: Before and After.* New York: Harper & Row, 1988, pp. 256–58.

22. Sandra Beaman Jordan, "The Facts About Fibroid Tumors." *McCall's,* July 1985, p. 62.

23. Ivan K. Strausz, *You Don't Need a Hysterectomy: New and Effective Ways of Avoiding Major Surgery.* Reading, MA: Addison-Wesley, 1993, pp. 93–94.

24. Estimated figures from the National Center for Health Statistics.

25. Robert S. Neuwirth, "Hysteroscopic Management of Symptomatic Submucous Fibroids." *Obstetrics and Gynecology,* Vol. 62, No. 4 (October 1983), pp. 509–11.

26. Strausz, op. cit., pp. 141–55.

27. Sidney M. Wolfe et al., *Women's Health Alert.* Reading, MA: Addison-Wesley, 1991, p. 69; Strausz, op. cit., pp. 171–210.

28. Niels Lauersen, *PMS: Premenstrual Syndrome and You.* New York: Pinnacle Books, 1984, p. 88.

29. Niels Lauerson and Eileen Stukane, *Listen to Your Body.* New York: Simon & Schuster, 1982, p. 61.

30. M. Greenberg, "Hysterectomy, Hormones and Behavior: Letter to the Editor." *Lancet,* Vol. 1, No. 8217 (Feb. 21, 1981), p. 449.

31. Lynn Payer, *How to Avoid a Hysterectomy.* New York: Pantheon, 1987, pp. 82–83.

32. "Hysterectomy," in *The Prevention Guide to Surgery and Its Alternatives.* Emmaus, PA: Rodale Press, 1980, pp. 287–328.

33. Payer, op. cit., pp. 85–86.

34. Strausz, op. cit., p. 139.

35. Lynda Madras and Jane Patterson, with Peter Schick, *Womancare: A Gynecological Guide to Your Body.* New York: Avon, 1981, pp. 386–89.

36. Payer, op. cit., p. 128.

37. Ranney and Abu-Ghazaleh, op. cit.

38. Richard Mattingly and John D. Thompson, *Te Linde's Operative Gynecology.* Philadelphia: Lippincott, 1985.

39. Niles Newton and Enid Baron, "Reactions to Hysterectomy." *Primary Care,* Vol. 3 (December 1976), p. 793.

40. The Boston Women's Health Book Collective, op. cit., p. 600.

41. J. L. Young, Jr., et al., "Surveillance, Epidemiology and End Results: Incidence and Mortality Data 1973–77." National Cancer Institute Monograph, 1981, p. 57.

42. Lauerson and Stukane, op. cit.

43. Joanne Tobachman, et al., "Intra-Abdominal Carcinomatosis After Prophylactic Oophorectomy in Ovarian-Cancer-Prone Families." *Lancet,* Vol. 3, Oct. 9, 1982, p. 795.

44. Wolfe, op. cit., p. 65.

45. Harriet Goldhor Lerner, "Good Advice. Hysterectomy: Was It Necessary." *New Women,* September 1991.

46. Public Citizen Health Research Group, *Medical Records: Getting Yours,* 1992. 2000 P St., NW, Washington, DC 20036. $10.

47. Sybil Shainwald, "A Legal Response to Hysterectomy Abuse." *The Network News,* Vol. 10, No. 3 (May/June 1985), p. 6.

23

HYPERTENSION, HEART DISEASE, AND STROKE

✦

BY ELLEN DORSCH

1994 UPDATE BY DIANA LASKIN SIEGAL WITH SPECIAL THANKS TO PATRICIA P. BARRY

RESOURCES FOR THIS CHAPTER ON PAGE 494

Many of us have had someone close to us become ill or suddenly die from cardiovascular disease, the leading cause of death in the United States. Cardiovascular disease, or disease of the heart and blood vessels, can damage every part of the body. Some of us have experienced a heart attack or a stroke. Many of us fear being well one minute and seemingly at death's door the next.

Although healthy habits are no guarantee that we can prevent cardiovascular disease, we do know that high blood pressure, smoking, eating foods rich in saturated fats and cholesterol, stress, and inactivity all increase our chances of developing it. We can decrease the probability of serious illness or premature death by reducing these risk factors, regularly checking our blood pressure, and knowing the early warning signs of heart attack and stroke.

HEART DISEASE *IS* A WOMAN'S DISEASE

In the past, heart disease was considered a man's disease. Most research until recently did not include women, so much of the information we have about heart disease is based on studies of men, assuming that they are the norm. In fact, heart disease is the leading cause of death in women over sixty today, and women who have heart attacks are more likely to die from them than men, possibly because they are older and have other serious associated diseases. We can no longer afford to ignore the impact of heart disease on women's health—more research is needed on women and heart disease.

Because heart disease is often regarded as a man's disease, many physicians pay less attention to symptoms in women than in men, and don't emphasize preventive steps, such as lowering cholesterol levels. Women often suffer needless discomfort because they or their physicians ignore or minimize early symptoms.

I was lying in bed at about 2:00 in the morning. I felt a pain in my chest, which I thought might be indigestion. Then the pain went into my arm and up to my neck and head. That really hurt. I jumped up and it seemed to get better, so I didn't tell my daughter. The next night it started again. I knew there was a problem, but it went away again when I jumped up. The next morning I told my daughter but I refused to go to the doctor. I knew what had happened. But after the pain stopped, I thought maybe nothing happened. I'm stubborn and we fought for two days. Then I went and the doctor put me in the hospital for fourteen days. [a seventy-two-year-old woman]

How the Heart Works

The heart, a four-chambered muscular organ, is divided into a left and right side. The right side receives through the veins blood that is low in oxygen and high in carbon dioxide and passes it to the lungs, where oxygen is added and carbon dioxide eliminated. The oxygen-rich blood from the lungs then goes to the left side of the heart, where it is pumped to all parts of the body through the arteries of the circulatory system. Valves in each chamber of the heart regulate this flow of blood. The circulating blood supplies nutrients and oxygen to all organs and tissues of the body. It picks up waste products from the cells and carries the waste to the kidneys or lungs to be eliminated. The pumping action of the heart is controlled by a bundle of nerves that acts as a natural pacemaker.

High Blood Pressure (Hypertension)

Hypertension, or high blood pressure, increases the risk of strokes and often contributes to heart attacks and other diseases. Most people who have hypertension experience no signs or symptoms; some may experience headaches, dizziness, fainting spells, ringing in the ears, or nosebleeds.

Blood pressure is the force of blood against the walls of the arteries and veins. The force is created by the heart as it pumps blood to every part of the body. Blood pressure is recorded with two numbers: for example, 120/70, read as "120 over 70."

- *Systolic,* the first or upper number, represents the blood pressure in the arteries when the heart is pumping blood;
- *Diastolic,* the second or lower number, is the pressure in the arteries when the heart is filling with blood for the next beat.

The American Heart Association (AHA) considers any systolic pressure over 140 to be abnormal. (Other researchers have defined hypertension in the elderly as blood pressure over 160/90.)[1] For people over sixty-five, systolic pressures of 150 to 155 are not uncommon, but the AHA suggests that they be lowered, if possible. If your diastolic pressure remains above 90 to 95, you are considered hypertensive.

A painless and simple test measures blood pressure. Taking blood pressure is an easy skill to learn. Since many women are under stress in a doctor's office, it may be preferable to check your blood pressure at home or at work. A family or a group could share the cost of the equipment. If you are a large woman, be sure that the cuff you use is big enough to fit around your arm, as one that is too small may cause a false reading. Don't rely on coin-operated machines that are available in drugstores and supermarkets; they are not always adjusted properly and can give false readings.

A diagnosis of high blood pressure should not be based on only one reading, because blood pressure varies with the time of day, activity, and stress, including the stress of having your blood pressure taken. At least three elevated readings, taken days or weeks apart while both sitting and standing, should be found before hypertension is diagnosed.

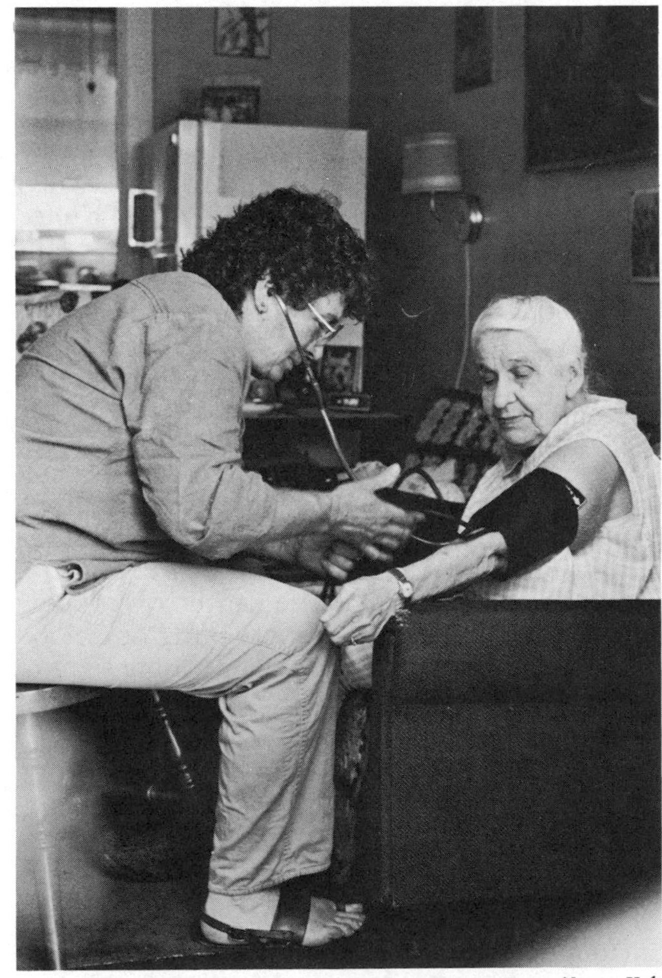

Norma Holt

Blood pressure, especially systolic, tends to rise with age and after menopause. About 50 percent of people over sixty-five have hypertension.[2] Women of color are more susceptible to hypertension than white women.

More black women than white women develop hypertension, and they develop it earlier in life, more severely, and suffer hypertension-related deaths more frequently. Death rates from strokes, in particular, are much higher among blacks than whites. Some researchers attribute these high hypertension rates to a genetic adaptation useful for survival in the African climate but not needed at colder temperatures. Others criticize this theory and state that these high hypertension rates are related to high-stress lives caused by poverty, diets high in salt and fats, and limited accessibility to health care.

I am a sixty-one-year-old black lady who has been diagnosed as having severe hypertension. For thirty-odd years I have tried hard to accept and cope with this problem: no salt, no fat, weight control, etc. It is very hard but if you want to live a fairly normal life, you have to try to do what's best. After having all kinds of tests and medication I have learned one of the best remedies for me is to try and not let things bug me. I try not to get upset over things which I have no control over. Sometimes it doesn't work, but I still keep on trying. My doctor has tried different medications and when something new comes along she will suggest it to me, tell me the side effects, and then leave the decision up to me. Usually I try these medications because maybe something will come along that will help me, or someone else.

WHAT CAN BE DONE FOR HIGH BLOOD PRESSURE?

If you have mild hypertension you may be able to lower your blood pressure without medication, or with less medication, if you adopt the following good health habits.

- Eat well for weight management.
- Exercise. If you are not accustomed to exercise, start by taking a walk each day. If you are not able to get around, see the section When Movement Is Limited, pages 72–74. Exercising also helps weight management. (See Weighty Issues chapter.)
- Reduce salt intake.
- Reduce stress and use relaxation exercises. (Read Aging Well chapter for a more complete discussion of these suggestions.)

MEDICATION/DRUGS FOR HIGH BLOOD PRESSURE

If your hypertension is severe, or if the above suggestions do not lower your blood pressure enough or soon enough, you may need medication to lower it. However, good health habits will contribute to your well-being and should be continued even if you take medication.

If medication is necessary, the first type of drug tried is usually a diuretic (often called a "water pill," because it reduces the amount of fluid in the body). Possible effects include a low potassium level and elevated uric acid and blood glucose levels, which can cause fatigue, muscle weakness, leg cramps, and other problems. Do not take over-the-counter diuretics without consulting a health-care provider. Anyone taking diuretics should be carefully monitored for signs of dehydration and urinary problems. If you are taking a potassium-depleting diuretic, you should eat four servings a day of potassium-rich foods.* If you cannot eat enough of these foods, you may have to take a prescribed potassium preparation.

If diuretic therapy alone is not effective, you may be given additional medications. *Beta-blockers,* such as propranolol (Inderal), metoprolol (Lopressor), nadolol (Corgard), and antenolol (Tenormin), lower the heart's demand for blood. Beta-blockers are not considered a good choice for treating hypertension in black people, some older people, or people with asthma or heart failure. For others, in low doses, beta-blockers effectively treat heart pain (angina pectoris) and irregular heartbeats (arrhythmias). Some women may experience other effects from beta-blockers, such as nausea, cold feet, insomnia, tiredness, depression, a slow heartbeat, or wheezing asthma. Sometimes, though not often, these medications may cause lowered sexual desire. Too high a dose can cause dizziness and fainting spells. If you are taking insulin for diabetes, you should carefully review any possible reactions with your health-care practitioner. ***Never stop taking beta-blockers abruptly;* you must taper off gradually.**

*Apricots, avocados, bananas, broccoli, cabbage, cantaloupe, dates, figs, raisins, grapefruit, molasses, mushrooms, oranges, peanuts, pineapple, plums, potatoes, prunes, pumpkin, radishes, rhubarb, tomatoes, watermelon, wheat germ, whole grains, cooked dried beans.

Calcium-channel blockers are increasingly used as the second step, rather than beta-blockers, in medically treating hypertension. Because calcium-channel blockers prevent spasms of the coronary arteries, they keep the supply of blood flowing into the heart and are useful when spasms play a role in causing angina pain. They also slow a racing heart rate.

Vasodilators are another kind of drug commonly taken for high blood pressure. These relax the blood vessel wall, allowing more blood to flow through. Some women who take them complain of headaches, swelling around the eyes, heart palpitations, shortness of breath, dizziness, or aches and pains in the joints. If these symptoms continue after the first few weeks, talk to your doctor about changing medications.

A combination of small doses of various hypertensive drugs is often more effective for older persons than a single form of medication. Attempting to lower blood pressure over a period of weeks or months, rather than suddenly, produces better results with fewer side effects.

Some General Suggestions for Reducing High Blood Pressure with Drugs

- Your pharmacist is a valuable resource. Ask her or him about generic or less expensive substitutes for your prescription; food and drinks to avoid; and best times to take medication.
- Don't mix drugs. Tell your physician and pharmacist about all drugs (prescription and over-the-counter), including vitamins and birth-control pills, you are taking and any drug reaction you have had in the past.
- Keep to your schedule for taking drugs. Your blood pressure is lowered only while the drugs are working, so you must keep a continuous supply in your body. Some people need medication for the rest of their lives; others may be able to reduce or stop medication if changes in life-style lower their pressure sufficiently over a significant period of time.
- Do not stop medication because your blood pressure is normal or because you feel okay. Remember, you have to *keep* your blood pressure normal.
- Drink little or no alcohol.
- Know your blood pressure. Keep a record of it. You can know your blood pressure only by measuring it, not by how you feel.

Arteriosclerosis/ Atherosclerosis

There are two conditions that underlie cardiovascular diseases. As people grow older, their arteries tend to lose elasticity, decreasing the amount of blood that can pass through (called "hardening of the arteries," or arteriosclerosis). Its effects are more serious if you have anemia, diabetes, heart failure, or the second of the underlying conditions, called atherosclerosis.

In atherosclerosis, over time the walls of the arteries become lined with deposits of a combination of fat (cholesterol) and calcium, called plaque, which can narrow or block the arteries leading to any part of the body, including the heart and brain. The deposits are likely to form where damage has occurred because of high blood pressure. The deposits can cause intense pain in the heart (angina pectoris) if there is partial blockage; heart attack, if total blockage occurs in a coronary artery; or a stroke, if the blockage occurs in arteries in the brain.

Angina can occur whenever less oxygen reaches the heart than is needed. Exercise, extremes of temperature, reactions to stress or strong emotions, or other causes, such as anemia, may cause angina. Some of us experience pain but can live full lives with it for many years, even when the cause is not clear.

In school and the early years of marriage and child rearing, I was always hurrying from one activity to another. I developed chest pains that the doctors diagnosed as angina. My blood pressure was never high. Now at age seventy-four the old problem is back and I live with it. I drive, work, clean, mow lawns, and go to meetings. I do get tired but I sleep well. My hands and feet get cold easily and I wear sweaters much of the year. My mother also had the same problem. She lived to be eighty-four and died of what the doctor called a tired heart.

Cholesterol is one of several blood fats (lipids) in the blood. Lipids must be combined with proteins, forming lipoproteins, to transport fat in the blood. High-density lipoprotein (HDL) contains the highest proportion of protein and is important in transporting fat away from body cells, preventing the accumulation of cholesterol and other fats within the artery walls. Women tend to have higher levels of HDL than men. Athletes also have high levels, especially long-distance runners. Smokers have lower levels of HDL.

Low-density lipoprotein (LDL) contains the largest proportion of cholesterol of any of the lipoproteins. LDL is a factor in the accumulation of fatty materials in the artery walls and is significantly related to risk of heart attack and stroke.

Lowering the cholesterol level in the bloodstream reduces heart attacks and heart-attack deaths. Every 1 percent drop in the cholesterol level means a 2 percent decrease in the likelihood of a heart attack.[3] Although women had not been included in most past studies, studies now show that women benefit more than men from low-cholesterol diets.[4]

In addition to food sources of cholesterol, the body also produces it. Blood cholesterol levels generally increase with age. An estimated 15 million American women have blood cholesterol levels of 260 milligrams per 100 milliliters (260 mg/100ml) or above, placing them at high risk of developing heart disease. Recommended levels of blood cholesterol vary among medical professionals—some set the desirable level under 200mg/100ml for adults,[5] while others suggest 100-plus-your-age (up to a maximum of 160) mg/100ml.[6] The average American adult consumes between 400 and 700 milligrams of cholesterol each day.[7] The American Heart Association recommends that Americans limit cholesterol intake from food to no more than 300 milligrams a day (a medium-sized egg yolk contains about 275).

PREVENTING CARDIOVASCULAR DISEASES

We can do a lot to reduce the factors that affect our chances of having a heart attack or stroke. The first step is understanding the role of hypertension and other risk factors. Then we can make changes to improve our health and reduce the risks.

SMOKING AND HEART DISEASE

Cigarette smoking definitely increases the risk of heart disease.[8] Women who give up smoking can lower that risk. Studies show that smokers who quit return to nonsmoker risk levels for heart disease within approximately ten years.[9] Some studies suggest that after age sixty-five the influence of cigarette smoking on heart disease declines,[10] though all the other negative effects of smoking continue.

Smoking affects the circulatory system in a number of ways. It damages the linings of the arteries, making it easier for plaque to build up in them. Nicotine from cigarettes overstimulates the heart to work harder to remove the carbon monoxide. Finally, smoking harms the respiratory system. (See pages 22–25 for help in stopping smoking.)

EXERCISE AND WEIGHT

Regular aerobic exercise helps regulate weight, raises beneficial HDL levels, and increases overall cardiovascular fitness by improving blood circulation throughout your body. Exercise is especially important for those whose bodies produce high levels of cholesterol. If you have cardiovascular disease, check with your health-care practitioner before starting an exercise program, to make sure you know the level of exercise suitable for you. (See Avoiding Injury on pages 74–75.)

Research shows that those of us who are very overweight are at greater risk for developing hypertension. Some studies show that increasing exercise to lose weight can be as effective as diet and drugs in controlling hypertension; others suggest that regular exercise is more important than weight loss.[11]

As we age, the eating patterns of our younger years tend to stay with us, but we often exercise less, causing an increase in fat in our bodies. Women who accumulate fat around the waist and abdomen are at higher risk of heart attack, stroke, hypertension, and diabetes than others who accumulate fat around the hips and lower extremities.[12]

DIET

Diet influences HDL and LDL levels in the blood and therefore influences the likelihood of developing heart disease. We can reduce this risk by: (1) replacing saturated fats with unsaturated fats, (2) eating less food high in cholesterol, (3) eliminating "empty calorie" foods with little nutritive value, and (4) increasing exercise to reduce the ratio of fat on the body.

Salt contributes to fluid retention, increasing the amount of energy the heart must exert. It also counters the effect of diuretics, which are often prescribed for hypertension. Take the salt shaker off the table and avoid most canned and packaged foods, baking soda, ketchup, relishes, and cold cuts, all of which contain high amounts of salt.

Eat poultry and fish rather than meat. Limit meat to lean cuts, trimming all visible fat. Replace butter and shortenings with vegetable oils. Eliminate coffee.[13] Reduce egg yolks to no more than three a week. Eat more garlic, onions, whole grains, fruits, and vegetables. Choose low-fat milk and cheeses, but take care not to eliminate calcium (which is found in dairy products) from your diet, since calcium is a factor in the prevention of both hypertension and osteoporosis.

Reports have indicated that eating fish two or three times per week reduces risk of atherosclerosis. Eating fish does reduce the number of high-cholesterol, red-meat meals you consume, but the omega-3 polyunsaturated fats fish oil contains do not appear to have beneficial effects on blood cholesterol and are not advised for persons with diabetes.[14]

Studies show a potential reduced risk of heart disease in women taking vitamin E supplements. However, recommendations about the widespread use of vitamin E should await the results of further research.[15]

DIABETES

Diabetes is a major risk factor for heart disease, even more important in women than in men.[16] If you have diabetes, keep it under tight control (see Chapter 25) and pay close attention to reducing as many of the other risk factors for heart disease as you can.

STRESS FACTORS

Although reactions to stress vary, most health practitioners agree that reducing emotional stress benefits general health and particularly heart disease. The Framingham Study, a long-term project that looked at various aspects of heart disease, found that women who work outside of the home have fewer heart attacks than women who do not. However, women who have children, work in stressful clerical jobs, and have unsupportive bosses and husbands are the most frequent victims of heart disease.[17] Some employers offer employees stress-reduction programs to reduce lost time on the job and prevent stress-related disease. Many community recreation departments, clinics, or hospital outpatient departments offer stress-management programs. (See Disarming Stress, pages 12–16.) Many of us, as we get older, need to balance rest and activity. Take a rest in the afternoon if you feel tired and can fit it into your routine.

HEREDITY

Some health practitioners believe there is a link between family history and the likelihood of developing cardiovascular diseases. Others think this link reflects family behavior more than inherited traits. We not only pass on genetic traits to our children but often also eating, smoking, and exercising habits, which may have greater effects than hereditary factors. Nonetheless, if several members of your family have died of heart attacks or strokes at a young age, you should pay particular attention to preventive measures.

AGE, GENDER, AND RACE

Although heart disease is not directly related to aging, there is an increase in heart disease after the age of forty. In women, the increase in disease runs about ten years later than in men and the increase in deaths runs twenty years later for women than for men. There is no drastic increase for women at menopause and it is not until age seventy-five that the rates of sudden deaths are equal in men and women. Black women younger than seventy-five years of age do have higher rates of heart disease and their chances of surviving a heart attack are poorer than white women's.[18]

HORMONES AND HEART DISEASE

The relationship between hormones and heart disease is not fully understood. The early oral contraceptives, which contained high levels of hormones, caused a twofold or greater increase in risk of heart attacks and strokes—an increase well beyond their blood-pressure-raising effect.[19] Smoking has an additional harmful interaction with hormone use. Women who use the current oral contraceptives and smoke are ten times as likely to suffer from coronary heart disease as nonsmoking women who take oral contraceptives.[20] Among a group of heavy smokers (twenty-five or more cigarettes per day), aged forty to forty-nine and currently using oral contraceptives, the risk of a heart attack was thirty-nine times greater than that of women who neither smoked nor used oral contraceptives.[21]

Because heart disease among women increases at about age fifty, the average age that menopause occurs, those researchers who stress the importance of estrogen assume that it offers some protection. Menopause, especially when caused by the early surgical removal of the ovaries, reduces estrogen and seems to remove some of our protection from heart disease. Estrogen use in women seems to reduce LDL cholesterol and increase HDL cholesterol, both effects that should protect against cardiovascular disease. Most observational studies show a reduction in heart-disease risk of about 50 percent and contradictory results about stroke in postmenopausal women taking estrogen.[22] Though further testing is under way, it is not yet currently recommended that women take estrogen for the prevention of cardiovascular disease or stroke. All the other things we can do to improve our health are of greater total benefit and do not have the risks of taking estrogen. Also, we cannot ignore the other controllable risks and think that estrogen alone will counterbalance them.[23] In fact, estrogen use among men increased heart disease.[24] The hormone progesterone (progestogens or progestin) may increase LDL cholesterol and lower HDL cholesterol, and it has been linked to an increased risk of heart attack and stroke.[25]

While one study that took cigarette smoking into consideration supported the hypothesis that the postmenopausal use of estrogen therapy reduces the risk of coronary heart disease,[26] another study published at the same time found no benefits from estrogen use but rather an increased stroke rate among nonsmoking estrogen users and an increased heart-attack rate among smoking estrogen users.[27]

More research is needed on the effects of postmenopausal hormones (both estrogens and progestogens) on cardiovascular diseases. Further research is under way, but 2 million to 3 million women in the United States are taking these hormones before all the long-term effects are known.

Because one study found that high iron levels are a risk factor for heart attacks in men, there has been speculation that the increased iron levels in women after they stop menstruating is what causes the increased risk for women after menopause.[28] This has yet to be proven.

The same group of women in whom the possible estrogen and vitamin E benefits were found were also found to benefit from small doses of aspirin. Again, no policy recommendation on its widespread use can be made without further study.[29]

HEART ATTACK

When the supply of blood to the heart is interrupted, because of narrowed arteries or a blood clot, part of the heart muscle dies from lack of oxygen and nutrients. This is called a heart attack, or myocardial infarction (MI).

HOW TO KNOW YOU ARE HAVING A HEART ATTACK

You will be the first one to suspect you are having a heart attack. Look for these signals:

- Uncomfortable pressure, fullness, tightness, squeezing, or pain in the center of your chest lasting two minutes or more. The pain may fade away and then return. Unlike the pain of angina, the pain of a heart attack does not go away after physical or emotional stress ceases.
- Pain that spreads to your arms, shoulders, neck, jaw, or stomach.
- Severe pain, dizziness, fainting, sweating, nausea, or shortness of breath.

Everyone does not experience all these symptoms. If you experience any of these conditions, try to stay calm. Do not panic, but do not wait. Get help immediately. The sooner you begin treatment, the greater your chances of surviving. Call your local emergency rescue number or go to the emergency room at a nearby hospital. In the emergency room, a health-care practitioner will take your history, give you a complete physical exam, take an electrocardiogram (EKG), and draw blood for lab tests.

DIAGNOSIS OF HEART DISEASE

A wide variety of tests exists to determine whether someone has heart disease or has had a heart attack. All tests are not necessary for everyone who suspects heart disease—some are expensive and should only be performed when necessary. Ask your doctor why a particular test is being ordered and what you will learn from it.

An *electrocardiogram (EKG)* to identify abnormal heart rhythms is usually the first test performed when heart disease is suspected. This can be done in a medical office or hospital.

Exercise testing, or *stress testing,* primarily determines the nature and cause of any chest pain and is useful in the early detection of coronary heart disease. Through graded exercise, the stress test determines whether the coronary circulation is capable of increasing the oxygen supply to the heart muscle. Unfortunately, the results for women often show damage when none exists (called a false positive result). Some physicians, therefore, always order thallium scanning (radionuclear imaging) along with stress testing for women. Other physicians, to avoid unnecessary testing and save expenses, order thallium scanning only if the stress test is positive.

Radionuclear imaging, sometimes called a *thallium test* or *thallium scanning,* is a technique in which a small amount of thallium, a short-lived radioactive substance, is injected into an arm vein. The thallium circulates with the blood and concentrates in the heart. There it gives off gamma rays that are translated by computer into a picture. The physician can tell if any areas of heart muscle have been damaged by heart attack, or if any part of the heart is not getting enough blood and oxygen, the cause of angina. This test may also be done while exercising.

Echocardiography uses sound waves to study the heart's structure and function. It is noninvasive (does not penetrate the body and therefore does not cause pain or discomfort). It can be helpful in identifying patients with disease of the heart valves, an often overlooked problem with the elderly.

A *Holter monitor exam* is a twenty-four-hour EKG. You wear a portable EKG machine for twenty-four hours. This gives the doctor a longer record of your heart's activity than she or he can get in the examining room.

Coronary arteriography, sometimes called *cardiac catheterization,* is a procedure in which a long tube, or catheter, is inserted in an artery and dye is passed through it. The dye allows X rays to show whether any arteries to the brain or heart are blocked. Catheterization is not recommended for everyone, especially not for the elderly. If your heart disease can be managed with medication, or if you are considered a high-risk candidate for bypass surgery, little useful information will be gained from performing a catheterization.[30]

Treatment for Heart Attack

Most people who have suffered a heart attack are admitted to a hospital coronary care unit (CCU) or intensive care unit (ICU). Here their heart is monitored, and life-saving services are available in case they are needed. For some people, however, the atmosphere in the ICU or CCU is itself tension-producing and may slow recovery.

Two kinds of drugs are prescribed for people who have suffered a heart attack: those that increase the flow of blood, bringing extra oxygen to the heart; and those that reduce the need for oxygen.

After a heart attack, the blocked artery that was responsible for the heart attack may need to be opened, allowing the heart to get adequate oxygen. New treatments to open blocked arteries have been developed. These use the same process as cardiac catheterization. One method involves injecting streptokinase, a clot-dissolving drug, through a catheter or directly into the artery. If used within a few hours after a heart attack, streptokinase will dissolve the clot within twenty minutes. It is not recommended for anyone who has a bleeding disorder or who has recently had surgery. Although streptokinase is no longer considered experimental by most physicians, it is not widely used, especially in small hospitals. Tissue plasminogen activator (TPA) is a newer drug with fewer adverse effects that is beginning to replace streptokinase. The sooner you get treatment after you suspect you have had a heart attack, the more likely it will be effective.

Another method used to clear a blocked artery is balloon angioplasty. In this treatment, a small balloon is inserted and is inflated at the site of the obstruction to clear a partially blocked artery. For some patients, this procedure is a less expensive alternative to coronary bypass surgery. It does not require the chest to be opened and involves shorter hospitalization, lower cost, and shorter recovery time. Over 300,000 were done in 1991. Laser procedures combined with angioplasty are more effective than angioplasty alone.[31]

Cardiac bypass surgery is sometimes performed when an artery is blocked and cannot be cleared with medication or balloon angioplasty. Surgeons use a vein, usually taken from the leg, or an artery from the chest[32] and construct a detour, or bypass, around the blocked artery. In bypass surgery, the chest is opened up and a heart/lung machine keeps the blood circulating while the new segment is attached to the heart.

I had a history of heart condition. You can imagine what it's like going someplace and never knowing what's going to happen. I was so tired and depressed all the time that I wasn't enjoying my retirement. After the second heart attack they suggested a bypass operation but I wasn't ready for it then. They tried all the medicines and nothing worked. After my third heart attack I decided that was enough, I would have the surgery.

I did quite well and had as much physical therapy as Medicare would pay for, but I didn't have as much as I should have had.

I do what I can to keep fit. I bought a stationary bike and ride it a half hour, five days a week. I walk a mile several times a week. I cut down on meat and stay away from cold cuts. I haven't had any bacon for two years. At the hospital where I had the surgery they said, "Be careful, but have it, don't crave it," so I have a hot dog once a year at a Labor Day cookout. I'm a good vegetable eater and since my operation I planted a garden. My cholesterol level was high for years but it is better now. My blood pressure is fine.

I get tired and have my limitations but I can do so much more than I could before. I have entered a three-mile walk this month for persons over the age of forty. [a sixty-nine-year-old woman]

Some women who have bypass surgery experience dramatic relief from pain and lead physically active lives again. However, bypass surgery primarily relieves pain; there is no proof that surgery increases life expectancy for most people. For only one group, those with obstruction of the left main coronary artery, does surgery improve chances of survival. Yet over 400,000 operations are performed each year.

Several studies have shown that a more conservative approach is as effective as bypass surgery for most people.[33] These studies suggest that bypass surgery could be avoided through the use of medication, exercise, diet, stress reduction, and smoking cessation. These changes must be made even with surgery or the bypass may clog.

Before having bypass surgery, you may want to consult with a cardiologist who specializes in the *medical* rather than surgical treatment of heart disease. This will ensure that you get opinions from two different perspectives. Finally, death rates for bypass surgery vary from hospital to hospital. Generally, medical centers with specialized surgical teams have the best records. The more often a team operates, the better their record. *Never consider undergoing bypass surgery at a hospital where fewer than two hundred procedures a year are performed.*

Many women are concerned about how their scars will look after surgery, and they should ask.

My scar starts above my ankle and goes almost up to my throat. I love to swim, but the scar turns blue when I get it wet. This summer I didn't swim or wear shorts. I don't care too much about my chest scar. They sewed it on the inside and it doesn't show as much as the scar on my leg. The men at rehab all bragged about their scars, whose was longer and meaner-looking. We didn't do that. Some women in the rehab program only wear turtlenecks or high-neck blouses, because they don't want anyone to see their scar. [a sixty-eight-year-old woman]

Some Other Surgical Procedures

Modern heart surgery may extend life and improve its quality. Unfortunately, it can also hold out false promises and be performed unnecessarily, at great cost to the individual and to society.

Pacemakers

A bundle of nerves in the upper-right chamber of the heart—our natural pacemaker—transmits electrical impulses that control our heartbeat. When these impulses slow down or become irregular or blocked, we may not experience any symptoms or we may experience weakness, breathlessness, slow pulse beat, lack of increased pulse beat when exercising, or even loss of consciousness.

No treatment is needed in many instances. In some instances, a battery-powered artificial pacemaker is used externally for a time or implanted permanently under the skin of the chest wall. The artificial pacemaker controls the heart rate by sending out rhythmic electrical impulses to activate the contractions of the heart. The implantation carries a risk, as does any surgery. The Food and Drug Administration reviews the safety and effectiveness of new models of pacemakers developed since 1976, but does not review so thoroughly those pacemakers that are similar to models developed before passage of the 1976 medical-device amendments to the Food, Drug and Cosmetic Act.[34]

As useful and necessary as pacemakers are in many instances, estimates of their overuse range as high as 75 percent. Controversy also continues about whether unnecessary or no-longer-necessary pacemakers should be removed.[35]

An artificial pacemaker's batteries usually last an average of four years, despite claims made by some manufacturer that theirs will last longer. Monitor your pacemaker by telephone with a pacemaker-monitoring company to detect problems before they are serious. Pacemakers should be checked more often and earlier than some manufacturers recommend. Medical insurance policies do not but should be required to cover the cost of monitoring pacemakers.

Valve Replacement

Some procedures, such as replacement of the valves in the heart, can affect positively both the length of life and its quality.

For at least two years I had progressively less strength and was feeling more and more tired. I couldn't do physical activity like gardening, which I loved. I also felt psychologically under a cloud, that my life was draining out. I wasn't feeling pain in my chest but I was feeling spasms, quivering, palpitations, and butterflies that I thought would go away. I kept attributing these symptoms to getting older, but when I had headaches, which I never had before, and couldn't do a lot of walking, I knew something was the matter.

I went to the doctor, where they did all the tests and said that I needed a valve replacement within a month. I read up on it a bit first and then went into the hospital for twelve days, five of them in intensive care. After I came home the stairs were difficult for a while and there were some days when I couldn't walk very far. I gradually went back to work. I started feeling really great after about six months. [a fifty-four-year-old woman]

Transplants and Artificial Hearts

Research in cardiology today often emphasizes sophisticated treatment of existing disease conditions at the expense of prevention and early intervention. Newspapers are filled with stories about patients receiving procedures costing $200,000 or more, while prevention programs go unreported and often unfunded. Insurance plans pay for heart transplants yet do not pay for us to attend a cardiopulmonary resuscitation (CPR)* course to learn how to save lives or support group meetings to help us change habits in order to lower our risk of developing heart disease.

Heart Failure

Heart failure occurs when the pumping action of the heart becomes inefficient. Sometimes it affects only one side of the heart, but when it affects both sides it is called congestive heart failure. Despite its name, heart failure is not an immediately life-threatening disease and does not result in the heart stopping suddenly, as can happen in a heart attack.

All of the same life-style changes (healthful food, exercise, cutting out smoking, adopting relaxation strategies) that help prevent hypertension and other heart and stroke conditions also help prevent heart failure.

Treatment of heart failure and any underlying condition that leads to heart failure may allow you to return to normal activities. There are many drugs, including some new ones, that are effective in extending both length and quality of life.

Even if you need to rest more, keep your legs in motion by frequently shifting your position or relaxing and contracting your leg muscles. The action of your leg muscles helps move the blood along. You will probably also need to cut down on salt intake.

Stroke

A stroke, sometimes called a "shock," occurs when the flow of an area of blood to the brain is disrupted. One of the most common forms of stroke, cerebral thrombosis, occurs when a clot develops in an artery damaged by atherosclerosis. In cerebral embolism, a wandering clot, or embolism, lodges in one of the arteries, blocking blood to the brain. In a cerebral hemorrhage, a burst artery floods the brain tissue with blood, causing blood loss to the brain and pressure on the brain tissue. This bleeding can be caused by a head injury or an aneurysm—a blood-filled pouch that balloons out from a weak spot in the artery wall.

Long-standing hypertension and having heart disease are major causes of strokes. Women with diabetes, especially those with hypertension, are at greater-than-average risk of stroke and should especially take action to keep their blood pressure normal.

How to Know You Are Having a Stroke

The following symptoms may be warnings that you are about to have a stroke or are having little strokes already. Even if they are temporary, you should not ignore them.

*CPR is an emergency procedure combining mouth-to-mouth resuscitation and closed-chest heart massage that can be peformed by a layperson while waiting for trained help to arrive. In Seattle, Washington, the extensive training of the population in CPR is credited with saving two hundred lives annually.

- Temporary weakness or numbness in the face, arm, or leg on one side of the body.
- A severe, persistent headache.
- Temporary loss of speech or difficulty speaking or understanding speech.
- Temporary dimness or loss of vision.
- Dizziness or unsteadiness, possibly causing you to fall.
- Memory loss.

I was frightened to realize that there were parts of three days I couldn't reconstruct. I usually have a fabulous memory; people call me for details from a meeting held seven years ago. And now I couldn't recall last week's appointments, phone calls, or letters. I was in a real panic by the time I got to my doctor's office.

A thorough examination turned up things I hadn't even noticed—a generalized weakness on my left side, the inability to make a fist, a little problem with my speech, and bruises on my left leg that suggested I'd been bumping into things. My blood pressure was very high. The doctor had me see a neurologist that same day. After many tests the final diagnosis was made—I'd had several strokes. [a sixty-year-old woman]

Little strokes, or transient ischemic attacks (TIAs), sometimes precede a major stroke by days, weeks, or months. These are generally warning signs of a major stroke to come. If you experience any of the symptoms listed above, *see your health-care practitioner right away*.

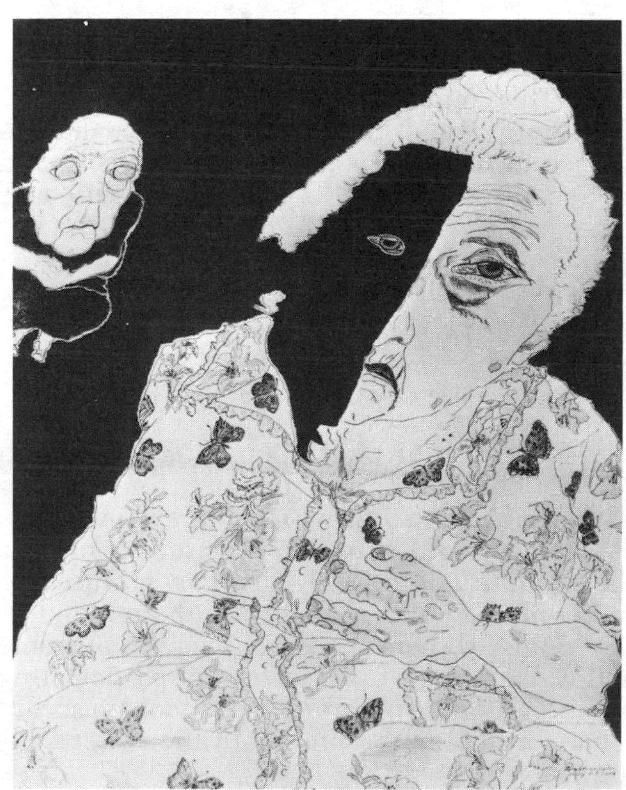

Elizabeth Layton

TREATMENT FOR STROKES

Treatment for strokes starts with treatment of those very conditions that are also risk factors for strokes: hypertension, cardiac disease, TIAs, high hematocrit (percentage of red cells in the blood), and diabetes. TIAs are treated with aspirin or other anticlotting medication to reduce the possibility of forming new clots.

None of what followed my stroke was easy. Getting my hypertension under control proved to be difficult. I found it hard to let my children and my friends do things for me. Most of all, I had to face my own feelings. I felt older. I was depressed and scared. Would I have another, more crippling, stroke? Just how much would my life have to change?

I continued to work and now, three years later, I'm about to take a new job. I don't forget anything important. I walk and use a stationary bike and have cut down on fats and sugars, so I feel great and thinner. My blood pressure was 130 over 70 yesterday. The amount of medication has been reduced over time. Taking it has become just one more thing I do regularly each day—like brushing my teeth. [the same sixty-year-old woman]

RECOVERY AND REHABILITATION*

After heart attacks, strokes, and surgery, people often reevaluate their lives and find new directions.

I now celebrate two birthdays—the day I was born and the day I had the surgery! [a sixty-nine-year-old woman after bypass surgery]

After surgery I took a trip to Europe. I felt well physically and I was beginning to think of alternative things I might do. Seeing people dress and think differently had an effect on me. New possibilities presented themselves. I felt a physical and emotional connection between my heart and my experience that I hadn't completely grasped before.

*Not all insurance plans cover rehabilitation, but Medicare covers some of the costs. In some states, Medicaid does not cover rehab programs, making it impossible for Medicaid recipients to get vocational services, which would in some cases lead to paid employment and help them get off Medicaid.

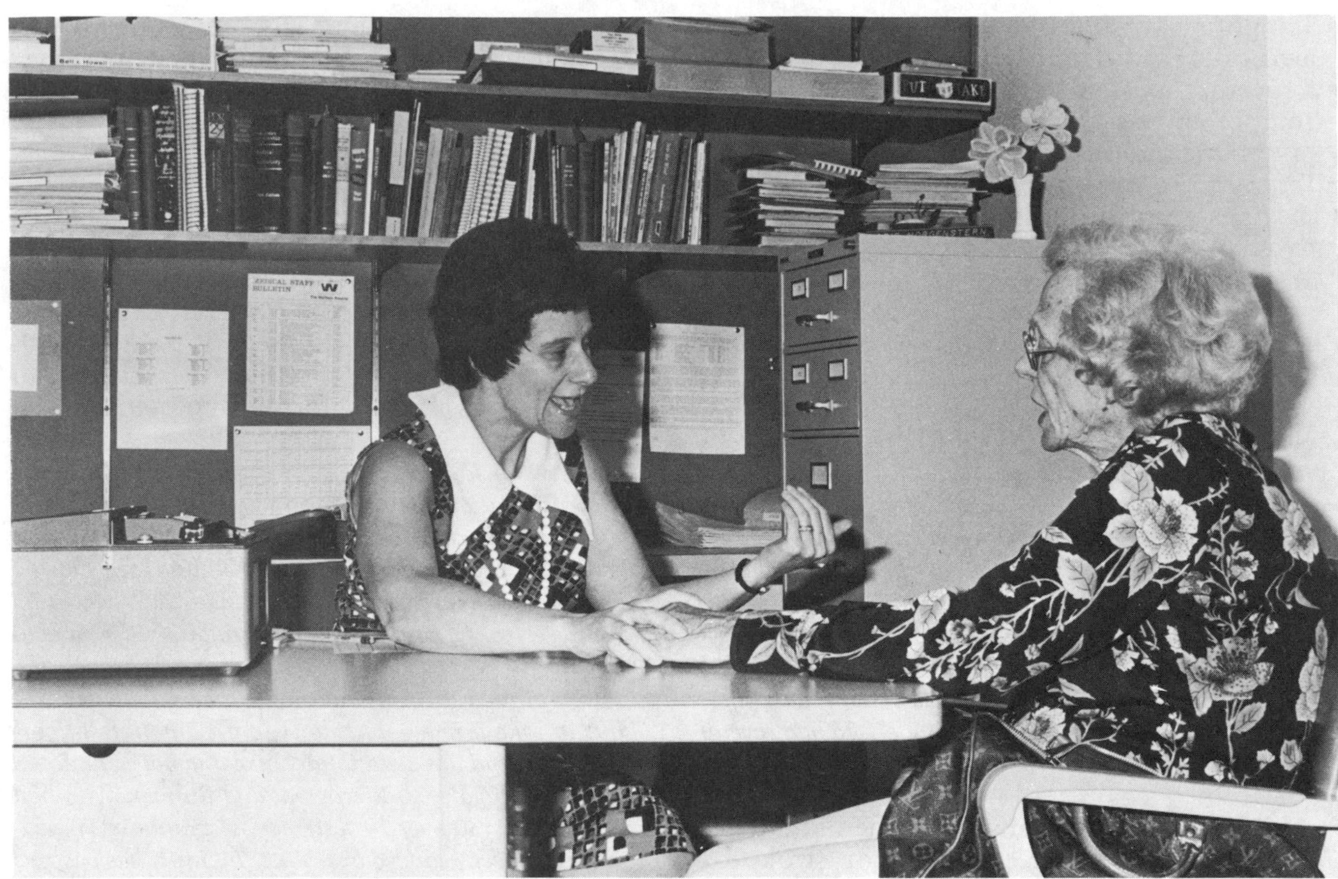

Mikki Ansin/The Picture Cube

When I came home I started seeing a therapist. She said, "Now you have a new life and you want to figure out what to do with it." One of my goals is to make more connections and to get involved in organizational and political work. I'd like to change my job to one where I can meet more people. I realize I'd be better off if I had more friends and more associations with other women. [the fifty-four-year-old woman who had a valve replacement]

Formerly, a person who had a heart attack was told to rest in bed for three weeks. Recent evidence shows that this can be harmful. Rehabilitation, or rehab, programs help people who have had a heart attack or cardiac surgery return to health. Persons with chronic stable angina and heart failure may also benefit. Many rehab programs begin in the ICU or CCU, where you can begin doing ankle circles and limited-range exercises while your heart is monitored. By the time you leave the hospital, you will be walking and climbing stairs. In a good rehab program you will learn exercises to continue at home and diet changes to follow. You should be fully informed about any medications you will be taking.

The second phase of rehabilitation is usually an outpatient program lasting about twelve sessions. This combines monitored exercise, discussion groups, and education. Here you have a chance to increase your physical capacity and talk about your concerns with people who have experienced a similar trauma.

After my heart attack, my morale was very low. In rehab, I was with people who had already gone through what I was going through. I felt encouraged. [a seventy-two-year-old woman]

Most rehab involves counseling, along with occupational/vocational therapy for patients who aren't able to return to their previous jobs.

A third phase of rehab programs continues the exercise component (often in groups and sometimes at a rehab facility) without monitoring. Some women choose to exercise at home and walk on their own, instead of participating in this part of the program. Other women stay in rehab for the support and motivation of exercising in groups.

Physical, speech, and occupational therapy

help people who have had strokes regain all the skills possible. A stroke can affect speech, behavior, thought patterns, memory, and ability to understand, and sometimes can cause paralysis. Only 20 percent of those individuals considered appropriate candidates for cardiac rehabilitation services actually receive them. New federal guidelines on cardiac rehabilitation will be available soon.[36]

In the past, rehabilitation stressed compensation for the disabled parts of the body, so the stroke victim depended more on the unaffected side of the body. Today's approach to rehabilitation emphasizes relearning control over the affected side.

She heard the doctor say as he left her hospital room, "There can be no hope of recovery from this." She could see everything; words were exploding in her mind but none escaped into sound. She couldn't believe the doctor's words. Would she be helpless for years to come? She was a photographer. Would she never take another picture?

"It isn't so!" The voice of the nurse reached her. She was leaning over the bed, her face very angry. "He shouldn't have said that!" The nurse was whispering furiously. Recovery was possible. She had seen it often in people who put their will into it. A tremendous sense of confidence welled up in her. Of course she knew the nurse was right. Relief flooded her, and she became possessed of a single thought: recovery. The nurse stayed with her for an hour, talked with her, encouraged her.

That night, she slept soundly, dreamlessly. The next morning she glanced down at her hand on the white sheet. Two fingers on her right hand flickered. Watching her hand, she willed it to happen again. Slowly her forefinger lifted, then her second finger. The little movements occurred slowly, bit by bit.

On the third day her speech returned. By the tenth day she was able to lift her right hand up to her chest. The next day she lifted both hands, a few inches below her heart. A deep sigh went through her. It would be all right, just a matter of time and effort. She wanted to tell her family, the nurse, everyone just what it meant to her to lift her hands in that gesture with just enough space to hold her camera. That was how she knew she wasn't finished. She could go back to work again. [a seventy-year-old woman]*

Families and friends should be included in the rehabilitation of persons who have had strokes. Not only must they be kept up-to-date about expectations for the patient, but they can help in the process by encouraging her or him to reach the highest level of independence possible.

*Adapted with permission from the section about Eleanor Milder Lawrence in *Gifts of Age: Portraits and Essays of 32 Remarkable Women* by Charlotte Painter and Pamela Valois. San Francisco: Chronicle Books, 1985, pp. 126–29.

WHAT ABOUT SEX?

A common myth about heart disease is that having sex will cause a heart attack or even death. This is not true. Nor does a heart attack or heart surgery or stroke mean an end to a satisfying sex life. Most women find that after their initial recovery, lovemaking is as pleasurable as before. (See Sexuality in the Second Half of Life chapter, especially pages 93–99.)

A massive stroke impaired my ability to function independently and seriously damaged my physical and emotional stability. Facing life was difficult. Learning to swim was one of my most effective coping techniques. Two swimming sessions weekly (forty-five minutes each) increased my strength and endurance. The constant verbal encouragement by the therapist and members of the group for even a tiny accomplishment provided enormous support and was a tremendous morale booster. We adopted the motto "Press on regardless." I discovered that working in a group was the most effective technique for helping me and my family cope with a long-term disability. [a thirty-eight-year-old woman]

NOTES

1. Franz H. Messerli, ed., *Cardiovascular Diseases in the Elderly.* Boston: Martinus Nijhoff, 1984, p. 65.
2. Ibid., p. 77.
3. John Langone, "Heart Attack and Cholesterol." *Discover,* Vol. 5 (March 1984), pp. 20–23.
4. "Study Says a Low Cholesterol Diet Does Little to Increase Longevity." *The Boston Globe,* Apr. 1, 1987, p. 11. Note that the headline states the finding for men at low risk for heart disease, not the different finding for women.
5. National Institutes of Health, *Lowering Blood Cholesterol to Prevent Heart Disease.* Consensus Development Conference Statement, Vol. 5, No. 7 (December 10–12, 1984), p. 5.
6. Nathan Pritikin with Patrick McGrady, Jr., *The Pritikin Program for Diet and Exercise.* New York: Grosset & Dunlap, 1979, p. 16.
7. American Heart Association, *An Older Person's Guide to Cardiovascular Health.* National Center of the AHA, 7320 Greenville Ave., Dallas, TX 75231, 1983.
8. Walter C. Willett, "Cigarette Smoking and Nonfatal Myocardial Infarction in Women." *American Journal of Epidemiology,* Vol. 113, No. 5 (May 1981), pp. 575–82.
9. R. Paffenburger, "Physical Activity and Fatal

Attack." In E. Amsterdam, ed., *Exercise in Cardiovascular Health and Disease.* New York: York Medical Books, 1977.

10. Francis D. Dunn, "Coronary Heart Disease and Acute Myocardial Infarction." In Messerli, op. cit., p. 156.

11. Jesse A. Berlin and Graham A. Colditz, "A Meta-Analysis of Physical Activity in the Prevention of Coronary Heart Disease." *American Journal of Epidemiology,* Vol. 132, No. 4 (1990), pp. 612–28. Unfortunately, most of the studies were done only on men.

12. Per Bjorntorp, "Regional Patterns of Fat Distribution: Health Implications," in *Health Implications of Obesity,* program and abstracts. National Institutes of Health Consensus Development Conference, February 11–13, 1985, p. 35.

13. Dag S. Thelle, et al., "The Troms Heart Study: Does Coffee Raise Serum Cholesterol?" *The New England Journal of Medicine,* Vol. 308, No. 24 (June 16, 1983), pp. 1454–57.

14. For a full discussion, see "Triglyceride, High Density Lipoprotein, and Coronary Heart Disease." Reprinted from NIH Consensus Development Conference *Consensus Statement,* Vol. 10, No. 2, February 26–28, 1992; also *Harvard Medical School Health Letter,* Aug. 5, 1989, p. 5.

15. Meir J. Stampfer, et al., "Vitamin E Consumption and the Risk of Coronary Disease in Women." *The New England Journal of Medicine,* Vol. 328, No. 20 (May 20, 1993), pp. 1444–49; and "Editorials," same issue, pp. 1487–89.

16. E. Barrett-Connor, et al., "Why Is Diabetes Mellitus a Stronger Risk Factor for Ischemic Heart Disease in Women Than in Men?" *Journal of the American Medical Association,* Vol. 265 (1991), pp. 627–31.

17. Suzanne Haynes and Manning Feinleib, "Women, Work, and Coronary Heart Disease: Prospective Finding from the Framingham Heart Study." *American Journal of Public Health,* Vol. 70, No. 2 (February 1980), pp. 113–41.

18. Patricia P. Barry, "Coronary Artery Disease in Older Women." *Geriatrics,* Vol. 48, Suppl. 1 (June 1993), pp. 4–8.

19. Nancy R. Cook, et al., "Regression Analysis of Changes in Blood Pressure with Oral Contraceptive Use." *American Journal of Epidemiology,* Vol. 121, No. 4 (April 1985), pp. 530–40.

20. The Boston Women's Health Book Collective, *The New Our Bodies, Ourselves.* New York: Simon & Schuster, 1992, p. 632.

21. Charles H. Hennekens, et al., "Oral Contraceptive Use, Cigarette Smoking and Myocardial Infarction." *British Journal of Family Planning,* Vol. 5 (1979), pp. 66–67.

22. Meir J. Stampfer and Graham A. Colditz, "Estrogen Replacement Therapy and Coronary Heart Disease: A Quantitative Assessment of the Epidemiologic Evidence." *Preventive Medicine,* Vol. 20 (1991), pp. 47–63; and Fanchon F. Finucane, et al., "Decreased Risk of Stroke Among Postmenopausal Hormone Users," *Archives of Internal Medicine,* Vol. 153 (Jan. 11, 1993), pp. 73–79.

23. Kathleen I. MacPherson, "Cardiovascular Disease in Women and Noncontraceptive Use of Hormones: A Feminist Analysis." *Advances in Nursing Science,* Vol. 14, No. 4 (1992), pp. 34–49; "Heart Disease: Women at Risk." *Consumer Reports,* Vol. 58, No. 5, pp. 300–304; and National Women's Health Network, "Proposed Cardiovascular Indication for Premarin." Testimony before the Food and Drug Administration, June 14–15, 1990.

24. Patricia A. Kaufert and Sonja M. McKinlay, "Estrogen-Replacement Therapy: The Production of Medical Knowledge and the Emergence of Policy." In Ellen Lewin and Virginia Oleson, eds., *Women, Health, & Healing: Toward a New Perspective.* New York: Tavistock Publications, 1985, p. 116.

25. Erkki Hirvonen, et al., "Effects of Different Progestogens on Lipoproteins During Postmenopausal Replacement Therapy." *The New England Journal of Medicine,* Vol. 304, No. 10 (March 5, 1981), pp. 560–63.

26. Meir J. Stampfer, et al., "A Prospective Study of Postmenopausal Estrogen Therapy and Coronary Heart Disease." The Nurses' Health Study. *The New England Journal of Medicine,* Vol. 313, No. 17 (Oct. 24, 1985), pp. 1044–49. See also Graham A. Colditz, et al. "Menopause and the Risk of Coronary Heart Disease in Women." *The New England Journal of Medicine,* Vol. 316, No. 18 (Apr. 30, 1987), pp. 1105–10.

27. Peter W. F. Wilson, et al., "Postmenopausal Estrogen Use, Cigarette Smoking, and Cardiovascular Morbidity in Women over 50." The Framingham Study. *The New England Journal of Medicine,* Vol. 313, No. 17 (Oct. 24, 1985), pp. 1038–43.

28. Lawrence K. Altman, "High Level of Iron Tied to Heart Risk." *The New York Times,* Sept. 8, 1992, pp. A1, C3.

29. J. E. Manson, et al., "A Prospective Study of Aspirin Use and Primary Prevention of Cardiovascular Disease in Women." *Journal of the American Medical Association,* Vol. 266 (July 1991), pp. 521–32.

30. Messerli, op. cit., p. 155.

31. Larry Tye, "Lasers Show Promise for Heart Patients." *The Boston Globe,* Jan. 20, 1987, p. 6. Report from the American Heart Association meeting held in Monterey, California, January 19, 1987.

32. Floyd D. Loop, et al., "Influence of the Internal Mammary-Artery Graft on 10-Year Survival and Other Cardiac Events." *The New England Journal of Medicine,* Vol. 314, No. 1 (Jan. 2, 1986), pp. 1–6.

33. Marcia Millman, *The Unkindest Cut: Life in the Backrooms of Medicine.* New York: William Morrow and Co., 1977; and Office of Technology Assessment, U.S. Congress, *Assessing the Efficacy and Safety of Medical Technologies,* GPO Stock No. 052-003-00593-0, 1978; and Kenneth M. Kent, "Coronary Angioplasty: A Decade of Experience." *The New England Journal of Medicine,* Vol. 316, No. 18 (Apr. 30, 1987), pp. 1148–50.

34. Esther R. Rome and Jill Wolhandler, "F.D.A. Is Lax in Enforcing Medical Regulations." Letter to the Editor, *The New York Times,* Nov. 30, 1985, p. 22. Information on pacemaker models can be obtained from the medical devices section of the Food and Drug Administration, (301) 443-4190.

35. "Correspondence: Complications of Permanent Cardiac Pacemakers." *The New England Journal of Medicine,* Vol. 313, No. 17 (Oct. 24, 1985), pp. 1085–88, in response to B. Phibbs and H. J. L. Marriott, "Complications of Permanent Transvenous Pacing." *The New England Journal of Medicine,* Vol. 312, No. 22 (May 30, 1985), pp. 1428–32.

36. AHCPR, *Research Activities,* No. 166 (July 1993), p. 12. See AHCPR on page 482.

24

CANCER

✦

BY SHARON BRAY AND DIANA LASKIN SIEGAL

BREAST CANCER BY JANE HYMAN

COLORECTAL CANCER BY EDITH LENNEBERG

SPECIAL THANKS TO NORMA MERAS SWENSON AND JANE JEWELL

1994 UPDATE BY DIANA LASKIN SIEGAL WITH HELP FROM GAIL GRAMAROSSA

BREAST CANCER BY RITA ARDITTI AND DIANA LASKIN SIEGAL

RESOURCES FOR THIS CHAPTER ON PAGES 494–97

Forty-nine years ago when I had my first surgery and radiation for ovarian cancer, people were so afraid of cancer that they couldn't use the word. They would say, "She has C." They lied to me but I knew they were lying when they gave me radiation. I'd read enough to know I had cancer. Today things are better, more open, people talk more. Now I visit other cancer patients and they mostly know. They can talk about it more now. [a seventy-five-year-old woman]

The diagnosis of cancer is not a death sentence; many live long lives with the disease and eventually die of other causes at a ripe age. Most of us know at least one person who has lived many productive years after a diagnosis of cancer. The same woman continues:

Eight years ago, at age sixty-seven, I developed colorectal cancer and had a colostomy. I went back to work afterwards and I wear a bag all the time. I do everything I did before. I'm in a relationship with a man and it doesn't make any difference to him. I walk a lot. I like to keep my shape. I tell my doctors, "I feel good, I just get cancer once in a while."

While it is true that most of us will never get cancer, one out of three of us will; so we need to know more about it for ourselves and for those close to us. We have heard stories of painful, lingering death and of treatments that sound more miserable than the disease itself. We may worry that we will lose a breast or go bald and be less attractive, less womanly. Cancer is still one of the most feared diseases. Although women's risk of death from heart and circulatory diseases is higher in older years, cancer causes the most deaths in forty-five- to sixty-four-year-old women, mainly from lung and breast cancer.

I HAVE HELD HANDS WITH FEAR

I have held hands
with fear;
We have gone steady
together.

Sorrow has been
my mate;
We have been bed-
companions.

The days of my night
have been long.
They have stretched
to eternity.

Yet I have outlived
them.
And so shall you.

Mitzi Kornetz

What Is Cancer?

We call it by one name, but cancer takes many forms, alike only on a basic biological level. The cancerous patch of skin removed from a forehead bears little resemblance to breast cancer or to leukemia until we understand how cancerous cells develop, grow, and spread through a living body.

Most cells in our bodies reproduce themselves and grow in order to repair or replace damaged organs and tissues. But sometimes the cells change so that they lose their ability to function properly, and they begin an abnormal process of uncontrolled growth. Scientists think this change begins as a result of contact with carcinogens (cancer-causing agents). While the process of normal cells evolving into cancer cells is not fully understood, it appears that the abnormal change happens in steps. Some carcinogens *initiate* the change and others *promote* the process. Some carcinogens may be both initiators and promoters. Others work as a destructive team, as when alcohol promotes mouth and throat cancers started by tobacco.

Some inborn factors may predispose a woman to developing a cancer, making her more vulnerable to carcinogens. Many experts now believe it is likely that everyone has some cancerous cells at one time or another, but our immune systems eliminate them before they develop sufficiently to cause problems. Virtually all experts agree that about 80 percent of all cancers are *environmentally* caused, that is, from toxic substances in cigarettes, air, water, or food, or from workplace hazards or medical treatment. Increasingly, women are banding together with neighbors and colleagues to fight for a safer environment. Since so many cancers are environmentally caused, prevention is a societal issue, not only a personal one.

How Cancer Grows

At its earliest stage, a cancer is limited to one location, one organ, perhaps one cell. The number of cancer cells may increase rapidly or very slowly. (Some cancers are not discovered until up to twenty years after the first cells change.) A cancer may affect one organ without ever spreading to other parts of the body—or it may spread.

One kind of spread occurs when the mass of cancerous cells in one organ (a "primary" cancer) touches another organ and begins to grow in it also. This regional growth (sometimes called a "secondary" cancer) should not be confused with a new cancer (called a second "primary") that grows in another place.

Another kind of growth occurs when cancer cells are carried to other parts of the body from the primary site by the blood or lymph system and begin to replace normal cells in other organs; the cancer has then become "systemic" or "metastatic." This may never occur, or may not occur until many years after cancer is first discovered. It also may happen simultaneously with the first growth of cells in the primary site. Many cancers are slow-growing, produce no symptoms, and are not discovered until many years after the cancer begins. Both regional spread and systemic distribution of cancer may be referred to as metastasis.

Several systems are used to describe the stages of cancer from localized to metastasized. When evaluating research and other people's experiences with various treatments, always take the type and stage of the cancer into consideration.

Risk and Prevention

Lists of cancer-risk factors are based on statistics and on scientific studies. Many risk factors are identified by the fact that, since so many people with a particular cancer have them, it seems unlikely to be mere coincidence. Some risks, such as exposure to asbestos, have also been studied in laboratory tests on cultured cells in dishes (in vitro) or in animals, where scientists have been able to observe the cancer-causing process.

If you know about some risk factors, you may decide to change your habits to reduce the risk. Those risks you cannot control—things that happened at work years ago, your family health record, where you live—may alert you to watch for symptoms and to be conscientious about regular checkups. Even though early cancer detection does not guarantee cure, it does help in many cases.

Some risk factors may involve things you do not want to give up. If you are eighty years old and love pickles and bacon, giving them up is not likely to make much difference in whether you will ever have cancer (though there are other reasons to avoid the salt and fat they contain). On the other hand, research has shown that giving up smoking, even for people who have smoked for fifty years, very quickly improves health.[1] **Smoking is the number-one controllable cause of cancer, causing at least 30 percent of cancer deaths.**

Anyone who has a history of cancer is at increased risk of developing another one. Reducing the risk factors, especially stopping smoking, may help prevent further cancers. Regular checkups with a health practitioner can help discover new cancers early.

Sometimes we make important choices for our bodies in spite of known future risks. For example, the immune system has to be suppressed in anyone receiving an organ transplant so that the organ from the donor will not be rejected. People who have had a kidney transplant have a higher risk of cancer than people who did not undergo such treatment.

THINGS YOU CAN DO TO REDUCE YOUR RISK OF CANCER[2]

In the list below, factors that minimize the risk of breast cancer specifically as well as other cancers in general are marked with an asterisk (*).

*1. Don't smoke. Avoid smoke-filled places. Smoking also markedly increases the risks from other carcinogens such as alcohol, asbestos, and industrial agents. Don't use smokeless tobacco products such as snuff and chewing tobacco, which also cause cancer.

2. Know the risks and follow the health and safety rules of your workplace. Where needed, wear protective clothing and use safety equipment. If your employer does not enforce safety rules, ask for help from your state's Department of Health or Attorney General.

3. If you are a professional artist or a hobbyist, be aware that many artists' materials are hazardous (oil paints, turpentine, potters' glaze, photography chemicals, fabric dyes, etc.). Wear protective gloves, goggles, and clothing, work in a well-ventilated room, and read labels carefully.†

*4. Avoid unnecessary X rays whenever possible. Don't hesitate to ask your doctor if an X ray is necessary, but do not refuse an X ray needed for a diagnosis because you fear cancer. If you need an X ray, be sure shields are used to protect other parts of your body, especially the trunk.

*5. Avoid taking estrogen except for severe symptoms that have not responded to other treatments. If you do take estrogen, ask about combining it with progestin, which reduces the risk of endometrial cancer. (Progestin offers no benefits if you no longer have a uterus, and does not reduce the other risks of using estrogens, such as gallbladder disease. Progestin may even increase the risk of breast cancer and heart disease. See box on page 129.)

6. Eat a well-balanced diet with a variety of foods (see Eating Well chapter).

- Eat a variety of whole grains, vegetables, and fruits rich in bran and fiber—grown without pesticides (if available and affordable).
- Eat foods high in beta-carotene and vitamin A: carrots, pumpkin, sweet potatoes, cantaloupe, spinach, winter squash, greens, apricots, broccoli. Eat soybeans and cruciferous vegetables such as kale, broccoli, cauliflower, cabbage, brussels sprouts, greens, bok choy, kohlrabi, turnips, and rutabagas.[3] Vitamin A pills are *not* a substitute for beta-carotene, and high doses can be toxic.
- Eat foods high in vitamin C: citrus fruits, sweet peppers, leafy greens, broccoli, cauliflower, tomatoes, fresh potatoes, berries, melons, bean sprouts. Eating the whole fruit gives you more nutrients than just drinking the juice.
- Eat foods high in selenium: brewer's yeast, garlic, onions, asparagus, tuna, shrimp, mushrooms, whole grains, brown rice. Eggs, liver, and kidneys contain selenium but are also high in saturated fat. Selenium can be toxic in high doses, so it is best to get it in foods instead of pills.

*7. Reduce the fat in your diet (see Eating Well chapter). Adding fish may be beneficial.

8. Minimize consumption of smoked, salted, or pickled foods, and avoid chemical additives, including food coloring.

*9. Limit or eliminate alcohol.

*10. If you are substantially overweight, try to take off weight by increasing exercise and by reducing fat and sugar in your food.

†Michael McCann, *Health Hazards Manual for Artists*. New York: Lyons and Burford, 1985; Siegfried Rempel, *Health Hazards for Photographers*. New York: Lyons and Burford, 1993; and National Association of Working Women, an affiliate of 9 to 5, *Health Hazards for Office Workers*. Cleveland, OH: Working Women Education Fund, 1981.

There is evidence that people who weigh more than 40 percent over recent recommendations have higher rates of cancer.

11. Maintain frequent and regular bowel movements by exercising, drinking water, and including fiber in your diet.
12. Avoid sunburn and excessive tanning, especially if you have light skin. You do need some sun for vitamin D, or foods or supplements with vitamin D such as cod liver oil, if you live in the North during the winter.

Most of the above are really basic cancer preventive-care measures that also promote general good health. Doing as many of them as your willpower, interest, and finances allow should make your body all the stronger to prevent cancer or to help you fight it. While quitting smoking, eating better, or making other changes will not guarantee you a cancer-free life, they will influence your statistical chances and should make you generally healthier. Some choices seem to be contradictory. Cancer experts may warn you against alcohol, while heart experts may advise that a couple of ounces a day is good for you. Fat women have higher cancer risk but lower risk of osteoporosis. The best you can do is emphasize moderation in life-style and understand your own body and health history.

Environmental and Occupational Risk Factors

It can be upsetting to read cancer statistics for your state or town if you happen to live in an area with higher-than-average rates of specific cancers. Rates that vary considerably from one year to another may be only chance variations. Contaminated water supplies, toxic-waste dumps, nuclear radiation, pesticides, electromagnetic fields, organochlorines, and other environmental factors, however, may contribute to higher-than-expected cancer rates. So does living or working in buildings without adequate ventilation. Individuals can be effective through organized community action to prevent, publicize, regulate, and clean up some of these problems. Actions against companies that pollute the air or water supply have been started by women who noticed something unusual.

Some higher rates of cancer may also be caused by natural environmental factors. If you have light skin, for example, the closer you live to the equator, the higher your risk of skin cancer related to sunshine.

There are clear links between certain occupational hazards and diseases. Many common household products contain carcinogens, and some studies show that housewives have higher-than-average rates of cancer. Artists, craftswomen, laboratory and medical workers, and others should seek information about the proper handling and ventilation of the materials they use. There is increasing evidence that chemicals used in the microchip industry can cause immune-system problems.[4] Always investigate the risks of any chemicals or equipment used at your work site.

Other Risk Factors You Cannot Control

Poverty. Poor people don't live as long with cancer compared with wealthier people. The five-year breast-cancer survival rate for white women earning less than $15,000 is 63 percent, compared with 78 percent for women earning more than $30,000. For women who did not finish high school, the rates were 64 percent for white women and 61 percent for black women, compared with 81 percent for white women who graduated from college.[5]

Age. The longer you live, the greater your chances of having some kind of cancer. Half of all cancers are diagnosed in people over sixty-five. The cancer incidence begins to rise at about age thirty-five for women (and a little later for men).

Gender and Race. A higher percentage of men than women, and blacks than whites, die from cancer. Controllable factors such as variations in smoking rates, access to health care, eating habits, and exposure to occupational hazards can account for some of the differences in these cancer statistics.

Family. Some cancers are found more often in people whose parents or close family members have had them. Be sure to inform your health-care providers if anyone in your family has had or has died from cancer. Some cancers can be prevented or detected early when family members are alert to a common environmental hazard or a familial disposition.

LET'S NOT BLAME THE VICTIM

Cancer patients face stigmas that have yet to be obliterated. Though few people still think cancer is "catching," many still believe that all cancers are inevitably fatal. These stigmas can lead to personal isolation and to discrimination in employment. Some protection is now available under the 1990 federal Americans with Disabilities Act (see page xxiv). We should also fight for state definitions of "disabled" to include people with cancer who require regular treatments over an extended period or who are unable to carry out major activities.

People with cancer often feel shame or guilt, wondering what they have done to be so punished. Sometimes they blame themselves, and others blame them also, for exposures to the risk factors that might have predisposed them to the disease. Many people still try to hide the fact that they have cancer—even from close family and friends. But the stigma will never go away until we all learn as much as possible, as well as talk much more to each other, about our cancer experiences. We should not accept isolation when we most need support.

Right after surgery, a lot of my friends came to cheer me up. But I had to put them at ease first. They didn't know what to say. The cancer was like a wall between us. So I just took a deep breath and started talking about it. Then it was all right. [a forty-year-old woman with breast cancer]

Much of what has been written about cancer ends up "blaming the victim." Particular personality traits have been attributed to persons with cancer, just as they were attributed in the last century to persons with tuberculosis.[6] Doctors themselves tend to hold patients responsible for their progress, giving great credit to "gallantry and grace in the face of hardship," and therefore by extension blaming those who do not get well for "not trying hard enough."[7]

There are two dangers in believing that your state of mind is the major influence on the course of your cancer: (1) You may suffer guilt and feelings of failure if your cancer advances in spite of your own efforts. (2) You might abandon medical therapies that might actually help you. It is very important to get the best treatment you possibly can. Periods of anger, fear, grumpiness, depression, hopelessness, and passivity are common, as you can discover by talking with others who have experiences with cancer. The success or failure of any treatment is not caused by the strength or weakness of your faith in it, by living right, or being a happy person. One study found no relationship between "psychosocial" factors such as marital status, other companionship, work and life satisfaction, and hopefulness and how people with advanced cancers responded to treatment or how long they lived.[8] Another study did find longer survival among women with breast cancer who were in support groups.[9]

People who are at all times full of courage, grace, faith, and endless, cheerful endurance are rare. On the other hand, we should not abandon all sense of control. We have many decisions to make about how we will live and what treatments we will choose. Sometimes both the person with cancer (or other chronic disease) and those in relationships with her or him take more control over their lives and are stronger than before.

CANCER RESEARCH

Money and institutional support for cancer research come from private organizations, individuals, and government agencies. Scientists as individuals and in groups ask for more funding than is given out each year. Decisions may speed up one researcher's projects while forcing another to delay or abandon research. Many factors go into deciding who gets how much money for which kind of research. Political considerations such as the state the applicant works in, the power of that state's senators and representatives, and the research institution's connections with decision-makers controlling funds do influence funding for cancer and other health research.

The special interests of politically powerful groups also influence funding of cancer research. Labor unions, for example, have demanded answers when their members have occupation-related cancers. The "right-to-breathe" antismoking movement has spurred research on links between smoking and various kinds of cancer. Women are now exerting more influence on what decisions are made. At the same time business and industry have used their economic and political power to block legislative action on substances and practices that seem to cause cancer or to limit the funding of relevant research.

DIAGNOSIS

Why find out early? With some cancers, early detection offers the possibility of cure or substantial remission with years—even decades—of symptom-free life. Many cancers are more easily treated and controlled when discovered early. Certain skin cancers, cervical cancer, and colorectal cancer are common and can be detected early and cured.

- Basal- and squamous-cell skin cancers are visible, grow very slowly, and cure rates approach 100 percent following removal.
- Cervical cancer, which grows unnoticed, can be stopped before it leaves the cervix. A Pap smear every one to three years will catch cervical cancer at its earliest stages. Discuss the appropriate interval with your health-care practitioner. Hispanic women have not received enough information on the importance of Pap smears.[11] Heterosexual women who are sexually active and whose partners do not use condoms should have regular tests. Not all abnormal Pap smears mean that cervical cancer will develop, however, and it is crucial to try to reverse changes in the cervical cells (dysplasia) before agreeing to surgery (see Hysterectomy and Oophorectomy chapter, especially pages 326–27).

Other, less common cancers may also be treated effectively if discovered early. Sometimes, however, early detection does not prolong life. It only bolsters statistics on survival rates because, while the person survives only as long as most others who have the same disease, the counting starts sooner. Many cancers cannot be detected earlier than the time when they produce symptoms.

Some women would rather not know they have cancer at all, especially if the symptoms are not likely to disturb their lives until a late stage shortly before death.

By the time my mother had cancer in her early forties, she had already had two close women friends about ten years older than her die of cancer. She was terrified of the disease and of the idea of death itself. So when her lung cancer was diagnosed, we didn't want anyone to tell her. But an X-ray therapist did anyway. She died about two months later, and it was as awful for all of us in the family as it was for her to die so young. [a forty-year-old woman]

PHYSICIAN, DO NO HARM!

Too often drugs or other methods for treating medical conditions are adopted without sufficient research; and too often they prove useless, and even harmful, only after many people have been exposed to them. Examples include radiation to pregnant women, resulting in leukemia in the child; radiation to the neck in childhood that leads to an increase in thyroid cancer in adulthood; DES (diethylstilbestrol) prescribed during pregnancy, leading to a rare cancer in female offspring and an increased risk of breast cancer in the mother many years later. Inform your physician if you had radiation to the upper body as a child, to increase the chance that any possible cancers can be diagnosed and treated early.

Use of DES (a synthetic form of estrogen) was approved by the Food and Drug Administration in 1942 to stop milk flow in mothers and to treat menopausal symptoms and vaginal inflammation (vaginitis) despite studies as early as the 1930s showing estrogens to be carcinogenic in laboratory animals. In 1947, the FDA extended approval of DES in even higher doses for use during pregnancy, even though there had been no studies to examine potential effects on the fetus or on the mother. Doctors commonly prescribed DES if a woman had a history of miscarriage, diabetes, high blood pressure, or slight bleeding during pregnancy. Some researchers and drug companies recommended DES as a routine preventive measure to avoid miscarriage even before there were signs of trouble.

Although studies showed conclusively as early as 1953 that DES was ineffective in preventing miscarriage, the FDA did not warn against using it in pregnancy until 1971, after its link to cancer was established. Even now, doctors still prescribe it for nonpregnant women who may be infertile or suffering some other gynecological problem.

If your mother or you were among the group of pregnant women for whom DES was prescribed, be sure you and your daughter are checked as needed. Some DES sons also show abnormalities. (See DES Action USA in Resources, page 495.)

Women who were given DES when pregnant have a moderately increased incidence of breast cancer[10] and cancer of the uterus, cervix, or ovaries, and noncancerous tumors of the uterus. If you are a DES mother, get a professional breast exam every year in addition to performing monthly breast self-examination. Be sure your health-care provider is informed of your DES history.

Others take steps immediately:

My second husband had cancer, but I remember so many good times in our all-too-short marriage when his treatments led to remission. So when my mammogram showed a suspicious shadow, I was very motivated to do something about it. Yes, I was scared, but I knew I could get some help. [a sixty-year-old woman]

If you have one of the following warning signals publicized by the American Cancer Society, tell your nurse practitioner or physician:

- *C*hange in bowel or bladder habits
- *A* sore that does not heal
- *U*nusual bleeding or discharge
- *T*hickening or lump in breast or elsewhere
- *I*ndigestion or difficulty in swallowing
- *O*bvious change in a wart or mole
- *N*agging cough or hoarseness

None of these is a sure sign of any disease, and all have other possible causes besides cancer. But you should at least talk it over with a practitioner you can trust.

DIAGNOSTIC METHODS

You may want to make choices about diagnostic methods in cases where several approaches are possible. Breast cancer is the most widely publicized disease where you can make these choices (see page 366). Ask your practitioner to explain exactly the methods she or he uses, whether there are others, and why those others are not suggested for your specific condition.

X rays, including mammograms, can suggest but not definitively diagnose cancer. Often cells are taken from a suspicious mass (the procedure is called a biopsy) to make a more certain diagnosis. A few cells can be removed and sent to a pathologist for examination. Needle biopsies can be done for breast, lung, or pancreatic tumors. A corkscrew-shaped needle (trucut needle biopsy) may be used to draw tissue out of a solid lump. A D and C (dilation and curettage) or an endometrial biopsy of the inside of the uterus yields cells to examine for endometrial cancer. Biopsies can be done through a small incision using an endoscope (a device consisting of a tube and an optical system) to reach polyps in the colon and stomach, and lung tumors.

Depending on the size and location of a lump, and whether there is more than one, the surgeon will recommend *incisional* or *excisional* biopsy. Incisional means taking a small slice, usually of a larger mass. Excisional means removing the entire lump (lumpectomy). The tissue removed is divided and prepared into permanent sections and sometimes frozen sections on glass slides for the pathologist to examine. Results from the frozen section are known quickly, while the permanent section, which is more accurate, takes at least twenty-four hours. Sometimes, as in abdominal surgery, the decision for additional surgery during the operation is made on the basis of the frozen section in order to avoid another operation. In other sites, such as breast cancer, there are good reasons to wait for the results of a permanent section before deciding on further treatment, so a frozen section is not needed.

The slides prepared from the sections become part of your medical record. Slides and X rays should be available if you want the opinion of another pathologist or radiologist.

Some women report complications of the diagnostic surgery itself, so make sure your surgeon is experienced in dealing with your specific condition and preferably has a reputation for conservative, but adequate, surgery.

LIVING WITH CANCER

"How long will I live?" is a frequently asked question. We fear death, and the statistics, showing little improvement in survival rates for many cancers, only compound the fear.

Every time a friend of mine dies of cancer, it's not necessarily the same kind of cancer as mine. It's not the same stage or in the same place, etc. But knowing that doesn't keep me from getting frightened. I wonder if I will keel over this afternoon or tomorrow. It's not intellectually sound but I do feel that way. [a fifty-seven-year-old woman now being treated for cancer]

How many stories have you heard about people who were only supposed to live two years . . . or one year . . . or six months . . . five years ago? We marvel to see them "still going strong at seventy-five." Stories like these, mostly true, are one reason why doctors hesitate to set time limits for survival with cancer diagnoses, even for very advanced cases. You might want to know how long you will remain active or will live because you have things to get done, relationships to mend or a book to finish, but what will you do as you approach that time limit?

Time limits for living with cancer come from two basic sources: statistics that count hundreds of thousands of people, and the individual physician's own experience with the specific disease. Remember that half the people live longer than the often quoted "median" figure for survival of any given cancer. Those who live longer can live anywhere from just a little longer to very much longer—maybe even decades longer.[12]

Doctors often use the word *cure* for what should be more correctly five- to ten-year survival rates. Statistics for remission (a temporary stopping of growth and of related symptoms and shrinkage of the cancer) and for cure (disappearance of all detectable signs of cancer) should never rule the outlook of an individual with cancer. Hope is essential, and many of us find that knowledge makes the reality of cancer easier to live with.

I feel very positive about recovery—wrong word—how about remission? My playful platelets are good and high, blood tests terrific and blood pressure down. I feel better than ever. [an active seventy-year-old woman with breast cancer]

Take Along a Friend

Whether you suspect that you have cancer or a diagnosis of cancer has been confirmed, you should consider taking someone with you whenever you go for diagnostic work, checkups, or treatment, particularly when decisions have to be made. You can probably use the moral support of someone who cares about you, and you may need help getting home after some procedures. It is useful to have a second person to ask questions and to listen to the answers, even to take notes, and to talk things over with afterward. The person you take could be your partner, your sister, a friend, or a volunteer from a women's group, the local Cancer Society, or other helping organization.

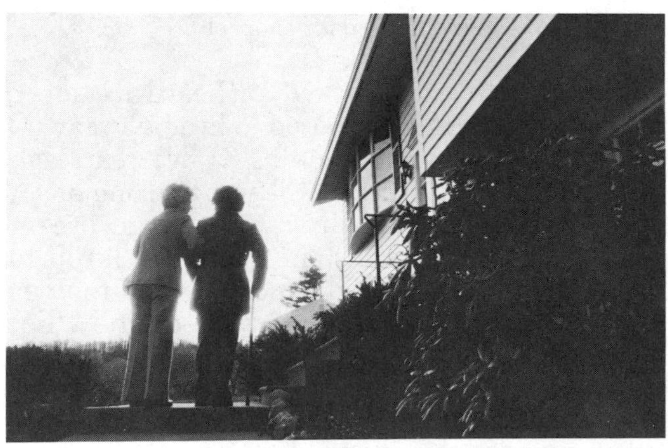

American Cancer Society/Massachusetts Division

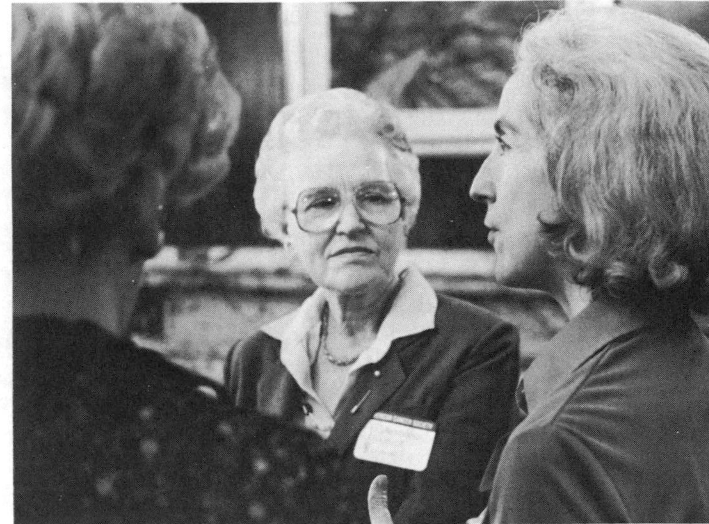

American Cancer Society/Massachusetts Division/Allen Smith

Everyone asks if you have any questions, but you just don't know what to ask when it's your first consultation. My doctor and the surgical nurse kept asking if I had any more questions and I really didn't just then. [a fifty-seven-year-old woman with cancer]

I had been to enough programs on women's health issues to know I should take someone with me when I went to hear the results of my mammogram. I took a woman I hired to clean my house and she turned out to be just the support I needed. [a sixty-year-old woman]

Support and Mutual-Help Groups

It has taken many years to break down the barriers keeping people with cancer from talking to each other. Only recently could a woman, rather than her physician, request the limited contact provided by the Cancer Society's Reach to Recovery Program. Groups dealing with specific problems such as ostomy and laryngectomy have a longer history. Many communities now have support groups. Because of the fears, silence, and misinformation about cancer, we especially need help when we face the diagnosis of cancer and the challenge of learning to live with it. Often, those close to us need support and information just as much as we do and can benefit from support groups. If none exists in your area, you can start one.

TREATMENTS

Each of us must be able to trust the decisions we make when cancer is found in our bodies or in our loved ones, in spite of the contradictory recommendations in the media and even within conventional medical circles. Gather all the information, advice, and support you feel you can use—but ultimately you will have to make the choices about which treatment to accept or reject.

I am their pet patient at the moment, though they learned to treat me rather gingerly after I refused to start chemotherapy until my incision stopped draining. Blew the young oncologist out of his chair when I remained firm, especially after he said he'd talk it over with my surgeon. To which I replied, "You can talk to her till hell freezes

QUESTIONS TO WHICH YOU NEED ANSWERS*

Select from this list the questions that pertain to you. *Similar questions will apply to other diseases.* Ask your health practitioners to give, or help you find, the answers. Use the resources listed at the end of this book and any others you hear of to give you this vital information for making decisions.

1. Exactly what kind of cancer do I have? Can you tell if it is slow- or fast-growing?
2. What therapies are available? Where?
3. How effective is each therapy? What is the probability of cure? What definition of *cure* is being used?
4. What benefits can I expect? Prolonged life by months? Years? Reduced symptoms? Reduced pain?
5. What percentage of people treated benefit from the therapy? How is that benefit measured?
6. Will I be able to continue my regular activities during therapy? What about sex? Working? Exercise?
7. Will the therapy require overnight stays in the hospital or can it be done on an outpatient basis?
8. What are the potential negative effects of the treatment? How serious are they? What percentage of people get them? Are they permanent? Are there any drugs that will help alleviate these effects? Do these drugs themselves cause any negative effects? How soon after treatment are symptoms likely to begin and how long do they usually last? (For example, does nausea generally start immediately, within twenty minutes, or several hours later? How long does it last?)
9. How long will the therapy last? Each session? How many sessions?
10. How many people get recurrences after this treatment? How soon?
11. Are there statistics on survival, cure, mortality, and remission rates for this therapy for my type of cancer, considering such factors as stage of cancer, age, sex, race, socioeconomic status, occupation, geographical location?
12. Who is my health-care provider while I am undergoing therapy? Whom do I contact, and how, if I have new symptoms while I am in therapy? After I finish the therapy?
13. What are the costs involved? Will my insurance cover all the costs? What part of the costs? Where can I get help to pay the costs?
14. May I speak with some of your other patients? Do you know of any local groups for people with cancer? Any groups for family members and friends?
15. Whom do I call, and when, if I have further questions?

You should take a written list of these questions with you to your practitioner's office and make notes, take a tape recorder, and have someone with you. This is a lot of information to assimilate at one time; it may take more than one question-asking session. But having these answers will make you a well-informed patient, and your physician will know it. Most health-care providers will respect you for asking such questions and will try to keep you informed of your progress.

*Adapted from the Boston Women's Health Book Collective, *The New Our Bodies, Ourselves.* New York: Simon and Schuster, 1992, p. 614.

over—this is not a medical decision; it is my personal decision since it is my personal body." The surgeon, a great woman, agreed. [a seventy-year-old woman]

One consideration in selecting a doctor is that you will also be expected to use the hospital in which the doctor practices. If possible, choose a hospital where there is a tumor board—an interdisciplinary committee that meets to review cases and treatments. This gives you access to other specialists instead of relying on one physician alone. In the past, surgeons controlled the treatment of cancer, but now treatments are more complicated, and it is important to have a team approach, the team including a surgeon or surgical oncologist, radiation therapists, and medical oncologists. (An oncologist is a specialist in the diagnosis and treatment of cancer.) Request a tumor-board review at the time of the initial diagnosis before you agree to any treatment and at all future decision points, such as the time of a recurrence .

I read everything I could find on cancer; so I could have rushed right in and told my doctor, "You're not doing the latest thing." I still read a lot on it. I'd be very disappointed if I found the treatments I've had aren't the best procedures. [a fifty-seven-year-old woman who had a mastectomy in 1977 and in 1986 was treated for metastases from the breast cancer to the bone]

Treatments for cancer range from high-technology radiation and chemical therapies to home remedies found in family herb gardens. All treatments for any disease are experimental to the extent that no one knows for sure exactly how *you* will respond to any given treatment or combination of treatments.

The three most common treatments for cancer are surgery, radiation, and chemotherapy (including hormone therapy and immunotherapy). These may cure the disease, slow it down, or relieve symptoms and make your life easier.

Surgery removes cancerous tumors, tissues, or areas where cancer cells have invaded normal tissue; or it can open up a blocked system or ease painful pressure on other body parts. You should try to find out as much as you can about your surgeon's and your hospital's experience and qualifications for doing the kind of surgery proposed.

After I had the tumor removed from my neck, I discovered that the doctor who did it had almost never done that kind of operation before. Had I known, I would have done what a friend at church did and gone to the medical center in a nearby city where they do similar surgery all the time and really know what they are seeing. [a sixty-year-old woman living in a small town]

Ask how the surgery will help your specific condition. Get second or third opinions, especially if a doctor suggests removing some healthy part of your body to prevent it from becoming cancerous. Breasts, ovaries, and uteruses have too often been removed just in case they might develop cancer someday; medical literature has no accounts of men having anything removed "just in case."

While your surgeon may urge you to decide immediately whether to have surgery and tell you a delay will allow the disease to spread, you always have time to get those additional opinions unless you have an emergency condition such as intestinal or bladder blockage. A cancer will rarely cause sudden life-threatening symptoms, but even if it does, you can get a second opinion within the hospital or from the tumor board.

Radiation therapy uses X rays or radioactive substances to destroy cancerous cells instead of cutting them out. Sometimes the radiation is used instead of surgery; often it is used before surgery to shrink a mass, or after surgery to destroy remaining traces of the cancer.

Radiation is also used for palliative reasons without curing—for example, to ease bone pain.

Radiation may cause nausea, diarrhea, fatigue, and burns, depending on the part of the body treated. But radiation therapy may also prolong active, meaningful life when used for some cancers, especially for Hodgkin's disease and some stages and forms of cervical, lung, nose, and throat cancers.

I just had modest side effects. I had a rash that developed after about the second or third week, a very itchy rash. I couldn't put anything on it because cream affects the way the beams go through. And I had a rash on the front that went all the way through so I had a sunburn on my back as well as on my front. The rash went away in a relatively short time. [a woman in her fifties]

In general, the more radiation, whether larger doses (more units of radiation—rads) or over a larger area, the more complications arise. Some of these do not show up for many years. Complications are minimized by dividing the therapy into several treatments. You might be willing to put up with more adverse effects if the radiation holds the possibility of cure than if it is only intended to make you more comfortable.

Radiation therapy often causes nitrogen and other nutrient deficiencies. You can prepare yourself by eating a high-protein diet with a good balance of vitamins and minerals before you start radiation therapy; and you can try to put on a little weight in case you become nauseous and can't eat.

Both radiation and chemotherapy aim to destroy the abnormal, cancerous cells. The aim is to do so without harming too many normal cells nearby or elsewhere in the body. Techniques are being refined to make cancer cells more vulnerable than normal cells to treatment or to restore damaged normal cells more quickly. One technique is to apply heat, especially to tumors near the body surface, as an adjunct to both chemo- and radiation therapy. Implanted heat sources may work on deeper tumors. A number of drugs are being investigated either to make the cancer cells more vulnerable or to reinforce normal cells, protecting them against radiation. Techniques to salvage and restore bone marrow are being tried.

Cancer cells tend to have less oxygen than normal cells (to be hypoxic) and tend to block the effects of radiation. So researchers are trying to find ways to oxygenate cancer tumors before irradiating them.

Large university or research hospitals are likely to have the most modern equipment and technology, plus well-trained personnel. You should always ask about the age of radiation equipment, when it was last inspected, and how often the therapists' training is updated. If the equipment is more than ten years old or you have doubts about the staff, contact the Cancer Information Service (1-800-4-CANCER) for the name and telephone number of the nearest university or research hospital with radiation therapy and oncology departments.

Chemotherapy—treating cancer with chemicals or drugs—is the only method that has the potential to reach cancer cells in every part of the body. It is called a systemic therapy. It is the basic treatment in cancers such as leukemia (cancer of the white blood cells) and a supplemental (or adjuvant) therapy to destroy cancer cells that are beyond the reach of primary surgical or radiation therapy. Chemotherapy sometimes has other effects, because anything strong enough to kill cancer cells damages other cells as well. Possible temporary adverse effects of chemotherapy are hair loss, nausea, diarrhea, and cessation of menstrual periods. Possible long-term and serious effects include permanent cessation of periods in premenopausal women over forty, kidney damage, heart disease, a weakened immune system, and leukemia. But many drugs and many combinations of drugs are used. Not everyone gets sick from them, and many people have been helped.

Have had two and about to have a third chemo treatment (injection of combined drugs) and NO side effects! Absolutely none. [a seventy-year-old woman]

When my hair grew back, it was all gray, and soft like a baby's hair. And curly! I had straight dark hair before. [a sixty-eight-year-old woman]

When a woman in my cancer support group said she was going to have chemotherapy, I told her that I had had the exact thing. No problems at all. But she turned out to be as sick as a dog. Now we both laugh about it, and we both know how different each person is. [a fifty-seven-year-old woman]

Your health practitioners should have enough experience with the chemicals they propose for your treatment to be able to explain exactly how they work, what could go wrong, and how well the treatment works on your specific cancer at the stage you are in. You should not have to carry a pharmacy textbook to the office or hospital to understand what they tell you. If they cannot be clear about the therapy, talk to another physician; get another opinion or two. You should also be aware that some therapies can actually *shorten* your life if given inappropriately.

Hormone therapy is slower-acting and generally less toxic than most chemotherapy. Hormones are substances that originate in one gland or organ of the body and are carried through the blood to stimulate another part of the body. Hormone therapy changes the hormonal environment in which the cancer is growing by removing the source of the hormone (surgically or medically), adding hormones, or using substances that block the action of hormones (antihormones), such as tamoxifen. Hormone therapy is used to treat breast, uterine, ovarian, and thyroid cancers as well as leukemia (cancers of the white blood cells), lymphomas (cancer of the lymph system), and other cancers. Corticosteroids (hormones from the adrenal glands) are also used to control nausea and vomiting caused by some chemotherapy and for treatment of tumors in the central nervous system.

Immunotherapy is an attempt to stimulate the body's immune defenses to recognize and attack cancer cells. Many substances and techniques are under study for their possible effectiveness.

Experimental/Investigational Therapies

New drugs or combinations of drugs are constantly being studied. You may choose to take part in an experimental or investigational cancer treatment program. Before you give your consent, you should understand all the potential risks as well as benefits, and the investigators should take all the time needed to answer your questions. They should explain how you were selected for the study, who is funding it, what outcomes they expect, what risks are known, and how the study could benefit you as well as others. They should tell you how the experimental treatments differ from the standard protocol (treatment plan) for someone with your diagnosis. In addition, they should tell you what any health practitioner should tell you about any treatment recommendation: how it works, what effects to expect, what your possibilities are for relief, remission, and/or cure.

Alternative Treatments

The things you can do to reduce your risk of cancer can also help the body fight existing cancer. Most alternative treatments have little or no statistical data to help you decide how well they have worked for large numbers of people like you with your specific cancer. You will have to judge them according to the kind of cancer you have, the experiences of people who have tried them, what you know about the practitioners who offer them, and by your own feelings about trying something outside the mainstream of current medical practice. We hope the Office of Alternative Medicine will investigate new approaches to healing and offer guidance.

Some alternative treatments may be combined with conventional treatments. But promoters of many alternative methods claim their treatments will not work if you have had radiation or chemotherapy because of the damage these therapies may have done to the body. If so, you might have to choose between an established therapy with only fair outcomes and a treatment that is severely questioned or totally rejected by your physician. However, some hospitals now offer alternative treatments along with radiation or chemotherapy.

Many alternative approaches were originally developed by physicians, but are either ignored or considered invalid by the medical establishment. Often these alternatives seem logical in their approach, and a great many people credit them with curing or controlling their cancers. The preventive diets now being tested by several medical research centers are based on the same principles as some alternative cancer therapies.

Some alternative therapies receive so much publicity that public demand forces the medical establishment to evaluate the treatment's safety and efficacy. One such case is that of Laetrile. Laetrile was finally tested and found to be useless after thousands of people with potentially controllable cancers spent their energy and considerable money traveling to foreign countries where the unapproved drug was available.

Many alternative therapies are simply another kind of chemotherapy, using natural or synthetic substances in different forms or amounts than in ordinary use. The contents of these foods/drugs range from herbs and citrus extracts to ground-up animal glands to industrial solvent. We need better investigation of all possibly beneficial substances and better protection than the FDA now gives us from those found to be worthless and even dangerous.

We do not know yet how to mobilize fully the body's self-healing capabilities and the mind's ability to influence the body's recovery. Many methods, such as the Simonton technique, whereby the body's strength and the treatments chosen are imagined (or visualized) to fight the cancer, are used both to treat symptoms of cancer and to enhance the effectiveness of the treatment (see Resources for this chapter). They have reportedly induced remission. Prayer, meditation, and religious rituals are especially useful as supplements to other treatment choices; sometimes they are credited with cure, and sometimes not with cure, but an enriched life.

The danger of relying solely on faith healers and psychics is that a person whose cancer has a chance of responding to medical treatment may forgo that treatment until her cancer has progressed to a stage that is much more difficult to treat.

Scientific Breakthroughs

The media frequently report new wonders of science that may help cure cancer. The sad reality for most people with cancer is that these reported discoveries are in the laboratory stage, at most being tested on animals. Even those that have had successful human trials are usually many years away from being available outside a few teaching and research institutions.

When you read or hear about something new that you think may help you or a friend, you can call your doctor, your local hospital, the closest medical school, the Cancer Information Service, or even the school or hospital mentioned in the report. You might also write to your legislators urging their support of the research if it sounds worthwhile to you.

Some of our most respected scientists and the public are becoming critical of the research. Because cures for most cancers are not likely in the near future, focusing so much money and energy on treatment research may be actually robbing us of the motivation and resources to try to prevent cancer.[13] In 1991, only 17 percent of the total budget of the National Cancer Institute was spent on primary prevention. Also, by focusing more on the quality of life than the quantity of life, we could better help those people who already have cancer to live with the disease constructively.

LUNG CANCER

There are several types of lung cancer, caused by different environmental conditions or carcinogens, but the most common one is bronchial carcinoma, caused by smoking. It is possible to get lung cancer if you never smoked or lived with a smoker, but more women now die of lung cancer caused by smoking than from breast or any other cancer. The chances of getting bronchial carcinoma depend directly on how much you have smoked and for how long. Quitting pays off—after only ten years your chances of bronchial cancer are the same as a nonsmoker's. Unfortunately, passive smoking (breathing the smoke from other people's cigarettes) also causes lung cancer.

Lung cancer is the best example of why prevention is superior to cure, because the disease is so difficult to detect until its advanced stages. A persistent cough is usually the only warning. Lung cancer is usually treated with a combination of surgery, radiation therapy, and chemotherapy. Only 13 percent of people with lung cancer live five or more years after diagnosis.[14]

I didn't feel well for a long time but a year ago nothing showed up on my physical. Six months ago I was down to 101 pounds and didn't care about eating. It was a blow to find out I had lung cancer. I had smoked since I started college—everyone did. Have you noticed how much smoking there was in the old movies? Katharine Hepburn, all the stars I admired, smoked in the movies. After the diagnosis I just stopped smoking even though I still have the urge. I got a lot of lectures from everyone. I get chemotherapy every three weeks. I lost my hair but I'm feeling better. My appetite has returned and I'm up to 115 pounds. I'm doing pretty well now but I wish no one else had to go through this. I've been to two funerals for women who have died of lung cancer in less than a month, and now my dental hygienist has lung cancer also. My faith and my friends are helping me. [a seventy-five-year-old woman]

What is diagnosed as lung cancer may also be a metastasis from a malignancy elsewhere in your body, even one that was apparently cured years ago. Many of these have a better prognosis if detected early in periodic follow-up examinations.

CANCER OF THE OVARY

Ovarian cancer is rare, and while the rate is declining, the number of women who die of it is going up because it is more common in women over age sixty. Because this disease has been so difficult to detect until considerably advanced, it is often fatal, with five-year survival rates of 39 percent for all stages combined.[15] There are no screening tests. Blood levels of CA125, thought to indicate the presence of a tumor, can be raised for reasons other than ovarian tumors. Early warning signs are usually intestinal upsets of different kinds. Ovaries feel swollen to the examining practitioner. Transvaginal sonography also shows ovarian enlargement but surgery is needed for diagnosis.[16]

For a long time a lot of things I ate would make me gassy, but I thought, "I'm just getting old, I can't eat the things I used to." I went to the doctor and he gave me fluid pills [diuretics] for the swelling I had, but he never examined me "down there." It wasn't until I started bleeding down there that I found out what I had. I nearly died in surgery, they couldn't get it all, and though the radiation made me sick, I'm a little better now. [an eighty-four-year-old woman, during remission, who later died of ovarian cancer]

Even though the risks of removing healthy ovaries clearly outweigh any benefit, many doctors believe the poor prognosis for ovarian cancer justifies the removal of healthy ovaries during other abdominal surgery. But ovarian cancer tissue can and does grow in the abdomens of some women after the ovaries are removed. (See Hysterectomy and Oophorectomy chapter.)

Researchers don't completely understand the causes of this cancer. The fewer children you have, the greater the risk, childless women being at greatest risk. There's an increased incidence among women who have taken fertility drugs and a decreased incidence among those who have used oral contraceptives for at least five years,[17] and women who have had tubal ligations. Women who already have cancer of the breast, intestines, or rectum appear to be at increased risk, as are women whose jobs involve electrical, rubber, or textile manufacture. The use of talcum powder is not recommended in the genital area. Cornstarch is a safe substitute for those bath powders that still contain talc.

Most recent studies are beginning to suggest that some of the same influences on breast cancer may also affect ovarian cancer. Women who are significantly fat, who have taken menopausal estrogens, or who have a family history of ovarian cancer also appear to be at increased risk. Estrogen overproduction is the central factor here. Treatment of ovarian cancer usually involves surgery, radiation, and chemotherapy, with surgery and chemotherapy currently showing the most favorable results.

COLORECTAL CANCER

Colorectal cancer (cancer of the large intestine) is the third most common cancer among women in the United States. Almost half of all people with this disease are cured, usually by surgery. Many experts say survival rates could be improved if the cancer were discovered earlier. Early detection not only improves the chance of survival but often makes it possible to save greater portions of the large bowel because the cancer has not yet spread so far.

Women should be examined for colorectal cancer, particularly if they are, for one reason or another, considered at higher than usual risk of developing this kind of cancer. Colorectal cancer grows slowly; it may take months or years before it causes symptoms. Bleeding or changes in bowel habits—such as constipation, more frequent movements, or diarrhea—may be the first symptoms.

You should see a physician as soon as possible if you notice that any of the symptoms described above persist or if you have abdominal pain that doesn't go away. In doing an evaluation, your physician or nurse will take a complete personal and family history, give you a physical examination (including a rectal exam), and perform laboratory tests; special attention will be paid to your large bowel, including tests for blood in the stool and looking into the bowel with an instrument (colonoscope or sigmoidoscope). X rays of the bowel are often taken; they require a barium retention enema. Your regular health-care provider may refer you to a specialist (surgeon or gastroenterologist) for more tests or treatment.

The major recommendations for the prevention of colorectal cancer are a well-balanced diet rich in fiber and low in fat, reduced alcohol consumption, and physical activity,[18] and never to smoke. Early detection is important and recent trials have shown some benefits from therapy for advanced cancers.[19]

WHO IS AT HIGHER-THAN-USUAL RISK?

1. *All people when they get older.* Up to age fifty, this risk is very low unless special circumstances are present (see 2 and 3 below). From then on, the risk doubles every ten years, peaking at age seventy. This is why the American Cancer Society recommends that people, *even if they feel completely healthy,* should routinely have certain tests beginning at age fifty. Such tests are: an examination of the rectum with a gloved finger (digital rectal) and a test for blood in the stool (guaiac test) annually, especially in women over age sixty-five; a "procto," which means inspection of the inside of the bowel with a flexible sigmoidoscope or with a flexible colonoscope (which allows examination of more of your bowel) every three to five years.[20] New flexible instruments cause less discomfort than the rigid instruments used in the past. These tests can be carried out by the family or primary-care physician, who would refer you to a specialist if any of the results suggest cancer, or if other kinds of problems are found.

2. *People with a personal or family history of colorectal cancer, breast cancer, or cancer of the endometrium* (lining of the uterus). Since such individuals have colorectal cancer more often than others—often at a younger age—doctors should take careful family histories and may do examinations every five years for colorectal cancer on blood relatives of these patients, beginning at age thirty-five or forty. In this situation, the whole bowel may be inspected by colonoscopy or a barium enema X ray. Inform your health-care provider of your family history. Thirteen percent of the people with colon cancer are estimated to have a gene thought to cause it and, perhaps, ovarian cancer. There is no way yet to test for the gene.[21]

3. *People with bowel diseases that are not cancer in themselves but often lead to cancer.*

(a) Inflammatory bowel disease (ulcerative colitis or Crohn's disease—sometimes called regional ileitis or enteritis). If one of these conditions exists for eight or ten years, the chance of developing colorectal cancer is increased.

(b) Familial polyposis. In this condition, the bowel is studded with polyps and examinations should begin much earlier, even in adolescence. The disease is inherited and leads to cancer in 50 percent of the cases. Close blood relatives of anyone who has this condition should also be examined early and periodically.

(c) Single polyps, especially of the cell type called "adenomatous," arc also associated with cancer of the bowel. These should be removed surgically (not a major operation), and the surgery followed by regular examinations.

4. *People who have ever smoked.* Unfortunately, the damage persists even when the person stops smoking.

Living with an Ostomy

When part of the intestine must be removed, the two cut ends are sewn together to maintain a passageway for food. When this is not feasible, an opening (a "stoma") is made in the abdominal wall, through which the undigested matter can pass into a pouch (appliance). The operation is called a colostomy when the stoma is made in the colon, and an ileostomy when the stoma is made in the portion of the small intestine called the ileum. People with colostomies may or may not return to a predictable time of bowel evacuation, depending on the location of the colostomy in the large intestine, on prior bowel habits, on the presence of other medical conditions, or on the use of medicines or other cancer treatments. Some people with a colostomy flush or irrigate the stoma with water to promote a bowel movement at a certain time of the day, others prefer to wear an appliance most of the time. Those with ileostomies must keep the bag in place all the time.

People often fear that a diagnosis of colorectal cancer leads automatically to a colostomy. This was never the case, and is even less true today with surgical techniques that reconnect parts of the large intestine after removing the cancerous section. Furthermore, living with an ostomy today is significantly easier than it was in the past. Women who have an ostomy can lead completely normal lives that include sexual relations. (See the pamphlet "Sex and the Female Ostomate" listed in Resources, page 461. See also the Sexuality chapter.)

I've always loved clothes and fashion. My lifelong ambition was to become a model. Two years ago I went to a modeling school to learn to be one—me and my colostomy with all the twenty-year-olds. Recently I went to the restaurant where I do informal modeling. I donned a dress which tied low on my right side and slipped into the bathroom to check it out in the mirror. One woman commented to another about my dress being the type she could wear because it had a tie to hide her right side.

COLOSTOMY

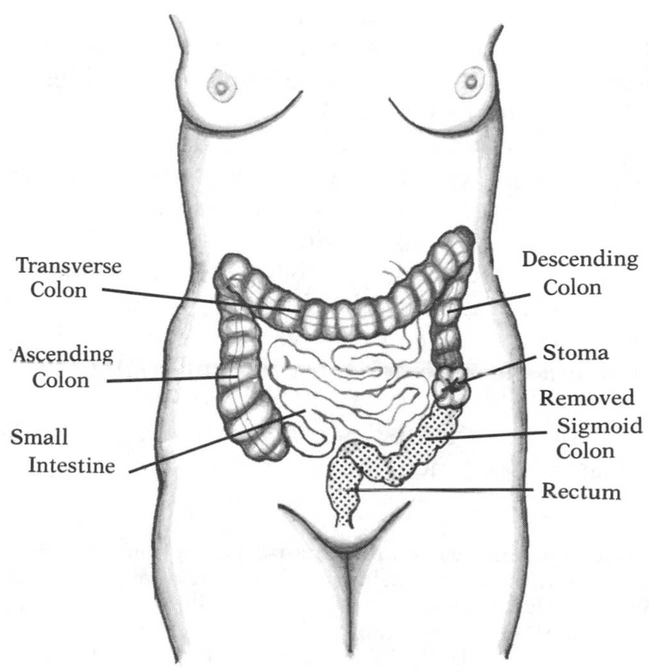

Then she said to me, "I wear a pouch, you know." To which I replied, "You do? Well, so do I!" I told her that if she was going to be in the restaurant a while longer, my next outfit was going to be a very brief bathing suit. The only kind of clothing I can't wear is a bikini. She only had the ostomy for three months and was wearing a tent dress so I thought it was very important that she see me in a bathing suit. That encounter really made my day as I'm sure it did hers. [a fifty-year-old woman]

To find help from those who have gone through the experience, contact a chapter of the United Ostomy Association (see your local phone book) or your local chapter of the American Cancer Society (see also Resources for this chapter).

I've been an ostomy hospital visitor for about nine years. I feel it is important for people to talk to others who have "walked the same road." [a fifty-year-old woman]

BREAST CANCER*

To women, breast cancer is perhaps the most familiar and the most frightening of all cancers. The older we get, the more we hear of friends and relatives who have the disease, and the more likely it is that we ourselves have experienced it.

Statistics on the disease cause us concern. Breast cancer was long the foremost cause of cancer deaths in women, and is now second only to lung cancer. Overall, one out of every eight women who live to age ninety-five develops it, but the risk of developing it before age seventy is less—one in fourteen. Breast-cancer incidence rises rapidly in women between thirty and fifty, then continues to rise, but more slowly, after age fifty.[22] Approximately 80 percent of all breast cancers occur in postmenopausal women, among whom rates continue to increase. It used to be more common in white women than in black women, but this is changing; among young black women, the rates have doubled so the incidence is now higher than that in young white women.[23]

But these statistics mask other facts about breast cancer, facts that are both reassuring and complex. Breast cancer is actually many different diseases, some aggressive and rapidly fatal, some so indolent and slow that they may not kill, and many between these two extremes. The rate at which breast tumors grow varies enormously, as does our immune systems' ability to fight them. Although many women with breast cancer die within a few years of diagnosis, others live as long as thirty or forty years before dying either of breast cancer or of other causes in old age. **Sixty percent of women with breast cancer live as long as their peers without the disease.**

Nonetheless, some researchers think that some or all breast cancers spread immediately, and as cancerous cells leave the breast through the lymph nodes or bloodstream, others remain in the breast to form a lump. But when breast cancer spreads, it does not necessarily kill. Whether or not a spreading breast cancer is fatal seems to depend on the same vital factors: How fast or slow is the cancer? Can the immune system keep it under control?

DETECTION

The Breast Self-Exam

Although most breast lumps are benign (noncancerous), a lump is the most frequent first sign of breast cancer, far more frequent than pain or nipple discharge. Unlike cancerous lumps in other parts of the body, a sizable lump in the breast is relatively easy to feel. For this reason, doctors usually encourage us to examine our breasts regularly for lumps in order to detect cancer "early" if it is there. But is the breast self-exam actually beneficial?

Researchers now know that breast cancer is in the body not months, but years, before it is detected through a lump in the breast. In most cases, by the time a lump is large enough to be felt, it has been in the body at least three to five years, more likely five to fifteen years, depending on its rate of growth. If it is going to spread at all, it has probably spread long before we can feel its presence.

But even if breast cancer has already spread, there are arguments for early detection: (1) removing the lump as early as possible leaves the immune system free to fight cancer cells that have spread rather than having to fight the cells in the lump as well; (2) the longer a cancerous lump remains in the body, the more time it has to

*Debate continues about the causes, detection, and treatment of the ever-increasing number of new cases of breast cancer. One excellent source of additional information about a range of important topics is "The Politics of Breast Cancer." *Ms.*, Vol. III, No. 6 (May/ June 1993), pp. 38–60.

populate the body with additional cancer cells, making it harder for the immune system or cancer treatments to fight them.

However, many women question the emphasis on breast self-exam and feel blamed if a cancerous lump is found and they didn't find it "early enough." A federal panel supported women's doubts by deciding that there is not enough evidence in favor of the breast self-exam to advocate it as a detection test.[24] It is unlikely, but still not definitely known, whether the practice of monthly breast self-exams can lengthen a woman's life. Statistics show that in fact most women do not examine their breasts regularly, partly out of fear of finding a lump and partly because, as healthy women, they don't want to look for disease. Other women like the idea of becoming familiar with their bodies by monitoring normal, cyclic changes in their breasts. They see regular or occasional breast exams as a way of knowing and taking care of themselves, and they examine their breasts when the time feels right for them.[25]

Mammogram Screening

A mammogram, an X-ray picture of the breast, is now the most widely publicized method of regularly checking or screening healthy women for breast changes. Its purpose is to locate a suspicious lump in the breast so it can be removed and examined under a microscope to see if it is cancerous. A mammogram itself cannot diagnose cancer and it is not a treatment.

Theoretically, the arguments in favor of breast self-exam hold true for the mammogram, with the advantage that, in some women, a mammogram can indicate the possibility of a small cancerous lump years before it is large enough to be felt. Large-scale studies in Sweden and in the United States show that **women over fifty benefit from regular mammogram screening, with 30 percent lower breast-cancer death rates.** The same advantage has not been shown for younger women. The National Cancer Institute recommends mammograms every one to two years for women over fifty but has stopped recommending screening mammograms for women under fifty.[26] Some researchers, however, believe that mammograms should still be given to women in their forties. The American Cancer Society still recommends that women in their forties be screened every one or two years.

Mammogram screening has its dangers. One is that radiation can cause breast cancer. Radiation is cumulative: many small doses over time equal one large dose. No one knows how large a radiation dose has to be to cause breast cancer, and the amount probably varies from woman to woman.* But the breast seems to become less vulnerable with age, the adolescent breast possibly being the most vulnerable to radiation. Since it takes ten to twenty years or more for radiation-induced cancer to appear, the older you are, the less risk.

Make sure that the radiologist uses the lowest feasible dose of radiation, if possible as low as 0.1 or 0.2 rads per examination. Also, it appears that screening only every two or three years, using a single X-ray exposure for each breast, may be just as beneficial as yearly screening with double exposure.[27] The practice in this country is to take at least two views of each breast, and some radiologists argue that this provides better accuracy.

Mammograms do not distinguish a cancerous lump from a benign one. Since some breast lumpiness is normal in women, many mammograms interpreted as "suspicious" lead to needless worry and to countless unnecessary breast biopsies. The breast biopsy rate is increased by physicians who are afraid of malpractice suits and who protect themselves by recommending biopsies "just to make sure."

Perhaps the most disturbing aspect of mammogram screening is that of overtreatment. A mammogram can find lumps so small they are difficult to diagnose correctly under a microscope. Some of these lumps are cancers that may not spread, called *in situ* cancers. Women with such cancers may be misdiagnosed and treated as though they have rapidly spreading disease. Also, these women will be called "cured," thus distorting figures on the supposed benefits of the mammogram and the treatment.

Mammograms also find fields of what are called microcalcifications, tiny spots of calcium

*Estimates for mammograms indicate that one rad (radiation absorbed dose) to the breast per examination can result in six cancers per one million women beginning ten years after exposure. Another estimate shows that approximately 788 cases of breast cancer per year are caused by X rays. However, this figure includes all X rays in which the breast was exposed to the rays, such as X rays of the chest and back, and CAT scans, as well as mammograms. These figures are more important for determining recommendations for population policies than they are for making individual decisions.

deposits that show up almost like grains of sand in the mammogram. While it is true that calcium deposits are often present in cancer cells and are one of the signs radiologists look for in the screening process, it is also true that 75 percent of microcalcifications are normal and do not indicate cancer.[28]

To date, mammography is the only imaging method of screening that can show benefit to women. Other forms of breast pictures, such as thermography, diaphanography, and ultrasound, are not yet reliable enough to be beneficial. Further study of effective screening methods that do not involve radiation is needed.

If You Have a High Risk of Breast Cancer

If you have already had breast cancer it is worth having regular mammogram checkups no mat-

THE "HIGH RISK" CONTROVERSY AND TAMOXIFEN TRIALS

Inquire carefully about any high-risk label assigned to you by your doctor. Inappropriate labeling may lead you to undergo unnecessary tests and procedures, as well as cause undue emotional stress. Of every one hundred women who develop breast cancer, less than 25 percent will have any risk factor as yet identified. Obviously, we do not know enough about what causes breast cancer and we do not know how to prevent it, or predict it.

Age. After fifty, a woman's age is the most important risk factor. The older we are, the more likely we will have breast cancer. It is important to stress that the majority of women in whom breast cancer is diagnosed and treated will live out their lives without a recurrence of the disease.

Personal History of Breast Cancer. Increases the likelihood of discovering new cancer (not a metastasis) in the other breast.

Family History. If a mother or a sister had a confirmed diagnosis of breast cancer *before age fifty* a woman's risk increases significantly, more so if the cancer was in both breasts. In a recent study, women whose mothers had breast cancer were 80 percent more likely to develop the disease; 130 percent more likely if their sisters had it. But this accounted for only 6 percent of all the breast cancers discovered. The majority of women who developed breast cancer had no familial disposition.[1]

Dietary Fat. One study showed an average fat intake of 39 percent and no reduction in breast cancer in those who reduced their dietary fat intake to 26 percent.[2] Animal studies, however, show a drop in breast tumors at 20 percent fat intake. Toxic substances such as pesticides are stored in fat tissue in the body and may be the culprit. Prospective studies now underway may yield more information about dietary factors in the next five years.[3]

Estrogens. Have been shown in numerous studies to increase the risk of breast cancer after menopause, particularly if taken for more than fifteen years. How much the use of progestins after menopause increase the risk of breast cancer is being investigated, but we will not have an answer for many more years.

Radiation, Diethylstilbestrol (DES), and Alcohol. Use of these has increased risk in a small number of women. Other environmental hazards have been ignored.

Delayed Pregnancy. Pregnancy leading to a birth (fullterm pregnancy) and nursing cause changes in the breast that seem to offer some protection from cancer. A first full-term pregnancy past the age of thirty-five seems to offer less protection than no pregnancy at all.[4]

An excellent resource for helping to determine your own breast cancer risk is *Understanding Breast Cancer* by Patricia Kelly (Philadelphia: Temple University Press, 1991).

Tamoxifen is useful in treating postmenopausal women with breast cancer. Many "high risk" premenopausal women are now participating in a questionable research project to test whether taking tamoxifen will reduce their chances of developing breast cancer.[5] While tamoxifen acts like an estroter what your age, since cancerous lumps often recur in the same or the other breast. Also, the benefits of mammogram screening probably outweigh the risks if you are over fifty and have a higher-than-average risk of breast cancer. If you are at high risk for breast cancer, but under fifty, have a mammogram every one or two years if it helps put your mind at ease, but remember that screening doesn't improve the longevity of women your age.

gen in parts of the body (increasing the likelihood of developing endometrial cancer), it acts like an antiestrogen on breast tissue, causes premature menopause, and can have other serious effects (liver or eye damage, and blood clots). Its effect on bone mass is not yet known.

Who benefits? ICI Pharma produces tamoxifen in the United States, charging $1.50 per pill, while tamoxifen can be purchased in other countries for only slightly over 20 cents. Wyeth Ayerst Laboratories (owned by American Home Products) produces Premarin, the estrogen prescribed most often to postmenopausal women. Premarin is now the second leading prescription drug sold in the United States.

1. Graham A. Colditz, et al., "Family History, Age, and Risk of Breast Cancer: Prospective Data from the Nurses' Health Study." *Journal of the American Medical Association*, Vol. 270, No. 3 (July 21, 1993), pp. 338–43; and "Correction." *Journal of the American Medical Association*, Vol. 270, No. 13 (Oct. 6, 1993), p. 1548.

2. Walter C. Willett, et al., "Dietary Fat and Fiber in Relation to Risk of Breast Cancer: An Eight-year Follow-up." *Journal of the American Medical Association*, Vol. 268 (October 1992), pp. 2037–44.

3. Walter C. Willett and David J. Hunter, "Diet and Breast Cancer." *Contemporary Nutrition*, Vol. 18, Nos. 3, 4 (1993), pp. 1–4.

4. Judy Foreman, "The Cancer Risk in Delayed Pregnancy." *The Boston Globe*, Sept. 27, 1993, pp. 27–29.

5. For more information: "Tamoxifen Prevention Trial Packet," National Women's Health Network, 1325 G St., NW, Washington, DC 20005. For a description of three studies now under way see Maureen Henderson, "Current Approaches to Breast Cancer Prevention." *Science*, Vol. 259 (Jan. 29, 1993), pp. 630–31.

If You Find a Lump

If you or your partner or health-care practitioner find a lump in your breast, keep in mind that 80 to 90 percent of lumps are benign (noncancerous). Breast lumps are common and normal in women, and most conditions causing change, lumps, or pain in the breast are not cancer. Probably the majority of older women have found one or more isolated lumps in their breasts through the years, and a general lumpiness of the breasts is common in half of all women. Many physicians call lumpiness or even one isolated lump "fibrocystic disease." But lumpy breasts are not a disease and do not increase our risk of breast cancer. For this reason, some physicians more appropriately refer to breast lumpiness as a fibrocystic condition.[29] Most benign lumps are related to the hormonal fluctuations of menstruation, however, so a new lump after menopause should be checked. There is no sure way of reducing noncancerous breast lumps, but some women find that reducing fat, salt, caffeine, chocolate, and cigarettes, while adding dietary supplements of vitamin E and evening primrose oil (available in health-food stores), has helped.

There is no harm in monitoring a lump yourself for a few weeks. If a lump fluctuates with your period, this is an indication that it is a harmless cyst, or fluid-filled sac. If you are past menopause, check the lump on the same date each month, since women continue to have cyclical changes in their breasts even after periods cease.

If your lump does not fluctuate and/or worries you, have an experienced physician examine your breast. Many women find that their own general practitioners or gynecologists do not know how to examine the breast properly, nor are they knowledgeable about how to distinguish a benign lump from a cancerous one. If possible, see a practitioner experienced in benign breast problems and breast cancer. A surgeon would be a likely choice for a first or second opinion. You can see a surgeon simply for a diagnosis of your lump. You do not have to plan on surgery or agree to it. Your physician should give you a thorough breast exam in both seated and supine (lying down) positions, palpate your underarms for swelling and your abdomen for suspicious masses, listen to your lungs, and take a complete blood count. These examinations are a precaution to check for cancer in the body. If your lump is large and feels like a cyst, your physician may try an immediate needle aspiration.

Diagnosis

Most breast masses are harmless. But in spite of the inconvenience and cost of testing many benign masses, you should consider a biopsy if you are in a higher-risk category of breast cancer or are past menopause. Certainly you should have one if other symptoms of possible cancer are present, such as hard, swollen glands in the armpit, a skin rash on the breast, bloody nipple discharge, or dimpling of the skin around the nipple or retraction of the nipple. The failure to diagnose breast cancer was the second most frequent reason for claims brought against physicians, most often by premenopausal women.[30] There are two basic diagnostic procedures to determine whether a lump is cancerous, both of them office procedures.

Needle aspiration: your physician inserts a needle into the lump. If the lump is a cyst, fluid is withdrawn and the lump collapses. If the lump proves solid, or if it is too small to insert the needle accurately into, the next step would be a surgical biopsy.

Surgical biopsy: the removal of the lump in order to examine it under a microscope. The surgery can usually be done under local anesthesia—unless you prefer general anesthesia, which entails risks and requires longer recovery time. Do *not* agree to a biopsy under general anesthesia just so the surgeon can remove the entire breast immediately should your lump prove cancerous. This "one-step procedure" is unnecessary and detrimental.

It is best to remove an entire solid lump (excisional biopsy), since some lumps are made up of both benign and cancerous cells. If only part of the lump is removed and proves benign, the part left in the breast could still be cancerous. The excised lump should be analyzed by permanent section, which will take a few days, but is more reliable than the quick-frozen section. There is no need of a bone scan or any further tests unless your lump is diagnosed as cancerous.

If you have a biopsy make sure your physician plans to order an immediate hormone-receptor test on the lump if it turns out to be malignant. This test will show how your tumor cells react to estrogen and progesterone. This test is vital to planning future treatment and must be done on the biopsied tissue without delay.

Fine needle aspiration of a solid lump and *trucut needle biopsy* are less common and are not definitive. If the needle shows only noncancerous cells, the cells remaining in the lump could still be cancerous. But if your lump is so large that removing it would greatly distort the breast, these procedures can help you decide whether or not to have further surgery.

Wire or needle localization biopsy may be used if a mammogram shows a suspicious area such as microcalcifications that can't be felt but that your physician thinks should be examined.[31]

While an X ray shows a picture of your breast, the radiologist inserts a fine wire or needle into the breast under local anesthesia, and points the wire to the area in question. The surgeon then follows the wire and removes the tissue at the end. Further examination is done to confirm that the correct area was removed.

A mammogram is not appropriate for diagnosing breast cancer. However, some physicians recommend a mammogram before a biopsy to see if there are other suspicious masses in the same or the other breast.

If Your Lump Is Cancerous

If your lump proves cancerous, there is no need to rush into action. Give yourself time to adjust to the powerful feelings you will have and to find out which treatment, if any, might be most beneficial for your special case. There is no harm in taking up to six weeks before making any decisions.

Making a Decision About Treatments

Since breast-cancer treatments are so controversial among physicians, and new studies are constantly clarifying treatment options, it is especially important to get second or even third opinions about the right treatment for you. Be sure to find out the results or trends of current studies, especially larger "randomized clinical trials."

You and your physician need to know as much as possible about your cancer in order to make a sound judgment on possible treatments. The first step is the hormone-receptor test. Your tumor cells may contain an estrogen and/or progesterone receptor (called an estrogen/progesterone-positive cancer, or ER+ and PgR+). This indicates a hormone-sensitive cancer, which is often a slower-growing one. It is most prevalent in postmenopausal women. The increase in breast cancer since 1960 has been mostly of the ER+ type.[32] The absence of this receptor is called an estrogen/progesterone-negative cancer, or ER– and PgR–. Estrogen/progesterone-negative cancers tend to be more aggressive than estrogen/progesterone-positive cancers.

As a second step, your physician may suggest removing a few lymph nodes from your armpit. The presence of cancerous cells in the nodes (called "positive nodes") is a sign that cancer may be elsewhere in the body and that your immune system, in which lymph nodes play an active role, is not successfully fighting the spreading disease. Conversely, cancer-free lymph nodes (called "negative nodes") indicate that your immune system is more successful in fighting the disease elsewhere in your body than if the nodes are positive. Lymph-node sampling is for diagnosis only, to help decide which treatment might be beneficial. Removing them does not help eliminate cancer from the body. Removing more than about ten nodes may cause arm problems later.

Two weeks after my outpatient nodal resection, I felt pretty good but could not raise my arm more than five inches from my side and had a lot of pain in my side when I tried. My cousin, a nurse, said the problem was muscle spasms in my back with referred pain to my side. The spasms were probably from the placement of my arm during the hour-long surgery. She massaged my back for an hour twice a day for three days and then showed my husband how to do it. After her first massage, I could raise my arm more normally and the pain in my side lessened. Five weeks after surgery I was able to raise my arm straight over my head, something that usually takes longer to regain. She said that since women are leaving the hospital right away, no one is telling them why their arm seems to be "bound" to their side and what to do about it. [a fifty-five-year-old woman]

Your physician should also do an abdominal exam and order blood tests, a chest X ray, and possibly a bone scan. These tests will show if the cancer has reached a detectable stage in a distant part of your body such as the bone or liver. Available treatments have helped some women have long remissions and live for many years with metastases. Furthermore, they have relieved uncomfortable or painful symptoms. The advantages must be weighed against the negative effects of the treatment.

Treatment Options

Local Therapies

The purpose of local therapies is to remove (surgery) and/or kill (radiation) cancerous cells at the site of the lump and in the surrounding area.

Lumpectomy. Lumpectomy is the surgical removal of the lump with varying amounts of surrounding tissue. If your biopsy included the entire lump and some surrounding tissue, this is considered a lumpectomy and you probably need no further surgery.

Women with tumors up to one and a half inches in diameter live as long with lumpectomy alone as with lumpectomy and radiation, or with mastectomy. This includes women with positive and negative nodes but with no evidence of distant spread. It also applies to women with obvious distant spread for whom systemic treatment would be added.

The possible adverse effects of a lumpectomy are some scarring and disfiguring of the breast.

Lumpectomy with Radiation. In this procedure, after the lump and surrounding tissue have been removed, the area surrounding the site of the lump is irradiated by X-ray beams and sometimes by temporary implants of radioactive materials (radiation implants). Radiation can evidently help prevent a cancerous lump from growing back again in the same breast, but it does not prolong life. Although radiation can have adverse effects, some women choose it to reduce the risk of a repeated lump and surgery in the same breast. However, this is a matter of choice. If you have a lumpectomy you do not have to agree to radiation also.

Adverse effects can include fatigue; dry, red, itchy skin; extreme sun sensitivity; muscle pain; and occasional cracked ribs or a temporary lung ailment similar to bronchitis. Theoretically, radiation therapy can also cause breast cancer, but this appears to be rare.

Black women treated at small hospitals and older women are less likely to be offered this option and may have to insist if they want it.[33]

During radiation treatment I used cornstarch several times a day, dusting it like powder on my breast, under it, and in the armpit. I didn't wear a bra but rather loose-fitting cotton clothing with sleeves to keep the area dry, cool, and not bind the breast in any way. [the same fifty-five-year-old postmenopausal woman. Her lymph nodes were clear. She decided on radiation after her lumpectomy, and then tamoxifen.]

Systemic Therapies

Chemotherapy. Drugs in the form of pills or injections attempt to kill cancer cells nesting or circulating in distant parts of the body. Premenopausal women with positive nodes live longer as a result of chemotherapy.[34] Women in this category who have one to three positive nodes or whose tumors contain poorly differentiated cells (cells in an undeveloped, embryonic state) seem more likely to be helped by chemotherapy than women who have four or more positive nodes or whose tumors have well-differentiated cells.[35]

A combination of drugs called CMF (cyclophosphamide, methotrexate, and fluorouracil) may work better than single drugs used separately, and a six-month regimen seems just as beneficial as longer use. Drug dosage, timing, combination, and duration of treatment are constantly under study. Studies show that chemotherapy can help premenopausal women with aggressive cancers but no node involvement.[36]

You will need to ask many questions to determine if you are likely to benefit from chemotherapy.

Hormone Therapy. Some hormones in the form of pills or injections aim to repress or eliminate estrogen in the body, thus curbing the spread of cancer. The hormones most commonly used are tamoxifen and male hormones.

Tamoxifen can prolong life in some postmenopausal women, especially those whose lumps have been diagnosed as estrogen-positive and whose nodes show signs of cancer. It is used also when the nodes are negative. Long-term use (two years or perhaps longer) seems to be more effective than shorter use. The drug evidently has few adverse effects on women past menopause except hot flashes and vaginal dryness. It is fairly expensive.

Physicians sometimes include tamoxifen in chemotherapy regimens. Adding chemotherapy to tamoxifen can be of value to postmenopausal women. No consistent evidence supports the addition of tamoxifen to chemotherapy in younger women. Ask your physician which drugs will be included in your regimen and why.

Postmenopausal women with estrogen-receptor-positive cancers benefit more from hormone therapy than do women with ER– cancers.

Outmoded and Rarely Necessary Treatments

Surgical Techniques to Limit Estrogen Production. These techniques include adrenalectomy (removal of the adrenals) and hypophysectomy (removal of the pituitary gland). The drugs discussed under hormone therapy can generally produce the same effects with fewer problems. Oophorectomy (removal of the ovaries) is sometimes used when tamoxifen is not effective.

Mastectomy. Mastectomy is surgical removal of the entire breast. This procedure, long thought the only way to treat breast cancer, is no more effective than removal of the lump alone. A mastectomy is probably necessary only if:

(a) Your breast is small and the lump so large that a lumpectomy would be more disfiguring than removing the entire breast; or

(b) The cancerous cells have not formed a lump but are diffuse in tiny clusters throughout the breast. In this case, many women and doctors want to "get it all out" by removing the entire breast, although there is no proof, even then, that a mastectomy prolongs life.

A radical mastectomy, also called the Halsted radical (removal of the breast, underlying muscle of the chest wall, and lymph nodes), is *never* necessary. However, some surgeons still recommend and perform it.

If You Have Had a Mastectomy

The mastectomy has been standard practice for over one hundred years. From 1970 through 1985 over one and a half million women had mastectomies of some kind, including the Halsted radical.[37] In the belief that time was essential, surgeons often performed the operation while the patient was under general anesthesia given for the biopsy. A woman awoke to find that she had cancer and had lost one or both breasts.

Most one-breasted women wear a prosthesis, a breast form made of foam rubber or silicone. Some have had surgical reconstruction to take the place of the amputated breast. Women's reports of problems with silicone-gel implants finally forced the FDA to withdraw them from general use.[38] If, on a warm summer day when light clothing would normally be worn, all women who had mastectomies decided not to wear a prosthesis, or could temporarily discard their reconstructed breasts, we would see in the streets, the shops, and beaches many one-breasted women.

Women who have lost one or both breasts face the emotional trauma of losing a part of their body strongly associated with sexuality and a sense of womanhood.

It's been a long process coming to terms with the loss of my breast. The mastectomy seemed unreal for a long time. I would look in the mirror and not believe it! I think it takes a lot of courage to say goodbye to a part of your body no matter what your age. But I was very young, and it seemed especially sad to lose my breast before I had lived with it and enjoyed it fully. I hadn't seen it get full of milk and breastfed with it; hadn't watched it age. Only long after the operation was I able to really say goodbye to my breast. [a thirty-nine-year-old woman]

For some women, the physical discomfort and pain resulting from a radical mastectomy are also a lasting concern. When the lymph nodes have been removed and the lymph and blood vessels cut during surgery, the lymph fluid in the arm cannot drain off and sometimes

GENES AND DISEASE*

by Ruth Hubbard

Many health conditions develop over time and therefore do not become evident until we get older. In addition, conditions such as high blood pressure, coronary heart disease, or cancer sometimes cluster in families, though they can also appear out of the blue. The Human Genome Initiative is a U.S.-led international effort to identify all the human genes, localize them precisely on our chromosomes, and analyze their composition. With new discoveries emerging, the media have recently been telling us about the identification of genes associated with colon, breast, and ovarian cancer in families in which unusual numbers of family members develop these cancers.

When scientists identify such genes, they can sometimes develop diagnostic tests to predict which family members are likely to develop the condition in question. The tests can never predict this with certainty, but they enable family members, who are predicted to be at risk, to undergo diagnostic tests more often than they otherwise might do so, while relieving the others of needless concern about this aspect of their health.

Our bodies and our health are always in a dynamic relationship with how we live. So it may actually be harmful to think that our fate is in our genes and that there is nothing we can do to improve our health, because, though many factors are beyond our control, we can sometimes make beneficial changes in our lives.

Not everyone feels positive about predictive tests. Some of us might want to live as healthfully as we can and take specific medical, or other, measures when we encounter health problems, without trying to foresee them. Others consider this kind of foreknowledge useful, even though it is never certain.

The situation becomes more problematic when predictive tests, developed by studying "high-risk" families, are generalized to the entire population. This can increase discrimination toward people carrying certain genes. Yet, it is never certain that genetic factors, identified in specific families, are relevant to everyone. Also, genes are never the only factors associated with these or any other health conditions. Our environment and other life circumstances—including chemical and radiation hazards at home and at work, the amount and quality of our food and water, the quality of the air, exercise and other forms of relaxation, emotional and physical stress and abuse—all affect the likelihood that any one of us will develop a chronic condition, irrespective of our genetic predispositions.

*For further discussion of this subject, see Ruth Hubbard and Elijah Wald, *Exploding the Gene Myth.* Boston: Beacon Press, 1993.

accumulates, causing swelling in the arm and even pain. At times, women who have had less extensive mastectomies, or only a lymph-node sampling, experience a similar, but milder, discomfort. There is no cure for this condition, called *lymphedema,** but there are ways of making it easier to live with. Wearing an elastic custom-fitted sleeve, and treatment with an inflatable sleeve (pneumo-massage), can alleviate discomfort. Some women find that exercise, especially under the instruction of a physical therapist, reduces the discomfort of lymphedema as well as any stiffness and numbness in the shoulder and arm (see Maggie Lettvin's book listed under Resources for this chapter). Talk with your physician or contact "Reach for Recovery" at your local American Cancer Society chapter or the Encore program at your local YWCA for more information.

New Developments—Women's Voices Will Be Heard!

Since our first edition, there have been several important developments that affect women's cancers, particularly breast cancer.

One is the work of the Human Genome Initiative, a $3 billion international project that is attempting to identify all human genes. (See box page 369.) Even if a gene that may confer greater susceptibility to radiation-induced breast cancer is discovered,[39] for example, reducing radiation exposure is still a necessity for everyone.

The second development is that women have found their voices and are organizing around such issues as breast cancer. Women are forming groups to demand new research directions, appropriate state and federal actions, and more education about hazards, treatments, and rights.

The third development is the mounting pressure for research on the environmental and economic causes for the growing breast-cancer rates in addition to the genetic and personal causes. Less than 25 percent of women with breast cancer fall into the currently defined high-risk categories. Therefore, there must be other ignored or unknown reasons for the increased number of women with breast cancer, especially in those areas with continued high incidence.

*Lymphedema can occur in the leg after lymph nodes are removed from the groin. Try the same methods mentioned above for the arm to alleviate discomfort in the leg.

One possibility lies in the use of organochlorines, a class of industrial chemicals made from chlorine. They include highly persistent and toxic subtances such as DDT, PCBs, and dioxin, plus thousands of lesser known chemicals. They persist in the environment and accumulate in living things, building up to higher and higher levels in food chains and in the bodies of wildlife and people. Many concentrate in the fat tissue of the body. Though Rachel Carson's 1962 book *Silent Spring* led to the ban of one organochlorine pesticide (DDT), the use of other organochlorines such as PCBs has increased and their possible link to breast cancer has been ignored.

Two lines of research led to organochlorines as being suspect. First, women with breast cancer seem to have higher levels of organochlorines in their tissues than women without breast cancer. Second, the rates and mortality in young women from breast cancer in Israel have dropped since the phase-out of all organochlorine pesticides there starting in 1978.[40]

An additional factor may be that low doses of radiation released from nuclear fission find their way into the air, the drinking water, and the fresh milk in surrounding areas. Studies of breast cancer mortality in the New York metropolitan area—including Connecticut, Westchester, and Long Island—show a correlation with the cumulative airborne releases from the nuclear plants in the area. This radiation appears to act synergistically with other carcinogens, such as ordinary air pollution, cigarette smoke, diesel fumes, asbestos, exogenous hormones, and organochlorines; that is, the effects of each are greater in the presence of the other.

Some researchers claim that the increases and decreases in breast cancer in other countries are explained by the increases and decreases in nuclear testing and the use of nuclear power, and in patterns of consumption of dairy products in those countries. They further claim that chronic exposure to the products of nuclear fission may be a factor in the increased incidence of most cancers in the general population in the United States since World War II.[41]

Another possibility is the risk posed by electromagnetic fields, including electric power transmission lines, blow-dryers, television sets, electric blankets, and other appliances. An EPA report is due in 1994.[42]

Special women's cancer groups include the National Breast Cancer Coalition, with 160 member organizations since its founding in 1991. The coalition succeeded in getting $400 million in

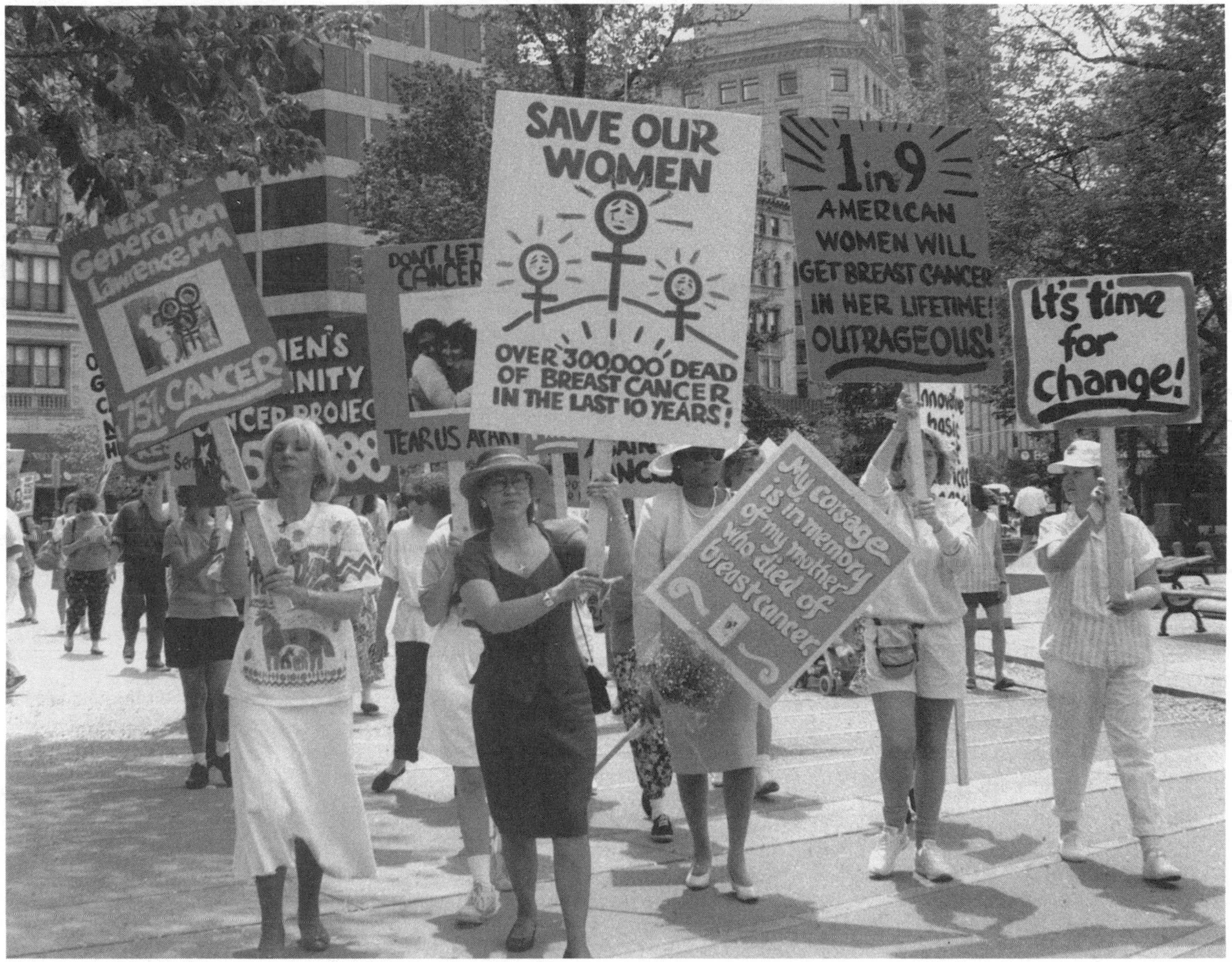
NEXT
Generation
Lawrence MA
75% CANCER
DON'T LET
CANCER
TEAR US APART
SAVE OUR
WOMEN
OVER 300,000 DEAD
OF BREAST CANCER
IN THE LAST 10 YEARS!
1 in 9
AMERICAN
WOMEN WILL
GET BREAST CANCER
IN HER LIFETIME!
OUTRAGEOUS!
It's time
for
change!
My corsage
is in memory
of my mother
who died of
breast cancer.

Ellen Shub

federal funds for breast-cancer research in 1992, double the amount for 1991. A sum of $25 million from the Department of Defense (DOD) budget was used to purchase mammography equipment to screen women in the armed services and to fund research on detection devices. The DOD budget was raised to $210 million in 1993 and women are speaking out to influence how it is spent.[43]

Another group is the National Coalition of Feminist and Lesbian Cancer Projects, which works to empower grass-roots women's cancer groups and speaks out on cancer issues within the lesbian-rights movement. Groups such as the National Women's Health Network are vocal on a variety of issues, including women's cancers.

Some state organizations have been formed. For example, the Massachusetts Breast Cancer Coalition, founded in 1991, has already succeeded in getting the state to regulate the quality of mammography equipment and the training of physicians who interpret mammograms. Area groups such as 1 in 9 Long Island Breast Cancer Action Coalition in New York, dissatisfied with the dismissal of environmental causes for the high rates of breast cancer there, are speaking out and conducting their own surveys.[44]

Many of the groups, such as the Women's Community Cancer Project, founded in 1989 in Cambridge, combine both the personal and the political. Members of the WCCP offer support groups, prepare materials for the media, educate the public through their publications, including brochures in several languages and a newsletter, and have developed broad support for *A Women's Cancer Agenda: The Demands to the National Cancer Institute and U.S. Government*.[45]

These activities mark the maturing of an important force within the women's health movement and include many older women.

NOTES

1. Robert L. Rogers, et al., "Abstention from Smoking Improves Cerebral Perfusion Among Elderly Smokers." *Journal of the American Medical Association,* Vol. 253, No. 20 (May 24/31, 1985), pp. 2970–74.

2. Adapted from the Boston Women's Health Book Collective, *The New Our Bodies, Ourselves.* New York: Simon and Schuster, 1992, p. 611.

3. Natalie Angier, "Chemists Learn Why Vegetables Are Good for You!" *The New York Times,* Apr. 13, 1993, pp. C1, C9.

4. Amanda Spake, "A New American Nightmare." *Ms.,* March 1986, pp. 35–42ff.

5. Jean Hardisty and Ellen Leopold, "Cancer and Poverty: Double Jeopardy for Women." *Sojourner: The Women's Forum,* December 1992, pp. 16–17; and M. Brinton Lykes et al., eds., *Unmasking Social Inequities: Victims, Voice and Resistance.* Philadelphia: Temple University Press, in press.

6. Susan Sontag, *Illness as Metaphor.* New York: Random House, 1979.

7. Marcia Angell, "Disease as a Reflection of the Psyche?" *The New England Journal of Medicine,* Vol. 312, No. 24 (June 13, 1985), pp. 1570–72.

8. Barrie R. Cassileth, et al., "Psychosocial Correlates in Survival in Advanced Malignant Disease." *The New England Journal of Medicine,* Vol. 312, No. 24 (June 13, 1985), pp. 1551–55.

9. David Spiegel, "A Psychosocial Intervention and Survival Time of Patients with Metastatic Breast Cancer." *Advances,* Vol. 7, No. 3 (1991), pp. 10–19.

10. T. Colton, et al., "Breast Cancer in Mothers Prescribed Diethylstilbestrol in Pregnancy." *Journal of the American Medical Association,* Vol. 269, No. 16 (Apr. 28, 1993), pp. 2096–2100.

11. Linda C. Harlan, et al., "Cervical Cancer Screening: Who Is Not Screened and Why?" *American Journal of Public Health,* Vol. 81, No. 7 (July 1991). Reviewed in *The Network News,* November/December 1992, p. 2.

12. Stephen Jay Gould, "The Median Isn't the Message." *Discover,* Vol. 6, No. 6 (June 1985), pp. 40–42.

13. Devra Lee Davis and David G. Hoel, "Figuring Out Cancer," pp. 447–53; and Samuel S. Epstein, et al., "Losing the 'War Against Cancer': A Need for Public Policy Reforms," pp. 455–69, including a refutation and a rebuttal. *International Journal of Health Sciences,* Vol. 22, No. 3 (1992).

14. American Cancer Society, *1992 Cancer Facts & Figures,* p. 13.

15. Ibid., p. 13.

16. Cornelius O. Granai, "Ovarian Cancer—Unrealistic Expectations." *The New England Journal of Medicine,* Vol. 327, No. 3 (July 16, 1992), pp. 197–99; and Maurice J. Webb, "Screening for Ovarian Cancer: Still a Long Way to Go." *British Medical Journal,* Vol. 306 (Apr. 17, 1993), pp. 1015–16.

17. Alice Whittemore, et al., "Characteristics Relating to Ovarian Cancer Risk." *American Journal of Epidemiology,* Vol. 136 (1992), pp. 1184–1203; Stephen A. Cannistra, "Cancer of the Ovary." *The New England Journal of Medicine,* Vol. 329, No. 21 (Nov. 18, 1993), pp. 1550–59.

18. Walter C. Willett, et al., "Relation of Meat, Fat and Fiber Intake to the Risk of Colon Cancer in a Prospective Study Among Women." *The New England Journal of Medicine,* Vol. 323 (1990), pp. 1664–72.

19. "Adjuvant Therapy for Patients with Colon and Rectum Cancer." *NIH Consensus Development Conference Statement,* Vol. 8, No. 4 (April 16–18, 1990).

20. Jane E. Brody, "Screening for Cancer of the Colon: Range of Options." *The New York Times,* Mar. 10, 1993.

21. Gina Kolata, "Cancer-Causing Gene Found, with a Clue to How It Works." *The New York Times,* May 6, 1993, pp. A1, B15.

22. "Lifetime Probability of Breast Cancer in American Women." National Center Institute, September 1992; and Jay Harris, et al., "Breast Cancer." *The New England Journal of Medicine,* Vol. 327, No. 5 (July 30, 1992), pp. 319–28; Part two: Vol. 327, No. 6 (Aug. 6, 1992), pp. 390–98; Part three: Vol. 327, No. 7 (Aug. 13, 1992), pp. 473–80.

23. Harris, et al., ibid., Part One, p. 320.

24. Michael S. O'Malley and Suzanne W. Fletcher, "Screening for Breast Cancer with Breast Self-Examination." *Journal of the American Medical Association,* Vol. 257, No. 16 (Apr. 24, 1987), pp. 2197–2203.

25. Anne Perkins, "Taking Our Breasts in Our Hands." *Sojourner,* Vol. 18, No. 11 (July 1993), p. 16.

26. Harris, et al., op. cit; statement released December 3, 1993, by the National Cancer Institute, Office of Cancer Communications, Building 31, Room 10A21, Bethesda, MD 20892.

27. L. Tabar, et al., "Reduction in Mortality from Breast Cancer After Mass Screening with Mammography." *Lancet,* April 13, 1985, pp. 829–32.

28. "Differentiating Benign Breast Conditions, Breast Ca[ncer]." *Ob. Gyn. News,* Vol. 20, No. 20 (Oct. 15–31, 1985), p. 41.

29. Susan Love, et al., "Fibrocystic 'Disease' of the Breast—a Non-disease." *The New England Journal of Medicine,* Vol. 307, No. 16 (Oct. 14, 1982), pp. 1010–14.

30. William L. Donegan, "Evaluation of a Palpable Breast Mass." *The New England Journal of Medicine,* Vol. 327, No. 13 (Sept. 24, 1992), pp. 937–42; Correspondence, *The New England Journal of Medicine,* Vol. 328, No. 11 (March 18, 1993), pp. 810–12.

31. Write for the material available from the Microcalcification Awareness Action Committee, c/o Women's Cancer Resource Center, 3023 Shattuck Avenue, Berkeley, CA 94705. Tel. (510) 548-9272. Their article was reprinted in *The Network News,* March/April 1993.

32. Harris, et al., op. cit.

33. Anid R. Satariano, G. Marie Swanson, and Patricia P. Moll, "Nonclinical Factors Associated with Surgery Received for Treatment of Early-Stage Breast Cancer." *American Journal of Public Health,* Vol. 82, No. 2 (February 1992), pp. 195–98.

34. Harris, et al., op. cit.

35. Edwin R. Fisher, "Pathologic Features as Prognostic Variables." *Adjuvant Chemotherapy for Breast Cancer.* National Institutes of Health Consensus Development Conference, 1985, pp. 26–27; and I. Craig Henderson, "Adjuvant Chemotherapy of Breast Cancer." *Journal of Clinical Oncology,* Vol. 3, No. 2 (February 1985), pp. 140–43.

36. Harris, et al., op. cit., Part three.

37. Figures from the National Center for Health Statistics.

38. Write to the Boston Women's Health Book Collective for a packet of materials on breast implant and reconstruction issues. P.O. Box 192, West Somerville, MA 02144.

39. Charles E. Land, et al., "Early-Onset Breast Cancer in A-bomb Survivors." *The Lancet,* Vol. 342, No. 8865 (July 24, 1993), p. 237.

40. Joe Thornton, *Breast Cancer and the Environment: The Chlorine Connection.* Washington, DC: Greenpeace, 1992; Andrea Della Monica, "The Lethal Connection: Environmental Contaminants and Breast Cancer." *New Directions for Women,* July-August 1993, p. 6; Michael McCarthy, "DDT and Breast Cancer." *The Lancet,* Vol. 341 (May 29, 1993), p. 1407; Rita Arditti with Tatiana Schreiber, "Breast Cancer: The Environmental Connection." *Resist,* #246 (May/June 1992); Tatiana Schreiber, "Environmentalists and Breast Cancer Activists Tell New York Commission: ACT NOW!" *Resist,* Vol. 2, No. 4 (April 1993): available for $1 from *Resist,* One Summer St., Somerville, MA 02143. Tel. (617) 623-5110; Mary S. Wolff, et al., "Blood Levels of Organochlorine Residues and Risk of Breast Cancer." *Journal of the National Cancer Institute,* Vol. 85, No. 8 (Apr. 21, 1993), pp. 648–52; David J. Hunter and Karl T. Kelsey, "Pesticide Residues in Breast Cancer: The Harvest of a Silent Spring?" *Journal of the National Cancer Institute,* Vol. 85, No. 8 (Apr. 21, 1993), pp. 598–99; "The Politics of Cancer." *Utne Reader,* November/December 1993, pp. 81–92.

41. Ernest J. Sternglass and Jay M. Gould, "Breast Cancer: Evidence for a Relation to Fission Products in the Diet." *International Journal of Health Services,* Vol. 23, No. 4 (1993), pp. 783–804.

42. Rita Beamish, "EPA Urges Study of Health Risks Posed by Electromagnetic Fields." Associated Press article in *The Boston Globe,* Feb. 27, 1993; "EMF." *Sojourner,* March 1993, p. 13H.

43. Susan M. Love, "Breast Cancer: What the Department of Defense Should Do with Its $210 Million." *Journal of the American Medical Association,* Vol. 269, No. 18 (May 12, 1993), p. 2417.

44. Susan Ferraro, "You Can't Look Away Anymore." *The New York Times Magazine,* Aug. 15, 1993, pp. 24–27, 58, 61.

45. Available in English or Spanish by sending a self-addressed stamped envelope to WCCP, c/o The Women's Center, 46 Pleasant St., Cambridge, MA 02139. Ask for their other materials.

25

DIABETES

✦

BY DOROTHEA F. SIMS

1994 UPDATE BY DOROTHEA F. SIMS WITH SPECIAL THANKS TO DARCY BACALL

RESOURCES FOR THIS CHAPTER ON PAGES 497–98

Diabetes is a major health challenge today. Statistics show it to be a leading cause of death in our country because it is the underlying cause of much heart and kidney disease.[1] In recent years, however, we have learned measures to prevent some diabetes and to allow those who have it to live fairly healthy lives. These measures include the same practices that also keep all of us active and healthy during and after midlife.

Diabetes is of special concern to women over forty. Women are more likely to develop diabetes than men.[2] Black and Hispanic women are even more at risk.[3] The disease is not only dangerous in and of itself, but also because people with diabetes often develop complications that result in severe disability and even death.[4] Because it involves our eating habits, those of us with diabetes may suffer from guilt as well as anxiety in connection with the disease.

For a long time I felt really guilty about being diabetic because doctors told me that what I ate was causing some difficulty in my body and that if I would take care of myself I would be in better shape. I think a lot of diabetics stay in the closet about their diabetes because of the guilt. [a fifty-three-year-old woman]

Anything to do with food and eating touches issues of "ideal body weight," dieting and body image, and our own needs in relation to our role as nurturer in our homes and in society.

WHAT IS DIABETES?

In diabetes the pancreas does not produce enough insulin. The pancreas is the part of the communication system in the body that directs the use and storage of energy from foods. This system is an awesome network of biochemical signals that maintains the body's energy balance whether we are at rest or running, hot or cold, old or young, sick or well. Appreciating this balance (called homeostasis) helps us to collaborate with our bodies, even when we are not healthy, instead of viewing our bodies as enemies.

Insulin is a vital link in this communication system. A slow trickle of insulin is normally produced in the body at all times, with larger amounts secreted when eating. Insulin facilitates the movement of fuels from the food we eat into our cells so that these fuels can be used for energy, growth, and healing. The main such fuels are glucose from carbohydrates, amino acids from proteins, and fats from the fat in our diet. When insulin is lacking, glucose builds up in the bloodstream because it is unable to enter cells, and we are short of energy. Some proteins then combine with the abnormally high level of glucose in the blood, blood fats are increased, and blood-vessel walls are damaged. This sequence of events causes further injury throughout the body's tissues and nervous system.

Insulin performs another important task. When we eat more than we can use right away, it promotes the storage of those extra calories for future use. The extra calories are stored in the liver and muscles as glycogen, and in fat cells as fat. That trait helped prehistoric people survive times when food was not available. However, today in our country, where most of us are able to eat every day, this trait is no longer so useful.

Two Types of Diabetes

Diabetes really should be thought of as a plural noun. There are at least four classes. The two main types differ in cause, inheritability, and treatment. They are now called Type I, insulin-dependent, and Type II, noninsulin-dependent. Type I usually occurs in young people and used to be called "juvenile-onset." People who have Type I are usually thin, no matter what age they are when it develops. Type II usually appears after the age of forty and used to be called "adult-onset." Eighty to 90 percent of people with Type II diabetes are fat.[5] It is now known that each type can occur at any age. We now know that as many as 25 percent of older people once thought to be Type II actually have slowly developing Type I, and will ultimately require insulin.

More than 14 million people in the United States have diabetes. It is estimated that 7 million of them have it and don't know it yet.[6] Most of those who are undiagnosed have Type II diabetes. Unlike those with Type I, they still have some of their own insulin available and so may not have any dramatic symptoms. The warning signs for *both* types of diabetes include fatigue, thirst, frequent urination, slow healing of cuts and bruises, urinary tract and vaginal infection and itching, steady weight gain or recent weight loss, dental disease, and difficulty with eyesight. In Type II, these come on gradually and can easily be mistaken for "just getting older." Some people have undiagnosed Type II diabetes for many years.

In both types of diabetes, not enough insulin is secreted by the pancreas to regulate the blood sugar within the narrow range (60 to 140 milligrams per deciliter) needed for normal health. However, there the similarity between the two types stops. In Type I diabetes, the cells in the pancreas that produce insulin have been destroyed. The pancreas fails to produce any insulin and the body is quickly starved. The person becomes rapidly and acutely ill and diabetes is easily diagnosed. Recovery is also rapid when insulin is given. Type I has been the most publicized kind of diabetes, but only 10 percent of the people with diabetes in this country have Type I.

Though some people do develop Type I diabetes as they grow older, middle-aged and older women are at more risk for Type II diabetes. As our population ages, Type II diabetes is increasing most rapidly in people over sixty-five. The most important thing to keep in mind about Type II diabetes is that people who have it still produce generous amounts of their own insulin. However, their bodies have become resistant to insulin, and they are not able to make enough insulin to compensate for this resistance. Though why this happens is not yet completely understood, it is clear that becoming overweight and relatively inactive has a lot to do with insulin resistance.[7] Unfortunately, insulin resistance does not extend to the storage of fat. So a sedentary life-style and a diet generous in fatty foods increase the likelihood of weight gain, further insulin resistance, and eventual diabetes. When fat accumulates in the abdomen, it is most likely to result in diabetes and its associated health problems. So our activity level and food habits have a lot to do with the increase in Type II diabetes.

Type II diabetes is inherited much more often than Type I. Knowing your family history is useful. People who are overweight often feel guilty because they have long been indirectly and unfairly blamed for their condition. Now science tells us that some people have genetic traits that give them a tendency to store excess calories as fat. They may also have another genetic factor in the way insulin influences the energy balance inside the cells of their body.

We develop diabetes because it is hereditary and it isn't because we have been "bad." It took me a long time to understand that I was OK. Actually it was when I went into the hospital for an eye operation and was talking to a doctor there about the cause of my blindness. He said, "You really sound very guilty." I said that I do feel guilty about the way I have taken care of myself and particularly the way I have eaten. And he said, "If you really think that diabetes is caused just by the way you eat, then practically every American should be diabetic because look at the diet of the average American—it is full of sugar." And it wasn't until that time that it occurred to me that, of course, there was something more to it than that. I certainly had been off sugar for quite a while at that point. [a fifty-four-year-old woman who lost her vision at age fifty]

Those who have inherited the likelihood of getting diabetes if they get fat are at an unfair disadvantage in our overfed society, especially if they were brought up in families where heavy eating was encouraged. In addition, people often use food as a comforting substitute when they are scared, lonely, or angry, and this can make it hard to change eating habits. Understanding how these environmental and cultural elements interact with inherited tendencies can relieve feelings of guilt and helplessness about diabetes. We should not be blamed for genetic defects, but we don't have to remain at their mercy. We should offer the same respect and support to those struggling to change eating habits as we do to those who have to inject insulin every day.

Type II Is Not "Borderline" or a "Mild" Form of Diabetes

Because people with Type II don't usually need to take insulin, it has been called a "mild" form of diabetes. However, it is now known that this is not the case. Type II diabetes can cause such long-term complications as large-blood-vessel disease and loss of vision and kidney function, just as Type I can.[8]

When my doctor discovered I had diabetes, he said, "But it is only mild." So I assumed it was not necessary to be careful and ate sweets anyway. Then I remembered my brother had been totally blind and had recently died of kidney and liver failure. His urine never showed any sugar. The first symptom he had was when he awakened one morning blind. The eye doctor said he had had diabetes for fifteen years to have such severe hemorrhage in his eyes. I hope these types of accidents can be prevented more now with the new light on Type II diabetes. [a sixty-eight-year-old woman from a family of ten, five of whom have diabetes]

There is a brighter side to this picture. When people with Type II diabetes lose weight and increase their physical activity to maintain a steady weight, their own insulin often comes back into healthy play. If so, they may be able to avoid the expense, inconvenience, and possible reactions of taking insulin or pills.

I have had Type II diabetes for several years. When I was fifty-six years old, I was on 34 units of insulin, my blood sugar was 180 and I weighed 210 pounds. Then I cut down my calories but kept the healthy foods such as ½ cup servings of vegetables. In three weeks I had to stop taking insulin because of reactions. My doctor knew I was doing this and has records on it. I had lost 20 pounds. I did some bike riding. I had had a heart attack a year before, but now my heart seems okay. One year later, my weight is 148, my blood sugar 125, and I'm walking five to ten miles a day, am insulin-free and feeling wonderful! [a fifty-seven-year-old woman]

People with Type II diabetes who have a great deal of difficulty in keeping to a treatment plan of diet and exercise may need insulin injections or the pills for diabetes called oral agents, either separately or in combination. However, neither of these interventions works without the diet and exercise aspects too. Diet and exercise are necessary to restore the body cells' sensitivity to insulin. In addition, there are some disadvantages to taking insulin without implementing a diet and exercise program as well. Insulin makes you hungry, so it's harder to keep calories down. This may lead to a cycle of weight gain that, in turn, increases insulin resistance and calls for higher doses of insulin.

The sixty-eight-year-old woman who had five family members with diabetes now reports:

I recently lost 10 pounds. For exercise, I never use the elevator, sometimes walk up five flights. I work as a Foster Grandmother at a school for the retarded. I push wheelchairs there. For a while I was taking one of the pills for diabetes, but it made me confused and gave me a low blood sugar. After talking with my doctor, I stopped. I am doing quite well.

Oral agents can be used in Type II diabetes for people who still produce their own insulin. They help to increase the body's insulin and make it more effective. Some of the oral agents that have been on the market for many years may soon be superceded by new agents being developed and in use abroad. They do not promote weight gain and act directly to reduce insulin resistance. Some of the new agents also lower harmful blood fats and help to normalize blood pressure. Within a year or so, some of them, such as metformin, should be available in the United States. Oral agents must be prescribed and utilized appropriately for each individual and be very carefully monitored.

HEED EARLY WARNING SIGNS

If you have a strong family history of obesity, gave birth to a baby with a high birth weight, or developed temporary diabetes during pregnancy, you may be able to prevent Type II diabetes both for yourself and your children by following the life-style recommendations in this chapter. You will have a good influence on your family's diet and exercise habits and you may be able to prevent further diabetes in your family.

Gestational diabetes is the "temporary diabetes" that sometimes surfaces during pregnancy. Even if we don't plan to have more children, or are past menopause, we can alert our daughters, granddaughters, and other younger women to the dangers of developing sugar in their urine during pregnancy. Pregnant women should be screened for gestational diabetes at about twenty-four to twenty-eight weeks of their pregnancy.[9] Sixty-five percent of women who have gestational diabetes and who *also* are overweight during pregnancy eventually develop full-blown diabetes.[10] If they can be persuaded to change their habits while they are still young, to keep their weight down, and to increase their activity, they may improve their chances of avoiding diabetes.

I was one of those women who had gestational diabetes. My blood sugar went high during a pregnancy and then was fine again. I was told that I might be a "borderline diabetic." "Be careful but you don't have to worry about it." Because no one ever told me what might really happen to me if I developed diabetes, I had absolutely no inkling of what would happen. Even though I had seen at least two doctors, they never gave me much information. So for years my weight went up and down with my age, with emotional stuff, with whatever. I was not really very careful until eight to ten years ago. I would eat sugar and just was not very good about my diet. Basically it wasn't until I became a vegetarian that I began to be a little more clear about diet. [the fifty-four-year-old woman who lost her vision at fifty]

My granddaughter just had a nine-pound baby and she showed some sugar while she was pregnant. She goes on gaining weight. I worry about it because I don't know if her doctor takes it seriously. He says that lots of people have sugar when they carry a child, but that it goes away later. My father had diabetes and so have I. I'm going to ask my diabetes doctor to visit with her. [a sixty-eight-year-old woman who developed diabetes in her fifties]

COMPLICATIONS OF DIABETES

The worst aspect of diabetes is that people who have undiagnosed or poorly managed diabetes are more likely to develop complications than those who keep control of their blood glucose. The most common of these are heart disease, stroke, kidney failure, visual impairment, sexual problems, and amputation of legs and feet. All of these problems are caused by inadequate circulation of the blood in both the large and small blood vessels. For example, diabetes causes one half of the fifty thousand leg and foot amputations performed annually because the blood flow in the arteries has been damaged. It is estimated that 50 percent of these amputations are preventable.[11]

I didn't take care of myself when I was told I had diabetes at age eighty. My husband was sick and I had to pay more attention to him. I didn't go on a diet, I would drink too much orange juice and have no exercise at all. After my husband passed away my diabetes came right down on me. It was then that I went to the hospital and was told I had no circulation in my leg at all so that's why I had to have my leg taken off. [an eighty-four-year-old black woman]

Women with diabetes and hypertension should take special care to keep their blood pressure normal (see pages 334–36) as well as their blood glucose level. When blood glucose is normal, the quality of all aspects of life improves. If your blood glucose is high, so is your urine glucose. Sugary urine turns the vaginal area into a perfect environment for infections and breakdown of the tissues. The resulting discomfort is a major barrier to sexual satisfaction for women with diabetes. However, there is now evidence that working hard at keeping your blood glucose level as close to normal as possible may minimize, postpone, or prevent these complications.

Diabetes is the leading cause of new blindness in adults in the United States. Too many physicians supervising diabetes fail to refer their patients for an annual eye exam. Many fail to do even a rudimentary eye exam themselves. **Every person with diabetes should have her eyes examined annually through dilated pupils by an ophthalmologist.**

CHANGES AT MENOPAUSE

Usually, as your levels of estrogen and progesterone decrease leading up to and after menopause, your insulin requirements will go down. Weight gain and lack of exercise, which are not healthful and which raise insulin requirements, could cancel out the decreasing insulin need. You can make these adjustments smoothly only by careful monitoring. There has not been enough research yet on the interaction of the various types of estrogens and progestins with diabetes. Therefore, the decision of a postmenopausal woman with diabetes about taking estrogen or hormone therapy requires consideration not only of all the factors discussed elsewhere in this book, but also careful discussion with her health-management team. Do not make the decision based solely on the recommendation of a gynecologist.*

SELF-CARE

Diabetes is the supreme example of the value of self-care, both in terms of prevention and health maintenance. The first principle in self-care is to stay in touch with trusted health professionals who are up-to-date on advances in all aspects of prevention and treatment, including oral agents, insulin-delivery and blood-glucose-testing instruments, and diet and exercise recommendations.

There is special value in the ability to test your own blood at any time of day or night to find out how well your treatment plan is working. It is more reliable than urine tests, in which high blood sugar may not show up because of changes in kidney function. A drop of blood is obtained with an automatic spring-loaded finger lancet† and the blood-glucose level is read from a test strip. The finger prick is practically painless if good equipment and the sides of the fingertips (rather than the central pads) are used. This self-blood-glucose-monitoring (SBGM) allows you to read your body signals with regard to food and exercise. It rewards you with immediate feedback. Self-blood-testing takes the mystery out of the daily chores of living with diabetes and puts the power of management of diabetes squarely in your hands. You can share your record with your supervising health professionals, who will help you stay up to date on new advances and make suggestions that fit your particular needs.

What are other daily tasks of self-care for the person with diabetes? They differ according to the type of diabetes. People with Type I have to take insulin injections two to four times a day, and they have to learn to match their food intake with their energy output and the dosage of insulin. There are many alternatives to choose from in accomplishing this difficult routine, including the use of insulin pumps, which are worn outside the body and can be programmed to give insulin automatically. The greatest daily hazard faced by people taking insulin is an unpredictable lowering of blood sugar (hypoglycemia) called "insulin reaction," which requires immediate ingestion of sugar. The symptoms of hypoglycemia may include hunger, cold sweats, clammy feeling, dizziness, shakiness, weakness, irritability, pallor, headache, personality change, slurred speech, and if untreated, seizures and unconsciousness. **People who have diabetes should carry medical identification at all times.**

Many people with Type II diabetes don't need to take oral agents or insulin unless their supply of insulin is so reduced that there isn't enough to overcome insulin resistance. However, those with Type II may need to take insulin temporarily during times of physical or emotional stress, such as before, during, or after surgery, or during a personal crisis. They are faced with the demanding task of losing weight and becoming physically active, sometimes after having been sedentary for years, and the lifelong task of remaining active and keeping their weight down.

Conquering these challenges is well worth the effort. People with either type of diabetes who succeed in effective self-care feel well most of the time and lead productive lives of normal length.

Support Groups

A support group of people with diabetes can be very comforting in keeping up courage, and a practical help too. The American Diabetes Association and many hospitals offer such groups.

See pages 18–21 for how to start a support group if one does not exist in your area.

*An excellent source is *A Friend Indeed,* Vol. X, No. 2 (May 1993). See Resources, page 466. See also Lorna Wissner Greene and Etah S. Kurland, "Managing Menopause Without Estrogen." *Diabetes Self-Management,* Vol. 11, No. 1 (January/February 1994), pp. 38–42; and Lois Jovanovic-Peterson, "Changing with the Change." *Diabetes Forecast,* February 1993, pp. 45–48.

†Precautions against sharing needles with other people also apply to these lancets.

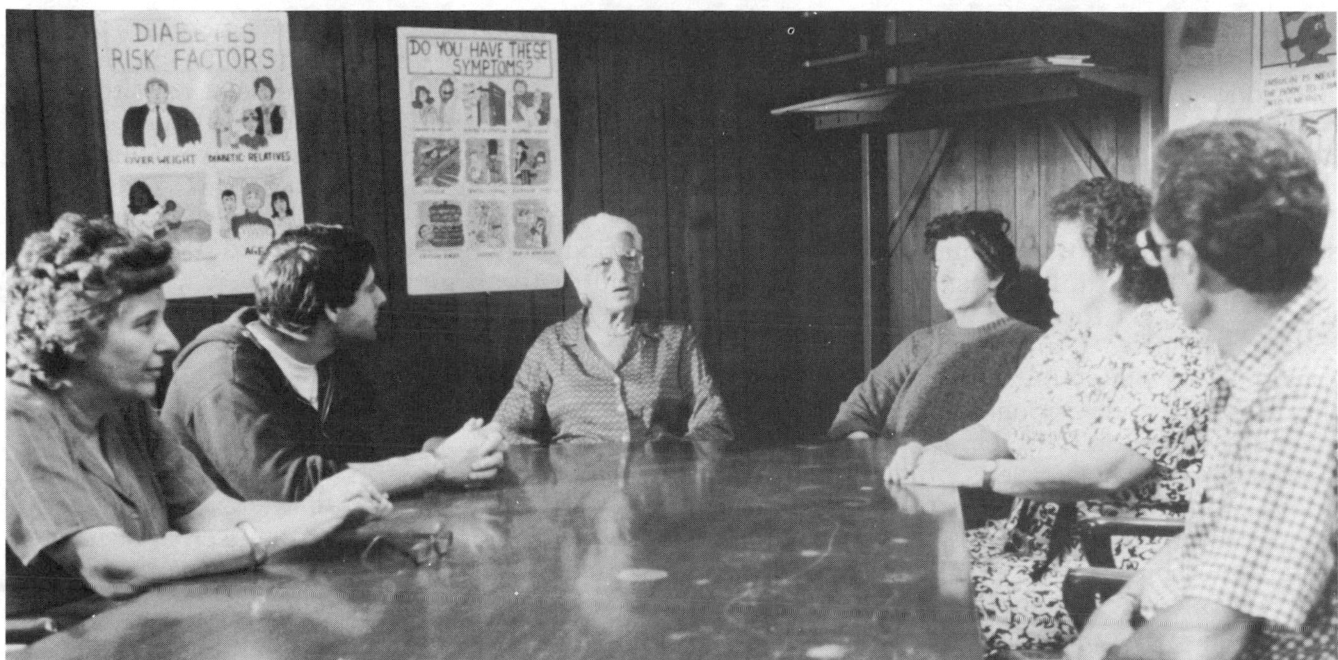

David Whittier/Greater Boston Diabetes Society

You don't always have to have a professional person there. We learn more from each other than any other way—like don't drink a diet soda between meals because the sweet taste starts up the hunger reflexes even if there aren't any calories in it. Salty snacks will do the same thing. Chew a carrot instead! We help each other to shop sensibly, too. We read the labels and consider the costs. Many of the so-called dietetic foods cost more than ordinary brands and are no more healthy. But in general, the supermarkets are offering better food today than even a few years ago. [a woman in her forties with diabetes]

Exercise

Exercise plays an important role in the self-care of people with diabetes. We are all familiar with the many reasons for remaining as active as possible throughout life (see Moving for Health chapter). In addition, persons with diabetes are at high risk for osteoporosis and must exercise in order to utilize the calcium in food to strengthen bones (see Osteoporosis and Fracture Prevention chapter). For those of us with diabetes, exercise brings the added benefit of increased sensitivity of the body's cells to the actions of insulin.[12]

The management of exercise as a vital part of self-care differs for the two types of diabetes. For Type I diabetes, this means that in order to avoid having too much insulin when exercising, each individual has to learn how much to reduce insulin dosage and increase food intake in order to exercise safely. For Type II diabetes, exercise not only burns unwanted calories but also helps to overcome the inherited resistance to insulin. In fact, there are many people with Type II diabetes who have normalized their blood sugar by exercise, even though they do not lose all the weight they had gained over the years.

If I forget my exercise for two weeks, I am depressed and tired. When I exercise, I feel fine because my blood glucose is within normal range. So it's worth it to keep at it, though I've had to accept the fact that my body will never be really slim again. [a fifty-two-year-old woman]

In addition, those who make the switch to a more active life find it has lasting psychological benefits, although the routine may not have been easy to establish.

For me, running has made a tremendous difference in this regard. This is not to say that I don't have to watch my diet. It does mean that I don't have to count every calorie. I no longer gain three pounds after one decent meal. My weight is at a fairly reasonable level and isn't constantly fluctuating five to ten pounds as under the starve/stuff routine. You soon disprove the old exercise-produces-increased-appetite myth. Right after and during exercise, food is the last thing on my mind, since the blood has been diverted away from the digestive system to the muscles. One of the primary fringe benefits is the psychological one. I can start out feeling anxious, depressed, fatigued and/or angry, and as I push myself it all dissipates. [a woman in her forties]

Diet

Everyone says that diet restrictions are the most irritating part of living with diabetes. Today, however, nutritionists are taking a new and more flexible approach to food for people with diabetes. Most nutritionists now recognize that social, cultural, and emotional habits of eating have to be taken into consideration, and that when people eat food, they are not necessarily thinking about nutrients. Diabetes organizations now make available meal plans that reflect ethnic, religious, and regional food preferences. You can adjust your diet to include your preferences as well as your caloric needs, but you will need to know about the components of foods to do so. The recommended balance among carbohydrate, fat, and protein is as follows: 55 to 60 percent of your calories should come from carbohydrate, 30 percent from fat, and 12 to 20 percent of your calories should come from protein. Restriction of fat in the diet is essential for people who are overweight and valuable for reducing risks of heart and other diseases in all people.[13] Your diet will vary depending on your age and general level of activity as well as general health and type of diabetes. For this reason, the services of a nutritionist can be of great value. Yearly follow-up visits are helpful to make sure your diet remains in tune with your body's needs as you age.

Most people who monitor their blood carefully and are willing and able to exercise regularly can eat at least a little of almost everything, but some people with diabetes must restrict their food choices and may feel severely deprived.

I was greatly surprised to find that I had Type II diabetes six years ago. I'm supersensitive to food and if I break my diet in the smallest way, it makes a difference in weight gain and blood sugar. I do get sick of it. It seems that everything that makes food attractive is what I can't have. After trimming the pork chop, cutting it up in pieces and weighing it, who wants to eat it, all by itself in the middle of the plate? Sometimes I feel that people who have Type I diabetes are lucky. They really need to eat to stay even with their insulin. [a fifty-two-year-old woman]

No Smoking

As well as adopting new diet and exercise habits, there is another vital self-care decision to be made. That is the decision not to smoke. Smoking does a great deal of damage to the body's circulatory system. Nicotine acts to constrict the smaller blood vessels and thus increases the risk of hypertension. Combining that hazard with the risk of damage to blood vessels from the high blood glucose and blood fats of diabetes is virtually inviting heart attacks, strokes, and other serious complications. It is difficult to quit smoking, especially because there is sometimes a period of increased appetite and possible weight gain in the beginning. However, it is a crucial investment in a longer and healthier life for everyone, but especially for those of us whose risks include diabetes.

USE THE HEALTH-CARE SYSTEM TO YOUR BEST ADVANTAGE

People who have diabetes themselves or in their families need to make the best use of the entire health-care system. Find a doctor who is up to date on diabetes and interested in working with you as an individual in coordinating your health care. Nurse practitioners are skilled at helping with management of diabetes. Since diabetes can affect all the body systems, you may also need the support and advice of specialists such as a dentist, a nutritionist, a podiatrist for foot care, and an eye doctor. A certified diabetes educator (C.D.E.) can teach the various aspects of diabetes care and assist you in integrating this new knowledge into your life-style. (See Resources for this chapter for locating C.D.E.s in your area.) Fortunately, health-insurance providers and health maintenance organizations are beginning to pay for these services to prevent costly complications requiring hospitalization and lost work days. Coverage varies from state to state and from plan to plan, so ask.

Since diabetes can complicate and slow down recovery from other illnesses, those of us with diabetes have to insist that our caregivers collaborate on their treatment suggestions. Inform any other doctor you use that you have diabetes and make sure that she or he is in touch with the doctor who manages your diabetes.

DIABETES AND STRESS MANAGEMENT

The way our bodies respond to stress goes back to prehistoric times when the threats were to life and limb, calling for quick energy for flight or fight. Chemical signals mobilize fuels stored in the liver and muscle and raise the heartbeat and breathing rates for rapid circulation of energy. This outpouring of glucose was fine when we had to run from a lion, but it is not useful or healthy for a person who is caught in a traffic jam or mad at her boss. Moreover, we don't need *extra* stresses like caffeine. The rise in blood sugar, with no way to compensate for it through physical action, is not good for those of us who have diabetes. We need to learn from other people who are coping successfully how to avoid stress and to minimize it when it develops.

Diabetes causes stress both for those of us who have it and for our families and friends. Maintaining the balance of food, activity, and insulin takes time and money and requires planning that limits freedom of choice and spontaneity. Diabetes is yet another challenge to test our native adaptability and lifelong experience. Others may not understand why we have to eat right on time or why we have to avoid certain foods. We need to let them know what we need and why. We must respect our personal needs and learn to meet them even when they differ from the needs of those who share our lives.

NOTES

1. National Diabetes Data Group, *Diabetes in America 1985.* NIH Publication 85-1468, National Institutes of Health, Rockville Pike, Bethesda, MD 20014.
2. American Diabetes Association (ADA), *Diabetes Facts,* 1992.
3. National Diabetes Data Group, op. cit., Chapter 8, p. 1, and Chapter 9, p. 1; and American Diabetes Association, op. cit.
4. National Diabetes Data Group, op. cit., Chapter 1, pp. 1–4; and ADA, op. cit.
5. ADA, op. cit.
6. National Diabetes Data Group, op. cit., Chapter 1, p. 1.
7. R. A. DeFronzo and E. Ferrannini, "Insulin Resistance: A Multifaceted Syndrome Responsible for NIDDM, Obesity, Hypertension, Dyslipidemia and Atherosclerotic Cardiovascular Disease." *Diabetes Care,* Vol. 14 (1991), p. 173.
8. National Diabetes Data Group, op. cit., Chapter 1, pp. 1–4; and ADA, op. cit.
9. R. S. Abrams and D. R. Coustan, "Gestational Diabetes Update." *Clinical Diabetes,* Vol. 8, No. 2 (March/April 1990), pp. 19–24.
10. J. B. O'Sullivan, "Gestational Diabetes: Factors Influencing the Rates of Subsequent Diabetes." In Sutherland and Stowers, eds., *Carbohydrate Metabolism in Pregnancy and the Newborn.* New York: Springer-Verlag, 1979, pp. 425–535.
11. ADA, op. cit.; Department of Health and Human Services, Centers for Disease Control, *The Prevention and Treatment of Complications of Diabetes: A Guide for Primary Care Practitioners.* Atlanta, GA, 1991, p. 27.
12. H. Kan, et al., "Exercise and Diabetes Mellitus," in E. S. Horton and R. L. Terjune, eds., *Exercise, Nutrition, and Energy Metabolism.* New York: Macmillan, 1988; JoAnn E. Manson et al., "Physical Activity and Incidence of Non-insulin-dependent Diabetes in Women." *Lancet,* Vol. 338, No. 8770 (Sept. 28, 1991), pp. 774–78; and S. Ackerman, "Exercise as Prevention." *Diabetes Forecast,* March 1992, pp. 35, 36.
13. ADA, *Physician's Guide to Diabetes,* 1988; and Dorothea Sims, "Food Is Central to Life," in *Diabetes: Reach for Health and Freedom,* St. Louis: C. V. Mosby Co., and American Diabetes Association, 1984, pp. 20–25.

26

GALLSTONES AND GALLBLADDER DISEASE

✦

BY GLORIANNE WITTES

1994 UPDATE BY CLARA A. LENNOX

RESOURCES FOR THIS CHAPTER ON PAGE 498

Gallstones are a common problem faced by many women in midlife. Gallbladder disease is at least twice as common in women as in men.[1] It is even more common in certain ethnic groups, notably Native Americans and Scandinavians; and groups with a high incidence of diseases with fragile red cells such as sickle-cell disease (blacks), thalassemias (Mediterraneans), and liver parasites (Southeast Asians).[2] Gallstones can be detected in almost 90 percent of Native Americans and others with Native American heritage (mostly women), such as Mexicans, and at a much earlier age than in whites. In one study, 35 percent of Mexican-American women had symptoms of gallstones by age sixty-five.[3] Such high rates in certain groups warrant special study and care.

Gallstones used to be disparagingly labeled by some physicians as an affliction of women who were "fat, forty, and flatulent." Some added "fertile" to the list. This label disclosed a bias against aging women in general and fat women in particular. Now that we understand better the causes and course of gallbladder disease, its occurrence in certain groups, including young women, and its relationship to estrogen, we can seek care from practitioners who are knowledgeable and not biased. Though the NIH Consensus Statement does recommend seeking safe, noninvasive cost-effective solutions, some of the money that is spent on developing equipment could be better spent on research into causes and prevention.[4]

THE GALLBLADDER, GALLSTONES, AND GALLBLADDER DISEASE

The gallbladder is a small sac located on the right side of the abdomen under the liver. It serves as a reservoir for bile, a bitter fluid that is produced in the liver. Following a meal, the gallbladder contracts to release bile into the duodenum (the beginning of the small intestine), where it assists in the digestion of food.

Bile is made up of cholesterol, lecithin, bile salts, and bilirubin (yellowish pigment). When this balance is disturbed and there is too much cholesterol or bilirubin in the bile, the excess separates out in the form of thickened material called sludge that can crystallize into stones. Seventy-five percent of stones in Americans and Europeans are cholesterol stones; the rest are pigment stones, made mostly of bilirubin.[5]

Eighty percent of people with gallbladder

DIGESTIVE ORGANS

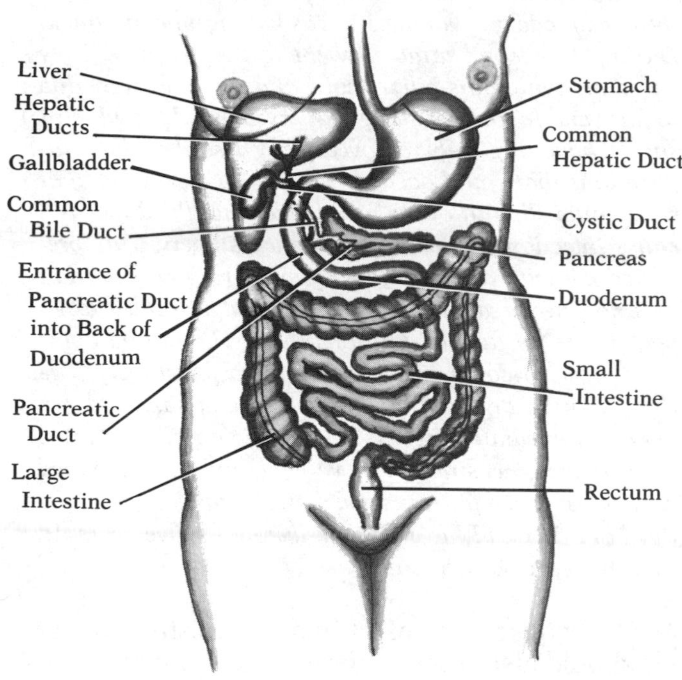

sludge or stones will not have symptoms for many years, and may never develop symptoms.[6] Many symptoms commonly attributed to gallbladder disease, such as indigestion, belching, bloating, intolerance of fatty foods, or pain after meals, are also frequently caused by other problems. They may be caused by irritable bowel syndrome, peptic ulcer disease, sensitivity or allergy to certain foods, and gastroesophageal reflux (acidic stomach contents back up into and burn the esophagus). The now-accepted definition of symptomatic biliary disease is *episodic, severe, steady pain in the right or mid-upper abdomen lasting one to five hours, often awakening the person at night.* In people found to have gallstones, these episodes will develop in about 10 percent within five years and in 20 percent within twenty years.[7] Some people will have typical pain episodes but will be found to have only sludge.

Serious complications of gallbladder disease occur within twenty years in up to 25 percent of people with such episodes. These complications include stones in the common bile duct; inflammation of the gallbladder, bile ducts, and pancreas (cholecystitis, cholangitis, and pancreatitis); and, though it is rare, gallbladder cancer. *Symptoms may include sudden, severe nausea, vomiting, jaundice, fever, chills, and pain in the right or mid-upper abdomen that may go through to the back or the right shoulder blade. This is an emergency* and must be treated immediately to prevent organ damage, infection, and even death. However, please note that it is unusual for a person with gallstones to develop severe complications until she has had typical symptomatic episodes for some time.

RISK FACTORS

Anything that increases the proportion of cholesterol or bilirubin in bile can increase the likelihood that sludge will form and tiny crystals will start to occur that can grow to form stones. Cholesterol and bilirubin levels in bile can be affected by greater output from the liver, by delays in emptying the gallbladder, or by decreasing bile salts, which keep cholesterol dissolved.

Estrogen is a major risk factor causing increased cholesterol output into bile by the liver, decreased bile acid production, and slowed passage of stools through the intestines (constipation), allowing more reabsorption of cholesterol.[8] Estrogen also decreases the vigorous action (stasis) of the gallbladder.[9] Conditions in which estrogen levels are increased include being female, pregnancy, use of some birth-control pills, and estrogen prescribed for postmenopausal women. The risk increases as the dose and duration of use increase, and does not decrease when estrogen levels return to normal since stones formed will remain.[10]

Biliary cholesterol output also increases with age and in Scandinavians and Native Americans. It does not correlate with total blood cholesterol levels but does correlate with decreased levels of HDL (the "good") cholesterol and with high levels of triglycerides.[11] It is also caused by excess alcohol intake, which blocks fat metabolism in the liver.

As mentioned, formation of sludge can result from delayed emptying of the gallbladder, which occurs by skipping meals, prolonged fasting, starvation, and rapid weight loss. It is also common in pregnancy. Any constipation slows down the passage of stools through the bowels and causes cholesterol reabsorption.

Decreased bile acid secretion occurs in Crohn's disease and in Native Americans.[12]

The likelihood of the need for gallbladder surgery is much higher in markedly fat women whose body mass index is in the highest fifth of the population.[13]

Red blood cell fragility leads to increased bilirubin levels and the formation of pigment stones in persons with sickle-cell disease, thalassemias, and other such conditions.[14]

Prevention

If you fall into a high-risk group, you might want to prevent gallstones before they develop. The mainstream medical establishment has paid very little attention to this issue so far.[15] Given what we now know about gallstone formation, consideration should be given to the following plan:

- *Low-fat diet*—to maintain a comfortable weight and keep the triglyceride levels low. Triglyceride levels are related to the amount of fat in our diets. (See Chapter 23 for the relationship between triglycerides and heart disease in women.)
- *Low alcohol consumption*—to avoid interfering with our ability to burn fat.
- *High-fiber diet*—to keep stools moving briskly and to decrease biliary cholesterol reabsorption.
- *Eating foods high in sulfur*—to stimulate the flow of bile. These are foods such as cabbage, asparagus, brussels sprouts, celery, cauliflower, onions, and radishes.

Some experts recommend adding supplements of lecithin, taurine and methionine (amino acids), copper, vitamin B_{12}, folic acid, vitamin C, and magnesium to a low-fat diet to increase the solubility of bile.

Herbalists use organic herbs, including dandelion root, burdock root, wild yam, and Oregon grape root to prevent and treat gallbladder disease.[16]

Eating frequent, small meals keeps the gallbladder emptying and prevents sludge formation. Eating breakfast is especially important since the gallbladder has stored up bile overnight.

Regular daily exercise should help by increasing HDL cholesterol, speeding up bowel action, helping to maintain optimal weight, and improving metabolism in general.

Markedly fat people (those with body mass in the highest fifth of the population) who are considering weight loss should choose a plan that results in very slow long-term weight loss and should especially avoid drastic weight changes and "yo-yoing." Regular exercise is important.

I had two attacks while away on holiday. The symptoms were excruciating. Pain in the upper abdomen and across the back made me wonder if I was having a heart attack. During the second attack I went to the hospital. They called my symptoms biliary colic and said they were due to fine sand [a form of stones] in my gallbladder, which I should have surgically removed. They described the complications that could occur if I didn't do so, that is, that sand could slip out of my gallbladder into the ducts and cause infection, requiring emergency surgery. This presented me with a terrible dilemma. Since my condition was not life-threatening at the moment I decided to go back home for further opinions there. The second opinion I received concurred with the need for surgery. The third opinion argued that the presence of sand did not require immediate surgery. This physician did not want to operate on me, since I was very fat, and recommended weight loss and a fat-restricted diet. I went along with the third opinion and have been well now for five years. [a fifty-five-year-old woman]

The consequences of increased estrogen levels should also be considered when planning the number of pregnancies you want and in considering the dosage and duration of use of any estrogen. States of increased estrogen, if chosen, should be balanced by as many preventive measures as possible.

Detection and Diagnosis

Many people who have not reported symptoms of gallbladder disease are often discovered to have gallstones when they undergo tests for other, unrelated reasons. Currently the most widespread diagnostic test is an abdominal ultrasound. A machine emitting sound waves is moved over the abdomen, and the rebounded echoes are recorded on a machine that shows an outline of the gallbladder and any sludge or gallstones bigger than 1 to 2 millimeters. If the ultrasound is normal but symptoms suggest gallbladder disease, oral cholecystography can show stones, polyps, or sludge, or may not show the gallbaldder at all if it is inflamed or if the cystic duct is obstructed. This test requires the person to take tablets containing a dye with iodine the day before the test. The material must be absorbed, processed by the liver, secreted into the bile, and then concentrated by the gallbladder. Sometimes it is deemed abnormal when the gallbladder is normal (called a false positive). This type of testing does require the use of X rays.

Nuclear scans are used to diagnose acute gallbladder infection (cholecystitis). Short-lived radioisotopes are used. This test can detect total obstruction of the gallbladder neck due to inflammation, but provides no data about gallstones.

Blood tests can show evidence of gallstones in the ducts (elevated amylase level) or acute cholecystitis (elevated bilirubin or liver enzymes).

Treatment Methods

The accepted standard of care once gallstones were discovered used to be prompt surgical removal of the gallbladder (cholecystectomy). Physicians were taught that they should give this advice to avoid being sued for malpractice.[17] The result was that removal of the gallbladder and the uterus (hysterectomy) were the most frequently performed unnecessary operations. Three quarters of the gallbladder removals were done to women.

Racial, ethnic, gender, age, and class biases affect treatment recommendations for gallbladder disease, as they do for other conditions. Some physicians assume that every complaint by a middle-aged woman is related to menopause and ignore gallbladder disease until surgery is necessary. The poor, less-educated, non-English-speaking, and people of color—most of whom are middle-aged women—treated at major teaching hospitals provide learning experiences for surgeons-in-training. In addition, removing gallbladders is a major source of income for surgeons. Physicians are still mostly male and involved in "old boy" networks with surgeons.

Surgery is usually not needed until a person has had several symptomatic episodes. Rare exceptions may include people with gallstones larger than 3 centimeters, gallbladder polyps larger than 1 centimeter, "porcelain" (calcified) gallbladder, and possibly Native Americans, due to their unique risk of gallbladder cancer.[18] If gallstones are found in children, people with sickle-cell disease, or people who will be isolated from medical care for a long time, removal of the gallbladder may also be recommended.[19] It is worth restating, however, that surgery is now not recommended in most cases until people develop symptomatic episodes.

The first phase of treatment, therefore, involves the management of gallstones in people who have never had symptoms. The ideal would be to dissolve the stones and prevent them from developing again. If this can't be done, then at least you will want to prevent symptoms or complications. All the measures listed under Prevention should be started with appropriate help.

Two and a half years ago, an X ray for a slipped disk showed a number of stones the size of chickpeas. An ultrasound confirmed the stones and a lot of sludge, and I was strongly advised to have surgery right away. In retrospect, I had been having symptoms of fatty food intolerance for a long time. I did not want to have major surgery, since I would be moving across the country to start a new job in a month. When I moved I found a family-practice doctor and told her that I knew I might face an emergency situation if a stone lodged in the duct and became infected. She encouraged me to wait until the balance of problems outweighed my not wanting to have surgery and encouraged diet changes. So I waited. At the end of the second year, I became sick with a fever and weakness and pain. That was the signal that the time had come. I had the surgery six weeks ago. I believe the surgery was then necessary and I am also glad I waited. [a forty-year-old woman]

There are no cheap, effective, safe, proven methods of dissolving gallstones.[20] There are drugs that dissolve some cholesterol gallstones and there are procedures that shatter gallstones (lithotripsy). With both methods, recurrent stones are a problem and long-term consequences are unknown.

The drug ursodiol causes decreased cholesterol manufacture and secretion into bile by the liver, less reabsorption of cholesterol in the bowel, and less crystal formation in bile. It works best in people with small gallstones that are floating in a functioning gallbladder. The cystic duct must be open. Treatment is expensive, takes six to twelve months, and can have a 60 to 90 percent dissolution rate (better for smaller stones). Gallstones may recur in up to 50 percent of people within five years, but symptoms will develop in only one in four people. This treatment option causes no increased risk of death, other major effects, or injury. Symptoms of gallbladder disease often decrease before the stones dissolve. If faster results are needed, a combination of two drugs, ursodiol and chenodiol, can be used, without the usual other effects of chenodiol. The major drawback to this medication is its cost. Long-term effects are not known.

Extracorporeal shock-wave lithotripsy involves the use of very strong vibrations (sound waves) to shatter stones. The tiny pieces can then flow out in the bile, through the ducts and into the intestines, and be eliminated. It requires a functioning gallbladder and open ducts. People must also take ursodiol to dissolve fragments. Forty-five percent of people treated will have typical gallbladder episode pain (some very briefly) as larger pieces pass through the ducts.

This technique works better with small numbers of small stones, which were cleared in up to 95 percent of people with just one noncalcified stone smaller than 20 millimeters, and up to 60 percent of people with three or fewer stones from 20 to 30 millimeters. It can be successful in people with pigment (bilirubin) stones. Complications are less frequent than when the technique was first developed. Stones recur in about 11 percent of people who have had this treatment.

Alternative Holistic Treatments

Some people who have gallstones find that treatments such as acupuncture and imagery have helped them (though not in emergency situations, when a stone is lodged in a duct).

An acupuncturist stimulates specific points on the body by inserting needles, applying heat, pressure massage (acupressure), or a combination of these methods.

During my acute gallbladder attacks my friend massaged my back to give me some relief from the agony I was experiencing. As she touched a certain point in my back I asked her to dig in deeply to reach the pain inside. She did so and the pain suddenly disappeared, totally and completely, in these few seconds of deep pressure. I embarked on a series of acupuncture sessions. This felt similar to the experience when pressure relieved my pain. The acupuncturist I chose said that acupuncture was unlikely to dissolve the stones, but could possibly rectify the bile imbalance and other physical dynamics that were forming them. I haven't been troubled by any gallbladder attacks since that series and I attribute it, in part, to this treatment, along with careful diet and imagery work. [a fifty-five-year-old woman]

Imagery is a technique that encourages one's mind and body to mobilize resources to restore and optimize well-being. Each person develops her own preferred image. There are many possibilities. One woman visualized her body as a strong heroine overpowering the disease. The same woman explains:

I was familiar with the use of imagery to fight cancer, and use imagery regularly myself to relax or envision how a design project will look when completed. It comes easily to me and I believe in it. So I imagined my bile salts armed with spikes shattering the stones that were plaguing me and excreting them effortlessly out of my body. I did this imagery work daily during the six weeks I was undergoing acupuncture. It made me feel less anxious about my condition because I felt I was doing something that could potentially cure me.

One holistic practitioner suggests that gallbladder pain can be due to spasms caused by food allergies, especially to eggs, and that this should be considered, especially if no gallstones are found.[21] Some holistic nutritionists suggest that the gallbladder can be stimulated to flush and clean out sludge, although this is not effective with large stones. Others say they will not supervise such a program because of the danger that a piece of stone will get lodged in a duct and require emergency surgery. Medical journal articles focus on surgery. Other methods, such as herbs, acupuncture, and imagery, are ridiculed and dismissed although they have not been adequately researched. Trials of such methods could reveal the effectiveness of these treatments, which some consider safe and effective. Most research is conducted by drug companies that will not spend the money required to meet FDA criteria unless they think they will make a big profit. Perhaps we could pass a law, as in Germany and England, permitting the time-honored use of herbs.[22]

Surgery

If a stone gets squeezed out of the gallbladder and through the cystic duct, and then gets stuck in the common bile duct, severe symptoms occur, due both to spasm and to backup of bile into the liver and sometimes into the pancreas. This is an emergency situation. The only safe course is removal of the stone by a procedure called Endoscopic Retrograde Cholangio-Pancreatography (ERCP). General anesthesia is required. A specialist passes an endoscope through the nose, down the throat, through the stomach, and into the small intestine (duodenum). The opening of the common bile duct is found and entered. The stone seen through the scope is removed either by enlarging the opening so the stone comes through into the intestine, or by grasping the stone with a tiny basket and pulling it through. In expert hands, this is successful 90 to 95 percent of the time. Stones in the common bile duct are found in 8 to 15 percent of people under age sixty and 15 to 60 percent of people over age sixty who have gallbladder surgery.

In 1991, 600,000 people in the United States had surgical removal of the gallbladder (cholecystectomy). "Open" cholecystectomy was the preferred operation until 1991. An incision is made below the right rib cage; the gallbladder is removed, and the abdomen is explored for other problems. Your surgeon should not remove your appendix unless you give your consent in advance. People stay in the hospital about five days, often have severe pain, and require three to six weeks to recover. A hernia may develop at the site of the incision. Complications depend on age, previous general health, surgeon's skill, and difficulty of the situation (with or without jaundice, infection, or stones in the common bile duct). Patients must be able to have general anesthesia and must not have serious heart or lung problems.

For years I was uncomfortable after eating the least amount of fat and had to watch myself like a hawk. Gallstones were never diagnosed. Finally, after a severe attack of biliary colic, my doctor suggested gallbladder surgery, though no stones visualized at all in my tests. The surgery revealed that sludge [fine sand] had lodged in the common duct and that the pancreas duct and gallbladder were also infected. I was furious that the diagnosis of gallbladder disease hadn't been made earlier, for if surgery had been done earlier I might have been spared all this infection and post-operative discomfort. [a fifty-six-year-old woman]

I could not face the possibility of ever again having an attack like this one. I dreaded the presence of little demons inside me threatening to strike again at the least expected moment. So I insisted on surgery, and do you know, I sailed through it with no complications, despite my age? They found thirty-two small stones in my gallbladder! Now I guess it took me longer to recuperate than a younger person with this same surgery, but that's to be expected at my age and with my medical problems. [an eighty-two-year-old woman]

Laparoscopic cholecystectomy was first done in France in 1987 and in the United States in 1988. Over the last three years it has increased dramatically in popularity, and is now used in about 80 percent of all cholecystectomies. People like it because, if all goes well, they get out of the hospital in one to two days, have only mild pain, and are disabled for only one to two weeks. Although hospitalization costs are reduced, total costs have risen because the number of procedures performed has increased alarmingly. Physicians are recommending it even for people whose symptoms are not considered serious enough for surgery.[23]

Under general anesthesia, small incisions (about ½ inch long) are made in the abdomen through which carbon dioxide gas is pumped and the scope and instruments are inserted. The organs are handled and viewed remotely on a TV screen via the scope. The gallbladder can be removed through one of the small incisions. It can be used in 90 to 95 percent of people with symptomatic episodes.

This procedure is more difficult than open cholecystectomy. Problems can occur due to unique anatomy, old scarring, or other difficulties, such as heavy bleeding, requiring prompt conversion to open cholecystectomy. This happens in about 5 percent of surgeries and should be considered a complication of laparoscopic cholecystectomy itself.

Complications include accidental damage to organs, blood vessels, and the common bile duct. Death, injury, and complications for this laparoscopic surgery are very low, as they are for open cholecystectomy, but include slightly more cases of damage to the common bile duct, liver, and pancreas.

A major concern is that injuries are much harder to spot than in open surgery, and are not being detected until later, when the person continues to have fever, pain, nausea, jaundice, bloating, or other problems. Major medical centers that have very low rates of bile duct injuries are already reporting an increased number of patients referred from other hospitals for treatment of such injuries. *Complications will continue to be discovered, since scarring from bile duct damage can take months to years to show up after surgery.* There are no long-term data about delayed adverse outcomes from laparoscopic cholecystectomy, and very little about standard open cholecystectomy. Current data on injuries discovered so far show that the outcome of laparoscopic cholecystectomy is greatly influenced by the training, experience, skill, and judgment of the surgeon.

Surgeons inexperienced in laparoscopic procedures tend to cause more injuries than experienced surgeons. Training in this difficult procedure has not been standardized, and may consist of only one or two days, sponsored by surgical equipment companies. Many hospitals have no requirements that must be met before surgeons are allowed to do new procedures. Always ask for the surgeon's complication rates, training, and experience to compare surgeons when deciding whom you want to perform the surgery.

I tried the drugs to dissolve the stones for one and a half years but then had a bad attack with severe pain at 1 a.m. I decided to have the laparoscopic procedure, so I checked out the surgeons. The one I chose had done it more than 275 times so I felt confident about his experience. I went home from the medical center the day after the surgery and was back to normal within two weeks. [a sixty-six-year-old woman]

There are common problems after either kind of surgery. People who continue to have various symptoms after surgery are said to have postcholecystectomy syndrome. Some of them had symptoms before surgery that were not typical gallbladder episodes but were attributed to their gallstones after tests for other likely causes were negative. After surgery, the same symptoms continue and may be due to irritable bowel syndrome. Some symptoms may be due to food allergies.

After its removal, the bile is no longer being stored in the gallbladder and released only after eating. Instead, it flows out of the liver constantly as it is produced and enters the small intestine. Some people develop bile reflux esophagitis as the bile backs up into the stomach and even into the esophagus and mouth causing heartburn and damage. Some people develop diarrhea, which may be episodic or constant. Sometimes the constant flow of bile salts irritates the intestines, causing pain. Those who may not have enough concentration of bile to digest their food may benefit from bile supplements.

As usual, our medical establishment has focused first on surgery, then on gadgets. Other approaches have been patronized, derided, or scorned. Mainstream medicine taught until the last few years that a person found to have gallstones should have her gallbladder removed to avoid potentially drastic complications. Current research has disproven this dogma.

NOTES

1. David E. Johnston and Marshall M. Kaplan, "Pathogenesis and Treatment of Gallstones." *The New England Journal of Medicine,* Vol. 328, No. 6 (Feb. 11, 1993), pp. 412–21.
2. Ibid.
3. Kenneth M. Weiss and Craig L. Harris, "All 'Silent' Gallstones Are Not Silent." *The New England Journal of Medicine,* Vol. 310, No. 10 (Mar. 8, 1986), pp. 657–58.
4. "Gallstones and Laparoscopic Cholecystectomy." NIH Consensus Statement, Vol. 10, No. 3 (Sept. 14–19, 1992), p. 3; and Alan G. Johnson, "Gall Stones: The Real Issues." *British Medical Journal,* Vol. 306 (Apr. 24, 1993), pp. 1114–15.
5. Johnston and Kaplan, op. cit.
6. NIH Consensus Statement, op. cit., p. 3.
7. Ibid., p. 6.
8. Johnston and Kaplan, op. cit., p. 412; and Kenneth W. Heaton, et al., "An Explanation for Gallstones in Normal-Weight Women: Slow Intestine Transit." *The Lancet,* Vol. 341 (Jan. 2, 1993), p. 10.
9. Personal communication from José Marçal, M.D.
10. Diana B. Petitti, Stephen Sidney, and Jeffrey A. Perlman, "Increased Risk of Cholecystectomy in Users of Supplemental Estrogen." *Gastroenterology,* Vol. 94 (1988), pp. 91–95.
11. Johnston and Kaplan, op. cit., pp. 412, 414.
12. Johnston and Kaplan, op. cit., p. 414.
13. Diana B. Petitti and Stephen Sydney, "Obesity and Cholecystectomy Among Women: Implications for Prevention." *American Journal of Preventive Medicine,* Vol. 4, No. 6 (1988), p. 327.
14. Johnston and Kaplan, op. cit., p. 412.
15. NIH Consensus Statement, op. cit., p. 20.
16. Rosemary Gladstar Slick, *Herbs for the Liver and Hayfever.* E. Barre, VT: Sage, no date; and personal communication.
17. Personal communication, Clara A. Lennox, M.D.
18. NIH Consensus Statement, op. cit., p. 7; and Johnston and Kaplan, op. cit., p. 416.
19. NIH Consensus Statement, op. cit., p. 6; Johnston and Kaplan, op. cit., p. 416.
20. Material on treatment taken from NIH Consensus Statement, op. cit.; and Johnston and Kaplan, op. cit.
21. Personal communication from Daniel Kinderlehrer, M.D.
22. Simon Y. Mills, *Out of the Earth: The Essential Book of Herbs.* New York: Viking, 1992.
23. "Laparoscopic Cholecystectomy: Too Much of a Good Thing." *Journal of the American Medical Association,* Vol. 270, No. 12 (Sept. 22, 1993), pp. 1469–70.

27

VISION, HEARING, AND OTHER SENSORY LOSS ASSOCIATED WITH AGING

✦

VISION CHANGES BY ELLEN BARLOW, DIANA LASKIN SIEGAL, FAIRE EDWARDS, AND PAULA B. DORESS-WORTERS

SPECIAL THANKS TO PENNY GAY AND JANE STRETE

1994 UPDATE BY JANE PENTHENY AND DIANA LASKIN SIEGAL WITH HELP FROM PAULA B. DORESS-WORTERS

HEARING IMPAIRMENT IN THE OLDER YEARS BY ELLEN BARLOW, PAULA B. DORESS-WORTERS, AND DIANA LASKIN SIEGAL

SPECIAL THANKS TO JUDITH CHASIN, JESSIE BUCK, AND LOIS HARRIS

1994 UPDATE WITH HELP FROM TAMAR KATZ, DIANA LASKIN SIEGAL, AND PAULA B. DORESS-WORTERS

RESOURCES FOR THIS CHAPTER ON PAGES 498–500

Our senses—sight, hearing, smell, taste, and touch—connect us to the world outside ourselves. There are substantial differences from one person to the next, but most of us can expect the acuity of our senses to dim somewhat as the years pass. Usually changes occur so slowly that we adapt without being aware of the differences in perception.

Someone else may be the first to point out to us that we don't seem to be hearing or seeing as well as we once did. Our sense of touch may become less dependable for such formerly rote tasks as fixing the clasp on a necklace, separating bills in a wallet, or turning pages.

While all of the above may seriously interfere with our efficiency and enjoyment, the most serious effects of sensory losses have to do with health and safety. Loss of taste or smell can lead to loss of appetite, and even to serious malnutrition. Changes in our sense of touch may result in burns due to failure to withdraw from a hot surface in time. Older persons are actually less sensitive to changes in temperature. As a result their body temperature may drop to a dangerous level (hypothermia) before they are aware of it. (See Resources for this chapter for more about hypothermia.) Changes in the sense of balance increase the risk of falling and injury.[1]

Some changes are genetically determined; some are influenced by injuries or environmental factors, such as exposure to noise; some are caused by illness or disease. Some change is inevitable with aging, but no one should settle for a medical dismissal of her concerns as "simply aging" without a careful diagnosis of the cause of any changes in vision, hearing, or other senses. There *are* things we can do when we recognize changes in our senses.

VISION CHANGES

At this very moment, your eyes and your brain together are producing the images you are now perceiving on this page. The eye has the ability to adjust to see near and far objects, shading and colors, and variations in lighting from almost complete darkness to sudden emergence into light.

Most people retain good vision into their older years and don't need to worry about losing their sight. For some of us, though, changes in vision, whether minor or quite serious, can bring troubling changes in our lives. Age-related changes in vision occur in two primary areas of the eye: the lens and the retina.

Presbyopia is the term used to describe slowness in changing the focus from far to near, stemming partly from the loss of elasticity in the lens.[2] The eye's ability to accommodate for near distances starts diminishing at age ten, but not enough for us to take notice of it until about age forty or so. According to medical textbooks, the loss in flexibility of focus is usually fixed by age fifty-five to sixty, though exercises may promote flexibility. Reading glasses, bifocals, and contact lenses can correct sight to normal vision.

I now wear bifocals—originally an embarrassment—and find reading increasingly tiring, a big problem for someone who has been a compulsive reader since childhood. [a fifty-year-old woman]

I really thought they had changed the size of newsprint. I complained that they were making the type size of phone books and the eyes of needles smaller to save money. I'd never had any problems with vision before, so it was a slow realization that it was really me that was changing. [a woman in her seventies]

If you need simple magnification in both eyes and have no other conditions that require correction, you may want to try over-the-counter reading glasses, which are now available in some states. Always begin with the weakest glasses with which you can read. This will reduce strain. Start with the highest number (32, the weakest magnification). Take something to read to test the strength you need. These glasses do not correct for any other visual problems, nor do they allow for differences in each eye.

Do not neglect regular eye exams: a complete eye examination is important to check for glaucoma and other serious eye diseases and may detect other undiagnosed systemic conditions such as diabetes and hypertension. Everyone over forty should have her eyes checked every two years by an ophthalmologist or an optometrist, and a test for glaucoma should be performed at every eye examination of persons over twenty-five. The intra-ocular pressure reading test takes only a few seconds. Good diagnostic procedure requires taking a family history, checking for structural abnormalities, and viewing the optic nerve with an ophthalmoscope, a flashlightlike instrument that allows the eye-care practitioner to see the optic nerve at the back of the eye. If you have a family history of glaucoma, or have had test results that are borderline or glaucoma-suspect, you should have your eyes tested at more frequent intervals.

Minor problems, such as excess tearing and dry eye, can become annoying as we age. Eyelid skin becomes thinner with age. Because the lid skin does not hug the eyeball as tightly as it once did, drainage function may be affected. Increased sensitivity to wind, light, and/or temperature can cause tearing. You can help yourself by more frequent blinking and other exercises to relax your eyes.[3] For dry eyes, by use artificial tear or lubricating drops and see page 499. Do not use drops that "get the red out" (vasoconstrictors). These are not helpful for dry eyes and can even lead to some types of glaucoma in predisposed individuals.

SELF-HELP ALTERNATIVE FOR HEALTHY EYES

Vision Therapy

A number of women have used vision therapy—that is, various eye exercises—as a form of self-help, and to improve their mental, as well as physical, focus and ability to relax. Vision therapy relaxes and focuses the mind and eye while keeping the muscles flexible. Though it cannot cure serious eye diseases and conditions such as those described below, it is a self-help technique for putting to full use the vision one has. It can alleviate eye strain and improve the ability of the eye to focus, in some cases making it possible to continue reading without glasses.

Advocates of vision therapy believe that by continuing to keep the muscles and other parts of our eyes relaxed and flexible as we age, we may even avoid cataracts. A young lens rarely develops cataracts. It is flexible and easily changes focus between distant and near objects. By regaining most of this flexibility, the lens is less likely to stiffen and deteriorate.[4] The eye, like every other part of the body, needs nutrients; relaxed, mobile muscles assist the flow of nutrient-rich blood to reach the lens through the aqueous humor—the fluid inside the eyeball.

To rest and focus your eyes, try:

Blinking: Blink about once per line when reading, and always when a change of focus is needed, as when looking up from reading or if you experience any momentary blur.
When Reading or Doing Close Work: Look off and focus on something at a distance for about five seconds, at least every five to ten minutes to keep your eye muscle from stiffening.
Palming: Lean your elbows on something to support them, then close your eyes and cover them with your palms. Breathe and relax. With your mind, either observe your breath, counting in-out cycles of ten, or visualize as clearly as possible pleasant memories and/or fantasies. Include as many of your senses as you can. Do this whenever your eyes feel tired, including once before you sleep.[5]

Nutrition for Healthy Eyes

Interest is growing in the role of nutrition as a factor in preventing eye disease. Studies have found a lower incidence of cataracts in people who ate a diet high in antioxidants—that is, vitamin E, vitamin C, and beta-carotene. However, no definitive recommendations are available as yet.[6]

EYE-CARE PRACTITIONERS

An *ophthalmologist* is a doctor of medicine (M.D.) who diagnoses and treats eye diseases and performs eye surgery; an *optometrist* is a doctor of optometry (O.D.) who is trained to examine, diagnose, and treat conditions of the visual system. Both can prescribe corrective lenses, but if you require surgical or medical treatment beyond what an optometrist is licensed to provide, the optometrist will refer you to an ophthalmologist. The role of the optometrist as primary eye-care provider is regulated by the states, and the scope of practice varies from state to state. An *orthoptist* specializes in diagnosis and treatment for problems of binocular vision (problems coordinating the use of both eyes). An *optician* fits and makes eyeglasses and in some states fits contact lenses from a doctor's prescription.

You can get a referral to an ophthalmologist in your local area from the National Eye Care Project Hot Line, sponsored by the American Academy of Ophthalmology. Call toll-free 1-800-222-3937 weekdays, 8 A.M. to 4 P.M. (Pacific Standard Time). The doctor will accept Medicare payment or will provide free services if you are over sixty-five and "economically disadvantaged." Cost of glasses, drugs, and hospitalization is not included.

DISEASES OF THE EYE

Four diseases are the principal causes of visual impairment and blindness in older persons: cataracts, glaucoma, macular degeneration, and diabetic retinopathy.[7]

Cataracts involve no pain or discomfort, just less clarity. Gradually the lens of the eye becomes cloudy until there is no longer enough light passing through to the retina to focus a clear image. Vision becomes hazy or blurred and sensitivity to light and glare increases. Risk is increased by diabetes, exposure to ultraviolet B sunlight, smoking, and alcohol. One drink a day quadruples the risk.[8] The most common type is associated with aging. More than 90 percent of Americans over sixty-five have some evidence of cataracts.

Not all cataracts develop to the point where removal is necessary. Some people can live with considerable loss of vision; others may have their livelihood or hobbies threatened by even mild vision loss. There is no need to have surgery unless you experience vision loss that seriously limits your activities. As with any surgery, you should seek a second opinion. Medicare and some private insurance plans require you to do so. Before agreeing to cataract surgery, be sure to ask whether other eye problems exist that could seriously interfere with vision. Cataract surgery should not be performed unless vision will be significantly improved.[9] Given a long life span, a person is more likely to undergo a cataract operation than almost any other surgery. And according to one report, no other operation in medical practice is as dramatically successful so much of the time.[10] Sight is restored after removal of the lens by implantation of an artificial plastic lens (during the same surgical procedure as the removal), or by wearing eyeglasses or extended-wear contact lenses. The contacts or implanted lenses restore a full field of vision; there may be some distortion with glasses. Cataract surgery is most often an outpatient procedure. Get detailed after-care instructions from your doctor. Have someone take you home and stay with you for at least one day after surgery.

Glaucoma is one of the more common and potentially severe eye disorders in people over forty.[11] Glaucoma occurs when there is too much fluid pressure in the eye, causing internal eye damage and gradually destroying vision. It is a myth that glaucoma inevitably leads to blindness. With *early detection* and *prompt treatment,* it can usually be controlled and blindness prevented.

Chronic Wide-Angle or Open-Angle Glaucoma (80 percent of glaucoma cases) seldom produces early signs, and usually there is no pain from increased pressure. Symptoms can include blurred vision that comes and goes, difficulty in adjusting to dark rooms, and reduced side vision. Testing for glaucoma should be part of every routine eye examination.

Chronic glaucoma is more common among blacks and people who are nearsighted, hypertensive, or diabetic.

I first noticed a spot six years ago. I thought it was a spot on my glasses but it was still there after I cleaned my glasses several times. I believe that eyes are precious and have always taken care of mine so I went right into an eye doctor's office that very day. He examined me and referred me to a special eye clinic, where I went the very next day. They said I had glaucoma in one eye and started me on medication, but it did not bring the pressure down enough. Laser therapy was new then but I was willing to try it. Then two years later the pressure started in the other eye so I had laser therapy in that eye also. The pressure is down now but I will have to stay on medication for the rest of my life. It's expensive but I don't want to lose my sight. [a seventy-one-year-old black woman]

Treatment for chronic glaucoma involves bringing down the pressure in the eyeball as quickly as possible with eyedrops and oral medication. This treatment continues throughout life and, with regular checkups to monitor progress, usually ensures that no further loss of vision will take place. If the drugs fail to reduce the pressure, the eye-care practitioner may recommend surgery (usually done with a laser beam) to create an artificial drainage channel.[12]

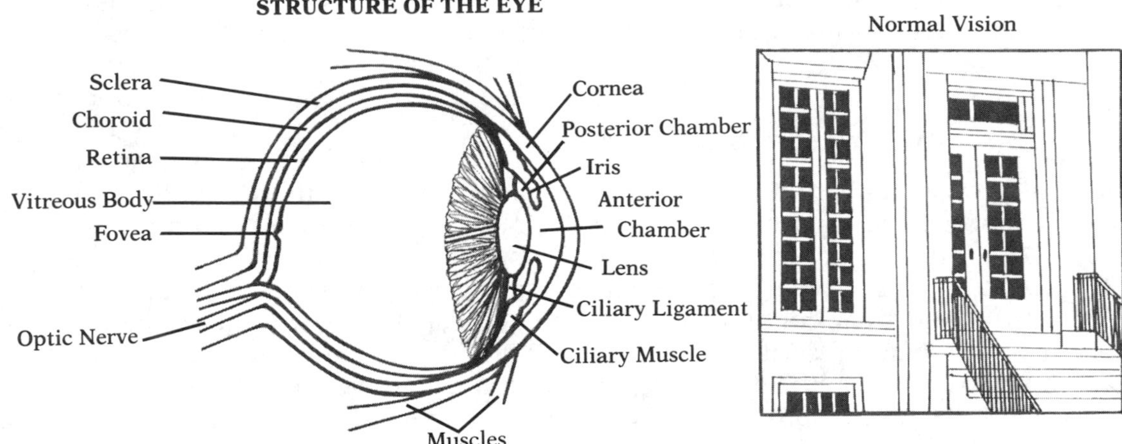

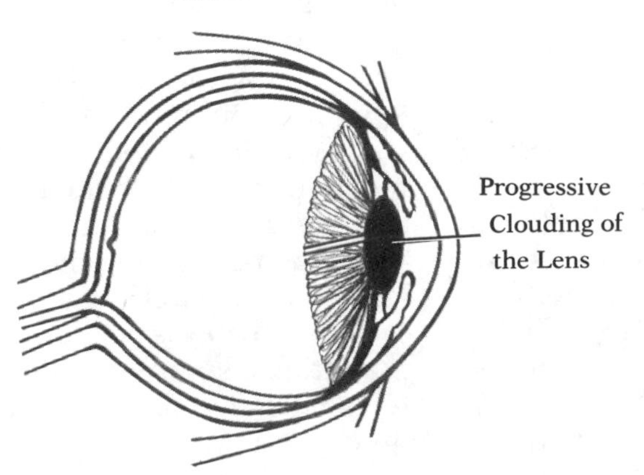

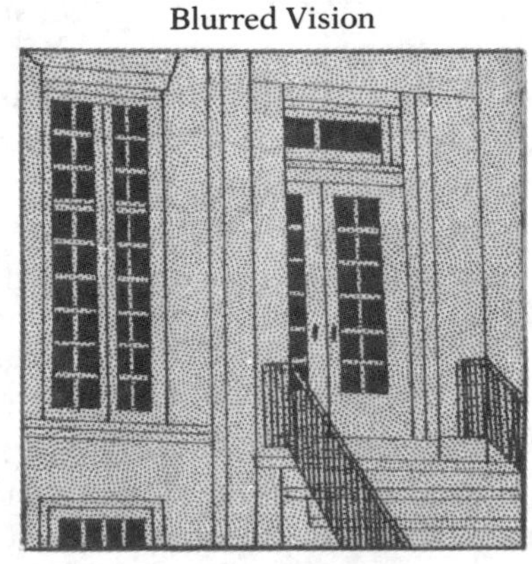

In **Acute Glaucoma** (about 10 percent of glaucoma cases), a sudden blockage occurs in the network of tissue between the iris and the cornea that is called the drainage angle. In farsighted people, Asians, especially Chinese, and people with small eyes, the distance between the cornea and the iris is shorter than normal and the drainage angle narrower, thus making it more likely for pressure to build up.

Sometimes preliminary (subacute) attacks occur, but usually with no permanent damage to vision. Early symptoms of acute or subacute glaucoma are foggy vision, colored rainbows around lights, sudden pain in the eyes, headache, nausea, and vomiting. In an acute attack, permanent loss of vision can occur, especially if treatment is neglected. Early treatment is essential. **If you experience such symptoms, go immediately to your eye-care practitioner or a hospital emergency room.** Emergency treatment consists of eyedrops to bring the pressure down, followed within a day or two by a surgical procedure called an iridectomy, in which a small piece of the iris is removed to relieve the pressure. This is usually done with a laser beam.[13] Laser therapy is sometimes done preventively in persons who may be predisposed to acute glaucoma because of an especially narrow drainage angle in the eye. There is time to get a second opinion if preventive laser therapy is recommended.

Retinal Disorders

The retina is a thin lining on the back of the eye made up of receptors that receive visual images and pass them on to the brain. Retinal disorders include macular degeneration, diabetic retinopathy, and retinal detachment. These are the leading causes of blindness in the United States.

Age-Related Macular Degeneration is the deterioration of the macula, a center spot in the

GLAUCOMA

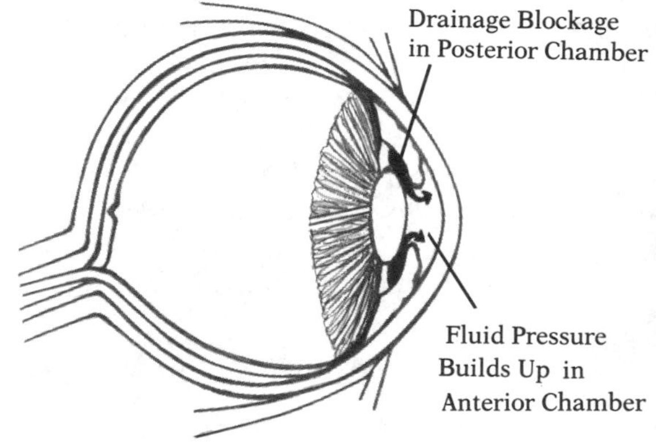

Blurred Peripheral Vision and Possible Blindness

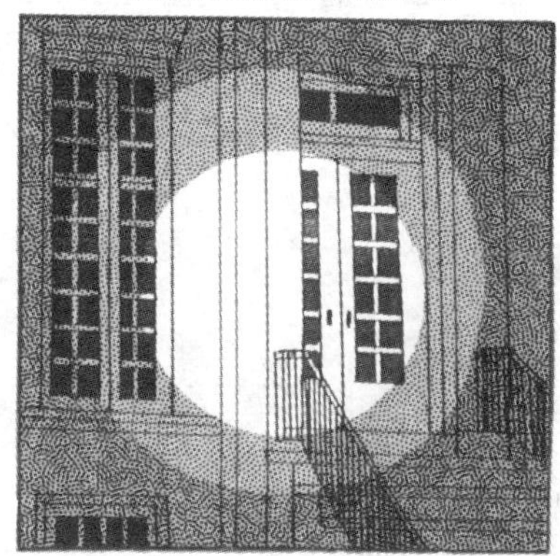

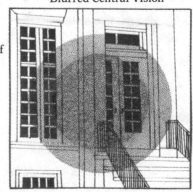

MACULAR DEGENERATION

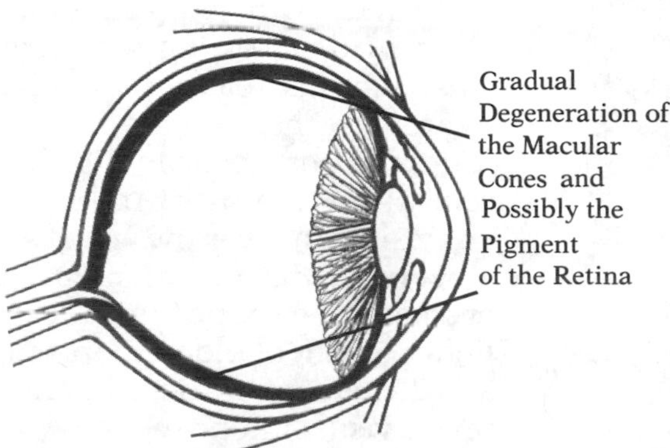

Blurred Central Vision

retina responsible for sharp color and fine-detail vision; it is more common in women than in men. It is the most common cause of vision loss in adults over fifty-five years of age. Side vision is usually retained. Macular degeneration is thought to be caused by a breakdown in the supply of blood to the retina. An early sign of macular degeneration is wavy distortion of horizontal or vertical lines. Check yourself periodically by looking for a few seconds at a line of print, a door, or a stairway to see if this occurs. Use an object with strong contrast such as light color against black.

There are two forms of macular degeneration, wet and dry. The wet kind is less common, but can result in more serious damage. Sometimes laser therapy can help with the wet form of macular degeneration, but it must be done promptly. A variety of low-vision aids (magnifying glasses, telescopic glasses, light-filtering lenses, and electronic devices) can in many cases compensate for visual difficulties.

Diabetic Retinopathy was uncommon a few decades ago. Improved survival rates for diabetes means that many people with diabetes live to suffer complications of the disease. Diabetic retinopathy is at present the leading cause of new blindness in the United States for adults ages forty-one to sixty. Careful control of the diabetes and early diagnosis increase the chances of controlling this eye disease.

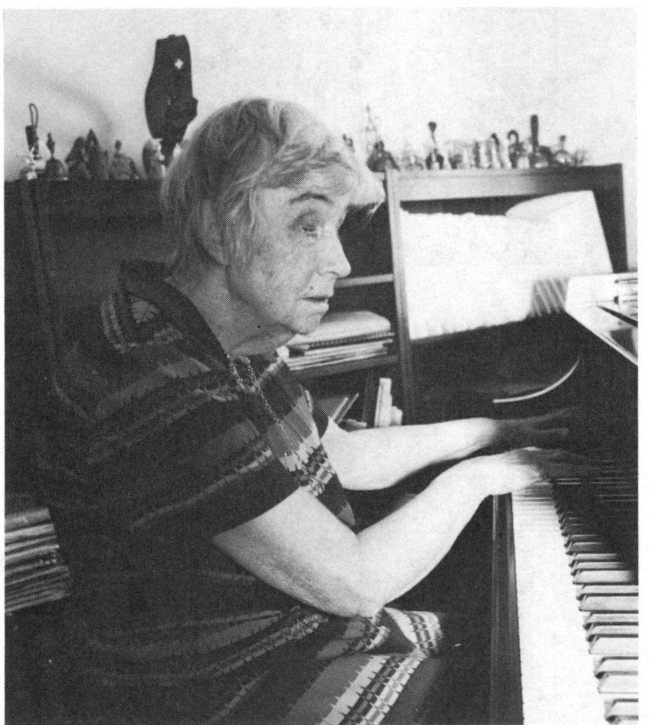

A 78-year-old pianist and composer, blind since birth.
Anne Chapman Tremearne

It never occurred to me that I would ever become blind. Even knowing I had diabetes and knowing it was a possibility, I still never believed that it would happen to me. [a fifty-three-year-old woman]

Many physicians specializing in diabetes control still fail to refer persons with diabetes to an eye-care practitioner for an annual eye exam, and many fail to do even a rudimentary eye exam themselves. Persons with diabetes should consult an eye-care practitioner annually.

Detached Retina is a serious eye problem that occurs more frequently in middle-aged and older persons, especially those who are nearsighted. This condition may be signaled by spots or "floaters" and/or flashes of light. Most floaters are insignificant, caused by changes in the eye's vitreous fluid. To alleviate floaters, glance up and down a few times. However, they *should* be reported to your eye-care practitioner. **Warning:** Sudden, new, or unusual floaters that do not move or flashes of light or loss of side vision may indicate a torn or detached retina. Get emergency medical attention at once, and have an eye-care practitioner make the determination.

I developed floaters in my eyes and was told I'm at high risk for detached retina. My father lost his sight in one eye. I'm a visual person, I love color and nature and beauty, and blindness terrifies me. I don't want to go crazy if it happens, so to compensate I'm learning touch typing, flute, and drums. [a fifty-four-year-old woman]

Degrees of Vision Loss

Very few people actually lose all their vision to the point of not seeing light or dark. Three primary degrees of vision loss are:

- **Low Vision:** Imperfect vision that cannot be improved with conventional eyeglasses or other medical or surgical means. Low-vision aids, such as telescopic lenses, can help the wearer use her remaining vision, but do not restore vision to near 20/20. Forty-eight percent of the almost 2 million Americans with low vision are over the age of sixty-five.
- **Severe Visual Impairment:** Inability to read ordinary newspaper print, even using glasses. Four percent of older people in the community and 26 percent of those in nursing homes have severe visual impairment.

- **Legal Blindness:** Defined as 20/200 vision (or less) in the better eye as corrected by glasses, or as having peripheral fields (side vision) of no more than 20 degrees diameter or 10 degrees radius.[14] Of the 1 to 2 million legally blind Americans, 70 percent are over the age of sixty.[15] Many resist being labeled "legally blind," yet it is a status that makes one eligible for tax exemptions, tax abatements, and certain services. Legally blind people may also be eligible for special financial benefits depending on their income level, such as Supplemental Security Income (SSI) or Social Security Disability Income (SSDI). SSDI has no financial-need requirement. The local Social Security office will have this information. (See Money Matters chapter for more information.)

Getting Help

You can learn skills to get around and manage on your own even with a loss of vision. The ability of eyes to adjust to changing amounts of light diminishes somewhat with age. Dark glasses reduce visibility; yellow shades cut glare without reducing visibility. Night driving can be a problem, but glancing at the right side of the road instead of at oncoming headlights, installing halogen headlamps, having an antireflection coating put on your eyeglasses, wearing yellow shades, and keeping the windshield clean can help. Having to give up night driving can be isolating if your community doesn't have public transportation or if you are reluctant to ask for help.

I had to learn patience. I used to wait until the last minute to jump into the car to do an errand or to meet someone. Now I have to make a lot of time for whatever I am doing because I either go on a bus or by cab or I have to ask someone to pick me up. These all take some time and some waiting. [a fifty-three-year-old woman whose vision loss started at age fifty]

Each state has a Commission for the Blind, which is a good resource, as it provides catalogues of low-vision aids and referrals to eye-care practitioners. However, in most communities, organizations that serve the legally blind cannot provide services to those with low vision or visual impairment who have not yet been declared legally blind. Even if the diagnosis clearly points to a future loss of vision, services are not available until the person qualifies as legally blind.

VISION Foundation is an organization founded by three women who were coping with the oncoming loss of their sight. Frustrated by their inability to get help from established organizations in learning how to manage the expected changes in their lives, they reached out for help by writing to the "Confidential Chat" (a readers' letter exchange of *The Boston Globe*), then banded together for mutual help.

Today, VISION Foundation is an information and referral organization for Massachusetts residents that provides telephone support and self-help groups. It is staffed primarily by persons with sight loss. Your local information and referral center or the National and American Self-Help Clearinghouses can refer you to a self-help group in your area. (See Resources—Self-Help Groups, pages 448–49, and Resources for this chapter, pages 498–99.)

Doctors often fail to refer people who are losing their sight to self-help organizations. Medical emphasis is on surgical solutions, which, unlike other areas of medicine, have had great success for elders. However, physicians may feel a sense of frustration and failure when surgery cannot succeed in saving sight. They may continue to have a patient come back every six months but do little to help the person learn to adapt to low vision, to find the resources she needs to learn new skills, and to find adaptive products, appliances, and other aids. Doctors in many states are not required to report loss of vision to the State Commission for the Blind, except when the patient is "legally blind," and even then they frequently fail to do so. Yet many older people can be helped to live with low vision.

Several states have radio stations that broadcast special programming such as reading daily newspapers. These can be heard on special radios. Inquire at your State Commission for the Blind.

Magnifying devices, self-threading needles, and other gadgets are available to aid near vision. Some sewing-machine stores or notions departments sell magnifiers to attach to your sewing machine. For people who are losing their vision, there is a wide variety of articles available, including talking watches, talking clocks, and other electronic items.

Our Association for the Blind sells aids to clients at cost. I bought a lamp which I can adjust to give me better lighting on my work table. The library loaned me a wonderful magnifier which included a light and lets me see work I do with my hands.

One lady's vision became so bad that it seemed as though she must go into a nursing home. The peer counselor from the Association came and taught her a lot of ways she might use to stay in her own home, including a dot of adhesive tape at the 350-degree mark on her oven control. Now she's still independent, with just a little help from her friends in the building. [an eighty-year-old woman]

Help in learning to manage household tasks, some of it free of charge, may be available from state services for the visually impaired or from your local Association for the Blind. Some associations also offer activities.

For people who are totally blind, and still have a good sense of touch, braille has a lot to offer. Others become very skilled at taking notes on tape recorders.

Large-print books are available from your public library or its regional lending service. Books and magazines on records and cassettes and the special equipment needed to play them are available to order by catalogue through the Libraries for the Blind and Handicapped; if you do not have one near you, your local public library can make the contacts for you. Don't give up on your library because of vision loss. Local libraries can be a wonderful resource for the visually impaired. If your librarian is not aware of these services, you can inform her of their existence and learn together.

Since I have become partially blind my life has become one of learning and study. Recordings for the Blind has all the best dissertations, scientific publications, all the classics, all the best poetry—so I can get anything. And the joy! What difference does the body make when you've got the joy of learning inside you? [an eighty-five-year-old woman]

HEARING IMPAIRMENT IN THE OLDER YEARS

As we reach our fifties and sixties it is increasingly likely that we will experience some degree of hearing loss. Hearing loss is the third most common chronic health problem of older Americans. Sixty percent of people over sixty-five and 90 percent of those over seventy-five have some degree of hearing impairment.[16] Severity of loss tends to be greater for men than for women.

Hearing loss is invisible; thus it is often overlooked by others, who would be more helpful if they were aware of the problem. Because hear-

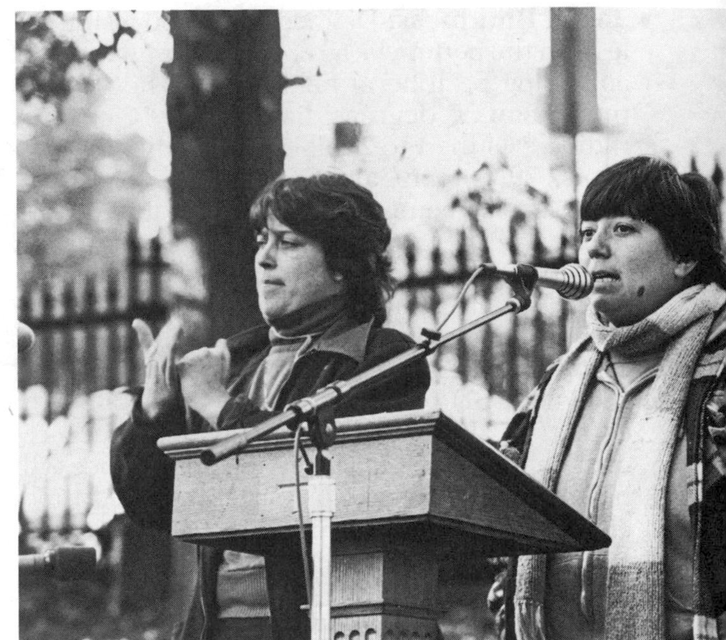

Ellen Shub

ing loss begins so gradually, we ourselves may not be aware of it for some time. We may gradually begin avoiding situations with groups and/or with a lot of background conversation or noise. We may appear to go on with our lives as usual but become progressively more isolated. Even a mild-to-moderate hearing loss can be isolating. We may go through a grieving process in stages similar to mourning a death before we can accept ourselves as having a hearing impairment.[17]

At first I stayed home by myself, until a friend came to talk with me. She said I didn't have to do that to myself. I decided to make myself come to groups—like this exercise group. I have to be willing to hear less. I can't hear half of what the other women say. I can hear R. [male leader] because he has a low voice. [an eighty-eight-year-old woman]

I have hearing loss and cannot hear speech when there is competing loud noise. That means I cannot talk to anyone in the clubs, a primary social gathering place for gay women. It has become an impossibility for me to carry on conversation in any public place (restaurant or club) where there is competing music in the background. The louder sounds mask or distort the voices of my companions. I am reluctant to go to these social gathering places and am becoming more of a stay-at-home. I feel increasing stress in wanting and needing social contact with other women and at the same time having to consciously avoid the very places where I am most likely to meet people. [a fifty-year-old woman]

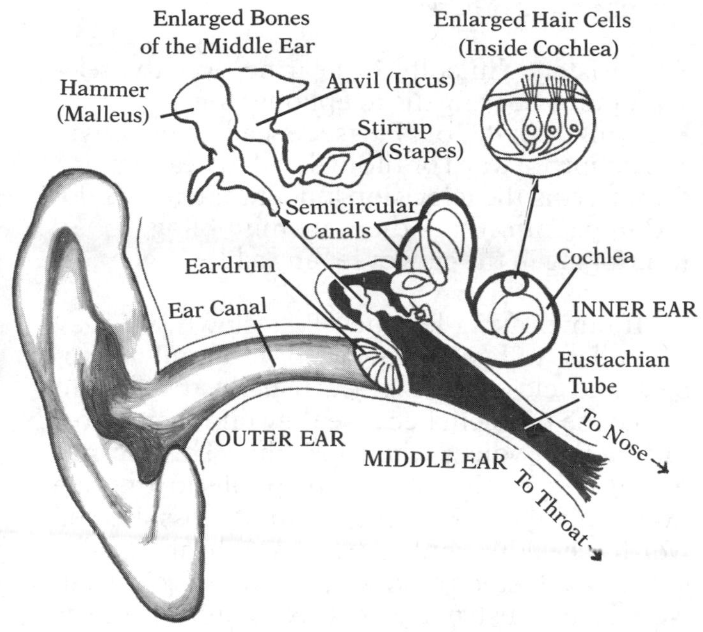

For those of us who have not experienced any hearing loss, it is difficult to comprehend the isolation and frustration experienced by someone who is losing one of her major sensory connections to society, and along with it, the consequent loss of access to information and social cues.

My two hearing aids help in communication, at least sometimes they do. Often the light, particularly enjoyable part of the conversation doesn't get through. The punch line of the joke gets lost. The resulting smile, if I produce one, is artificial. I may use the occasion to educate my hearing friends. Other times I don't. At least my judgment of others is tempered as I remember how often I was thoughtless about hearing problems before I had one of my own.

And I think of various ways by which I can experience lightness, relaxation. Since my sight is adequate, foreign movies with English subtitles are a godsend for me. There we are, all of us, whether we can hear well or not, using those subtitles together. It makes me feel more part of the group.

Perhaps most important of all are small mutual support groups. In the intimate, caring atmosphere of such groups, communication between hearing and hearing-impaired persons can flourish. Each can truly be at ease. [an eighty-two-year-old woman]

Sensitivity on the part of others is crucial. Those of us who have hearing loss, and others of us who have close friends or family members with hearing loss, have learned a variety of skills to improve communication. We must advocate that all cultural and political events be signed for the hearing-impaired. More of us should learn sign language to communicate with deaf people of all ages. It may help us if we lose hearing as we get older.

THE STRUCTURE OF THE EAR AND HOW IT WORKS

The ear is an intricate structure that can process and distinguish over 350,000 different sounds. Sound is funneled into the ear canal and transmitted by vibrations to the eardrum, where it is pushed along through the middle ear by bones known, because of their shapes, as the hammer (malleus), anvil (incus), and stirrup (stapes). It is the stirrup that starts the fluid in the cochlea of the inner ear vibrating. The hair cells then convert sound energy to electrical impulses that

TIPS FOR TALKING WITH A PERSON WITH A HEARING DIFFICULTY[18]

1. Don't talk from another room or from behind her.
2. Reduce background noise. Turn off radio or TV if possible.
3. See that the light falls on your face so she can use visual clues.
4. Get her attention before speaking. To help her focus attention, address her by name and state the subject before beginning: "Marge, we are discussing plans for the picnic. Will you bring salad?"
5. Face her directly, and on the same level if possible.
6. Keep your hands away from your face. Avoid speaking while you are smoking or eating.
7. Don't shout. Speak naturally but slowly and distinctly—and continue that way without dropping your voice.
8. She may not hear or understand something you say. If so, try saying it in a different way rather than repeating.
9. Recognize that she will hear less well if tired or ill.
10. Be patient. Even hints of irritation or impatience hurt.
11. Be an attentive listener. It's probably easier for her to talk than to listen.

telegraph sound interpretations through the nervous system to the brain.

The cochlea looks like a spiral seashell and has approximately twenty-five thousand sensitive hair cells lined up on its membrane. The mechanism by which pitch is discriminated can only be theorized at this time, but it seems to depend on which hair cells are stimulated. Those cells near the base of the cochlea are the high-note cells and those farther along are the lower-frequency ones. Changes in the inner ear, particularly the loss of hair cells associated with high-frequency hearing, have been shown to accompany the aging process. Loss of hair cells is irreversible and occurs throughout our lives from exposure to jet takeoffs, loud music, machinery, and a myriad of other recreational and occupational noises we encounter.

The loud sound systems at rock concerts and in clubs really impair hearing, and should be a health concern for everyone. Tests of hearing in the population at large show that the hearing of people in their twenties and thirties has already begun to deteriorate, and is often as impaired as that of older people. Unless young people take steps to protect their hearing, hearing impairment in old age will increase even more in the decades to come.

Recognizing and Acknowledging the Signs of Hearing Loss

As a slight hearing loss progresses to the point where we become aware of missing much of what is going on, we may react to the first signs of hearing loss with disbelief and denial. Before we can act to help ourselves we must come to terms with our feelings of loss and the consequent change in our image of ourselves.

I can't say exactly when it started. Hearing and understanding telephone conversations is the first difficulty I recall. I found myself asking people to speak up: "This is a poor connection." Sometimes an abrupt silence followed my comment, indicating it had not been entirely appropriate. "I must be more attentive. It's not considerate of the other person for me to let my mind wander while talking." The next clue was that I could hear when someone spoke to me from another room but I could not understand what was said, and it made no difference how loud the person was speaking. A year or two or three passed and these two problems became worse before I took action. [a woman in her fifties]

Signs of hearing problems to look out for in ourselves and others:

- Consistent difficulty in hearing over the telephone or hearing the telephone ring;
- Saying "What?" or "Please repeat" frequently;
- Leaning forward or tilting head to hear better;
- Preferring the television louder than others do;
- Complaining that others are mumbling;
- A ringing in the ears or feeling a blockage.

If our hearing loss develops slowly, we may be the last to become aware of it. Family members and close friends are usually the first to notice the problem because they find themselves raising their voices when speaking. The advance of the loss is almost imperceptible to the one experiencing it. But even a mild loss is well worth checking out. There are hearing aids geared to all kinds of losses, and hearing specialists who can instruct us on ways to improve overall communications.

The degrees of hearing loss are:

Mild	Difficulty hearing faint speech
Moderate	Frequent difficulty hearing normal speech
Severe	Can understand only very loud or amplified speech
Profound	Cannot hear very loud or amplified speech

A common misperception is that hearing loss is a simple reduction in the volume level of sound. This is true for a conductive loss—but not for the type of loss caused by very gradual but irreversible changes in the inner ear.

The main types of hearing loss are:

Conductive Hearing Loss, which involves blockage or impairment of the structures of the outer or middle ear so that sound waves are not able to travel properly. Packed ear wax, extra fluid, abnormal bone growth, or infection can cause this condition. The symptom: Your own voice sounds abnormally loud and other voices sound muffled. Flushing the ear, medication, or surgery may correct the condition.

I started going deaf at about age thirty-six. I was examined by an ear, nose, and throat specialist and by an audiologist and both thought it was nerve deafness, which my mother also had. I didn't know to question the diagnosis at that age. I tried several kinds of hearing aids, which helped only a little. I had four or five really tough years until another audiologist told me she didn't think it was nerve deafness and suggested that I go to another physician. What I had was otosclerosis—a tiny growth which prevents the stirrup from vibrating and so causes conductive deafness. I had an operation called a stapedectomy in one ear when I was forty-two. At that time they used an artificial material to replace the stirrup. When they did my other ear last year they actually used a bit of my own ear lobe. I had a little dizziness for a week or two each time and then it went away. I can hear normally now. [a fifty-eight-year-old woman]

Sensorineural Hearing Loss, caused by damage to the inner ear and/or the nerve pathways to the brain. A high fever or severe infection, head injury, use of certain drugs, vascular problems, and lengthy exposure to loud noises are among the causes. This condition cannot usually be treated medically or surgically. A hearing aid can improve hearing of those with sensorineural loss but won't restore hearing to normal. For some, speech reading (lip reading) and aural rehabilitation can be beneficial.[19] Aural rehabilitation classes teach how to use one's remaining hearing to best advantage by positioning oneself with the better ear toward the speaker, using light and vision effectively, etc. This can be done with or without a hearing aid.

Some hearing loss is temporary and may just go away. Aspirin in large doses (20 to 30 per day), sometimes prescribed for arthritis, may cause a temporary hearing loss. Switching to a non-aspirin product will often remedy the problem. Discuss this with your physician.

Age-Related Hearing Loss (Presbycusis), a sensorineural hearing loss, and the most common type among older persons. As we grow older, many of the hair cells of the inner ear disappear or wither, causing words to sound mumbled. In most cases there is an increasing loss of sensitivity to high-pitched sounds.

I went to a violin and piano concert and I only heard the piano! [a woman in her eighties]

The symptoms vary, but often people with presbycusis have a problem with "speech discrimination," or the ability to understand words when spoken loud enough to be easily heard. For example, the words *sail, fail,* and *tail* all begin with high-pitched consonants; with this type of hearing loss, it would be difficult to tell them apart.

Manipulating the Environment

Once we get used to the idea of having a hearing loss, we can learn to help ourselves by arranging the environment to enhance the hearing we still have.

For many of us hearing is not a problem in an ideal quiet environment with well-articulated face-to-face conversation. At home we can sit facing others and can use soundproofing materials such as carpets and drapes to improve the acoustics. Also, there are many sound-amplifying devices that can be attached to the telephone, television, radio, alarms, doorbell, etc. In addition, visual signaling can be used when you can't depend on hearing. Devices such as a "moonbeam alarm clock" or smoke alarms that light up your bedroom may be ordered by mail. A special device costing about $200 can be installed to enable you to receive closed-captioned television programs. Ask your audiologist or hearing-aid dispenser how to order such devices.

Manipulating the outside environment is more difficult. What we can do is to physically position ourselves to maximize lighting and acoustics.

At home or away, we can ask people we are conversing with to repeat sentences more clearly and slowly, and to emphasize consonants. We can learn to deal with impatient people, be persistent in our requests for clear speech, and learn to listen better ourselves.

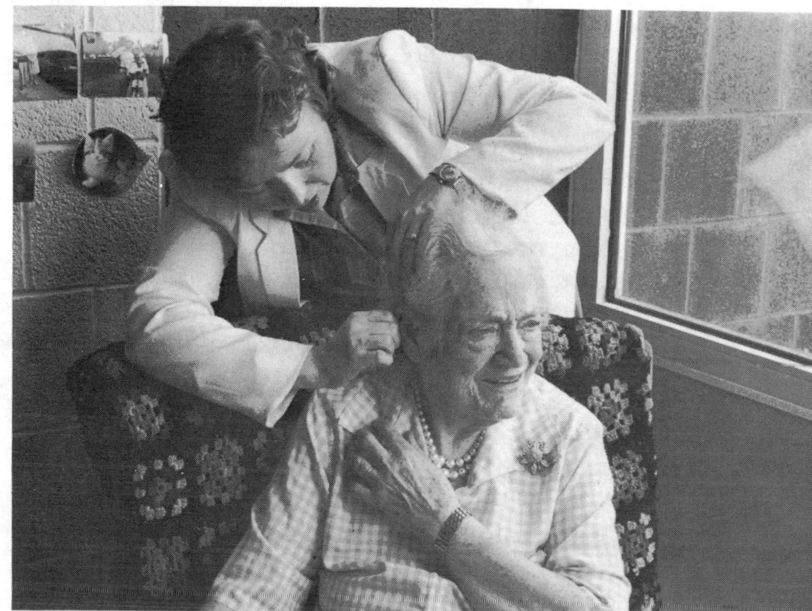

Norma Holt

I began confronting the reality that my hearing acuity was less than normal. I quietly but firmly informed friends, relatives, peers, supervisors, and clients that I had a partial hearing loss and needed them to face me, to speak more slowly and distinctly and in lower tone ranges.

Prevention

As part of a regular physical checkup, insist on a routine hearing check. The primary-care physician should routinely screen everyone over age fifty for pure-tone sensitivity as part of the general physical examination.[20] Too often, people with remediable ear disease fail to get proper attention until the condition is beyond medical help. If you already have some hearing loss it is still important to have your hearing checked regularly and to act on changes in your hearing.

Where and How to Seek Help

If you suspect that you may have some hearing loss, have a medical evaluation by a licensed physician, preferably an otologist (one who specializes in diseases of the ear), or if none is available in your community, an otolaryntologist (ENT), specializing in ear, nose, and throat. Ear specialists can diagnose the different types of hearing impairments and can tell you whether the problem can be treated with surgery, medicine, or by use of a hearing aid or rehabilitation. The importance of establishing the cause and type of loss, and thus the treatment, cannot be overstated. In some cases, particularly where surgery is recommended, you may want to seek a second opinion. Once medical or surgical treatment is ruled out or completed, the ear specialist can refer you to an audiologist for tests and recommendations.

Audiologists are professionally trained and in some states must satisfy specific requirements for a license. They are certified by the American Speech-Language-Hearing Association, and the initials CCC-A after their name indicates a Certificate of Clinical Competence in Audiology.

The principal testing instrument is an audiometer, which emits carefully calibrated pure tones as well as recorded or live voice speech. It precisely measures and records a patient's hearing threshold, the quietest level at which a person can hear a specific sound stimulus 50 percent of the time. Physicians may use audiological test results to diagnose specific hearing problems. This testing is particularly significant because it can be repeated over time to detect changes in hearing.

The audiologist may help the physician evaluate test data to determine whether you would benefit from a hearing aid and in some cases may recommend a particular type. For example, some hearing devices amplify only those frequencies that you need to have amplified. If you tried a hearing aid in the past and were not able to use it, you may want to try again, as they have been improved a great deal in recent years, especially in their capacity to screen out background noise.

Role and Responsibilities of the Dispenser

A dispenser sells or rents hearing aids. The dispenser may or may not be a medical doctor or an audiologist. A dispenser's functions include giving the patient hearing tests for selection and fitting of hearing aids, encouraging prospective users to try amplification, making impressions for ear molds, counseling hearing-impaired people on adapting to a hearing aid, and repairing damaged hearing aids.

In most states hearing-aid dispensers are licensed under standards of competence and a strict code of ethics. The National Hearing Aid Society has a voluntary certification program for qualified dispensers.

An FDA regulation effective August 25, 1977, imposes conditions for the sale of hearing aids to help prevent misrepresentation and to assure adherence to proper medical standards. Hearing-aid dispensers must obtain a written statement from the patient signed by a licensed physician stating that the patient's hearing has been medically evaluated and that the patient is considered a candidate for a hearing aid. This medical evaluation must have taken place no longer than six months before the date of sale. The dispenser must give you written instructions for using the hearing aid selected and must make sure you understand them.

Dispensers must also advise patients to consult a physician or ear specialist promptly if the dispenser finds any of several conditions, such as conductive hearing loss, dizziness, or sudden fluctuating loss of hearing, which may indicate a medical problem.

Patients eighteen or older may waive the medical evaluation requirement, but the dispenser is required to warn them beforehand that it is not in their best health interests. The dispenser must avoid encouraging patients to waive the medical examination. Whenever a patient chooses to waive, the dispenser is required to obtain her or his signature on a waiver statement. The dispenser must keep a copy of each patient's medical evaluation or a signed waiver on file for three years.[21]

Adapting to a hearing aid can be trying because, in most cases, all sounds are amplified—not just the sounds you want to hear. It takes time and practice to learn when and where and how to use your hearing aid.

The first few weeks almost convinced me that I wanted only to retreat into "my silent world" and manage as best I could. It was like living in a noisy factory. It was a constant bombardment of sound, and all of it too loud! Finally all the fine adjustments were made and now I can enjoy movies and concerts and theater again. I can hear my grandchildren as they learn to make sounds and form words and conversation.

All is not as before though. Large gatherings of people are simply noisy confusion. Driving my car with the window down is very tiring emotionally because of the assault of noise, and I must regularly visit the audiologist to adjust the aid. [a fifty-eight-year-old woman]

It may be hard to get used to the increased volume level. The new digital programmable hearing aids help with background noise. They increase the volume of high frequencies and decrease the volume of low frequencies.

An ethical hearing-aid dispenser will allow you thirty days to try out a hearing aid, and will charge you only for the ear mold and/or a fee for her or his time if you are unable to adapt to it and must return it. You may have to try out several hearing aids before finding the one that works for you.

Hearing aids don't help everyone. Many hearing-aid dispensers offer trial rentals or a money-back guarantee if you are not satisfied with the hearing aid. This is a good indication that they will take the time to serve you properly. Be sure to ask this in advance. Beware of mail-order hearing aids. Proper fit means molding and adjusting the device to the individual. You may need several appointments to adjust and adapt. Find someone who is patient and will work with you. Most require that you pay when you pick up your hearing aid, but will give you a partial or full refund if it is not satisfactory. Some have payment plans with no finance charges. Find out all the details at or before the first visit. Other questions to ask include: Does the cost include an ear-mold fitting, if needed? How long will the dispenser provide free service? How long do the batteries last and what do they cost? This can vary greatly and can become an expensive item. Will the dispenser provide you with a loaner hearing aid if your aid needs repair?

Rehabilitation

Rehabilitation includes a broad range of services, such as occupational services—finding alternative employment and/or adaptations to enable you to continue in your present occupation.

I became aware that if my hearing loss continued I'd not be able to function in the same way, especially at work. I am a registered nurse and just a year or two earlier had completed the education and certification to qualify me as a nurse practitioner. Bedside nursing or ambulatory care—it really didn't matter which: I had to be able to accurately hear the patient's complaints, history of illness, breath sounds, abdominal sounds, heart sounds, doctors' instructions and orders—I had to hear! Having also been recently divorced, I was supporting myself entirely. I struggled to not hit the panic button.

I decided the time had come to plan the necessary changes before complete hearing loss inflicted change in my life—perhaps at a time when I would be at a disadvantage.

I consulted the local office of the State Rehabilitation Commission for guidance. First a complete medical exam of my ears and a full audiological evaluation. Then conferences with my nursing director and the administrator of the health-care facility where I am employed. Amplifier headsets were added to telephones I had to use, and an electronic stethoscope (extremely sensitive to even the slightest sound) was purchased for my use. [a fifty-seven-year-old woman]

Rehabilitation also includes help in discriminating sounds and speech reading, sometimes called lip reading. Classes may be available at low cost in your community. See Resources for this chapter for referral sources, or call your local Council on Aging.

"Why a lip-reading class?" my friends ask. The reason is a gradually increasing hearing loss I have had for several years. Unless I'm in a room with good acoustics and with people who speak clearly, I have trouble following the conversation.

In the meantime, here I am in the lip-reading class of our community education program, learning a lot about how to face up to hearing difficulties. The mutual support of the group is reassuring.

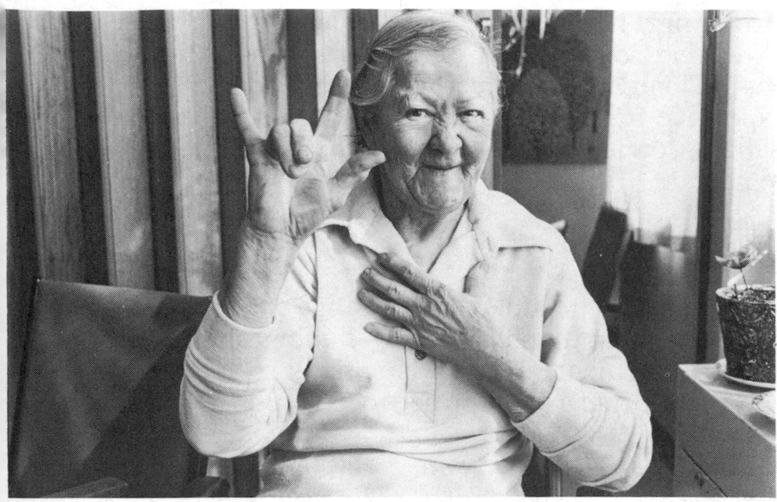

Marianne Gontarz

While there is no magic cure, hearing aids, signing, and lip reading can help. Lip reading is hard work. Many sounds can't be seen, so we are learning to be aware of other body clues and are improving our visual skills in general.

We are also planning strategies for better community understanding: distributing a leaflet titled "Tips for Talking to the Hard of Hearing" and doing a skit demonstrating some of the problem issues. [an eighty-year-old woman][22]

Policy Issues

Hearing loss is one of the most common conditions of the older years, one that can lead to social isolation and withdrawal, yet little is done about it. Most services are medical and surgical, yet these are not helpful for the kind of hearing loss that affects most older people. Fragmentation of services seriously limits the ability of older persons to get help for hearing impairment—medical doctor for checkups, audiologist for hearing-aid evaluation, and in some cases a hearing-aid dispenser to get the hearing aid. Many accept the dispenser as the primary provider of hearing-related services and never go back to the physician for regular care of the ears. Some of us cannot afford hearing aids because neither Medicare nor Medicare supplementary insurance will cover the costs. In some states Medicaid will pay for hearing aids. Charitable organizations, such as the Lions Club, sometimes help purchase hearing aids for those who cannot afford them. Our patchwork system of health-care delivery must be changed so that all who need hearing aids and rehabilitation services can have them as a matter of right. You can join with advocacy organizations such as the AARP (see General Resources) and coalitions such as the Campaign for Women's Health (see Women's Health and Reforming the Medical Care System chapter) to fight for a comprehensive and integrated national health-care program.

Notes

1. Jeffrey R. M. Kunz, *The American Medical Association Family Medical Guide.* New York: Random House, 1982, pp. 720–21.
2. Gay Becker, et al., *Vision Impairment in Older Persons,* Policy Paper No. 9, 1984. Aging Health Policy Center, University of California, San Francisco.
3. Personal communication, Ro G. Gordon, D.B.O. (Diploma of British Orthoptists), vision therapist.
4. Ibid.
5. Ibid.
6. Cataract Management Guideline Panel, *Cataract in Adults: Management of Functional Impairment.* AHCPR Pub. No. 93-0542. Rockville, MD: Agency for Health Care Policy and Research, Public Health Service, U.S. Department of Health and Human Services, February 1993, p. 20.
7. Becker, op. cit., p. 10.
8. Cataract Management Guideline Panel, op. cit., pp. 18–21.
9. "Cataracts." *Health Letter.* The Public Citizen Health Research Group (see General Health Resources, p. 483), Vol. 3, No. 3 (March 1987), pp. 1–6.
10. T. J. Liesegang, "Cataracts: What They Are, What to Do About Them." *Mayo Clinic Proceedings,* Vol. 59, August 1984, pp. 556–622.
11. Kunz, op. cit.
12. Ibid., p. 322.
13. Ibid., pp. 320–21.
14. Fran A. Weisse and Mimi Winer, *Coping with Sight Loss. The VISION Resource Book.* Watertown, MA: Vision Foundation, p. 3; and Jane Porcino, "Vision Capacity of Women Over Forty," in *Growing Older, Growing Better.* New York: Crossroad Continuum, 1991, pp. 301–2.
15. Personal communication, Annette Maleson, Massachusetts Commission for the Blind.
16. AARP, "Facts About Hearing Loss." *Disability Initiative: Fact Sheet,* 1992.
17. Beatrice A. Wright, *Physical Disability: A Psychological Approach.* New York: Harper, 1960. Quoted in Maurice H. Miller, "Restoring Hearing to the Older Patient: The Physician's Role." *Geriatrics,* Vol. 41, No. 12, December 1986.
18. Reprinted with permission from the Boston Women's Health Book Collective, *The New Our Bodies, Ourselves.* New York: Simon and Schuster, 1992, p. 543.
19. *Aging Notes,* U.S. Senate Special Committee on Aging, January 8, 1985, p. 2.
20. Maurice H. Miller, "Restoring Hearing to the Older Patient: The Physician's Role." *Geriatrics,* Vol. 41, No. 12, December 1986.
21. *FDA Consumer,* HHS Publication No. (FDA) 80-4024. Washington, DC: U.S. Government Printing Office, May 1980.
22. Reprinted with permission from the Boston Women's Health Book Collective, op. cit., p. 543.

28

MEMORY LAPSE AND MEMORY LOSS

✦

BY JANE HYMAN

SPECIAL THANKS TO GUILA GLOSSER

1994 UPDATE BY MARILYN S. ALBERT

RESOURCES FOR THIS CHAPTER ON PAGES 501–2

As we grow older, some of us find ourselves becoming more forgetful. We notice that we cannot remember names as easily, forget errands, or misplace keys or household items. Frequently what we notice is not a memory loss but a memory lapse. It simply takes us longer to retrieve names, addresses, and dates from our memories than it used to. When this happens in our older years we may see it as a sign of age and become flustered, frustrated, embarrassed, or angry with ourselves. We may even think this forgetfulness could be a sign of senility.

When I'm with friends my age and I forget a name of something—we laugh. That makes it easy. Not so when I'm with younger people. For example, when I'm giving information to a salesperson—I know *where I live but occasionally I have to think a minute to remember my address. And I always feel as though they're looking at me thinking, "Oh, this senile old thing." I'm* not *senile! Now I just say to myself, someday they'll be my age and they'll know what this is like.* [a seventy-three-year-old woman]

The dictionary definition of *senility* is "a loss associated with old age, of mental faculties." But the word has no real meaning, because it has become a catch-all term for any forgetfulness or mental disorder experienced by an older person. Until recently physicians assumed that senility was an inevitable part of old age. This assumption kept them from identifying and treating true memory disorders.

Alzheimer's disease is gradually replacing senility as a specific focus of our concerns. Media coverage of Alzheimer's can lead to unnecessary fears over signs of forgetfulness. This emphasis on the negative—on potential losses as we get older—can make us feel that forgetting names or misplacing objects is more significant than our interests, our knowledge, and our wisdom gained over the years. It also obscures research that shows that some intellectual abilities often increase with age.[1] It is important to put memory changes into perspective and to understand the differences between normal forgetfulness and memory disorders. We want to stop feeling uneasy about forgetfulness—but we also want to know when to seek help.

There are three categories of memory lapse or memory loss associated with age.

1. Normal forgetfulness, *benign senescent forgetfulness,* is part of the normal aging process. But it does not necessarily worsen with the years and does not interfere with our lives in any significant way or endanger our health.

2. Memory loss may be related to disorders or conditions such as depression or malnutrition. These conditions and the resulting memory loss are reversible and can and should be diagnosed and treated.
3. A disease of the brain, *late-life dementia* or *senile dementia,* is not normally part of the aging process. It is irreversible and progressive, preventing the individual from carrying out even simple responsibilities. Late-life dementia needs medical diagnosis and special care. The most common form of late-life dementia is Alzheimer's disease.

The difference between normal forgetfulness and the early stage of Alzheimer's disease is not always clear-cut. But in Alzheimer's disease memory loss becomes progressively worse and is accompanied by a general decline in intellectual abilities and changes in behavior.

Benign Senescent Forgetfulness

Throughout much of our adult lives the brain loses nerve cells that are not replaced through regeneration. From around age fifty and on, parts of the brain can show other signs of change, such as cell tangles (abnormal protein substances in nerve cells, also known as neurofibrillary tangles) and senile plaques (degenerated nerve cells that form scars). These changes can be accompanied by a decline in memory, but for many of us such a decline never occurs, and we can continue to live well into our eighties and beyond experiencing little or no change in our mental vigor.[2]

It is not known why some of us experience a decline in memory and others do not. But our brains, like other parts of our bodies, differ from person to person because of genetic factors and in response to emotions and to physical and environmental changes.

Throughout our lives, including our older years, fatigue, anxiety, inattention, stress, and depression can cause moments of memory lapse or periods of memory decline. As we grow older we also become particularly vulnerable to changes in our social situations. Deaths of loved ones, relocation to an unfamiliar place, or increased social isolation can bring about emotional changes that trigger forgetfulness, confusion, and disorientation. Diseases and physical disorders can be accompanied by emotional distress that can lead to increased forgetfulness, especially when treatment in an unfamiliar place, such as a hospital or nursing home, is required. A loss of sight or hearing contributes to mental confusion by restricting a person's knowledge of the world around her and by putting additional stress on already weakened learning abilities and memory. Eye and ear impairments can also worsen a sense of social isolation or actually cause us to avoid social contact, possibly bringing about depression and a decline in mental functioning. These causes of forgetfulness, confusion, and disorientation are reversible, and mental capacities can return to normal after an adjustment period with proper medical treatment or sometimes with the help of friends and family.

Helping Ourselves Remember

Often we notice ourselves being forgetful for no apparent reason. Our memory changes can become bothersome to the point that some of us develop strategies for remembering. We avoid interruptions when concentrating on a task, knowing that distracted attention can be detrimental to our work. We write lists and notes to ourselves instead of relying on our memories. We adjust our surroundings to help us find objects (including our lists) more easily.

In the morning when I wake up I go through what I call a name exercise. I have various friends whose faces come before me, and then I go through that exercise of recalling the names I need for the day, up to ten or twelve at a session. I find that very useful. Sundays before going to church, I try to recall many names of church members who may be present so that they're fresh in the front of my memory. I do this same exercise before I go to meetings or social gatherings. In my bedroom I have my closets organized so I can find things. I even organize my refrigerator! [an eighty-six-year-old woman]

An orientation area can also be helpful: a room or corner with a calendar and bulletin board for written reminders, and a place to keep essential items such as glasses, keys, umbrella, and writing accessories. Such a special area can save energy we would otherwise waste in being upset over forgetting, losing, or misplacing something.

Some of us may want to seek outside help offered in the form of memory clinics, which are often affiliated with hospitals. Such clinics offer memory-skill training and individual and group

Organize, Don't Memorize[1]

What to buy and tasks:

Make a list rather than relying on your memory. Keep a pad available to jot down items as needed.

Taking medication:

Place medication in a special receptacle each night for the following day. When you see the receptacle is empty, you know you have taken the medication.

or

Use containers (paper cups, saucers, an empty egg carton, or boxes sold for this purpose), each marked for the day of the week. This is especially helpful if you take different medications on different days. (Caution: Do not leave medications within the reach of children.)

Turning off the stove, removing the laundry, leaving on time for an appointment:

Use a timer with a bell, or wear a watch with a timer. Set it for the appropriate time, and take it with you around the apartment or house so you will be sure to hear it.

Names and ages of grandchildren, names of friends and acquaintances:

Write the grandchild's name and date of birth under each photo in a photo album or frame. Write names under pictures of friends. Periodically look through your address book to refresh your memory or to recognize a name you are trying to think of.

Paying bills:

Place all bills to be paid in one place. Mark on your calendar the date on which to pay the bills. Cross off the reminder after you pay the bills.

Ask your local librarian for books on techniques for remembering. And remember: *You don't have to remember everything.*

1. Adapted from Florence Garfunkel and Gertrude Landau, *A Memory Retention Course for the Aged: Guide for Leaders.* Washington, DC: National Council on the Aging, December 1981.

counseling concerning emotional issues related to memory. They can also help to reduce stress and fear concerning memory changes.

Disorders and Drugs that Can Lead to Memory Loss

A number of specific disorders and drugs can lead to memory loss and mental confusion. These effects are not limited to the elderly, but the older brain is more vulnerable to them. *Most of them are reversible and should be identified and treated.* Correct diagnosis is extremely important, since the mental symptoms of these disorders often resemble those of Alzheimer's disease and can be misdiagnosed as Alzheimer's or as "senility" and left untreated.

Depression

Some of the symptoms of depression include a slowing of movement and speech, slowing of thought, changes in sleep and eating habits, decreased pleasure in activities, underestimation of one's true capacities, and low self-esteem. Depression is probably the disorder most commonly misdiagnosed as Alzheimer's disease, particularly when low self-esteem causes poor results on mental status tests. The profound changes in thinking and memory sometimes associated with depression have been called *pseudodementia.* However, thorough neurological and neuropsychological examinations usually differentiate depression from dementia. The two are different in both onset and behavior. The onset, or beginning, of depression is usually more sudden than the slow and gradual process of Alzheimer's disease. And a depressed person is more likely to exaggerate her or his difficulties, while it is common for a demented person to minimize them and not be aware of declining mental abilities. In many cases of pseudodementia there is a previous history of depression. There are currently a number of very effective treatments for depression, and a mental-health clinic or provider with experience in treating older persons should be consulted if this is suspected.

Drugs and Alcohol

As we grow older our tolerance for drugs (including prescription medicines and over-the-counter preparations) and alcohol decreases and our reactions to drugs may differ greatly from those

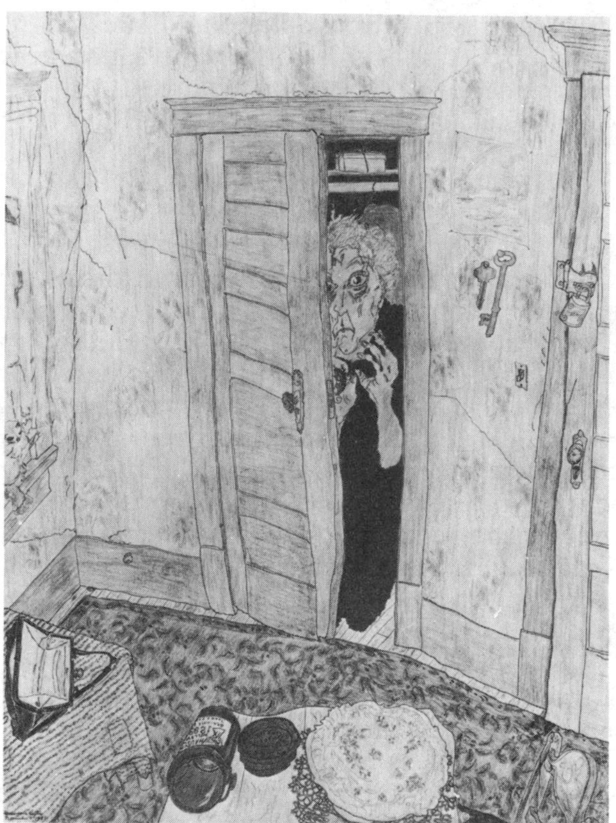

Elizabeth Layton

of younger people. Certain drugs alone, as well as alcohol alone, can affect mood, memory, and speed of reactions. Alcohol can worsen depression, and drugs or alcohol can worsen the symptoms of Alzheimer's disease. Chronic, long-term alcohol abuse may lead to serious decline in memory and other cognitive functions. Drugs that diminish or inhibit acetylcholine, a chemical in the brain, can produce significant memory loss in the elderly.[3] Such anticholinergic drugs include several prescription medications and over-the-counter remedies for diarrhea, nausea, and coughs. The older we get the more likely we are to be taking numerous drugs simultaneously to treat medical conditions or chronic diseases. Estimates show that in the United States most people over seventy-five take up to eight prescription drugs at the same time.[4] The brain is very vulnerable to drug interactions that can produce symptoms similar to those of dementia. Drugs are often necessary and valuable, but we need to be aware of the possible negative effects of any drug, *including over-the-counter remedies,* and of what the effect may be when we take two or more drugs at the same time, or combine a drug with alcohol.

Nutritional Deficiency and Anemia

As we age we may develop health problems that can cause malnutrition and anemia. Also, some of us develop poor nutritional habits because of physical infirmity or loneliness. A restricted budget can limit our choice of fresh and wholesome food, and weakness, frailty, or infirmity can make us reliant on others for transportation, food shopping, and food preparation. One or a combination of these factors can lead to malnutrition. Malnutrition (especially a vitamin B_{12} and folic acid deficiency) or anemia (a shortage of red blood cells and/or low hemoglobin content of these cells) can cause a person to appear disoriented and confused, to have severe memory lapses, and even to appear delusional. These deficiencies can be ruled out by blood tests and corrected by an adequate diet and supplements and by treating any underlying health problem.

Diseases and Other Health Problems

Some diseases and physical conditions can cause memory loss and mental confusion. These include thyroid disease, diabetes, kidney or liver problems, lung disease, gallstones, and syphilis. Other health problems, such as heart and lung ailments, feverish conditions, and even constipation, can cause mental confusion. Generally speaking, as we grow older we are less likely than before to develop specific symptoms when we become ill. We may become confused or withdrawn instead.

Brain Disorders

Disorders of the brain or central nervous system that can lead to memory loss include Parkinson's disease, a single stroke, brain tumor, trauma to the brain, subdural hematoma (bleeding in the brain because of trauma), and hydrocephalus (abnormal increase in the fluid surrounding the brain). Often these disorders can be treated, and timely treatment can prevent further damage.

Late-Life Dementia

Late-life dementia refers to a group of diseases of the brain that most frequently afflict those over sixty-five. The dementia influences all aspects of behavior, not only memory but also judgment, temperament, and social interaction. Late-life dementia is a neurological disorder (a disorder of the nervous system), not a psychological disorder, and it has nothing to do with a person's previous intelligence, education, or mental health. An estimated 90 percent of all late-life dementias are primarily caused by two irreversible conditions: multi-infarct dementia and Alzheimer's disease.[5]

MULTI-INFARCT DEMENTIA

Multi-infarct, or vascular, dementia is a condition of the brain caused by many small strokes. A stroke is a rupture or blockage of a blood vessel in the brain, which stops the flow of blood and destroys an area of brain tissue by depriving that area of oxygen and other necessary nutrients. The accumulated damage of many small strokes leads to an inability to function in various ways, depending on which parts of the brain are damaged. The mental and behavioral symptoms of multi-infarct dementia usually come on more suddenly than those of Alzheimer's disease. Multi-infarct dementia may also involve early signs of physical dysfunction, such as impairment of vision or sensation and muscle weakness or paralysis. The condition may begin abruptly and can be episodic, with short-term improvements and exacerbations. (This contrasts with Alzheimer's disease, which is hardly noticeable at first and progresses gradually.) Risk factors for multi-infarct dementia include atherosclerosis, previous strokes, heart attacks, severe chest pains (angina pectoris), high blood pressure, and diabetes. High blood pressure and diabetes should be treated in order to prevent further small strokes (see Hypertension and Diabetes chapters).

Multi-infarct dementia is preventable to the extent that we can prevent heart disease, strokes, and diabetes by not smoking and by drinking alcohol only in moderation, exercising regularly, eating well, and getting early treatment for high blood pressure.

Multi-infarct dementia alone makes up almost half of late-life dementias.[6] It can also occur in conjunction with Alzheimer's disease.

ALZHEIMER'S DISEASE

I'm going to fight it. Now what I do is write down everything I want to do. As I get them done I mark them off. Also I read a lot. This is the way I'm fighting it. It makes me so mad that every day I pound the table with my fist, because I don't want to be like this. I'm going to fight it every way I can. I'm stubborn. [a seventy-two-year-old woman in an early stage of Alzheimer's disease]

Since Alzheimer's disease, alone or in conjunction with multi-infarct dementia, makes up an estimated 75 percent of cases of late-life dementia, the term *Alzheimer's disease* has come to be the term most frequently used for late-life dementia. Often abbreviated as SDAT (Senile Dementia of the Alzheimer Type), it afflicts an estimated 5 percent of those over sixty-five, rising with age to 25 to 50 percent of those over eighty-five.[7] The incidence is expected to triple as the number of elderly people increases within the next three generations. It is more common in women than in men (two to one), although this seems to be a result of women's longer life span. Alzheimer's disease ranks as the fourth or fifth leading cause of death in the United States.[8] Currently dementia, of which Alzheimer's is the major cause, afflicts an estimated 4 million people.

Abnormalities in the chemistry of the brain and changes in the structure of brain cells prevent nerve cells from functioning. The cell tangles and senile plaques that occur in normal aging (see page 404) are more frequent and widespread in Alzheimer's disease. As more and more cells degenerate and parts of the brain die, the person's functioning deteriorates.

Stages of Alzheimer's Disease

At the beginning of the disease relatively few brain cells are affected, and the symptoms of memory loss may be noticed only by the victim herself* or, more typically, by a partner or employer. The victim may begin to forget once-familiar names or where she has put things, have difficulty finding words, become withdrawn, lose energy, anger easily, or avoid the unfamiliar. These can be signs of the first stage of Alzheimer's disease. But since an increase in forgetfulness can also be a part of the normal aging process, it should not cause concern unless it grows progressively worse and is accompanied by other symptoms that noticeably reduce the person's ability to carry out everyday activities.

Have you ever had a lamp with a loose wire? Sometimes when you switch it on it lights up and sometimes it does not. That's what my father was like. I never could predict whether he would know or remember something, or not. [a sixty-one-year-old woman]

*Since more women than men have Alzheimer's disease, the afflicted person is referred to as "she" throughout the text although the information applies to men also.

I first began to suspect my mom might have Alzheimer's when I noticed a marked change in her personality. I was getting all kinds of nasty notes and telephone calls from her. She would call me thirteen times a day asking the same question. She couldn't remember what day it was and couldn't remember to take her medication. She was getting angry, frustrated, and more and more forgetful. [a thirty-eight-year-old woman]

When forgetfulness *is* a sign of Alzheimer's it will eventually be accompanied by rambling and repetition in conversation, lack of concentration, difficulty with orientation and travel, and spatial disorientation. These symptoms signal a more advanced stage of the disease. At this stage most people will no longer consciously recognize the symptoms and may deny them, since their reasoning and judgment become impaired. However, some people may have periodic insight into their deficiencies and become depressed or frustrated by them. The depression, frustration, or anxiety can, in turn, complicate the symptoms.

As the disease progresses the person may forget the names and faces of intimate family members; become disoriented in the home, or wander off and get lost; become unable to drive a car; become emotionally unstable and irritable; become incontinent; and eventually forget how to speak, eat, dress, and use a toilet. Some become agitated and occasionally abusive and assaultive while others may become increasingly withdrawn and apathetic. At this stage the person is completely dependent on others for basic human needs and can no longer survive without full-time care.

For unknown reasons, during the later stages of the disease the patient often loses weight. Muscle control diminishes, making any form of exercise difficult or impossible. The person may eventually become confined to a wheelchair or become bedridden. The immobile or inactive person becomes more vulnerable to disease, infection, or heart attack. Pneumonia, viral infections, and heart attack are the most frequent secondary causes of death, the primary cause being Alzheimer's disease itself. The disease shortens life expectancy, but many people live for years in the final stages. Survival after the earliest symptoms varies anywhere from four to twenty years. The average survival is seven to ten years. In most cases the person will eventually require twenty-four-hour nursing-home care unless the caregiver(s) can provide or hire private assistants around the clock.

Diagnosis

As larger numbers of the population become eighty-five and older, incidence of Alzheimer's disease will increase. Research on the disease has become more urgent and extensive, but to date there is no cure for Alzheimer's disease, nor any treatment to reduce its intensity or halt its progression. Nonetheless, careful diagnosis is extremely important in order to rule out treatable disorders that can cause mental confusion as well as other forms of dementia such as multi-infarct dementia, viral dementia (such as Creutzfeldt-Jakob disease or sometimes AIDS), and hereditary dementia (such as Huntington's disease). Diagnosis is also important in order to help the person who has the disease and to help future caregivers understand what they are dealing with and obtain the necessary social, psychological, and medical support. When the afflicted person and her family finally know she has Alzheimer's, the disease is recognized as the reason for changes in behavior. This may alleviate the anger family members feel toward the afflicted relative and soften the blame they sometimes place on her for inappropriate behavior. It may also help to alleviate the victim's own embarrassment and self-blame.

My mother has Alzheimer's disease, but she was first diagnosed as having "geriatric depression." We went through years of her behavior getting worse and worse and driving me up the wall. If only we had had an earlier correct diagnosis, it would have saved us so much emotional pain and strain and turmoil. Now that the disease has been diagnosed it makes it easier for me to at least put a reason to her behavior. When you know what Alzheimer's disease is all about, the diagnosis is a relief—and not a relief. [a thirty-eight-year-old woman]

For diagnosis and future care, look for a physician who specializes in treating dementia or the elderly in general, such as an internist specializing in geriatrics, a neurologist, or a geriatric psychiatrist, and look for a gerontological nurse practitioner. The Alzheimer's Disease and Related Disorders Association (ADRDA) in your area, the American Association for Geriatric Psychiatry, the American Geriatrics Society, or the Gerontological Society of America may help you find a suitable physician (see Resources for this chapter). If you cannot find a physician in your area who specializes in geriatrics, or if you do not feel comfortable with her or him, the ADRDA will be able to give you names of internists, neurologists, or psychiatrists interested and experienced in treating the elderly, or hospitals that have set up special clinics to treat diseases of the Alzheimer type.

To date, the only definitive diagnosis of Alzheimer's disease is a postmortem examination of the brain. The only direct means of diagnosing the disease during the person's lifetime is the surgical removal and examination of brain tissue, a procedure too dangerous to perform routinely. Therefore, diagnosis takes place through the careful elimination of all other possible causes of a person's mental changes. Diagnostic tests should include a complete history and physical examination, a neurological and a psychiatric examination, neuropsychological and neurodiagnostic tests, and a functional evaluation to discover how much the person can do for herself.

The physical exam should include diagnostic tests for endocrine, hormonal, liver, kidney, and heart problems. The physician should also ask about family history and any history of mental disturbances, as well as the patient's social and occupational background, including education and exposure to toxic chemicals. The possibility of a fall or accident within the last six months should be explored. The way in which the symptoms came on and how they progressed over time is important to determine. The neuropsychological examination tests functions such as a person's ability to remember, to concentrate, to do abstract reasoning, to do calculations, and to copy designs.

Neurodiagnostic tests are procedures to evaluate brain function and include a brain-wave recording (electroencephalogram, or EEG) and a CAT or CT scan (computerized axial tomography), which forms a picture of the brain from X-ray images. The CAT scan can also locate possible brain cell loss, and can rule out the possibility of a stroke or brain tumor. Magnetic resonance imaging (MRI) may be used to assess structural changes in the brain, and the SPECT scan (single photon emission computed tomography) is sometimes used to evaluate the metabolic activity of the brain. MRI and SPECT scans are valuable in research on Alzheimer's disease but are as yet too experimental to be useful in routine diagnosis.

Extensive diagnostic testing can be an exhausting trial. It is important to find healthcare personnel who understand the condition, and who will not upset or exhaust the person by forcing too much testing at one stretch.

Treatment of Alzheimer's Disease

There is currently no treatment that cures, halts the progress of, or has a predictably and reliably helpful effect on Alzheimer's disease. However, many studies are under way. There is much false information in the media concerning possible cures. This misinformation takes advantage of our understandable need for encouraging, hopeful news. It is important to get reliable information on the results of new research.* Your physician, nurse, or social worker and the Alzheimer's Disease and Related Disorders Association nearest you can be of help. There are now twenty-eight major federally funded research centers in the United States. Some large hospitals and research centers are conducting studies of drugs that may help treat Alzheimer's and related disorders. You may want to consider entering the affected person in such a study if one is being conducted near you. (Contact the national headquarters of ADRDA, listed under Resources for this chapter, for information on these studies.)

Some symptoms of Alzheimer's disease, such as uncontrollable agitation, sleeplessness, night wandering, and hallucinations, are extremely hard on the caregiver; drugs to control these behaviors without harming the stricken person are urgently needed. Sometimes sedatives will make the stricken person's behavior more tolerable. However, all drugs, especially those that alter mental function, can have negative effects. It is important that drugs be administered under the care of a knowledgeable physician. In general, it is advisable to be cautious with all tranquilizers and to begin with the lowest possible doses, advancing slowly. Caregiver and physician should closely watch the stricken person for positive as well as adverse effects of all prescribed drugs, and they should frequently reevaluate the need for continued doses.

Environmental adaptations may help with troublesome behavioral changes.[9] For example, keeping lights on may diminish the agitation that some people with Alzheimer's exhibit at sundown, and serving menus consisting of finger foods will be more convenient for those who no longer recognize or use eating utensils.

*If you wish to aid future research on Alzheimer's disease, you can plan ahead for an autopsy of the afflicted person by contacting the nearest autopsy representative. (Call the national headquarters of the ADRDA, listed in Resources, page 501.) The purposes of an autopsy are to provide families with a posthumous, definitive diagnosis of Alzheimer's and to provide brain tissue for research.

Cause and Prevention

It is not clear whether there is a single cause of Alzheimer's disease; instead, many contributing factors may work together to lead to the development of the disease. Since the cause or causes are not known, prevention is also a matter of speculation. The aging of the brain may in itself be a main contributing factor, accelerated and augmented by other factors such as head injuries, smoking, environmental toxins, hormonal changes, nutritional deficiencies, stress, a slow virus, hereditary and familial predisposition, or malfunction of the immune system. Research showing concentrated forms of aluminum in the brains of Alzheimer's victims has led to speculation that exposure to aluminum contributes to Alzheimer's disease. However, there is no higher incidence among aluminum workers than among the general population; and exposure to aluminum in daily life—for example, through cookware—does not lead to higher aluminum concentration in the body. It is equally likely that higher brain levels of aluminum are a consequence rather than a cause of the disease.

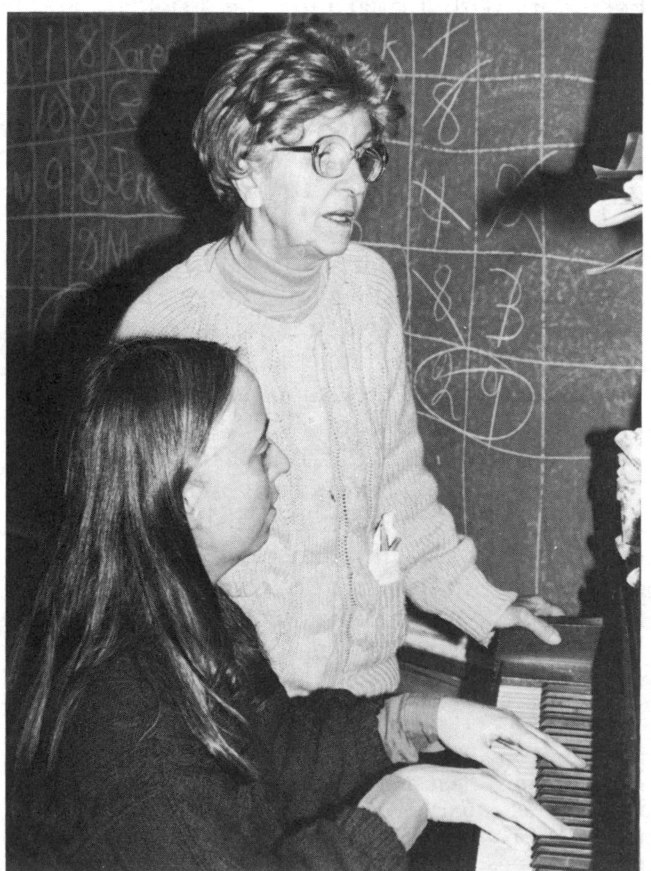

Anne Chapman Tremearne

A small group of people develop Alzheimer's disease earlier—between the ages of thirty-five and sixty-five. At least two genes (one on chromosome 21 and one on chromosome 14) have been identified as having a major effect on susceptibility to this form of the disease. Chromosome 19 has been linked to the form of Alzheimer's disease that develops after the age of sixty-five. It is therefore likely that a number of genes play a role in the development of Alzheimer's disease. Statistics tell us that a person with an immediate family member with Alzheimer's disease has at least a four-times-greater risk of developing the disease than a person without a history of Alzheimer's disease in the family. It is also true that many people with these genes do not develop the disease, so research is needed to clarify the many other factors that affect one's likelihood of developing the disease.[10]

Counseling for Caregivers and Persons with Alzheimer's

Group or individual counseling sessions can be important for the caregiver. They also are sometimes offered for the afflicted person, but only people in the early stages of the disease do well in counseling sessions. To find out about counseling programs, consult your physician or get in touch with local hospital and mental health centers that might offer such sessions. The ADRDA chapter nearest you will also know about types and locations of help available.

- *Respite:* In adult day health centers, people with Alzheimer's take part in activities according to their own abilities within a supervised, structured program. These provide the ill person with attention and social interaction, and provide caregivers with much-needed intervals of rest and relief. Respite in-home services, weekend assistance programs, and long-term (one to two weeks) respite care programs are also starting to develop in some hospitals and nursing homes.
- *Family Treatment:* In group sessions, partners, relatives, children, or close friends who are involved in caring for a person with Alzheimer's come together with a therapist to discuss fears and frustrations, deal with family crises that arise when a family member is diagnosed with dementia, ask questions, and exchange ideas for solving practical management problems.
- *Caregivers' Support Groups:* Caregivers meet

regularly to talk about their situation and exchange information informally or with a group leader. Such groups offer the caregiver practical information and ideas, emotional support, and social contact.

- *Support Groups for Persons with Alzheimer's Disease:* Persons in earlier phases of the disease meet without family members but under the guidance of a therapist to discuss the fears, embarrassments, and needs of their daily lives; to talk about what may happen in the future; and to exchange ideas for coping and support.
- *Reality Orientation or Cognitive Training:* Memory training sessions are offered in which an impaired person practices using association to remember information such as important names and addresses, and is repeatedly reoriented as to date, time, and place. It does not appear that such methods actually help the memory of the person with Alzheimer's, but in the early stages of the disease the sessions provide human contact and a supportive, structured environment. For people in the later stages, such sessions are generally not helpful.

The caregivers' support group certainly has been one thing that has kept my sanity together. Some group members are up to date on all of the resources for care and support agencies and are tremendously helpful. Also, I think just the feeling that you're not the only one in the circumstances is helpful. We're there to support each other with whatever knowledge and information we have or to hand out tissues to those who are in tears. [a fifty-seven-year-old woman]

Impact on the Stricken Person

Personal Impact of Alzheimer's Disease

Alzheimer's disease and other progressive dementias perhaps cause more stress and change in the stricken person and within the home than any other conditions. This is because of the devastating personality change and loss of control that the stricken person experiences.

I feel like half a person. Where's the rest of me? I really hate this and I'm frightened. Maybe listening to me will open a world that's closed to a lot of people. Nobody knows what it's like. They just don't understand. [a seventy-two-year-old woman in the early stage of Alzheimer's disease]

With the disease, both recent and remote memory are eventually lost. Losing recent memory means forgetting what happened an hour or even a minute ago and being unable to learn new information or lay down new memories. For the person with Alzheimer's, life is like continually walking into the middle of a movie, with no idea of what happened before, and no understanding of what is happening now. She may forget the names and faces of recently met friends and acquaintances, forget recent births and deaths in the family, and forget that she has just eaten and ask when dinner will be ready.

Losing remote memory means forgetting the past, including what we learned as children. This includes activities we take for granted—brushing our teeth, taking a bath, getting dressed, holding a conversation, using the toilet. As the disease progresses the victim regresses. She may forget how to use eating utensils, forget how to dress, forget the sensations of hot and cold, forget how to control bowel and urine, forget what food is, and how to chew and swallow. She may forget inhibitions learned in childhood and may expose or touch her sexual parts in public. The person with Alzheimer's loses a sense of time and can no longer look forward or back, or turn to the collected knowledge of her life for help. With such helplessness, partnerships between adults slowly change to parent/child-type relationships, or an adult child may have to become responsible for a stricken mother or father.

I miss having a partner. Max used to go to the office and stay all day five days a week. Now he doesn't go anywhere at all without me, and that makes a difference in my home life, because I'm very conscious of this individual who is solely dependent on me. And going to parties—well, anywhere—Max used to go to church with me some, and he always did the driving—he was an excellent driver. I find that I've lost the independent mind and gained a dependent one. [a seventy-six-year-old woman]

The stricken person's response to dementia is complex, changes as the disease progresses, and varies greatly from person to person. During the early stages the person may notice the changes within herself and be frightened and depressed by them. She may lose her job because she is progressively incompetent or because of personality changes unacceptable to those around her. She may be aware of her changed role within the household, as more and more responsibilities are taken from her.[11]

It's like being in a ship by yourself. I can't function as I did before and I feel as if I'm odd. I'm so different from everybody else and I wonder if they like me. I'm so forgetful that I'm afraid when I'm with other people I'm going to sound stupid. But when friends ask me out, I go. And I find I'm much more relaxed once I'm with them. They're very kind to me. [a seventy-two-year-old woman in the early stage of Alzheimer's disease]

Throughout the course of the disease, but especially in the early stages, the stricken person may notice changes in the way others treat her and react with anxiety and embarrassment at her own behavior. But usually she is unaware of her declining capacities and may blame the caregiver for hiding things she cannot find or for keeping dates and names a secret. She may become angry with the caregiver who prevents her from driving or managing her bank account.

Impact on the Caregiver

I think Alzheimer's disease is probably harder on the caregiver than it is on the victim. But I wouldn't change places for anything. [a seventy-eight-year-old caregiver]

Caring for someone with Alzheimer's disease takes a tremendous physical and emotional toll on the caregiver. In addition to the usual strains of caring for anyone with a long-term illness, unlimited patience and self-control are needed to cope with repetitive or unintelligible conversation, with complete silence, with extreme agitation, sudden aggression, or assault, or with any other of the possible changes in a stricken person's character. Along with this comes anger at the stricken person and inevitable feelings of guilt for becoming impatient, angry, and resentful—and showing it.

If I'm a little tired and Bob pursues a subject until—you have no idea how people like that can pursue a subject—I can feel myself getting tense and angry. Occasionally, only when I get really angry, does he stop. But I don't like to get angry like that. It's hard on me, and I feel that I've got to work something out to help. I've thought about biofeedback that lets you know how tense you are so I can learn to relax. That might help me, relieve me. [a seventy-seven-year-old woman]

We literally had to watch Mother minute by minute because she was active enough then to put an empty pot on the stove and turn it on. She wasn't sleeping at night so at midnight she thought it was morning, would dress herself in several layers of clothing, and walk down the stairs and out the door. We were chasing her all night long. I didn't have the emotional energy to think out some of the solutions like having a bell on the door which would buzz when she went out. All those things you figure out when you have enough leisure to think them through, but when you're in the middle of it you're so exhausted, so overwhelmed, that you're just sort of getting through the next second. We were all just grimly going step by step, putting one foot in front of the other. [a woman in her forties]

Mourning to Do

The new year and a fresh fall of snow,
The new year and mourning to do
Alone in the lovely silent house,
Alone as the inner eye opens at last—
Not as the shutter of a camera with a click,
But like a gentle-waking in a dark room
Before dawn when familiar objects take on
Substances out of their shadowy corners
And come to life. So with my lost love,
For years lost in the darkness of her mind,
Tied to a wheelchair, not knowing where she was
Or who she had been when we lived together
In amity, peaceful as turtledoves.

Judy is dead. Judy is gone forever.

I cannot fathom that darkness, nor know
Whether the true spirit is alive again.
But what I do know is the peace of it,
And in the darkened room before dawn, I lie
Awake and let the good tears flow at last,
And as light touches the chest of drawers
And the windows grow transparent, rest,
Happy to be mourning what was singular
And comforting as the paintings on the wall,
All that can now come to life in my mind,
Good memories fresh and sweet as the dawn—
Judy drinking her tea with a cat on her lap,
And our many little walks before suppertime.
So it is now the gentle waking to what was,
And what is and will be as long as I am alive.
"Happy grieving," someone said who knew—
Happy the dawn of memory and the sunrise.

*May Sarton**

The caregiver may feel deserted as she takes on more and more responsibilities in the home and perhaps becomes the sole means of financial support. Unlike people with diseases that mainly affect the body, a person with Alzheimer's disease often gives little or no thanks or recogni-

*"Mourning to Do" is reprinted from *Letters from Maine, New Poems* by May Sarton, by permission of the author and W. W. Norton & Company, Inc. Copyright © by May Sarton.

tion. The caregiver may feel resentful at the lack of reward for constant care. This resentment can be fed by a feeling that she is caring for a stranger—for someone whose behavior has become odd and embarrassing and who no longer knows or loves her. Added to this may come further feelings of guilt, as the caregiver feels love dying under the strain, and perhaps wishes for the death of the stricken person.

Caregivers of sexual partners experience a loss of companionship and intimacy and often turn to others for close friendship. They have to decide whether such relationships will include sex. Painful conflicts between loyalty to an ailing partner and one's own needs often result.

The strain of caring for a demented person leads to a high rate of stress-related disorders. Over 50 percent of caregivers show symptoms of anxiety and depression, including insomnia, headaches, irritability, and increased blood pressure.[12] The caregiver can become increasingly forgetful under stress, and fear that she or he too is developing the disease. In addition, when whole families are involved in the caregiving process, family life may virtually cease under the burden.

When we took my stricken dad in to live with us, supper table conversation became nonexistent. When you've got relationships within a family, you've got to have time to get together as a family, go away together—just have a meal together and talk together. I have two college-age daughters. One is saying, "I can't wait to get away from this place." The other is saying, "Home's the most awful place in the world." I feel terribly guilty and also frightened that they will never want to come home; that they won't remember home with enough pleasure to want to spend time with me. [a woman in her forties]

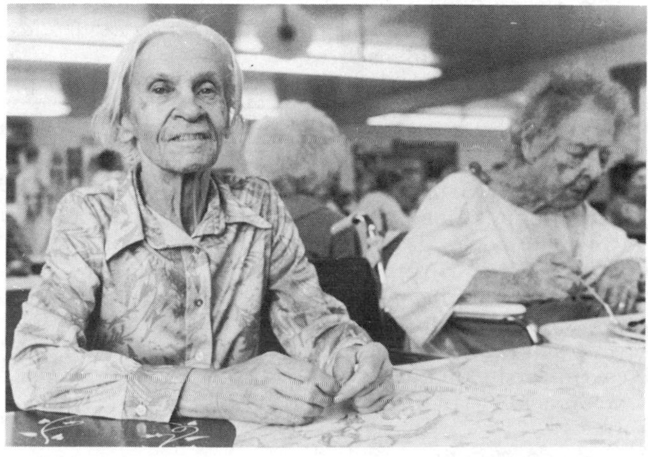

Marianne Gontarz

In addition to the burden of caring comes the insult of a medical-insurance system that ignores the victim's and the caregiver's urgent needs. At present neither Medicare nor supplementary insurance covers the cost of long-term care at home, in respite programs, or nursing homes. Only those eligible for Medicaid receive long-term-care benefits. An estimated 80 percent of the cost of all long-term care both at home and in a nursing home is provided by the caregivers and by informal community support, not by public funds.[13] The financial burden can be ruinous for family members, especially elderly partners.

The Special Role of Family and Friends

In such a difficult time, the support of friends and relatives becomes more important than ever. With Alzheimer's disease such support is difficult to sustain, since the stricken person loses the social traits that drew others to her: a sense of humor, kindness, special interests and talents. She also loses control over language as a means of communication. The stricken person becomes a stranger to relatives and friends, who may react with withdrawal and avoidance, appalled at the loved one's condition. In addition, visits can be difficult to manage since the victim is often confused by any changes in the daily routine and embarrassed by her inability to remember who the visitors are. The resulting isolation of the victim may also lead to isolation of the caregiver.

As relatives or friends of Alzheimer's disease victims, it is important for us to remind ourselves that the stricken person still needs and recognizes affection even if she may neither remember nor return it. Often just quietly holding the stricken person's hand will help. We should also keep in mind the caregiver's needs for social contact, a change of scene, and an understanding ear. However, our instinct to withdraw is understandable, since many of us fear becoming demented more than we fear any other illness or infirmity that may come with age. Understanding as much as we can about the disease may help alleviate our anxiety, especially when we know that in most cases the increased forgetfulness that many of us experience is not a sign of disease. For those of us who do not have friends or relatives with Alzheimer's, understanding the disease will help us give support to those who do. It will keep us from isolating stricken people and their caregivers out of fear.

CARING FOR THE CAREGIVER

Public discussion of the need for care, information, and financial aid is increasing. Several states have established commissions or task forces on dementias related to aging, and some have authorized further, but still inadequate, state funding for long-term care. But state funding cannot compensate for the lack of a national funding policy. Many of us who are caregivers have become vocal in demanding more help and are working with others through local ADRDA associations.

We need:

- Health professionals who are trained in the diagnosis and care of Alzheimer's disease and related disorders, and who will take the time to listen and talk to us.
- Current, reliable information about research on the cause, prevention, and cure of Alzheimer's disease.
- A supportive community of persons sharing their caregiving experiences.
- Regular periods of relief from daily caregiving—relief in the form of adult day care or aides in the home.
- Regular one- to two-week periods of respite from caregiving in order to maintain our own physical and mental health. Government-funded respite centers and home nursing are needed to make this possible.
- Nurse practitioners who can make home visits to prevent unnecessary disease complications.
- Medicare and private insurance coverage for long-term care within the home, in day-care centers, and in nursing homes.
- Hospital and nursing-home staff trained in caring for the demented who will treat our loved ones with dignity and with respect for their humanity.
- Help of lawyers trained to advise us when a victim becomes legally incompetent.
- Financial guidelines to protect assets from being completely depleted by the cost of full-time care.
- Police and fire department personnel who are informed about Alzheimer's disease and related disorders to help lost and wandering afflicted persons and to intervene in serious crises.
- Support of family and friends.

NOTES

1. K. Warner Schaie and James Geiwitz, *Adult Development and Aging.* Boston: Little, Brown, 1982, pp. 217–39.

2. Some studies show that approximately 33 percent of those between eighty and eighty-five show no decline on neuropsychological tests, including tests of memory, compared with younger age groups. A. L. Benton, et al., "Normative Observations on Neuropsychological Test Performances in Old Age." *Journal of Clinical Neuropsychology,* Vol. 3, No. 1 (May 1981), pp. 33–42; and Paul Verhaeghen, "Facts and Fiction About Memory Aging: A Quantitative Integration of Research Findings." *Journal of Gerontology,* Vol. 48, No. 4 (1993), pp. 157–71.

3. "Memory Loss May Follow Use of Anticholinergics." *Medical World News,* Aug. 12, 1985, p. 51.

4. Robert N. Butler, "Clinical Needs Assessment Studies Can Benefit Research on Aging." *Hospitals,* Vol. 55, No. 8 (Apr. 16, 1981), pp. 94–98.

5. Barry Reisberg, *A Guide to Alzheimer's Disease: For Families, Spouses, and Friends.* New York: The Free Press, 1981, p. 14.

6. Ingmar Skoog, "A Population-Based Study of Dementia in 85-Year-Olds." *The New England Journal of Medicine,* Vol. 328, No. 3 (Jan. 21, 1993), pp. 353–58.

7. This estimate is from the *Report of the Secretary's Task Force on Alzheimer's Disease,* U.S. Department of Health and Human Services, September 1984. However, accurate statistics on Alzheimer's are relatively new and in the process of revision.

8. U.S. Department of Health and Human Services, *Alzheimer's Disease Handbook,* Vol. I. San Francisco: Aging Health Policy Center, University of California, April 1984, p. 2.

9. Uriel Cohen and Gerald Weisman, *Holding on to Home: Designing Environments for People with Dementia.* Baltimore: Johns Hopkins Press, 1991.

10. Judy Foreman, "A New Picture of Alzheimer's." *The Boston Globe,* Feb. 15, 1993, pp. 25, 30.

11. John Bond, "The Medicalization of Dementia." *Journal of Aging Studies,* Vol. 6, No. 4 (1992), pp. 397–403.

12. J. R. A. Sanford, "Tolerance of Debility in Elderly Dependents by Supporters at Home: Its Significance for Hospital Practice." *British Medical Journal,* Vol. 3, No. 5981 (Aug. 23, 1975), pp. 471–73.

13. Lisa Gwyther, "A Statewide Family Support Program Mobilizes Mutual Support." *Center Reports on Advances in Research,* Vol. 6, No. 4 (December 1982), p. 2. Duke University Center for the Study of Aging and Human Development.

29

DYING AND DEATH

✦

BY MARY C. HOWELL, MARY C. ALLEN, AND PAULA B. DORESS-WORTERS

SPECIAL THANKS TO JANE STRETE

1994 UPDATE BY PAULA B. DORESS-WORTERS WITH SPECIAL THANKS TO ANNE ARSENAULT

RESOURCES FOR THIS CHAPTER ON PAGES 502–4

In many cultures, preparing for and making sense of death is the work of women, especially of old women. Whether or not it's fair or best, women in most societies, including our own, still act as the nurturers, caregivers, and custodians of those near death. Even with the removal of death to the institutional sphere, dying remains the province of women who work in those institutions.

The last person most of us see on earth is a woman—the nurse's aide (significantly one of the least paid and least valued workers in our society). . . . These are, in a sense, the midwives of death.[1]

Thus, it is most often women who meet the emotional and pragmatic needs surrounding death.

By the age of fifty-seven I had nursed my husband through terminal cancer, lived through widowhood, and been close to two dear friends who died. I assisted one friend and supported her family through the process of her committing suicide. I feel that my middle years have been significant in bringing me into close and familiar contact with dying and death.

BEREAVEMENT AND GRIEF

Grief is a normal reaction to the stress of losing someone. It is not a pathological reaction that needs to be "cured." According to Phyllis R. Silverman, founder of the widow-to-widow movement, we may go through several phases of grieving the loss of someone we care deeply about. At first, we may feel numb or dazed, unable to believe that such a grievous loss could have happened. That numbness often carries us through the first days and weeks, allowing us to function. Gradually, we begin to come to terms with the reality of the loss, realizing that we can no longer live as before. Eventually, when we can remember our loved one with less pain, most of us accommodate to our loss. Then we restructure our lives to make room for new roles and relationships.[2]

The following is excerpted from a woman's journal recording her feelings about her lover's death over a period of years:

In what later seemed to be extraordinary word usage, the doctor called me to say the operation on Karen was "successful." They resectioned her colon and took out the

tumor; she would not need a colostomy. But the tumor has metastasized and she will die; six months to two years is all they give her. No real hope.

It is 2:30 A.M. and I can't sleep because of rage at God, and then because of guilt. And because of fear for myself. How will I live without Karen to tell me I am brilliant and beautiful?

Images run through my head. Her hand warming my asthma-congested chest. Her step—quick, strong, fast up the stairs. As I remember that sound, I smile; the pain recedes. But if I shut my journal, the pain will return.

Does everyone who is dying look bewildered? Her head in my lap; her body spooned in pain. Dying means dependency. Pain. Listlessness. Fever. Exhaustion. Dying is frightening.

Death is final, but dying can drag on and on and on, destroying everyone. It saps the strength of the healthy and makes them sick.

My first birthday without her. Our anniversary. Her first birthday dead. My first Christmas and first New Year without her. One year it was the greatest New Year of my life, and the next year the woman who gave it to me was dead.

Each marker brings Karen to me and takes her. Soon my first spring without her. My first summer. Then a year since I last saw her will pass. A year since her death; a year since her funeral. And I will put a headstone in my heart: Karen, my dearest.[3]

Any one loss can remind us of all the other losses we have known—especially the earliest ones, which might not have been fully understood or explored.

When my lover died I was fifty-six. Over the next two years I relived, in a way, all of the other great sadnesses of my life—when my father left us when I was little, my mother's death, the endings of other love affairs. I don't think I had realized how much there was for me to mourn! [a sixty-two-year-old woman]

Acceptance of death can come only after a full experience of mourning that may last many months or even years.

My daughter died almost forty years ago, when she was ten. I'm still angry, and I still miss her. But for years after she died I couldn't quite believe that it had really happened—I kept thinking I heard her in the house. Now I can accept what happened, even if I don't like it. [a seventy-eight-year-old woman]

My husband died eighteen years ago and even though today I have a happy, full life, I still miss him. I am often reminded of what he is missing, especially at happy moments, such as the children's high school and college graduations, which are tinged with the wish that he were alive to share the joy. [a fifty-four-year-old woman]

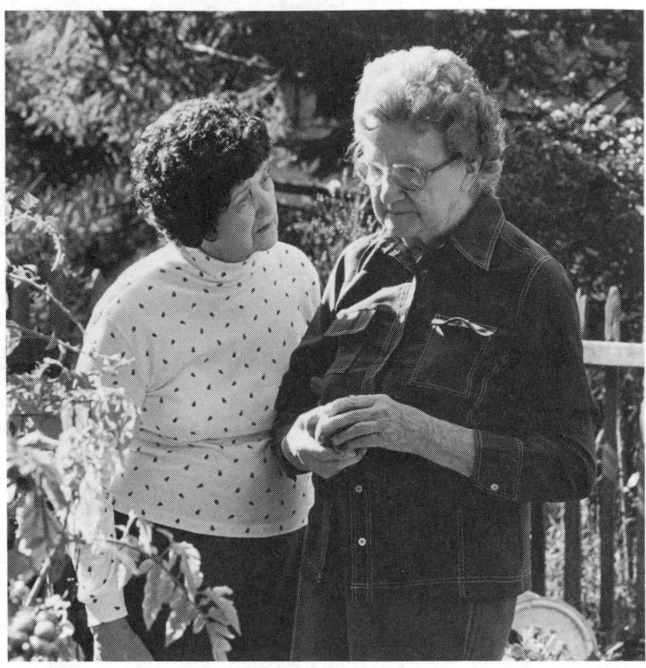

Deborah Kahn

Mental-health experts have observed that "troubled mourning" can be a principal reason for unhappiness and problems later in life. Mourning can go wrong in a variety of ways. We may be unable to grieve at the time of loss, feeling too numb to cry or to express our feelings in any way at all. We may begin to grieve but cut the process short, because of pressure to appear self-possessed for a job or family or friends. Or we may suppress our grief, drive it underground, in which case it is likely to erupt again, perhaps with surprising intensity, at the time of some later loss.

In these cases, we may try to protect ourselves from the pain of grief by adopting a self-protecting mask of composure that allows us to carry on with life as usual. Sometimes a physical illness may appear, or self-destructive behavior such as drug or alcohol addiction, an eating disorder, or repeated involvements in unsatisfactory relationships. One or more aspects of mourning can become exaggerated. We may dwell on guilt, self-blame, anger, anxiety, or sadness until we become completely incapacitated and such feelings take the place of grieving.

In each of the above cases, the underlying problem is that the person who mourns has in some way not completed the mourning process.

Sometimes friends or relatives, in a misguided desire to be helpful, urge us to "get on with it," when in fact what we need is to honor the urgency and depth of our feelings for as long as we need to do so. Paying attention to our feelings and talking about them with friends or relatives is extremely important.

When my husband was dying people helped us so much. They came to visit and brought food so that I could spend more time with him. They gave flowers and hugs, gave the children extra attention. Some people were too frightened to visit and I understood. But the friend who came fifteen hundred miles to see him before he died, the friend who came five hundred miles to hold my hand during the funeral, and the friend who stayed at the cemetery to cover his grave after the service will forever have my gratitude.

I was comforted by the notes and cards people sent me. I read them over and over again for many months, nurtured by the care, sympathy, and support they provided. Best of all were the handwritten notes that included something about the writer's relationship with my husband or memories of times together—sometimes things that were new to me. I received notes from people I had not known and was strengthened by their consideration. Even the printed cards and the simplest notes indicating that someone was thinking of me comforted me. Nineteen years later, I still have all the messages in a box so our now-grown children can share with their children how the grandfather they will never know touched the lives of so many others. [a fifty-four-year-old woman]

When my husband died it was like I was paralyzed socially for months after. My two good friends did me a great service just by sitting with me. Sometimes I would cry and sometimes I'd just be angry. Sometimes I was so sad I could hardly talk. They'd come over to visit me at least twice a week, and they stayed with it for more than a year. When I felt better I could be a good friend to them again. [a sixty-four-year-old woman]

I learned a lot about anger after my mother died. Somehow, when I was mourning, lots of anger came out that I didn't know was in me. My daughter suggested beating a pillow with a stick to get the anger out, and finally I got so I could talk with my husband and also with my daughter about some of the reasons why I felt so much anger at my poor mother. [a forty-three-year-old woman]

Observing religious and/or cultural traditions, writing about our feelings in a journal, talking to family and friends, meditating, reading poetry, watching emotion-evoking movies or plays, and singing or listening to familiar songs can all help us feel our grief as deeply and fully as we need. Joining a self-help group of people who are grieving, such as a widow-to-widow group or a hospice group, can be a great comfort. Such groups help us realize that what we are feeling is "normal" and is shared by others.

For some of us it is useful to get professional help—from a clergyman, for example, or perhaps from a bereavement counselor—to deal with the process of mourning.

I functioned extremely well most of the time (everyone always said how well), but I felt like I was just going through the motions, waiting for my husband to come home. Three times in the past four years I've arrived at the point where I felt a need for counseling. Each time I've learned more about myself. The counseling has helped me grow and find new meaning in my life. [a woman in her fifties]

The loss of a child or grandchild can be particularly painful. If death is caused by a sudden, unexpected accident that allows little or no time beforehand for preparation, as is often the case when someone we love dies young, the loss may be even more difficult to come to terms with. We cannot comfort ourselves by saying, "Well, she's lived a long and full life and it was her time to die." Even if we lose a child in her or his middle

HOW TO HELP A DYING OR RECENTLY BEREAVED PERSON

- Give them the time and quiet listening to express their feelings. Express your own sadness and regret, but do not presume to tell a bereaved or dying person that a death is "for the best," even if after a long illness. We don't really know how someone feels unless she or he tells us.
- Offer distractions, other topics of mutual interest, but be comfortable with silence and resist the need to fill every minute with words. Your very presence will help.
- Take care of a dying or bereaved person; do not expect her or him to take care of you. Bring food if you visit someone's home.
- Do send cards or notes if you can't visit.
- Offer help, and be specific in your suggestions. Say, "I have two hours free on Saturday. Do you want me to shop for you, or is there something else I can do that would be helpful?"

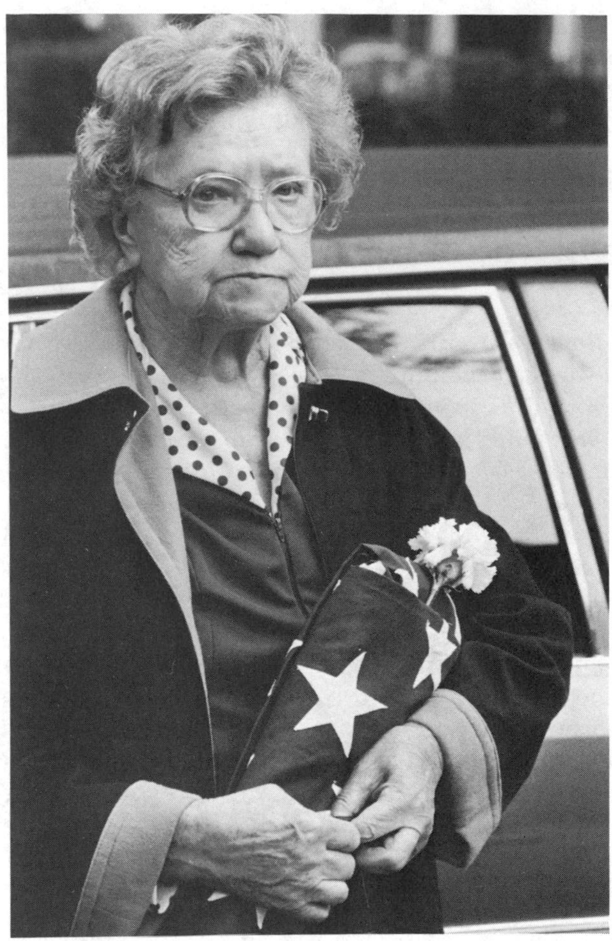

Deborah Kahn

or late years, we may feel a sense of unfairness, as if the natural order of things has been violated. This was not a loss we expected to sustain.

Losing my only daughter to AIDS was the hardest, most heartbreaking thing that has ever happened in my life. I kept trying to make sense of it. I couldn't get over my guilt. Why did I have to get sick? Why didn't I make her stay where she was instead of coming here to take care of me? Who would have known that she would fall in love with a man who would give her AIDS? He shot between his toes and hidden places on his body so she wouldn't notice the tracks. Only my faith in God and the help of my therapist carried me through my anger, my guilt, and wanting to die myself. Finally, I was able to accept her death and to cherish the happy years we had before she passed on. [a sixty-nine-year-old woman]

When death is expected, not only the person who is dying but also those who expect to be survivors have time to make some preparations, get relationships and business affairs in order, and reminisce and say good-bye.

My father died of a heart attack and my mother died of cancer. My father's death was a surprise and a shock, and my mother's death was a long ordeal. I know that people sometimes think that a sudden and quick death is easier, but for me it was important to talk with my mother and even just to sit and hold her hand, and though those last weeks and months were hard I'm grateful we had them. With my father there was no time to say good-bye. I wish there had been. [a forty-nine-year-old woman]

When we are faced with the shock of a sudden, unexpected death, we often console ourselves with the knowledge that the person we loved did not suffer. While having time to prepare for a death may be easier on our survivors, many of us would choose an unanticipated and painless death for ourselves.

When death comes at the end of a prolonged and chronic illness, our feelings may take longer to sort out. We may have already grieved, years ago, for the loss of the whole, well person we used to know.

My sister developed the first symptoms of Alzheimer's when she was sixty-two. I took care of her, moved into her apartment for five years so she could stay in familiar surroundings. Then I had to put her into a nursing home, where I visited her twice a week. I never missed a week for nine more years until she died. There was very little that anybody could do for her. It was very hard to see her become just a thin little curled-up ball in her bed. For the last seven years she didn't recognize me or even talk at all. She was my only sister, and it was terribly sad for me. [a sixty-two-year-old woman]

We may feel a sense of release for ourselves and for the person who died after prolonged suffering. But later, intense, renewed feelings of loss may surface.

Even though I thought I had prepared myself mentally for the inevitable, I found I was terribly shocked, even surprised, when my mother finally did die. I understand now that shock after a death is common among those close to a person, even when the death was expected.[4]

Coming to Terms with Our Own Deaths

One of the important developmental tasks of the second half of life is coming to a personal understanding, perhaps even an acceptance, of death. Some of us continue to feel ambivalent and scared about acknowledging death.

A few of my friends have died young. We all knew each other for so long. (We had a card-playing group.) Three of them were my age. One of them I met recently and recognized her name from elementary school, and so we were the same age. Another one was a few months older, so we were all in the same age bracket. Now my sister-in-law just died and she was only sixty-three. This has been on my mind so much lately, you know, reaching this point that people my age are starting to go. I never used to think of these things before. Like if an aunt or an uncle died that's one thing, but now it's cousins! One cousin my age died this summer, so I start to think "It's our turn" and in what order are we going? [a sixty-seven-year-old woman]

Intellectually, I'm very glib about it, but in my gut I can't accept that one day I won't be here. [a seventy-four-year-old woman]

Maybe no one can ever be fully "ready" for death in the sense of knowing about and fully accepting the experience in advance. But we can prepare ourselves in a variety of ways.[5]

I feel a greater awareness of a mystery and beauty in life since I have accepted death as a personal eventuality for me. I don't remember exactly when that awareness came. Before then, I had thought of death "out there," and now I know that one day it will be a reality for me. Eventually I am going to die. In a way, that has released me for more vivid living. [a seventy-eight-year-old woman]

I've dealt with losing loved ones many times in my life, and after seventy years of repetition of that experience of grief I find the thing that's so hard to deal with is that some person who has been a reality in your life no longer exists. When you're a kid, you learn how to separate fantasy from reality. But then, when you get older, you have to learn how to let go of a reality—that person no longer exists. I've got a handle on that from years of experience with it. So I no longer worry about my own personal death. [a seventy-three-year-old woman]

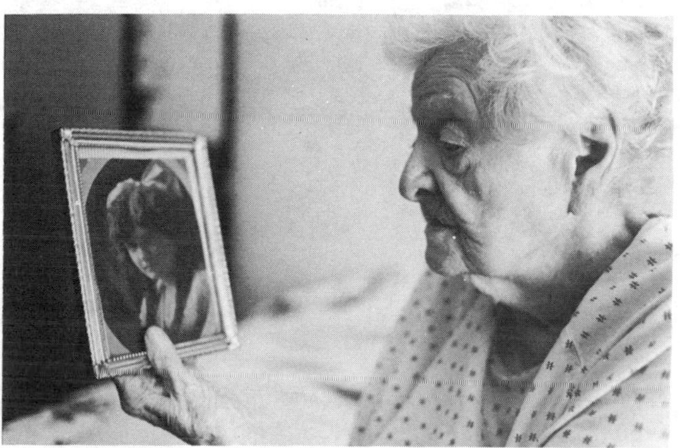

Marianne Gontarz

Some of us are comforted by religious, spiritual, or humanistic beliefs about life and death.

I believe that I am not just a body which is perishable but I am a spirit which is eternal. I believe that death is only an exit from this temporary life of unreality into a glorious new life of reality. I hope, therefore, that there will be only rejoicing, not grief, at the time of my release. I am trying to avoid being "earthbound" by releasing my attachments to material objects and persons before I enter this transition. [a ninety-two-year-old woman]

What I've been aware of lately because of a number of instances of my being thrown up against death is that I have a different perception of relationships. Death is not a termination of my life because my influence will continue until the last person who knew me has died. [a woman in her fifties]

Living each moment as fully as possible is probably the most important way to help ourselves become less fearful of death.

I do not look to the future with dread. It has to be shorter than my past but it does not have to be less rich. I'm more relaxed. I don't try to do everything.

That means I can take time for quiet, for meditation, alternate this with activity, and see how I can keep a moving, living balance between the two. [a seventy-eight-year-old woman]

*Death, I am learning through my own experience, need not be frightening. After all, we are all born terminal cases, because we will all die, at one time or another. Death is part of life. I have lived life fully and enjoyed it greatly, which makes it easier to consider bowing out than if you feel that you have missed out on a lot.**

Providing support to others can also help us come to terms with death. We can serve as resources for one another and create supportive networks that give us the strength and companionship we need to get through hard times.

On the day before her fifty-eighth birthday, my friend Maggy Krebs died in a Boston hospital. Maggy was a fem-

*Tish Sommers, age seventy, in a letter to members of the Older Women's League about her expected death. Tish founded and led the twenty-three-thousand-member organization after her cancer was diagnosed.

inist artist. * *Her humor, her drawings and paintings, and her music had filled many lives with joy. Because I believe that the final months of her life and her death were models for all independent women, I want to tell you part of the story.*

For months, Maggy gathered around her a group of her friends, who tended to her at her home and at the hospital. In addition to caring for Maggy, we met each other regularly, often weekly, to share our grief and anger at the anticipated loss of a friend, to find ways to share the responsibility of taking care of her and to support one another. We became a family for Maggy and for each other.

One of Maggy's legacies to us is the pride we feel that we were able to give her the comfort and love she needed. But Maggy also left a legacy of hope to all women who feel themselves to be alone by teaching us that we can support each other through the depths of illness, exhaustion, fear and loss.[6]

Sharing the responsibility as this women's group did avoids the guilt women sometimes feel when they can't do everything by themselves. An illness support group allows each woman to participate to the extent she is able to do so.

In the last four years I have come from the depths of despair to feeling that life is good and that there still is a reason and a need for me to be in this world. Helping to train hospice volunteers continues to be therapeutic for me. With the death of my husband, things which I'd only read about in books or heard others talk about became very real and personal to me. Much of my own grief work was done with the volunteer training classes, where the volunteers gave me the opportunity to talk about my experiences and my life, and the aloneness I felt at the loss of my best friend and life's companion. [a woman in her fifties]

Most of my friends are gone. You just have to say to yourself that it's something that's going to happen. But it's not easy. It helps to do all you can for your friends while they're living. I do a lot of calling on the telephone. I have a friend I call every day. He's been in the hospital a long time. I have another friend who lives down in another town who's quite sick that I call at least once a week. Death used to be scary to me. Four or five years ago, if I thought of dying, I'd push it out of my mind. But now, I think, after all, I've lived out my days and I know I've got to go. [a woman in her eighties]

Some Day This Flesh

Some day some atom of this flesh shall be
commingled with a tree,
Will taste the resinous sap spicing its veins;
Wrestle with tempests; dance with silver rains;
And stand a singing tower against the sky.

My lapping blood existence will partake
with some far, hill-girt lake,
will cherish water-lilies on its flood;
Will shadow winging bird and dreaming cloud;
And hold the evening star within its cup.

I have so joyed in campfire's comradeship;
Have felt such grip
of awed delight at dogwood's miracle;
Such rapture in the living slope of hill;
Surely I shall be fire and flower and grass!

Fear? Fear transfiguration glad as this?
Such loveliness?
With these I have so loved, to be enfurled,
inwoven in all the beauty of the world?
Perhaps—who knows?—My very heart shall be
for one mad hour of flaming ecstasy
a sunset!

Florence Luscomb

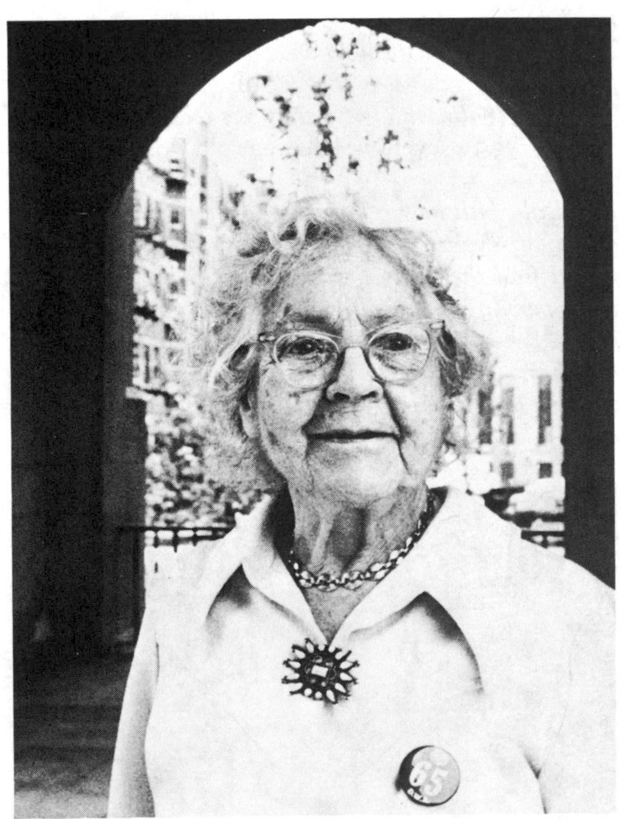

Florence Luscomb, suffragist, labor organizer, civil-rights and peace activist. Died in 1985 at age ninety-eight. *Ellen Shub*

*See pages 192 and 206 for cartoons by Maggy Krebs.

Another way to prepare ourselves for dying is to take care of any unfinished business in our lives. Most of us have unresolved relationships—some that go back quite far—that we may want to work out or perhaps just make a final statement on. We can seek out people with whom we have unfinished business and see to it that some old unforgiven hurts are healed—and recognize that some can't ever be healed. Those who have made the effort to do this say it is very important.

Before her death my sister asked to see each of her five brothers and sisters. We talked about the ways we had been close and trusting with each other, and we also talked about some of our long-standing fights and grudges. I know that the hour that she and I spent going over our times together was very important to me. It was one way to say good-bye. And I think it was important and healing for her, as well. [a forty-seven-year-old woman]

THE MEDICALIZATION OF DEATH

Understanding death has become more difficult and complicated because, in our culture, death is often a medical event. Most people in the last stages of life are in hospitals and nursing homes, and are thus "out of sight." Life-threatening situations at any age often take place in a hospital. Institutional methods of caring for the sick and dying make it difficult for us to experience and understand death as a natural end to life.

I can remember the day my grandfather died, in a tractor accident on the farm. The men brought him in from the field to the house, and my grandmother, my mother, and my aunt bathed and dressed him. It was a loving act, and a ritual, and I was terribly *impressed. I was eight at the time. My own father went from the hospital bed where he died to a funeral home, and I know my mother doesn't feel like she was a part of his dying. I'm trying to understand that difference, and what I myself want to do in that regard.* [a sixty-seven-year-old woman]

In some cultures, death is understood to be a natural transition at the end of life. Among some Native American tribes, for instance, each life is seen as a road that is expected to come to an end. The healers in those societies see themselves as "keepers of the road," guardians of health for as long as the journey goes on—not as persons who work to prevent the journey from ending in its expected transition.

But in our contemporary culture, we invest heavily in science and want to believe that through it we can control all the events of our lives. We have hope that the discoveries of science will allow us to prolong life and prevent death. These attitudes make it hard to look on death as the natural, expected end of life, and make it harder to accept the inevitability of death.

Physicians often use every possible means to prolong life without regard for its quality. The result can be feelings of anguish and helplessness on the part of the dying person, relatives, and friends.

When my husband had his heart attack I thought I should rush him to the hospital. The ambulance came right away but by the time they resuscitated him he already had a lot of brain damage. He never recovered consciousness. Everyone in the ICU [Intensive Care Unit] worked very hard to save his life, and he did live for another two weeks, but as far as I'm concerned he wasn't really alive—just a body attached to a lot of tubes and machinery. I wish now that I had just held him, cradled his head, when he first fell. I could have said good-bye that way. [a sixty-five-year-old woman]

As some medical professionals are beginning to recognize, focus on the inappropriate pursuit of a cure when the situation is clearly beyond hope can lead medical personnel to make a person's last days more painful and difficult than necessary. Of course, there are situations of acute emergency in which one cannot be sure whether recovery is possible; it is very hard to know the right thing to do in such a case. But some medical treatments designed to cure, such as chemotherapy and radiotherapy, may increase the dying person's discomfort.

Many of us may feel more secure in a hospital when we are very ill. Or we may feel we want to try, or should continue to try, medical remedies on the chance that one may heal us.

My daughter died of breast cancer at age forty-two. We thought she wanted to die at home and we were ready to take care of her there. But in the end the doctors urged her to try one more round of treatment with chemotherapy and she went back into the hospital. She never came home again, and for the last week she was so sick and in such pain that she didn't even want her teenage children to visit her. [a sixty-eight-year-old woman]

Discomforts such as pain, shortness of breath, weakness, nausea, and vomiting often precede death. The last days of living can be eased by concentrating on comfort rather than cure. (See *Dealing with Pain* in the chapter

Habits Worth Changing, pages 35–36.) Occasionally, treatments such as radiotherapy or even surgery may be used to bring relief of pain and discomfort, though it is more common to use high doses of pain-relieving drugs.

We were lucky enough to find a doctor who was willing to come to the house and could prescribe drugs for Grandma's pain and also for the nausea. We heard about the doctor because she had performed the same service for a neighbor down the street, and she made a hard time much easier than it might have been. [a thirty-six-year-old woman]

TAKING CONTROL OF OUR OWN DEATHS

Many of us would prefer not to be subjected to machines and tubes and complex technological procedures that may extend life a few extra days, weeks, or months at the expense of whatever quality it may be possible to achieve. Some of us who have such thoughts, however, will surely die in the very circumstances we deplore. How does this happen?

We tend to forget experiences that most of us have had as patients, like being moved from one treatment to another with little explanation of what is really thought to be wrong, how the treatment is supposed to work, and what to expect next, as if once we become patients we have given over the right or desire to make choices. The physician often doesn't present alternatives from which we can choose; the alternatives of *no* treatment or of treatments such as acupuncture or herbal remedies are rarely discussed. This failure to present alternatives makes it difficult for the ill person to make informed decisions. Being a patient can feel like being on a slippery slide you can't easily get off.

My daughter spent the last months of her life going to the hospital for outpatient treatments, and feeling terrible. I won't ever do that. I'm not saying it's any better to be sick from the cancer, but at least you'd feel like it's your body and your life. I'd want to have some time to myself to live a little if I thought I was going to die soon. [a fifty-nine-year-old woman]

Here are some things to remember about doctors and dying:

- Physicians cannot actually predict recovery, death, or future disability for any single patient; they can only make broad, educated guesses based on statistics for large populations. They deal in group probabilities.[7]
- Many people whose death was predicted with firm certainty by medical experts have recovered; this happens with sufficient regularity to remind us that illness is not fully understood by science.
- Each individual has a right to say how she or he will live out the last days of a soon-to-be-ended life. If living outside a hospital or without the discomfort of medical treatment is what you want, your right to do so ought to be honored.

Ten years ago, when I was forty-five, I was told I had breast cancer. For the next year I had chemotherapy and radiation—I was sick and worried the whole year. But now I feel that when the cancer comes back I just want to live with it, except for painkillers when I need them. I feel that if I'm going to live on, or die, I want to be able to experience each day as my day. *I've written letters to each of my children to let them know how important this is to me.*

Even when we try to stay in control, an illness can become overwhelming and may deplete our energy reserves, especially if we do not have a dependable support system. Though we may aspire to a serene death for ourselves or a loved one, surrounded by familiar faces, we must recognize that humans have never been able to control or predict death.

I felt like I was in a dream. I had promised my husband I wouldn't send him back to the hospital, but I was up for twenty hours each day taking care of him and I just couldn't go on. He agreed to go back because I promised him that I would live there with him. The last ten days he didn't talk but he seemed to be comfortable. They were giving him morphine intravenously. The doctor woke me at 3 A.M. to tell me he had died while I was sleeping. It bothered me that I was sleeping when he died because I had promised him that I would be with him. I don't know if he would have said anything if I had been awake. No matter how hard you try, it doesn't always work out the way you want. [a woman in her sixties]

Advance Medical Directives

If you decide that in some circumstances you would prefer to have no treatment, or treatment for comfort only, you have a right to refuse treatment. In every state, constitutional and common law support the right of any competent adult to refuse medical treatment in any situation.[8] However, writing your wishes in an advance medical directive can protect your right to refuse treatment, make it clear to your family members and health-care providers what you want, and help them to comply with your wishes.

A new federal law requires hospitals, nursing homes, HMOs, and home health agencies serving persons covered by Medicaid or Medicare to provide information upon admission about advance directives and to explain your legal rights and choices. If they will not honor your wishes they must tell you, so that you can select another institution. State laws vary on this, and may have provisions for doctors who, for reasons of conscience, will not comply with certain choices. Check with your state attorney general's office. They may be able to provide you with appropriate forms as well.

Advance medical directives can be stated in a living will or in a durable power of attorney for health care. In a living will you give directions for your future medical care, stating what you want and don't want. A durable power of attorney for health care is a document in which you appoint a health-care agent or proxy to represent you in the event you become unable to communicate your wishes. If possible, discuss your wishes with your health-care proxy or representative and give her or him copies of all relevant documents.

As of June 1993, all fifty states and the District of Columbia authorize either living wills or the appointment of a health-care agent. Three states, Massachusetts, Michigan, and New York, authorize only the appointment of a health-care agent, and two states, Alabama and Alaska, authorize only living wills.[9]

Living wills are valid only in cases of terminal illness—that is, when a person is expected to die in the near future, usually within six months, as a direct consequence of injury or illness. They are not honored in situations when a person has a slow degenerative disease or when a very old person has "multiple systems failure." In these situations, appointing a health-care proxy through a durable power of attorney may be more effective.

Another drawback of the living will is that it operates primarily for treatment refusal. If you want all possible treatments tried, a durable power of attorney is more useful[10] and may serve for treatment refusal as well.

Assuring that you get adequate medical treatment if you are severely ill may take more than writing out your wishes. The cost-containment emphasis in medical care has resulted in people being discharged from hospitals when they still hope for recovery and want treatment. Older persons, especially those with limited funds, are at an especially high risk of being discharged prematurely against their wishes.

Dying at Home

At one time, almost everybody could have expected to die in their own homes—even in their own beds. Now, death more often occurs in a hospital or nursing home. Recently, however, more people are insisting that they be allowed to die outside of these institutions.

I don't want anyone to tell me what to do. I lived all these years with my eight children, and made decisions, right or wrong, about how we'd live. I want to decide for myself now. I've no need for medicine, drugs, or hospitals, never have, and I don't want to start now. I want to die with dignity. *I'm comfortable in* my *home among my own things and with my family around me. They'll care for me. They'll respect my wishes. I can see who I want in my own home. I can eat what I want to eat. I know my own body and what it needs or can handle. I'm a private person. There's no privacy in the hospital. I want my children around me. I need their touch, their love.* [a seventy-six-year-old woman]

Mom needed to be hostess and be in charge in her home even while dying. She continued to direct and guide her children about her care. While we held a cup to her mouth, she would urge, "Eat with me." When she needed more care, we hired hospice workers. When I introduced my mom to the new worker, Mom was already in her "withdrawal from the world stage." But she drew herself together from her fetal position under the blankets to peek at this new person, and, in her weak, raspy voice, said, "Welcome to my home." These were her final words to the world. What a magnificent, feisty, independent woman this mother of mine was. She showed us how to live and how to die. Mom passed on as peacefully as possible considering her pain and weakness. [a fifty-seven-year-old woman, the daughter of the woman quoted above]

A woman who is a midwife wrote the following account of her mother's death:

This past year brought serious illness to my mother, Marion Cunningham. We sought conventional medical attention, plus an array of alternative healing practitioners. After months of misdiagnosis, Marion diagnosed herself as dying. We admitted her to the hospital and, alas, the diagnosis of lung cancer was finally acknowledged. My brother, my sister, and I stood in disbelief at her side.

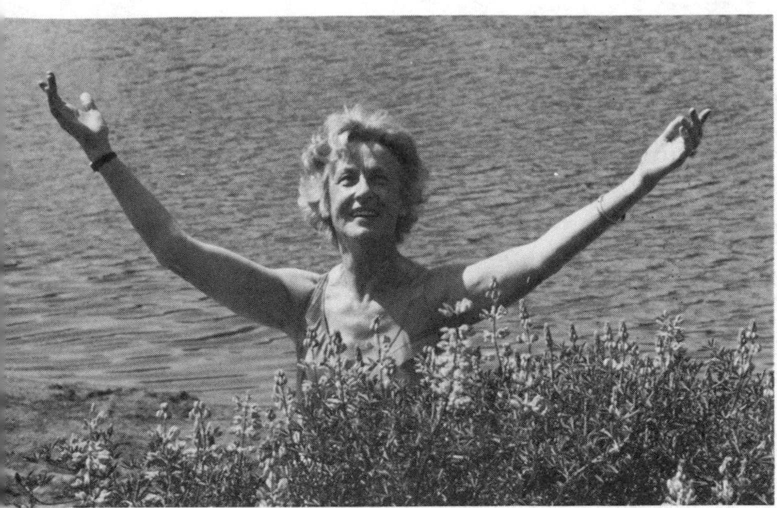

Marion Cunningham — Roxanne Cummings Potter

A pioneer in natural childbirth and in single parenting, she had always been our source of strength and inspiration. We all cried together that day. Then Marion spoke to me, words which would affect our caring of one another in the months to follow: "Why don't they have midwives for what I've got?" We decided to care for her at home.

One night at midnight I received a call from my brother . . . "Mom says she will die today and that you all should come."

And thus it was that we gathered round. My brother requested that I sing "The Goodbye Song," which I had written just a month before.

I'll see you in the babies' faces
I'll feel you in the wind
I'll hear you in the quietest places
I'll hold you in my friend.

I played on my guitar and sang to Marion, and in the midst of the song I could hear her breathing relax and I knew she would die. We watched one tear roll down her face and then she took her last breath.[11]

Hospices

A relatively new institution called the hospice has developed in response to the growing interest in dying at home. The hospice is modeled after medieval way stations that accommodated both travelers and those who were dying (death being, metaphorically, another form of travel).

Contemporary hospice agencies started out as coalitions of volunteers who were trained to visit and offer help to dying people in their own homes. Most hospice agencies now also have specially designed inpatient buildings where people can get short-term help managing uncomfortable symptoms and then go back home. The services of medical professionals are a relatively minor part of the care offered by hospices. They also provide trained volunteer visitors, visiting nurses, nurses' aides, homemakers, and bereavement counseling for family and friends.

One of the major goals of a hospice program is to maintain the quality of life through spiritual and emotional support, medication, and methods such as meditation and visualization for pain control. They will also provide temporary relief for caregivers.

Our son died of Hodgkin's disease two years ago. Toward the end he said he didn't want to go back into the hospital, no matter what. We called the hospice and they sent a volunteer who came to visit John two days a week at first and then, at the end, every day. He was almost like a member of the family, and the help he gave made a big difference to all of us—especially to John. [a seventy-six-year-old woman]

Some of these services have always been available from visiting-nurse and home-care agencies, clergy, church-visitation committees, and other local sources. But a hospice program coordinates all these services. Medicare, Medicaid, and some other insurance plans may pay part of the bill. Not all communities have hospice agencies, however. If you want to locate the hospice nearest you, call a visiting-nurse agency or a local hospital's social service department. (See Resources for this chapter for the two national hospice organizations.) A local Social Security office can also tell you which hospice programs are Medicare certified.

Choosing the Time of Our Death

Two years ago my mother, who was then eighty-three, told me that she planned to end her life by taking an overdose of pills. Her health was failing rapidly and she was going blind. She didn't want to become weak and dependent. She had always been a fierce and active woman. She wrote her intentions in a letter to me—I was her only close family member—and she told two friends and her doctor. We all told her that we would not help her accumulate enough pills to do the job. And I think we all worked very hard to help her find new reasons to be happy to be alive. But finally I understood that she really wanted to do what she had planned, and in the end, after she gathered together enough pills and took them, I sat with her for the last thirty-six hours as she slipped away. I can't tell you how many of her friends and acquaintances told me how graceful my mother was in her life to the very end. For my mother, given her personality, staying in control of her own life made her graceful. [a forty-one-year-old woman]

There is a great difference between someone, terminally ill and in pain, who says, "I've lived a full, long life and I think this is my time to die," and someone who is viewing life through the fog of depression and says, "I don't want to go on living." For a depressed person, a suicide attempt may be a call for help in finding resources to regain pleasure in living. You can get help for such a person through a suicide-prevention organization like the Samaritans (see Resources for this chapter).

It is very difficult to know what to do when a loved one wants to end her or his life. Talking with this person can help us distinguish temporary feelings of discouragement from the conviction that a life of pain and deterioration would be unbearable.

Laws vary from state to state, but nearly everywhere, a person who helps a dying family member or friend commit suicide risks prosecution as an accessory to a crime. To protect their loved ones, some dying persons have chosen to go off by themselves and take a fatal substance. They have had to do without the loving support and the talking and planning that would have eased the transition for everybody.

Claiming the right to control the end of our lives in no way minimizes the seriousness or the finality of the decision, nor the pain and grief of those we leave behind. A number of organizations, such as Choice In Dying, now publicize these issues and can help us deal with them personally (see Resources for this chapter).

Practical Matters

Before we die, some of us may want to arrange to donate vitally needed organs, such as kidneys and corneas, for transplant purposes. We can also plan the kind of funeral or memorial service we want. Helpful, practical information on these matters is available from the Older Women's League as part of their "Living Will Packet" (see Resources for this chapter).

A growing number of people today want to keep matters relating to death under the control of their immediate circle of friends and family. Preparing the body for burial, the burial or cremation itself, and last rites and memorial services can all, within broad limits, be designed to suit the wishes of the person who has died and her or his survivors.

The person I talked to about renting a place for the memorial service told me sharply that I had no business planning a memorial while my mother was still alive. But I am very thankful that we did plan it when we did. First of all, I was amazed to find that I was in absolutely no condition to make sensible plans after she died. . . . Planning the forms of the memorial beforehand helped me face the reality of my mother's death. Thinking about and writing what I would say brought the love we had shared back to me once more. Participating in the memorial gave me a kind of peace and acceptance I hardly dared hope for.[12]

If you have preferences about your burial, it will be much easier for your family and friends to carry out your wishes if you make them known in writing. This will also protect your loved ones from having feelings of guilt, because they will be assured they are following your wishes.

Remember that the funeral business is just that—a profitable business. There are some regulations, varying from state to state, that govern this industry. You can learn about them by calling your state attorney general's office.

I found out later that the funeral director lied to me when he said state law required a cement lining for my husband's grave, contrary to our personal and religious beliefs. [a fifty-five-year-old woman]

Those of us who are struggling to come to a better understanding of the great, universal transition at the end of life have many opportunities to ponder the matter. Experiences such as watching persons we are close to approach death, becoming aware of symptoms that might signal the beginning of life-threatening illness, putting our affairs in order in a written will, working as a volunteer in a hospice agency, or being part of a supportive network for a dying friend or relative, all can help us come to a peaceful, personal understanding of death.

NOTES

1. Tish Sommers, *Death—A Feminist View.* Paper presented at Drake University Law School, Des Moines, Iowa, March 27, 1976.
2. Phyllis R. Silverman, *Helping Women Cope with Grief,* Beverly Hills: Sage Publications, 1981.
3. Carolyn Ruth Swift, unpublished manuscript.
4. Mickey Spencer, "Plan Ahead." *Broomstick,* Vol. 7, No. 6 (November–December 1985), pp. 40–42.
5. J. W. Worden and William Proctor, *Personal Death Awareness.* Englewood Cliffs, NJ: Prentice-Hall, 1976.

6. Swift, op. cit.

7. See Stephen Jay Gould, "The Median Isn't the Message." *Discover,* Vol. 6, No. 6 (June 1985), pp. 40–42.

8. George Annas and Joan Dennsberger, "Competence to Refuse Medical Treatment: Autonomy vs. Paternalism." *University of Toledo Law Review,* Vol. 15 (1984), pp. 561–96.

9. Choice in Dying, Inc., (see Resources for this chapter), *State Statutes Governing Living Wills and Appointment of Health Care Agents,* June 1993.

10. Barbara Mishkin, "Making Decisions for the Terminally Ill." *Business and Health,* June 1985, pp. 13–16.

11. Roxanne Cummings Potter, "To Life—To Death." *California Association of Midwives Newsletter,* Spring 1984, p. 7.

12. Spencer, op. cit.

30

CHANGING SOCIETY AND OURSELVES

✦

BY TISH SOMMERS

SPECIAL THANKS TO LAURIE SHIELDS AND FRANCES LEONARD

1994 UPDATE BY PAULA B. DORESS-WORTERS WITH SPECIAL THANKS TO FRANCES LEONARD

RESOURCES FOR THIS CHAPTER ON PAGES 504–5

What kind of an older woman do I want to be? That's a good question to ask. Too often middle-aged and older women feel that it is too late to plan for the future, to make important changes in themselves, to have significant impact on the world around them. Not so. At forty we can expect half our adult life to be still before us. Sometimes the things that happen to us that we can do little about—like the death or desertion of a spouse—may trigger a whole new look at our priorities. Sometimes our way of life is curbed by a serious health condition, and this may also touch off a reordering of what is really important to us and may spur us forward. Even the shadow of impending death can be a stimulus to helping us put our lives in order.

Growing old is not easy, especially if you are poor and alone, as is the case with too many aging women, many of whom slip into poverty in their later years. It takes a lot of internal strength to cope with increasing infirmities or chronic pain, and the loss of choices brought about by reduced finances and physical limitations. It also takes preparation well before the calamities strike, and deciding as early as possible what kind of older woman you want to be. Will you go into a shell or be able to push past obstacles to make the last half of life as rich as the first? And what impact will you have on the people around you and the world at large?

You may decide to become an advocate, as some of us have. Pushing the establishment to be more in tune with the needs of those who are hurting—including yourself—can be as rewarding in your seventies as in your thirties. Contributing to something important beyond ourselves can keep us feeling that what we do still matters. And it can be a great impetus to personal growth.

I strongly believe that the advocacy work women do benefits the whole of society. It throws light on injustices and then eventually changes are made that help men too. [Annette Smail, advocate for ex-wives of military personnel]

STARTING WITH OURSELVES

The image of older women is changing. What we do today, both as role models and as forces for change in public policy, will greatly influence our daughters' futures. The present road to aging, especially for women, is a rocky one. But we, the old and the soon-to-be-old, can change that in our lifetimes. We can develop new ways of providing mutual help in our communities, and we can work together to assure that public policies do not neglect the needs of the aged. To achieve *interdependence* we need the wherewithal to be *independent,* which is why we must fight so hard to keep the entitlements and social programs that maintain dignity. The two—advocacy for rights and benefits, and working to create new forms of interdependency or mutual help—go hand in hand. As we improve the road to aging, we ourselves are changed in the process. We remain to the end of our lives contributing, caring, and creative members of society. As we change ourselves, we continue to make waves in the world around us.

AFTER SIXTY

The sixth decade is coming to an end
Doors have opened and shut
The great distractions are over—
passion . . . children . . . the long indenture of marriage
I fold them into a chest
I will not take with me when I go

Everyone says the world is flat and finite
on the other side of sixty
That I will fall clear off the edge
into darkness
that no one will hear from me again
or want to

But I am ready for the knife slicing into the future
for the quiet that explodes inside
to join forces with the strong old woman
to throw everything away and begin again

Now there is time to tell the story
—time to invent the new one
Time to chain myself to a fence outside the missile base
To throw my body before a truck loaded with phallic images
To write Thou Shalt Not Kill
on the hull of a Trident submarine
To pour my own blood on the walls of the Pentagon
To walk a thousand miles with a begging bowl in my hand

There are places on this planet
where women past the menopause
put on the tribal robes
smoke pipes of wisdom
—fly

*Marilyn Zuckerman**

*Marilyn Zuckerman, *Poems of the Sixth Decade,* 1993. Garden Street Press, P.O. Box 380055, Cambridge, MA 02238.

Ageism is as much a part of the fabric of society as sexism and racism. Think of all the conscious and unconscious ways we disparage our aging. "You're sixty-two? You certainly don't *look* that old. You shouldn't tell anyone because you could easily pass for forty-five." Or, "That dress makes me feel *old.*" Or, "All those old people together. I find it depressing."

Just telling your age forthrightly can be an act of defiance and a blow against ageism. Remember Gloria Steinem's rejoinder to a reporter who said she didn't look forty: "This is what forty looks like. How would you know? We've been hiding our age so long."

When Maggie Kuhn, founder of the Gray Panthers, was introduced by President Gerald Ford as a "young lady," she stood up and said, "Mr. President, I am not a young lady. I've lived a long time. I'm an old lady."

Age is part of our identity. To deny it is to say to the deepest layers of ourselves, as well as to the world, "I am unacceptable." Denial of age slowly erodes our self-esteem. The Older Women's League consciously selected its name—despite objections from many who said "mature" would be more acceptable—to help women take

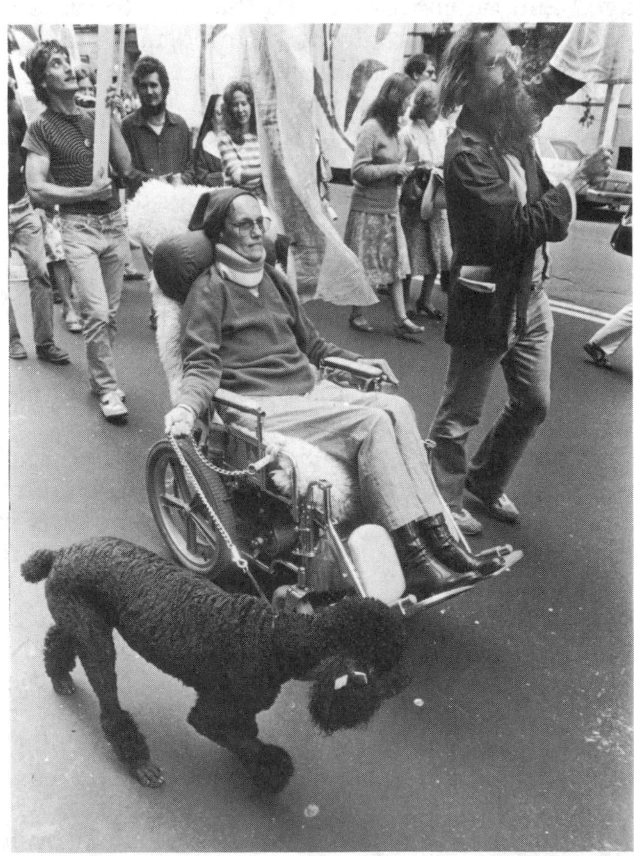

Jerry Howard/Positive Images

a conscious stand on the age question, to come out of the closet on age, so to speak.

Liberation from the shackles of ageism starts with learning to like ourselves and other older women. We must recognize the strength and beauty of our own age group. We have been separated from each other by our dependency on men, and many of us because of ageism and sexism have avoided the company of older women. Polls show that older people hold the same negative opinion of their peers as do the rest of the population. Yet older women like ourselves can provide us with great support in our later years. And if we are going to make changes on our own behalf and that of other older women, we must find each other. In the process we will discover our potential power.

Whatever our age or degree of disablement, feeling *connected*—being part of a family, either biological or a family of choice, or both; feeling part of a community of older women, but not isolated or alienated from other folks; having a sense of the continuity of generations—is essential. When we have this, growing older can be as rich and productive as any other time of life, especially if it is enjoyed in good company.

Advocacy organizations like the Older Women's League (OWL) and the Gray Panthers, women's support groups of all kinds, and local women's projects all provide opportunities for developing friendships and linkages. We need each other, especially as we grow old.

We also need to feel useful, productive, and self-realized. It's not enough to be part of a larger group if we don't feel we're contributing to it and to society as a whole. Because older people, if they are not careful, are relegated to the trash heap, this takes initiative. Determine early to "keep on keeping on." Then explore the many ways to do that in accordance with your own talents, desires, and opportunities. Paid and unpaid work, personal and group advocacy, any project in which you feel passionate interest, whether it's a garden or the government—can be rewarding. For example, there was never a better time of life to get on boards and commissions, which regulate a great deal of the way things function. If one-to-one helping makes you feel more connected and involved, by all means become involved in personal service.

I have been a volunteer for the last three years at Rosie's Place—a shelter for poor and homeless women in Boston. We provide meals for many women, beds for a few each night, clothing, and most importantly, respect, caring, concern, and love. I started doing this after the death of my grandmother, who took care of me while my mother worked. She and I were always very close. My volunteer work is a way for me to continue giving direct care to women on a regular basis. [a woman in her fifties]

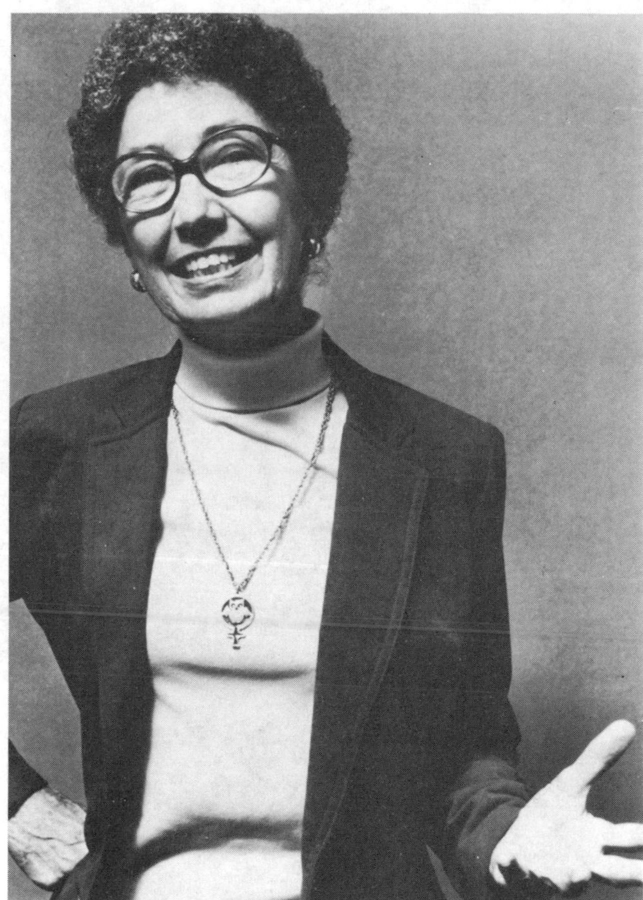

Tish Sommers, founder of Older Women's League
Janet Beller

Hope is the most important ingredient in a meaningful old age. Is the glass half full or half empty? In old age it may seem only a quarter full, but ah—how precious those few remaining drops can be! Hope is never out of season. It is the fuel that keeps the furnace going. We need to cultivate it, treasure it, and keep it alive when it seems most fragile. The second half of life is different from the first. There are losses: physical limitations can curb one's life-style, and the specter of death is present. But even when all seems lost, we can find new incentives for making each day count.

Too many women *endure* old age rather than *enjoy* it. Preventive measures taken while we still have time to prepare for our old age could mitigate some of the problems of growing older as a

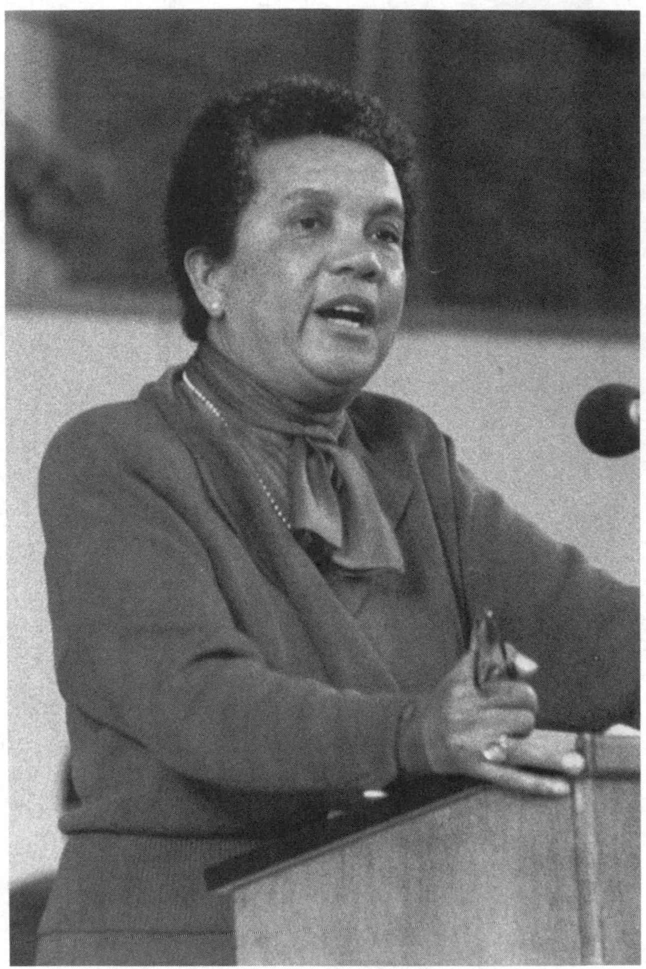

Marian Wright Edelman, advocate for America's children, Director of Children's Defense Fund Ellen Shub

woman. Many of us have been touched by the women's movement—positively, in that we are seeking new solutions and greater independence, and negatively, in that traditional homemaking roles of women to which so many of us have devoted years of our lives have lost status. We often feel caught in the middle.

We are all affected by role models, both positive and negative. Our mothers and grandmothers may or may not have been women of strength and courage. Strong role models decrease the fear of aging, so if we don't have them in our own families we should look for them elsewhere. Strong role models also help change the generally negative public image of older women. Think of Elizabeth Cady Stanton and Susan B. Anthony, both of whom were vigorous fighters to the end of their days. Susan B. Anthony continued to actively campaign into old age, making her final speech to a Woman's Rights Convention in 1904, when she was eighty-six years old. Mother Jones, the heroic fighter for unions and the oppressed, was ninety-three when she addressed the convention of the Farmer-Labor Party, telling them:

. . . not today perhaps, not tomorrow, but over the rim of the years my old eyes can see the coming of another day.[1]

And there are plenty of role models in today's society. Look around; choose one or more to draw substance from. Then decide to become a role model yourself. The changes we make in ourselves will not only warm our own lives but will have a ripple effect on the lives of others. Each of us in our own orbit influences others, combating the effects of ageism. Over the rim of the years we will see the coming of another day together.

FORMS OF ADVOCACY

Whatever our situation as we grow old, there is usually some way we can play an active role in making changes in our lives and in society. Some things we can do for ourselves, some we accomplish as individual advocates for another person, some we accomplish best when we have support from a group with similar concerns, and some need sustained organizational effort. Each kind of advocacy is important and contributes to the others. Social change does not come quickly, but over time the glacier does move. Awareness of the plight of older women is much greater than it was ten years ago.

Here is an example of personal action, the first kind of advocacy. A woman experiences age discrimination on her job. She is consistently bypassed for promotions, works in a back room, and notices that this is the pattern in the company. All newly hired persons are young people. Finally a manager lets slip that the company wants a "young image" and wants the employees to reflect this. That is a "smoking gun"—evidence of intentional discrimination!

I filed a complaint with the EEOC [Equal Employment Opportunity Commission]. I also filed one with the state agency which is responsible for employment discrimination. It was a long, hard battle and my employer did everything he could to make me quit. My workplace was pretty unbearable and I was expected to handle heavy boxes. But I knew he couldn't fire me without making a lot of trouble for himself so I stuck it out. After three long years I finally won my case. I was upgraded in my job and received $12,560 back pay. It finally was worth it!

Although many others will have to go through the same ordeal to make combined age and sex discrimination less pervasive in the job market, the woman who fights for her own rights makes a contribution to all of us.

In the second kind of advocacy one individual advocates for another.

Bonnie M. lived in an apartment house by herself and became acquainted with some of the other tenants, one of whom, Marianne, lived on disability benefits. One day Bonnie met her friend in tears.

Marianne showed me a letter which said her disability benefits would be cut off because she was not totally disabled and therefore presumed able to work. But she is sixty, she has no skills, and she has crippling arthritis. The poor woman felt completely at a loss about how she would survive because she has practically no assets and no relatives close by. In fact she was seriously thinking of doing away with herself. I read that letter again and saw that she could request a hearing. I said, "What do you have to lose? I'll go with you. Let's fight it." I helped her collect all the necessary medical data and tried to calm her down, and I could see that just having someone help her meant a lot. Well, the administrative judge overruled the decision and she got her monthly payments back. I wasn't too surprised, because I knew that a very large proportion of such decisions are overruled if they are challenged. I haven't been a social worker for nothing. In this system, the squeaky wheel gets the grease.

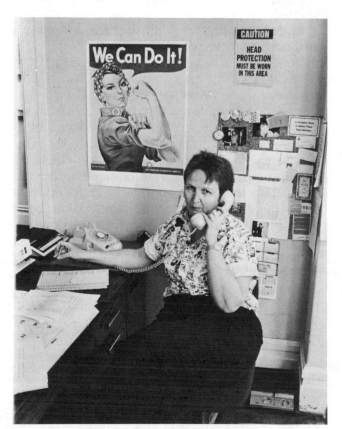

Cathy Cade

Bonnie became an advocate who in effect saved a life; the woman with the disability learned that when an injustice is done, it can be challenged. Neither woman will ever be quite the same again.

Cooperative caring is a kind of advocacy that is not so dramatic but equally important in the overall plan of making things happen. Older women can take the lead in breaking down generation barriers to foster mutual understanding and support among women. For example, the Seattle chapter of the Older Women's League decided to hold a workshop to help women of all ages strengthen their relationships with each other. They also wanted to encourage women to discuss more deeply and honestly how they feel about aging and to help women of different generations see what they have in common. They called their workshop "What Kind of Older Woman Do I Want to Be?" To make sure that there was a good balance of young, middle-aged, and old who attended, the admission "ticket" was five dollars *and* a woman of another generation. The talk was lively and very revealing.

I brought my grandmother, who is seventy-nine. We've talked before but never quite like we did in the small group where we were discussing how we felt about the age we are now. She said she was afraid of dying but even more afraid of being a burden to me. Hearing other women also talk about their fears made it easier. We all seemed to help each other and by the end of the day there was a lot of hugging.

That workshop was so successful that it was copied by other chapters of OWL and has been incorporated into *Wingspan,** an advocacy training manual for transforming personal problems of older women into social issues. That is how influence spreads and how intergenerational solidarity can be built.

This brings us to the fourth form of advocacy, organizational and legislative efforts. Midlife and older women can build bridges between the dynamic advocacy of the women's movement and the well-organized constituency of seniors. Conventionally, women are seen as joining a new category on reaching sixty or sixty-five. They are

*1994 update in press. See Resources pp. 443–44

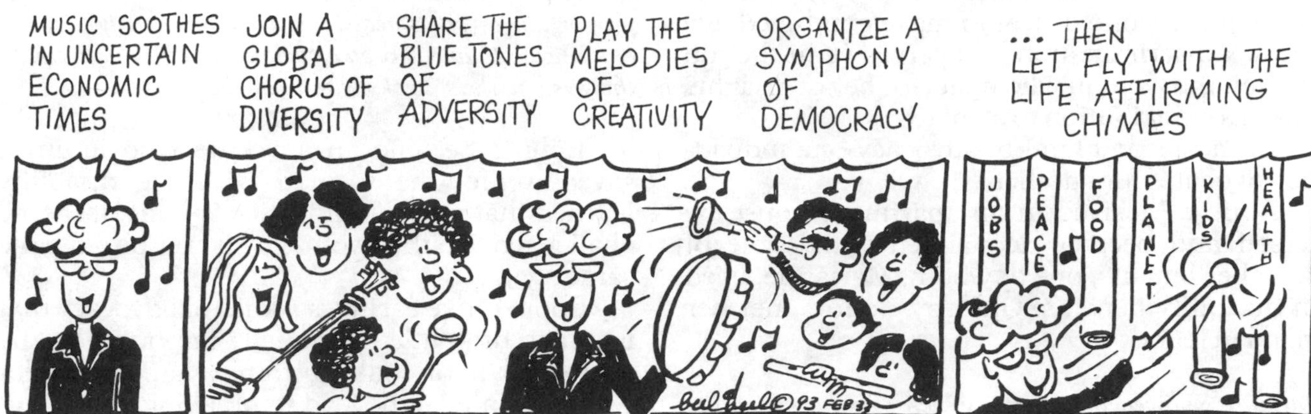
MUSIC SOOTHES IN UNCERTAIN ECONOMIC TIMES
JOIN A GLOBAL CHORUS OF DIVERSITY
SHARE THE BLUE TONES OF ADVERSITY
PLAY THE MELODIES OF CREATIVITY
ORGANIZE A SYMPHONY OF DEMOCRACY
... THEN LET FLY WITH THE LIFE AFFIRMING CHIMES
JOBS
PEACE
FOOD
PLANET
KIDS
HEALTH

no longer seen as women but as "seniors" or "senior citizens," without gender distinctions. Government policies are devised without recognition of significant differences between aging women and men, and women's organizations, until quite recently, tended to avoid issues of aging. Consciousness has been raised to some extent in both arenas, but only the active voice of older women speaking about their own special concerns can catch the ear of either constituency.

I belong to a senior group—all men, mostly from the trade union movement. They're real sexist. But they are working on issues like Social Security and Medicare, and it's important for them to realize how women will be doubly hit by the proposed cuts. I talk about their wives as widows—something they don't like to think about, of course—and their sisters and mothers, and I give them all the facts and figures about how poor older women are. They are beginning to see the light. Now they want me to testify for the organization.

My NOW chapter is made up mostly of younger women. In fact I'm the only member over forty. They are real concerned about abortion and of course the ERA, and so am I, but I had a terrible time getting them interested enough to do something about the Retirement Equity Act. At first they just couldn't think that far ahead, but I kept saying that NOW was supposed to represent all women and that they were the ones who would benefit most from passage of this legislation when they themselves are ready to retire. They finally got the message and really got behind it.

Building a bridge between the women's and seniors' organizations has enormous potential for positive change in society. If women's organizations recognize the extent to which aging is a women's issue, and if organizations of the elderly come to the same recognition, we will make great strides in finding new solutions to the problems of growing old in a youth-oriented society.

Women of color have the additional task and opportunity of building bridges between their cultural group and the concerns of older women.* Too many older black women live on very low incomes and have not benefited proportionately from the programs that have generally improved the situation of the elderly. Women who worked in jobs that were not covered by Social Security, such as domestic work, or who raised their children as single parents, still suffer the effects of poverty.

Marching in a Martin Luther King Memorial demonstration in Washington, D.C., Dorothy Pitts of California carried a sign, "One Half of All Older Black Women Are Poor—Why?"

A year later, Dorothy Pitts organized a conference for Older Women of Color to which she invited representatives of twenty-four black women's organizations. It was the first conference in the San Francisco area in which the problems of older black women were addressed. Aileen Hernandez delivered the keynote address: "Our whole survival has depended on being strong black women. . . . What we have done, we have done for our families. Now is the time to do for ourselves as older black women."

Sometimes when women get together at a conference or meeting, an idea emerges that inspires continued involvement. Jane Porcino was involved in such a group and reports on its emergence:

*The fifth national OWL convention focused on acknowledging diversity in the way women's issues are presented. See *Women of Diversity: Coming Together—A Report of a Multicultural Conference,* February 1993. Available from OWL. See pages 443–44

Hot Flash, *the quarterly newsletter of the National Action Forum for Midlife and Older Women, was conceived during a national conference on the health issues of women over forty. Following the three-day meeting, funded by the Administration on Aging, a group of twenty-five women remained to follow up on the enthusiasm generated by the conference. They envisioned a national newsletter to address the myriad health issues which affect all women in the second half of their lives. Traditionally, the physical and mental-health concerns of aging women have been shrouded in mystery, fear, and silence. This health newsletter would openly acknowledge the issue of aging and bring information to women which would help empower them in their lives. The name* Hot Flash *was unanimously chosen, since hot flashes are experienced by most women, but rarely publicly acknowledged or celebrated. Twelve years later that project is still going strong, distributed nationwide and in fourteen other countries.* *(See General Resources page 446 for subscription information.)*

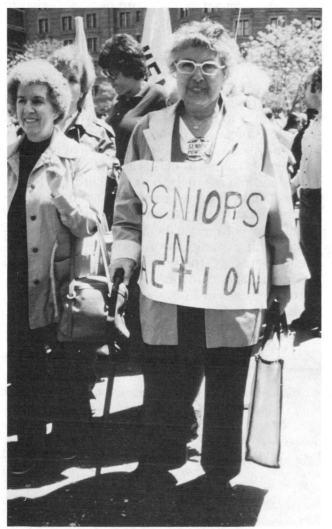

Ellen Shub

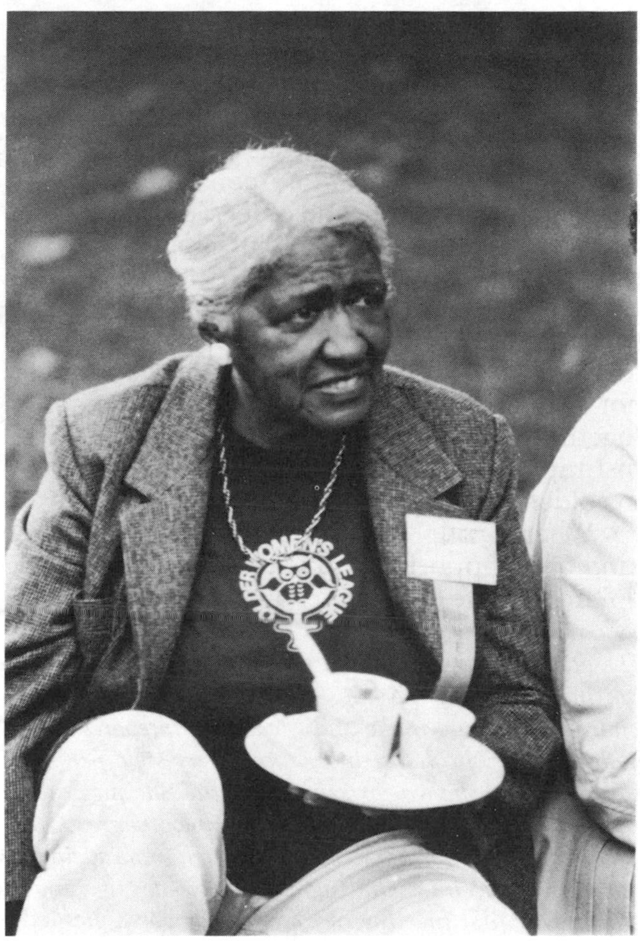

Eugenia Hickman, member of OWL's founding board of directors. *Faire Edwards*

Supports We Need to Overcome the Barriers We Face

Support groups (see page 18) are especially useful to women facing a crisis. Many support groups have already been described in earlier chapters. Widowhood, serious illness, or any situation that requires a major life adjustment are times when we need all the help we can get from each other. Widow-to-widow groups, caregiver-support groups, cancer-support groups, and chapters of the Alzheimer's Disease and Related Disorders Association are all examples of mutual-help groups that have emerged to fill a very real need. Not all, but most of these, are women's groups. For women who are not in crisis but interested in getting connected with other women, consciousness-raising groups for older women can be a useful starting point, either organized independently or formed in conjunction with organizations such as the Older Women's League. Job hunting can be so difficult in later years that support groups are helpful for that too.

Support groups are also stepping-stones to advocacy, or can be, if a leader or member of the group moves forward in that direction. Organizations like OWL promote consciousness-raising groups for midlife and older women in which feelings are shared and participants feel renewed. When women begin to recognize that their problems are not just personal, but have societal implications too, then they can move on to consider what can be done to tackle the cause, not only in their own lives but by taking action together with other women to change the social institutions and laws that penalize us for growing older.

Where your community doesn't have the kind of a support group you need, what do you do? You create one. Here is an example:

The doctor gave me the bad news—a recurrence of cancer, incurable, but perhaps controllable. There were so many decisions to make and I was so unprepared. But I had a friend who had cancer too, a very solid person. I called her and she was extremely helpful. She suggested a doctor for a second opinion, she gave me other resources to call, and she was an anchor when I felt more adrift. We talked several times and agreed we needed a support group. Our first meeting of four people was a picnic by the bay. We set the "rules": a women's group; we would help each other as much as we could, but [would] understand that at times we might not be up to it; we would meet monthly or more often to tell how we were doing, to share ideas and resources, and to talk freely about problems we are facing. The cancer-support group has been going now for over five years. We have lost some members, which has grieved us, but the group made their last days less painful. We had one wonderful retreat and are planning another. Our members, now twelve, have become resource persons who have appeared on television, spoken at conferences as cancer patients, and carried a message of hope wherever we go. Many cancer victims and their families call us for advice and support. We even sent a delegation to Kaiser Hospital to suggest changes in handling of cancer patients, which was well received. All those who are part of the group are grateful to it and to each other.

Any kind of support group has the potential for advocacy. The members of the cancer group above started out only helping each other, but as they became more knowledgeable and recognized that medical treatment of the disease left much to be desired, some of the members moved beyond the limits of personal support to become advocates for changes in the medical system. Some had all they could do just to cope with the illness. Others felt that fighting to improve the lot of others like themselves was a strong incentive to stay alive. The group accommodated both sentiments.

Another group that performs both functions—mutual help and social advocacy—is the Displaced Homemakers Network. Women, participating in support groups designed to help them become self-sufficient in the job market, find the small groups essential for gaining the confidence to begin a whole new life. In larger groups, members move to the bigger issues and begin to take part in social and political change, beginning with such immediate concerns as working for support of Displaced Homemakers programs. The extension, despite budget cuts, of such programs is largely the result of advocacy by those most directly affected, including those who have moved on to jobs. All of these women have taken steps outward from personal crisis to mutual help to advocacy.

BECOMING AGENTS FOR CHANGE

Our past experience can be very useful in bringing about social change. If you have experienced a problem, you may be the best advocate. When Annette Smail was divorced from her military husband she lost access to the medical care that had been available to her as a service dependent. In midlife, and not in the best of health, she found, as have many other women who are dependents on another's insurance coverage, that individual policies are both very expensive and grossly inadequate, with exclusions for "existing conditions." Feeling strongly the injustice of this unequal treatment, she convinced her Congressman to introduce a bill in Congress to continue medical benefits for ex-wives of military personnel. She says:

My own experience triggered my action. I had a background in community organization and I knew I could organize this community of women to accomplish something on this problem. I had looked for a job without success, so I appointed myself to this job and had to raise the money to do it. First I made the problem visible through the local newspaper, so that other women in the same straits would call me. And then I went national, urging other women to speak out as well. It's been the most marvelous experience in my life. I needed a challenge and here was a big one. And I met it. It required head work and homework—meeting people and learning how the system works. Most of all it required persistence. The Medical Rights bill was finally passed and triggered advocacy on other issues of ex-military wives.

How do you choose an issue and then begin to work on it? Chances are, if you have a problem, other women are likely to have it too, but first you must find them. Perhaps some of your friends share your problem and would be interested in a support group or study group. You can reach out to other women through community bulletin boards or organizations. A women's center may be willing to help you call a meeting to reach out to others who share your concern. Recognizing the common problem and talking about it together is the first step toward turning a problem into an issue. A group can begin by defining the problem very clearly and planning how to work together toward a solution. When the group comes up with a solution that it will support and work for, you are ready for the next step—broadening your constituency by publicizing your concerns.

The media offer the best opportunity for doing this. A little initiative can often lead to a radio or TV interview or a story in the local paper, which can provide a means for others to contact you. Then you can hold a public meeting to attract new participants and plan together how to deal with the problem.

If your group decides to work for passing legislation, be aware that timing is very important. When budgets are tight and lawmakers feeling stingy, a bill with a large price tag is not likely to pass. On the other hand, Congress passed the Retirement Equity Act even though at the time legislation on women's concerns was getting nowhere; this was because the bill required no appropriation and both Democrats and Republicans were vying for the favor of women voters. This important piece of legislation improves the women's chances of receiving a pension. For more information, contact the Older Women's League, listed under General Resources.

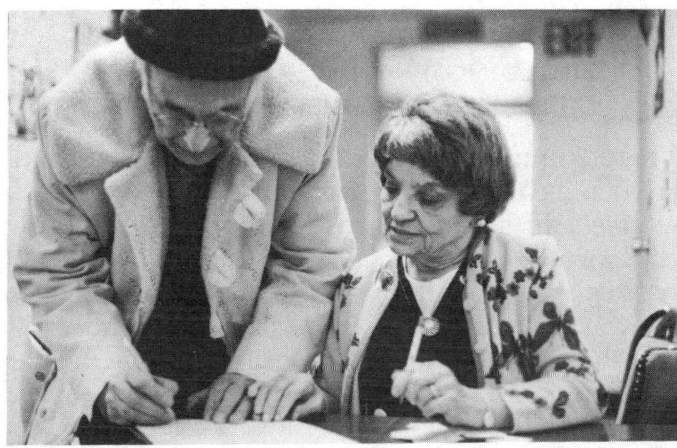

Norma Holt

Passing legislation can be difficult. It helps to take time to define your issue in a way that will appeal to the public and to get some experienced person's help in writing the bill. A group of women in California reported:

We had been meeting together for some time as Jobs for Older Women, trying to help each other and trying to alert the public to our difficulties in finding jobs. But we weren't making a great deal of progress. We decided we needed some legislative help. Fortunately there was a young lawyer working with us at the time so we asked her to write us a bill. But first we needed a name to describe our problem, something that would get their attention. We decided to call ourselves "displaced homemakers" and our model bill (into which we put everything but the kitchen sink) we called a Displaced Homemakers Bill. From that moment we had a handle with which to organize. We got a version of that bill passed through our state legislature in 100 working days, almost a record for that kind of lawmaking.

Laurie Shields, a widow in her mid-fifties, had never been involved in political action beyond driving people to the polls on election day. But she was energetic, a natural organizer, and ready to go when the first model displaced homemakers bill was written. She had experienced the problem of women long out of the work force and of the ageism in her field (advertising). She discovered and developed talents she was not aware of and made use of all her former work experience, paid and unpaid, when she became head of the Alliance for Displaced Homemakers.

Crisscrossing the country in my tennis shoes, I met thousands of women who, with disquieting unanimity, greeted the message of the legislation with a teary "My God, I thought I was all alone." . . . I built up a relationship with many of these women that transcended our shared problems. I came to know them as friends; I found myself deeply moved by their quiet courage in the face of real adversity. Sharing their lives, however briefly, and observing their battles against loneliness and despair gave new meaning to the importance of the legislation and the work we were collectively doing. . . . I would never have believed I could do it or accomplish so much. For myself and for the others, there is a new awareness of the truth and hope spelled out in Doris Lessing's words:

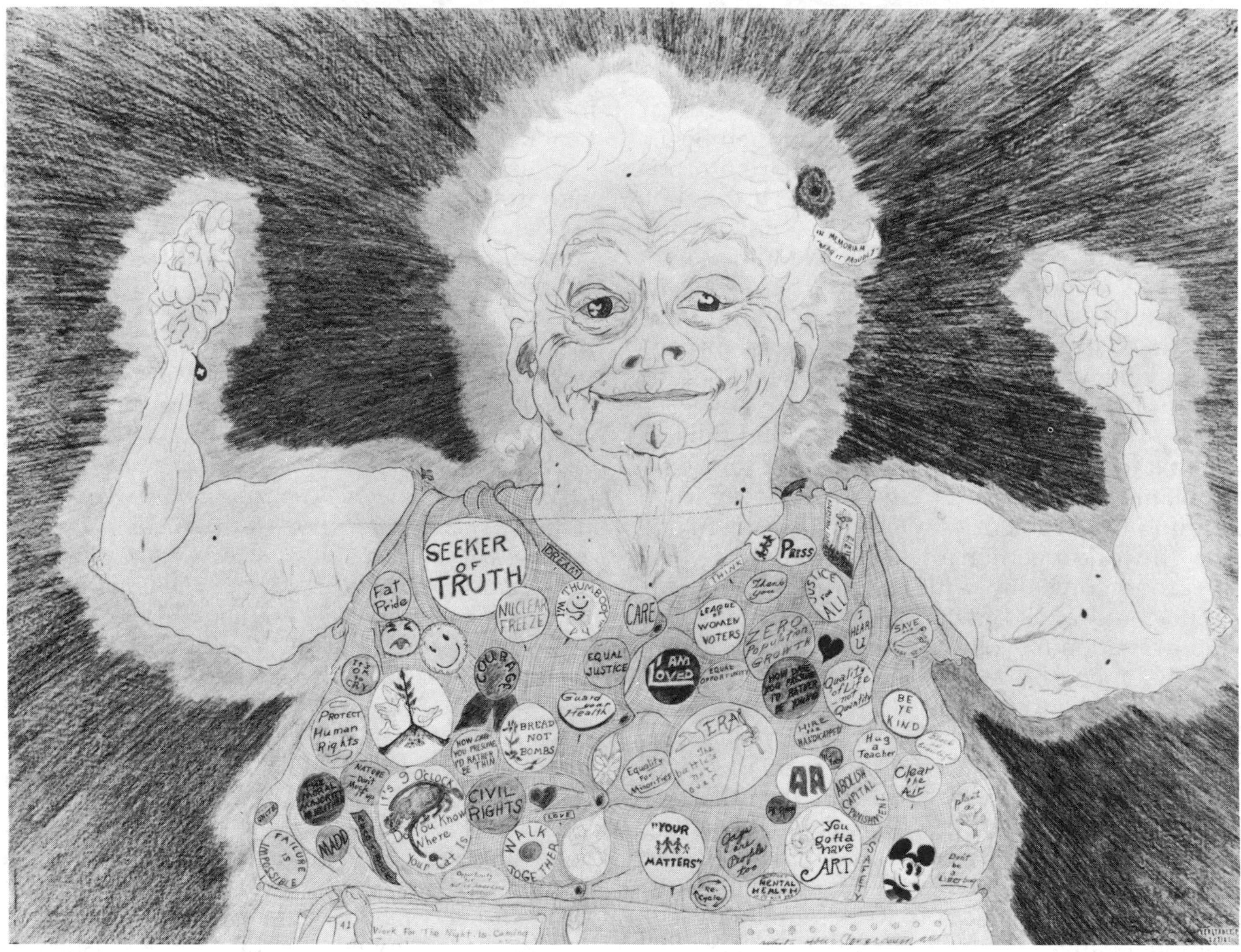

"Her strength is in her principles." *Elizabeth Layton*

"Any human being anywhere will blossom into a hundred unexpected talents and capabilities simply by being given the opportunity to use them."[2]

The effects of becoming an agent for change can be very dramatic. For example, Rosemary Bizzell of Jeffersonville, Indiana, a widow with seven sons and eight grandchildren, had never been involved in community affairs. In 1981 she joined OWL. Three years later, she had become an important figure in the statehouse and city council. She wrote:

My self-image as an older woman has improved tremendously, in spite of much rejection in job hunting. Apparently I was supposed to count my blessings and not expect to advance. Well, becoming involved in OWL has certainly challenged me. . . . I cannot thank the OWLs enough for opening up a whole new world for older women. I am proud of the opportunity to be part of it.

The later years can indeed be a time to have an impact on the world instead of being put on the shelf. Working to build a movement or an organization that works for a better future for all of us and for those coming along behind puts excitement into the later years.

BUILDING THE ORGANIZATIONAL FORMS FOR SOCIAL CHANGE

There is much we can do as individuals, both as advocates and as role models. We can work collectively in small groups and carry out significant projects on a local level or through court battles. But inevitably we come up against the "power structure" and the laws of the land. How can older women have a significant voice in the making of public policy? How can we be assured that we will be heard on matters that affect our lives? To accomplish that purpose we need organizations with large enough memberships to impress legislators, and the skills to use that voice effectively. See General Resources for activist organizations that advocate for women, for older persons, and specifically for older women.

The women's movement has produced national organizations in the form of the National Organization for Women (NOW), National Women's Political Caucus (NWPC), the National Women's Health Network (NWHN), and many others. There are traditional women's organizations, such as the League of Women Voters and the National Council of Negro Women, which are often influential in policy-making circles.

Older people have developed organizations of impressive size, notably the twenty-four-million-member American Association of Retired Persons (AARP), the union-based National Council of Senior Citizens (NCSC), and the more professionally oriented National Council on the Aging (NCOA). A smaller but more activist organization, the Gray Panthers, is intergenerationally structured.

A "new kid on the block" of activist organizations is the Older Women's League, which focuses on the specific problems of midlife and older women and bridges the gap between organizations in the aging field and women's groups.

All of these organizations have representatives who testify at hearings on the national and state level and mobilize support for issues of concern, as well as working with administrative bodies. If it seems that despite all this the needs of women and the aged are given short shrift by government, consider how much worse the situation would be without their input.

Organizations work both singly and in concert. Coalitions are built in support of, or in opposition to, specific measures, or to speak for a whole spectrum of organizations.

Specialized support organizations like the Pension Rights Center in Washington and the National Senior Citizens' Law Center (NSCLC) contribute to the cooperative advocacy efforts of the others. Families USA (see General Resources) is a foundation that provides technical assistance and information to organizations at the grass-roots and national level advocating for health care and economic issues.

Very important, however, is building harmonious working relationships between organizations so that they can join forces when necessary and move forward as a united front on an important issue. The strong underlying current of desire for peace and for a national health-care program,* concern about the military budget, and cuts in social services and entitlements designed to address human needs—all these offer common ground for collective action.

How can midlife and older women build alliances without losing our special goals? We can work as a "Concerns of Older Women Committee," raising issues within organizations with diverse membership, or we can work in our own independent organizations, and then in coalitions with others.

There are direct advantages to older women having their own established organization that can work as an equal in alliance with other organizations. This was a primary reason why the Older Women's League was formed as an independent entity. In a coalition of groups, a group with a proven constituency, such as OWL, is listened to quite differently from one with a good cause but no followers.

Working inside an established body with a broader base and forming an independent organization with our own specific focus are not mutually exclusive. In fact, both types of advocacy work best in unison. A close working relationship with the Older Women's League can make a "Concerns of Older Women Committee" more effective. For example, the "Women's Initiative" within the American Association of Retired Persons has been working toward increased recognition of the special issues of women after retirement.

In advocacy work we need to judge where we fit in. We may have special skills that come from wide experience, and we may have our own style or styles of organizing. Sometimes an older woman feels out of place in a feminist organization with a primarily young membership. Some women work more effectively with their own peers while others prefer the company of a mixed-age group. In trying to reach out to women older than ourselves, or to any women whose background and experience may be different from our own, it is important to respect "where they are coming from." Avoid downgrading the role of homemaker, when the real problem is the lack of recognition for homemakers, the inadequacy of Social Security, and the absence of other bene-

*The Campaign for Women's Health is a broad-based coalition of eighty national, state, and local women's organizations, unions, and health-care organizations spearheaded by OWL and representing 8 million persons. The Campaign works on behalf of women's interests in health reform. See Resources page 484.

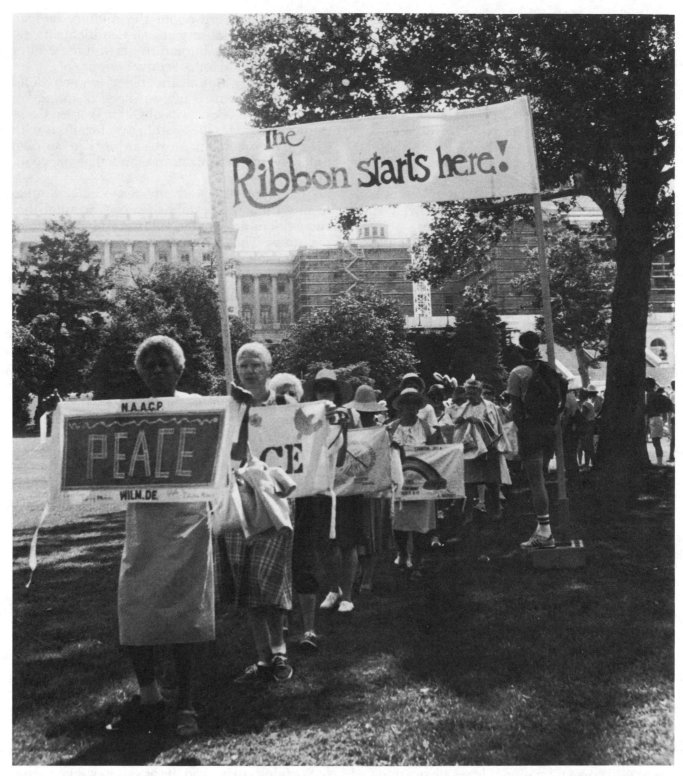

Women gathered in Washington, DC, carrying homemade banners, encircle the Pentagon demonstrating for peace. (For more about the "ribbon demonstration," see Marianne Philbin, ed., The Ribbon: Celebration of Life: The Remarkable Ribbon Around the Pentagon, A Unique Worldwide Plea for Peace. *See Resources, page 505.)* *Ellen Shub*

fits. Rather than disparaging a traditional style, it may be better to adapt that style to new content. We all start on the road to liberation from a particular point, wherever that may be. The important thing is the direction that road is taking.

Often, as former excluded groups enter the mainstream, we all learn and benefit from their special insights and experiences. As older women we have benefited from the experience of the black movement, the women's movement, and the elder advocates. We reject the demeaning images of older women and the exclusion of older women from policymaking for elders. We proudly claim our age and experience as demonstrating our right to define who we are and what we need to live lives of dignity, activity, and involvement in our communities: decent health care and housing; an income sufficient to enjoy, rather than simply to endure, our later years; and the recognition that we are important members of society with much to contribute.

EPILOGUE

Our later years, when we have a lifetime's worth of experience, and possibly lighter work loads to carry, can be a time to bring things together and to find spiritual and ethical coherence. Maggie Kuhn is a beautiful role model of someone who has contributed greatly to a better future through social and political involvement. Only after she formally retired did Maggie convene the Gray Panthers, calling upon young and old to join forces to work for a better world. This "little old woman" with white hair and arthritic fingers is an articulate voice for right and justice, the epitome of an "elder of the tribe," as she calls old people. Social and political involvement can be a fine way of making life meaningful to the very end. In Maggie's words:

In this age of self-determination and liberation many groups are struggling for freedom. All these struggles are linked in the worldwide struggle for a new humanity. Together they have the potential of a new community-based social justice system of human compassion and selfhood. Old people have a large stake in this new community—in helping to create it and extend it. The winds of change are impelling and empowering. They can free us or destroy us.

And I, Tish Sommers, age seventy, concur with all my heart. This summer, as in the past, I plan to go on a white-water river-rafting trip in Idaho. For me, rivers are a symbol of an activist's life. Last year our little raft was dashing down this churning cauldron, the young boatpersons yelling directions, the river about to make a figure S, and right in the middle of it a great big rock. Would we wrap around it or pass on through? We did flash by, but another boat was not so lucky. Then all the people descended on it to get the boat peeled off that rock and the passengers out of danger. No one was hurt. But for those few days, when the only concerns were the next rocks up ahead, I realized how lucky we are to be testing our strength and skill against the raging river of this period we are living in. There are lots of rocks and plenty of danger and it's very difficult to row upstream. But we can all learn to read the river, scout out the rocks ahead, find the eddies where the water moves upstream, and we can throw out a line if things go wrong. How much better to be in there with all the excitement than moping on the bank!

NOTES

1. *Autobiography of Mother Jones.* Chicago: Kerr & Co., 1972.
2. Laurie Shields, *Displaced Homemakers: Organizing for a New Life.* New York: McGraw-Hill, 1981.

AFTERWORD BY LAURIE SHIELDS*

Tish Sommers died at home, as she wished, on October 18, 1985. Her death was neither unexpected nor unplanned—for she had lived with stage four (meaning widespread) cancer for almost six years. During that time she practiced what she preached—she "kept on keeping on." She spent time with friends and colleagues, said her good-byes, but more to the point, gave each of them a "job to do for OWL." She taped two messages—for two events she knew she would not be attending—the December board meeting, at which she would propose Lou Glasse to take over the presidency of OWL, and OWL's 1986 convention in September. She completed a proposal that would, she hoped, fund a project to develop model state legislation dealing with health-care problems of older women. She even planned her own memorial service!

Tish consistently acted upon her belief that personal problems can be turned into public issues. She viewed her experience with cancer as affording an opportunity to help other women. Because *she* found it helpful, she advised other

*Laurie Shields died in 1987, the third of OWL's founding staff of five to die from breast cancer.

women to "question authority" and not accept, for example, a doctor's advice simply because it came from a doctor. She felt that patients, rather than doctors, were apt to be inventive about "make do" matters. A case in point: When she had a supra-pubic catheter inserted just before going on a river-rafting trip, the doctor insisted she not swim, indeed, not even take tub baths. In her journal she records wondering about this. "Why should I accept that dictum? Why couldn't I find a way to waterproof the area?" With the help of a public-health nurse, she did just that and won grudging approval from the doctor.

Tish strongly advocated staying in control of one's life to the very end. She pushed hard for national legislation that would give durable power of attorney to those entrusted to follow the wishes of a terminally ill patient. She and I had such documents in our medical files and, under the laws of California, felt reassured that we would each follow the other's wishes.

Tish regretted that she had not been a strong advocate for hospice services until she needed them herself. When she realized all that program gave, not only to the terminally ill but to their caregivers, families, and friends, she extracted a pledge from me that such advocacy would be a primary target for my organizing efforts.

In her final messages she made it clear that death was a part of what life is about, and that because of her own life she could say, "I face my own last transition with the sure knowledge that you will all go on to complete the tasks we have set for ourselves. And that is why I feel such joy and love."

And now it is we who must "keep on keeping on." Knowing that we have her assurance we can. "I bequeath to you," she said, "and to my fellow fighters for a better life, my faith in the future, even when things seem impossible and out of kilter." All it takes, as she knew, is caring, communication, and commitment.

RESOURCES

✦

General Resources

Following is a list of organizations and publications that pertain to women and aging in general, or that relate to more than one of the subjects covered in the book. **When you look for the resources for a particular chapter, remember to review these general resources also.**

Organizations

Area Agencies on Aging (sometimes called Triple As) are good centralized sources of information about services and agencies in your area. Set up by the Older Americans Act to provide information and referral, advocacy, and planning, they are federally funded but often receive additional money from local or state governments and may be located in a state, county, or private agency. Senior centers, councils on aging, and other elder groups are other possible sources of information for elders.

Advocates Senior Alert Process (A.S.A.P.)
1334 G St. NW
Washington, DC 20005
Tel. (202) 737-6340

Fourteen national senior organizations (many of which are listed below) have joined together to provide an information and action network for politically active advocates. Participants receive information on many issues at no charge. In return the participants agree to mobilize at least five other persons and to act on important issues affecting older persons by writing letters, making phone calls, and initiating other activities to influence the legislative process.

American Association of Retired Persons (AARP)
601 E St. NW
Washington, DC 20049
Tel. (800) 424-2277; (202) 434-2277

Membership for age fifty and up. Has Women's Initiative and Disabilities Initiatives programs and local chapters. Provides information, services, and advocacy for issues concerning older and retired people. Publishes *Modern Maturity,* a bimonthly magazine, *AARP News Bulletin,* a monthly newspaper, *Perspectives in Health Pro-*

motion and Aging, a quarterly newsletter, and a list of excellent bibliographies, books, and pamphlets.

Asociación Nacional Pro Personas Mayores (National Association for Hispanic Elderly)
3325 Wilshire Blvd., #800
Los Angeles, CA 90010
Tel. (213) 487-1922
Membership, publications, and projects.

Boston Women's Health Book Collective
240A Elm St.
Somerville, MA 02144
Tel. (617) 625-0271
Authors of all editions of *Our Bodies, Ourselves;* their Women's Health Information Center includes an extensive collection of books, periodicals, and clippings on such subjects as sexuality, women's health, menopause, and reproductive rights, feminism, and women in Third World countries. This collection is available to the public by appointment. The files and books used to compile *Ourselves, Growing Older* form the basis of its collection on women and aging. Information requests by mail or phone are answered for a nominal fee or donation to cover costs.

Families USA Foundation
1334 G St. NW
Washington, DC 20005
Tel. (202) 628-3030
Provides information, financial support, and technical assistance for grass-roots projects and national organizations around issues of health care, long-term care, and economic security. Sponsors A.S.A.P. for individuals to be informed and to make their views known to Congress.

Gray Panthers
2025 Pennsylvania Ave. NW
Washington, DC 20006
Tel. (202) 466-3132
An intergenerational organization of women and men opposed to ageism and active on behalf of world peace, a universal health-care system, and issues of social justice. Write to the national office for information on how to join or start a local chapter. Members receive *Network,* a quarterly newsletter.

League of Women Voters
1730 M St. NW
Washington, DC 20036
Tel. (202) 429-1965
Encourages informed participation of citizens in government. Membership is open to all. The League was founded right after women won the vote by suffragists who wanted to educate women on how to use their newly won clout effectively. They expected that in ten to fifteen years all the major social reforms would have been passed and they could disband the organization. The League has been around for over seventy years and does not appear to be running out of work.

Legal Services Corporation
750 First St. NE
Washington, DC 20002-4250
Tel. (202) 336-8800
Has affiliates in most major cities. Check your phone book under "Legal Assistance," or under "Elder Services—legal," or call your local bar association for the name of the organization in your community that provides free legal services for qualified low-income persons. For those over sixty, it is easier to qualify, and advocacy services are also available for dealing with Medicare, Medicaid, and the Social Security Administration. Or contact the national office.

National Asian Pacific Center on Aging
1511 Third Ave., Suite 914
Seattle, WA 98101
Tel. (206) 624-1221
Professionals concerned with improving and ensuring services to elders of Pacific/Asian ancestry.

National Association for Lesbian and Gay Gerontology
1853 Market St.
San Francisco, CA 94103
Tel. (415) 626-7000
An organization of seniors and professionals in gerontology, promoting responsible research, education, advocacy, and the development of services for aging lesbians and gay men. Their local program, Operation Concern—Gay and Lesbian Outreach to Elders, is an example of the services they promote. Publishes quarterly newsletter and *Resource Guide (1991).*

National Caucus and Center on the Black Aged
1424 K St. NW
Washington, DC 20005
Tel. (202) 637-8400
Formed in 1971 to research and advocate for

black elders, especially those whose employment formerly had not been covered by Social Security and who have inadequate retirement income.

NATIONAL COUNCIL ON THE AGING (NCOA)
409 THIRD ST. SW, SUITE 200
WASHINGTON, DC 20024
TEL. (202) 479-1200
A membership organization for professionals, volunteers, and caregivers. Membership, at reduced rates for elders and students, includes subscription to *Perspective on Aging,* membership in one of the seven affiliates, and a variety of other discounts. Send for list of resources.

NATIONAL COUNCIL OF JEWISH WOMEN
53 W. 23RD ST.
NEW YORK, NY 10010
TEL. (212) 645-4048
A national volunteer women's organization working in the areas of education, community service, and advocacy in response to community needs. Two of their six priority areas are women's issues and aging issues. For information, including their program on "The Sandwich Generation," write to the Program Services Department at the above address; for information on local chapters, write to the Field Membership Department at the above address.

NATIONAL COUNCIL OF NEGRO WOMEN
1667 K ST. NW, #700
WASHINGTON, DC 20006
TEL. (202) 659-0006
A coalition of thirty-one organizations in forty-two states dedicated to ameliorating the problems of black women and their families and to promoting their participation in the political, cultural, social, economic, and civic life of the United States. Membership can be acquired either directly or through organizations, and student memberships are available.

NATIONAL COUNCIL OF SENIOR CITIZENS
1331 F ST. NW
WASHINGTON, DC 20004-1171
TEL. (202) 347-8800
This organization's assertively activist orientation may stem from its labor-union connections. NCSC's forty-eight hundred local clubs provide a network for grass-roots advocacy efforts on behalf of legislation at the national, state, and local levels. Persons of any age may join, but certain benefits have age requirements.

NATIONAL INTERFAITH COALITION ON AGING
409 THIRD ST. SW, 2ND FLOOR
WASHINGTON, DC 20024
TEL. (202) 479-6689
Advocates the inclusion of gerontology in religious education; seeks to expand the role of church and synagogue in improving the quality of life and the spiritual well-being of the aging.

NATIONAL ORGANIZATION FOR WOMEN (NOW)
1000 16TH ST. NW, SUITE 700
WASHINGTON, DC 20036
TEL. (202) 331-0066
A membership organization working to bring women into full participation in the mainstream of American society, exercising all the privileges and responsibilities thereof in truly equal partnership with men. Works in a variety of areas such as economic rights and pay equity, lesbian and gay rights, eliminating racism and violence against women. Their legislative task force sometimes works on issues affecting older women, such as divorce and Social Security.

NOW LEGAL DEFENSE AND EDUCATION FUND
99 HUDSON ST.
NEW YORK, NY 10013
TEL. (212) 925-6635
Studies and litigates on issues relating to women's rights. Work includes a family-law project, ERA impact study, gender-neutral insurance, and legal cases, such as affirmative action.

NATIONAL SENIOR CITIZENS' LAW CENTER
1815 H ST. NW, SUITE 700
WASHINGTON, DC 20006
TEL. (202) 887-5280
Operates a legal services support center and advocates for poor elder clients. Sponsors conferences and workshops on areas of law affecting elders. Maintains a library. Publishes weekly newsletter, monthly *Nursing Home Law Letter,* various handbooks, guides, and testimony.

NATIONAL WOMEN'S POLITICAL CAUCUS (NWPC)
1275 K ST. NW, SUITE 750
WASHINGTON, DC 20005
TEL. (202) 898-1100
NWPC's goal is to get more women elected and appointed to political office.

OLDER WOMEN'S LEAGUE (OWL)
666 11TH ST. NW, SUITE 700
WASHINGTON, DC 20001
TEL. (800) TAKE OWL; (202) 783-6686

National organization with chapters in nearly every state. Focuses on issues of concern to midlife and older women. The 1993 agenda includes health-care reform, pension and Social Security reform, housing, discrimination in the workplace, violence against women and older persons, and staying in control of our death and dying. The bimonthly newsletter, *The Owl Observer,* contains excellent coverage of older women's issues. Issues special reports, a series of "Gray Papers," and annual reports on Mother's Day. Local chapters educate and advocate for a range of older women's issues.

SENIOR ACTION IN A GAY ENVIRONMENT (SAGE)
208 W. 13TH ST.
NEW YORK, NY 10011
TEL. (212) 741-2247
Ask for their resource list of lesbian and gay aging groups.

THE SILVER-HAIRED LEGISLATURE A grass-roots nonpartisan body composed of elder citizens, elected at Councils on Aging by their peers. Its purpose is to educate elder activists about the workings of a legislative body and to make recommendations to the legislature about issues of concern to elders and their communities. Twenty-three states have some form of Silver-Haired Legislature. Inquire at your area Council on Aging or your state legislature.

WORLD INSTITUTE ON DISABILITY
510 16TH ST.
OAKLAND, CA 94612
TEL. (510) 763-4100
Coalition of disabled individuals who do research, advocacy, and policy making on personal assistance services for people with disabilities. Referral to 200 Independent Living Centers nationally which can help individuals plan to meet their needs for assistance and accessibility.

Books and Articles

Aglietti, Susan L., ed. *Filtered Images: Women Remembering Their Grandmothers.* Orinda, CA: Vintage '45 Press, 1992.

Alexander, Jo, Debi Barrow, Lisa Domitrovich, Margareta Donnelly, and Cheryl McLean. *Women and Aging: An Anthology by Women.* Corvallis, OR: Calyx Books, 1986. Delightful collection of fiction, poetry, journal excerpts, photographs.

Allen, Jessie, and Alan Pifer, eds. *Women on the Front Lines: Meeting the Challenge of an Aging America.* Washington, DC: The Urban Institute Press, 1993. Compilation of the Project on Women and Population Aging of the Southport Institute for Policy Analysis. The authors explore many issues confronting women in an aging society.

Ascher, Carol, Louise DeSalvo, and Sara Ruddick. *Between Women.* New York: Routledge, 1993. Biographers, novelists, critics, teachers, and artists write about their work on women.

Banner, Lois W. *In Full Flower: Aging Women, Power, and Sexuality.* New York: Vintage, 1993. Authoritative, lively, and empowering.

Baruch, Grace K., and Jeanne Brooks-Gunn, eds. *Women in Midlife.* London: Plenum Publishing, 1984. Informative collection of scholarly articles.

Bowman, Meg, and Diane Haywood, eds. *Readings for Older Women: A Compilation of Wit and Wisdom.* San Jose, CA: Hot Flash Press, 1992.

Brown, Judith K. *In Her Prime: A New View of Middle-Aged Women.* South Hadley, MA.: Bergin & Garvey, 1985. Reports of women from diverse cultures.

Browne, Susan, Debra Connors, and Nanci Stern. *With the Power of Each Breath: A Disabled Woman's Anthology.* Pittsburgh: Cleis Press, 1985.

Building Community: A Manual Exploring Issues of Women and Disability, 1984. Groundbreaking manual clarifies the connections between gender and disability. Also, *Bridging the Gap: A National Directory of Services for Women and Girls with Disabilities,* 1990. More than three hundred listings. Produced by the Women and Disability Awareness Project. A program of Educational Equity Concepts, Inc., 114 E. 32nd St., New York, NY 10016. Tel. (212) 725-1803, Voice only; Fax (212) 725-0947.

Buss, Fran L. *Dignity: Lower Income Women Tell of Their Lives and Struggles.* Ann Arbor, MI: University of Michigan Press, 1985.

Butler, Robert N. *Why Survive? Being Old in*

America. New York: Harper Colophon, 1973. A classic on aging and ageism.

Choices and Challenges: An Older Adult Reference Series. Elizabeth Vierck, Series Editor. Santa Barbara, CA: ABC-CLIO, 1992. This series includes titles such as "Housing Options and Services for Older Adults," "Older Workers," "Paying for Health Care After 65," "Legal Issues for Older Adults," and "Caregiving of Older Adults," all clearly written and printed in readable type.

Cohen, Leah. *Small Expectations. Society's Betrayal of Older Women*. Toronto: McClellan and Stewart, Ltd., 1984. Analysis of the discrimination against older women drawn from interviews of women in Canada, the United States, and Great Britain. Highly recommended.

de Beauvoir, Simone. *The Second Sex*. New York: Vintage, 1974. First published in 1952, this is an early classic of modern feminism.

Delaney, Sarah, and Annie Delaney, with Amy Hill Hearth. *Having Our Say: The Delaney Sisters' First Hundred Years*. New York: Farrar, Straus & Giroux, 1993. Secrets of longevity and survival from two centenarians who achieved an impressive string of first and seconds pioneering in professions previously closed to blacks and women.

Durable Dauntless Dykes. San Francisco: Gay and Lesbian Outreach to Elders, 1987. Selected writings of older lesbians published in connection with the National Association for Lesbian and Gay Gerontology (see page 442).

Friedan, Betty. *The Fountain of Age*. New York: Simon & Schuster, 1993. Friedan takes on the "mystique of aging" with the same gusto that she brought to the liberation of women. She celebrates active old age in which women and men discover new possibilities for intimacy and purpose.

Grambs, Jean D. *Women Over Forty: Visions and Realities*. New York: Springer Publishing, 1989.

Hemmings, Susan. *A Wealth of Experience: The Lives of Older Women*. London and Boston: Pandora Press, 1985.

Hickman, Martha Whitmore. *Fullness of Time: Short Stories of Women and Aging*. Nashville: Upper Room Books, 1990.

Jacobs, Ruth Harriet. *Be an Outrageous Older Woman—a RASP.* Manchester, CT: Knowledge, Ideas & Trends, 1991. A fun and empowering book.

Koppellman, Susan, ed. *Between Mothers and Daughters: Stories Across a Generation*. New York: Feminist Press at the City University of New York, 1985.

Leonard, Frances. *Money and the Mature Woman*. New York: Addison-Wesley, 1993. Strategies for surviving gender bias in economic laws and policies.

Markson, Elizabeth W., ed. *Older Women*. Lexington, MA: D. C. Heath/Lexington Books, 1983. An excellent collection of articles that capture the social diversity of women growing older. Sections cover changes beginning at midlife, occupational and retirement patterns, variations in families and life-styles, and selected health issues.

Martin, Del, and Phyllis Lyon. *Lesbian/Woman: Twentieth Anniversary Edition*. San Francisco: Volcano Press, 1992. A twenty-year history placing the lesbian struggle in the context of other movements. By the founders of the first lesbian organization, Daughters of Bilitis.

Martz, Sandra Haldeman, ed. *When I Am an Old Woman I Shall Wear Purple,* 2nd ed., 1991, and *If I Had My Life to Live Over I Would Pick More Daisies*. Watsonville, CA: Papier-Mache Press, 1993. Essays, stories, and poetry by diverse women.

Miller, Jean Baker. *Toward a New Psychology of Women*. Rev. ed. New York: Harper & Row, 1986. A critique of sex inequality with an appreciation of women's traditional strengths and their value for women and men today.

Myerhoff, Barbara. *Number Our Days*. New York: Touchstone/Simon & Schuster, 1978. A moving account of the lives of elderly Jews in Venice, California, and how they affected the author, a prominent anthropologist.

Nickerson, Betty. *Old and Smart: Women and Aging*. The author's essays about her own life and her observations on aging. U.S. and Canada: All About Us Books, 1991. U.S. orders: 443 Adams St., Eugene, OR 97402; $19.95 U.S. dollars.

Canadian orders: RR#3 Ladysmith, B.C. Canada VOR 2EO; $23 Canadian dollars.

Painter, Charlotte, and Pamela Valois. *Gifts of Age: Portraits and Essays of 32 Remarkable Women.* San Francisco: Chronicle Books, 1985. A visually beautiful book.

Porcino, Jane. *Growing Older, Getting Better: A Handbook for Women in the Second Half of Life.* New York: Crossroad Continuum, 1991.

Reinharz, Shulamit. "Friends or Foes: Gerontological and Feminist Theory." *Women's Studies International Forum,* Vol. 9, No. 5 (1986), pp. 503–14. An excellent article analyzing the relationship between feminist and gerontological concerns and what each can offer the other.

Reyes, Karen Westerberg, and Lorena Fletcher Farrell, eds. *Emotional and Spiritual Guide for Gays and Lesbians Who Are Growing Older.* North Hollywood, CA: Newcastle Publishing Co., 1993. Good chapters written by old lesbians and a very thorough resource list.

Rubin, Rhea Joyce. *Of a Certain Age: A Guide to Contemporary Fiction Featuring Older Adults.* Santa Barbara, CA: ABC-CLIO, 1990.

Salber, Eva J. *Don't Send Me Flowers When I'm Dead: Voices of Rural Elderly.* Durham, NC: Duke University Press, 1983.

Sang, B., et al. *Lesbians at Midlife: The Creative Transition.* San Francisco: Spinsters Book Co., 1991. Essays, personal narratives, poetry, and research reports.

Simon, Barbara Levy. "C'est La Vie: Never Married Old Women and Disability, A Majority Experience." In Michelle Fine and Adrienne Asch, eds., *Voices from the Margins: Lives of Disabled Girls and Women.* Philadelphia: Temple University Press, 1987.

Steinem, Gloria. *Revolution from Within: A Book of Self-Esteem.* Boston: Little, Brown, 1992.

Walker, Barbara G. *The Crone: Woman of Age, Wisdom & Power.* San Francisco: Harper & Row, 1985. One woman's spirituality and the historic role of female elders. Offers a key to respect for older women today.

Wilson, Emily Herring. *Older Black Women of the South.* Philadelphia: Temple University Press, 1983.

Other Publications

Broomstick: A Bimonthly Feminist Periodical By, For and About Women Over Forty. Options for Women over Forty, 3543 18th St., San Francisco, CA 94110. Ceased publication autumn 1993. Some back issues may be available.

Disability Studies Quarterly. Excellent overview of new research about people with disabilities by a leading advocate. Order from Irving Kenneth Zola, Sociology Dept., Brandeis University, Waltham, MA 02154. $30 per year.

Encore: A Magazine for the New Woman of Age. P.O. Box 1599, Mariposa, CA 95338. A bimonthly magazine "celebrating the return of the crone." A resource to help women uncover and neutralize sexism and ageism in society.

Hot Flash: A Newsletter for Midlife and Older Women. c/o National Action Forum for Midlife and Older Women, Box 816, Stony Brook, NY 11790-0609. Contains articles and news about health and social issues. Quarterly. $15 per year.

Sojourner: The Women's Forum. 42 Seaverns Ave., Boston, MA 02130. Feminist monthly newspaper. $15 per year.

Older Women's Presses

The number of women's presses is too long to publish here. They are listed in reference books such as the *International Directory of Little Magazines and Small Presses,* Paradise, CA: Best Books, 1993–94. Check your library.

CRONES' OWN PRESS
209 WATTS
DURHAM, NC 27701
This press specializes in publishing and distributing writings of older women.

Audiovisual

A few films are listed under specific chapters. The following libraries and distributors rent or sell films or videos of interest to older women. See your library for local and other sources.

FANLIGHT PRODUCTIONS
47 HALIFAX ST.
BOSTON, MA 02130
TEL. (617) 524-0980

Their catalogs feature films about a range of health education issues such as, chronic illness, gerontology, disability and special needs, mental health, and choices about dying and death.

FILMMAKERS LIBRARY
133 E. 58TH ST.
NEW YORK, NY 10022
TEL. (212) 355-6545

Films and videos can be viewed in their office by appointment.

THE OLDER WOMEN'S FILM PROJECT
131 CONCORD ST.
SAN FRANCISCO, CA 94112
TEL. (415) 496-7532.

Produced *Acting Our Age,* a documentary film showing women in their sixties and seventies from diverse ethnic groups in the context of aging in America today.

THE PENNSYLVANIA STATE UNIVERSITY
AUDIO-VISUAL SERVICES
SPECIAL SERVICES BUILDING
1127 FOX HILL RD.
UNIVERSITY PARK, PA 16803-1824
TEL. (800) 826-0132 OR (814) 865-6314

Request their catalog, *Films and Video about, for, and by Women.*

TERRA NOVA FILMS
9848 S. WINCHESTER AVE.
CHICAGO, IL 60643
TEL. (800) 779-8491 OR (312) 881-8491

Distributes videos including *Women of the Georgian Hotel,* about four women, ages eighty-three to 107; *Whisper: The Women,* about seven older women of varied race and culture; and *Whisper, the Waves, the Wind,* about 154 women, ages sixty-nine to ninety-nine who talk about their lives at an art performance on a beach.

WOMEN MAKE MOVIES
462 BROADWAY, 5TH FLOOR
NEW YORK, NY 10013
TEL. (212) 925-0606

Has catalog of many films and videos by and about women. Covers a wide range of topics and styles.

AGING WELL

AGING AND WELL-BEING

The General Health resources starting on page 482 include entries that are also relevant to aging and well-being.

STRESS MANAGEMENT

Books

Benson, Herbert, and Eileen Stuart. *The Wellness Book.* Secaucus, NJ: Carol Publishing Group, 1993. How to maintain health and treat stress-related illnesses. Includes basic meditation techniques.

Birkedahl, Nonie. *Older and Wiser: A Workbook for Coping with Aging.* Oakland, CA: New Harbinger Publications, 1991. Practical steps for negotiating the challenges of aging in a workbook format.

Borysenko, Joan. *Minding the Body, Mending the Mind.* Reading, MA: Addison-Wesley, 1987; and *Fire in the Soul.* New York: Warner Books, 1993.

Louden, Jennifer. *The Woman's Comfort Book: A Self-Nurturing Book for Restoring Balance in Your Life.* San Francisco: Harper, 1992. How to nurture yourself through bathing, massage, music, herbs, and silliness.

Mason, Marilyn J. *Making Our Lives Our Own: A Woman's Guide to the Six Challenges of Personal Change.* San Francisco: Harper, 1991. Recognizes women's nonlinear growth patterns. Challenges myths of women as all-giving. Addresses issues such as substance abuse and sexual-spiritual integration in women's lives.

Scheller, Mary Dale. *Growing Older, Feeling Better in Body, Mind, and Spirit.* Palo Alto, CA: Bull Publishing Co., 1993. Self-care and wellness through spirituality and healing techniques such as breathing exercises, yoga, and acupressure.

MASSAGE

Organizations

To locate massage therapists in your area, contact:

AMERICAN MASSAGE THERAPY ASSOCIATION
820 DAVIS ST., SUITE 100
EVANSTON, IL 60201
TEL. (708) 864-0123
This professional organization certifies massage therapists and sets educational standards for training progams.

Or try massage therapy schools, physical therapists, massage collectives, women's centers, holistic health, fitness, and yoga centers, chiropractors, or acupuncturists in your area.

Books

Benjamin, Ben E., with Gale Borden. *Listen to Your Pain.* New York: Penguin, 1984. Self-help book for coping with injuries.

Berkson, Devaki. *The Foot Book: Healing the Body Through Reflexology.* New York: Barnes & Noble, 1979. Includes work with older adults, and treatments for specific conditions such as lower backache, arthritis, and high blood pressure, in addition to standard reflexology.

Downing, George. *The Massage Book.* New York: Random House/Bookworks, 1972. Good basic introduction to massage.

Lawrence, D. Baloti, and Lewis Harrison. *Massageworks: A Practical Encyclopedia of Massage Techniques.* New York: Phantom Publishing Group, 1983.

Lindell, Lucinda, et al. *The Book of Massage: The Complete Step-By-Step Guide to Eastern and Western Techniques.* New York: Simon & Schuster, 1984.

Maxwell-Hudson, Clare. *The Complete Book of Massage.* New York: Random House, 1988.

Prudden, Bonnie. *Myotherapy: Bonnie Prudden's Complete Guide to Pain-Free Living.* New York: Ballantine Books, 1985. And *Pain Erasure, The Bonnie Prudden Way.* New York: Ballantine Books, 1980. Describes trigger-point therapy.

Struik, Monika, with Connie Church. *Self-Massage: Touch Techniques to Relax, Soothe and Stimulate Your Body.* New York: Simon & Schuster, 1983.

Tappan, Frances M. *Healing Massage Techniques: A Study of Eastern and Western Methods.* Reston, VA: Reston Publishing Co., 1980.

West, Ouida. *The Magic of Massage.* New York: Putnam, 1983. A holistic approach that combines acupressure with Swedish strokes.

SELF-HELP AND SUPPORT GROUPS

Organizations

AMERICAN SELF-HELP CLEARINGHOUSE
ST. CLARES-RIVERSIDE MEDICAL CENTER
25 POCONO RD.
DENVILLE, NJ 07834
TEL. (601) 625-7101
Publishes *The Self-Help Source Book: Finding and Forming Mutual Aid Self-Help Groups.* $8. Send for complete publication list.

NATIONAL SELF-HELP CLEARINGHOUSE
25 W. 43RD ST., ROOM 620
NEW YORK, NY 10036
TEL. (212) 642-2944
An information and referral center to self-help regional clearinghouses and self-help groups around the country. Publishes a newsletter, runs research projects, and provides technical assistance.

SENIOR HEALTH AND PEER COUNSELING CENTER
2125 ARIZONA AVE.
SANTA MONICA, CA 90404-13998
TEL. (310) 828-1243
Offers access to counseling for those who may not be able to afford it. In addition, the peer counselors benefit from the training, the stimulation, and the satisfaction they receive. Contact the center for information about their peer-counseling program for persons fifty-five and over.

THE SUPPORTIVE OLDER WOMEN'S NETWORK (S.O.W.N.)
2805 N. 47TH ST.
PHILADELPHIA, PA 19131
TEL. (215) 477-6000

Helps older women in the Delaware Valley through support groups and other outreach services. Their lively, chatty newsletter may be helpful in starting a similar project in your area.

Books and Other Publications

Jackson, Maggie, and Zeb Harel. "Social Support Networks of the Elderly: Racial Differences and Health Care Implications." *Urban Health,* September 1983, pp. 35–38.

Jacobs, Ruth. *Older Women: Surviving and Thriving,* 1986. Order from Family Service America, 11700 W. Lake Park Drive, Milwaukee, WI 53224. A manual to help older women build self-esteem and solve practical problems. Twelve workshop sessions with handouts for participants on subjects such as health care, housing, community involvement, and sexuality.

Jerrome, Dorothy. "The Significance of Friendship for Women in Later Life." *Aging and Society,* Vol. 1, No. 2 (1981).

Lidoff, Lorraine. "Sharing a Common Concern." *Perspective on Aging,* Vol. 8, No. 1 (January/February 1984), pp. 26–27.

McGuire, Kathleen. *Building Supportive Community—Mutual Self-Help Through Peer Counseling.* 3440 Onyx St., Eugene, OR 97405. Tel. (503) 342-1033. $14.95. Self-help for creating a support network. Includes such techniques as peer counseling, empathic listening, conflict resolution, and consensus decision making.

Reissman, Frank, et al. *Self-Help and the Elderly. Considerations for Practice and Policy.* Washington, DC: National Council on the Aging, 1982.

Silverman, Phyllis R. *Mutual Help Groups: Organization and Development.* Beverly Hills, CA: Sage Publications, 1980. A guide to starting groups.

Other sources of information on self-help and support groups in your area include referral services (often operated by the United Way), community activity lists in the newspapers, and women's centers. The National Council on the Aging (see page 443 for address) also has a directory of self- help groups.

For books and articles on friendship, see Resources for Relationships in Middle and Later Life, pages 468–71.

SELF-DISCOVERY AND LIFE REVIEW

Books

Cameron, Julia, *The Artist's Way: A Spiritual Path to Higher Creativity.* New York: Jeremy P. Tarcher/Perigee Books, 1992. A course for discovering and recovering your creative self.

Hagan, Kay Leigh. *Internal Affairs: A Journal-Keeping Workbook for Self-Intimacy.* New York: HarperSan Francisco, 1990.

Houston, Jean. *A Course in Enhancing Your Physical, Mental, and Creative Abilities.* Los Angeles: J. P. Tarcher, 1982.

Maas, James. *Fifteen Past Seventy: Counsel from My Elders.* Berkeley, CA: Shameless Hussy Press, 1986. Profiles of women and men who, regardless of their life situations, relish their present and look forward to their future.

Metzger, Deena. *Writing for Your Life: A Guide and Companion to the Inner Worlds.* San Francisco: HarperCollins, 1992.

Robey, Harriet. *There's a Dance in the Old Dame Yet.* Boston: Atlantic/Little Brown, 1982. Author tells of her journey of self-healing and self-discovery in her later years.

FEMINISM, RELIGION, AND SPIRITUALITY

Books and Other Publications

Broner, Esther. M. "Blessing the Ties That Bind." *Ms.,* Vol. 15, No. 6 (December 1986), p. 50. And Hattie-Jo Pursglove-Mullins, "New Rites, New Rituals," p. 51. Rituals by older women to celebrate their ages. Includes an annotated list of materials from many traditions.

Christ, Carol, and Judith Plaskow, eds. *Womanspirit Rising: A Feminist Reader in Religion.* San Francisco: Harper & Row, 1979. A comprehensive look at feminist theology in Christianity, Judaism, and goddess-centered religion.

———. *Weaving the Visions: New Patterns in Feminist Spirituality.* New York: HarperSan Francisco, 1989. Selected key writings from a wide range of traditions.

Daly, Mary. *Pure Lust: Elemental Feminist Philosophy.* Boston: Beacon Press, 1984. Includes the visionary wisdom of older women.

Davis, Susan E. "Editor's Bookshelf." *New Directions for Women,* Vol. 22, No. 4 (July–August 1993), p. 42. An annotated list of seventeen books on women's spirituality from diverse religions and cultures.

Demetrakopoulous, Stephanie. *Listening to Our Bodies: The Rebirth of Feminine Wisdom.* Boston: Beacon Press, 1983.

Fine, Irene. *Midlife: A Rite of Passage and the Wise Woman, A Celebration.* Women's Institute for Continuing Jewish Education, 4126 Executive Park Drive, La Jolla, CA 92307. $8.95 plus $3 postage and handling. Jewish ritual that can be used by anyone. Catalog available from WICJE.

Gray, Elizabeth Dodson, ed. *Sacred Dimensions of Women's Experience.* Wellesley, MA: Roundtable Press, 1988. Feminist theological reflections, including a chapter by Jeanne Brooks Carritt on aging.

Iglehart, Hallie. *Womanspirit: A Guide to Women's Wisdom.* San Francisco: Harper & Row, 1983. A guide for individuals or groups to learn meditation, dream-work, mythmaking, and healing, and to create new rituals.

Mariechild, Diane, with Shuli Goodman. *The Inner Dance: A Guide to Spiritual and Psychological Unfolding.* Freedom, CA: The Crossing Press, 1987. Includes a celebration ritual for menopause.

Peters, Erskine. *African Openings to the Tree of Life.* Norwood, PA: Norwood Editions, 1987. Life principles from African philosophy and religion. These principles pertain to the person, the social group, and the community.

Sewell, Marilyn, ed. *Cries of the Spirit: A Celebration of Women's Spirituality.* Boston: Beacon Press, 1991. Sourcebook of diverse poetry and prose organized around themes central to women's experiences.

Spretnak, Charlene. "Essay: Wholly Writ." *Ms.,* Vol. III, No. 5 (March/April 1993), pp. 60–62. An essay with suggested readings on women's spirituality.

Starhawk. *The Spiral Dance: A Rebirth of the Ancient Religion of the Great Goddess.* New York: Harper & Row, 1979. Manual for the practice of a woman-centered, goddess-centered religion. Rituals and exercises designed to aid women in reclaiming their power.

Woman of Power: A Magazine of Feminism, Spirituality and Politics. P.O. Box 2785, Orleans, MA 02653. Tel. (508) 240-7877.

Habits Worth Changing

AARP (see page 441) has publications including *Is Drinking Becoming a Problem? Older Women and Alcohol; So Many Pills and I Still Don't Feel Good;* and *If Only I Could Get a Good Night's Sleep! A Self-Help guide for Understanding and Overcoming Insomnia.*

Smoking

Organizations

Action on Smoking and Health (ASH)
2013 H St. NW
Washington, DC 20006
Tel. (202) 659-4310

A national citizens' organization concerned with policy issues, regulations about smoking, and nonsmokers' rights.

The American Lung Association, the American Heart Association, and the American Cancer Society have literature and free or inexpensive group programs to help you stop smoking. See your local or state chapters.

Group Against Smoking Pollution (GASP), Box 15463, Kenmore Station, Boston, MA 02215; and Americans for Nonsmokers' Rights, 2530 San Pable Ave., Berkeley, CA 94702 are two of the organizations that work to protect the rights of nonsmokers to clean air in public places and in the workplace through nonsmoking ordinances. Similar organizations in other states may be found through ASH (see above).

Books and Other Publications

Useful materials are available from several U.S. government agencies: Office for Smoking and Health, Centers for Disease Control and Prevention, 1600 Clifton Rd., NE, Atlanta, GA 30333; Office of Cancer Communications, National Cancer Institute, Bldg. 31, Rm. 10A21, Bethesda, MD 20892; and the Environmental Protection Agency, 401 M St. SW, Washington, DC 20460.

American Cancer Society. *Cancer Facts and Figures.* 3340 Peachtree Rd., NE, Atlanta, GA 30026. Published annually. Contains statistics on smoking-related illnesses, treatment, and education.

Delaney, Sue. *Women Smokers Can Quit: A Different Approach,* 1989. Available from Women's Healthcare Press, 500 Davis St., Suite 700, Evanston, IL 60201. $6.95.

Whelan, Elizabeth. *A Smoking Gun: How the Tobacco Industry Gets Away with Murder.* Philadelphia: George Stickey, 1984.

Audiovisual

The Feminine Mistake: The Next Generation. Distributed by Pyramid Films and Video, P.O. Box 1048, Santa Monica, CA 90406. Thirty-minute 1989 videocassette about women and smoking.

The Lady Killers. A 40-minute British documentary featuring Bobbie Jackson, author of two books on women and smoking. Explores why women smoke and barriers to their quitting. Available from Communications Media, Yale Medical School, 333 Cedar St., New Haven, CT 06510.

ALCOHOL

Organizations

AL-ANON AND ALATEEN
AL-ANON FAMILY GROUP HEADQUARTERS
P.O. BOX 862, MIDTOWN STATION
NEW YORK, NY 10018
TEL. (800) 356-9996 OR (212) 302-7240

Al-Anon is a self-help group that can be of great value to family and friends of alcoholics, and Alateen is for teenagers whose parents or friends drink. Call the national office if they are not listed in your local phone book.

ALCOHOL HELPLINE. A nationwide 24-hour telephone referral service. Free of charge, run by Doctors' Hospital, Worcester, MA. Tel. (800) 252-6465.

ALCOHOLICS ANONYMOUS (AA)
GENERAL SERVICE OFFICE OF AA
BOX 459, GRAND CENTRAL STATION
NEW YORK, NY 10163
TEL. (212) 870-3400

AA is the most successful self-help group in the world and is listed in every phone book. Admission to AA is free, and a list of meeting times and locations in thousands of cities and towns can be obtained by calling any office. Though some meetings are open only to previously self-proclaimed alcoholics (the list of meetings indicates those for which this is the case), many others are open to anyone. Members of AA consider it part of their responsibility to offer newcomers transportation to and from meetings. A phone call to the closest office is all it takes to arrange a meeting. There are also women-only, and lesbian and gay AA meetings. Publications include *Alcoholics Anonymous* (the Big Book) and *AA for the Woman.* Send for their materials.

AMERICAN COUNCIL ON ALCOHOLISM, INC.
WHITE MARSH BUSINESS CENTER
5024 CAMPBELL BLVD., SUITE H
BALTIMORE, MD 21236
TEL. (410) 931-9393

Publishes educational materials and has a referral list to alcohol treatment centers. Members include individuals and treatment centers.

MOTHERS AGAINST DRUNK DRIVING
MADD NATIONAL HEADQUARTERS
511 EAST JOHN CARPENTER FREEWAY, SUITE 700
IRVING, TX 75062
TEL. (800) GET-MADD

Funded by donations. No charge to victims. Literature and materials for adults and youth.

NATIONAL ASSOCIATION OF ALCOHOL AND DRUG ABUSE DIRECTORS
444 N. CAPITOL ST. NW, SUITE 642
WASHINGTON, DC 20001
TEL. (202) 783-6868

Provides information on organizations and treatment programs. You can also find this information through your state alcohol and drug agencies; check the phone book.

NATIONAL ASSOCIATION OF LESBIAN AND GAY ALCOHOLISM PROFESSIONALS (NALGAP)
1147 S. ALVARADO ST.
LOS ANGELES, CA 90006
TEL. (213) 381-8524
Write for a list of programs specializing in the treatment of lesbian and gay alcoholics.

NATIONAL CLEARINGHOUSE FOR ALCOHOL AND DRUG INFORMATION
P.O. BOX 2345
ROCKVILLE, MD 20847-2345
TEL. (800) 729-6686
Call to order free federal government materials. Tel. (800) 662-HELP for treatment referrals.

NATIONAL COUNCIL ON ALCOHOLISM (NCA)
12 W. 21ST ST.
NEW YORK, NY 10010
TEL. (212) 206-6770
A nonprofit organization with information and publications on alcohol. Consult your phone book or write to their national office for their 190 local and state affiliates.

NATIONAL COUNCIL ON ALCOHOLISM
1511 K ST. NW, SUITE 926
WASHINGTON, DC 20005
TEL. (202) 737-8122
The District of Columbia Office of the NCA concentrates on public-policy issues and has effectively lobbied for warning labels on alcohol products.

WOMEN FOR SOBRIETY
P.O. BOX 618
QUAKERTOWN, PA 18951-0618
This organization has many local self-help groups that address the special needs of women alcoholics. Write for materials.

Books and Other Publications

Black, Claudia. *It Will Never Happen to Me.* Denver: MAC Printing and Publications Division, 1982. About children of alcoholics and the effect alcohol has on their lives.

Fishel, Ruth. *The Journey Within: A Spiritual Path to Recovery.* Pompano Beach, FL: Health Communications, Inc., 1987.

Ford, Betty. *Betty: A Glad Awakening.* Garden City, NY: Doubleday, 1987. A personal memoir of her addiction problems.

Kasl, C. L. *Many Roads, One Journey: Moving Beyond the Twelve Steps.* New York: HarperCollins, 1992. Primarily for women.

Kirkpatrick, Jean. *Turnabout: Help for a New Life.* New York: Doubleday, 1978. Alternative self-help program for women.

Larimore, Helen. *Older Women in Recovery.* Deerfield Beach, FL: Health Communications, 1992. Older women tell their own stories of recovery.

Nellis, Muriel. *The Female Fix.* Boston: Houghton Mifflin, 1980.

Pinkham, Mary Ellen. *How to Stop the One You Love from Drinking.* New York: Putnam, 1986.

Roth, P., ed. *Alcohol and Drugs Are Women's Issues.* Volumes I and II, Metuchen, NJ: Women's Alliance and Scarecrow Press, 1991.

Sandmaier, Marian. *The Invisible Alcoholics: Women and Alcohol Abuse in America.* 2nd ed. Blue Ridge Summit, PA: Tab Books, 1992.

Sober Days, Golden Years: Alcoholism and the Older Person, 1982. Johnson Institute, Inc., 1205 Ohms Lane, Edina, MN 55439. 48 pp. $2.75. Tel. (612) 831-1630. Also has films, other books, and training materials.

Swallow, Jean, ed. *Out from Under: Sober Dykes and Our Friends.* San Francisco: Spinsters Ink, 1983.

Wegscheider-Cruse, Sharon. *Choicemaking,* 1985. Health Communications, Inc., 3201 SW 15th St. Deerfield, FL 33442. Tel. (305) 360-0909.

Woititz, Janet G. *Adult Children of Alcoholics.* Deerfield, FL: Health Communications, Inc. (address above), 1983.

———. *Struggle for Intimacy.* Pompano Beach, FL: Health Communications, Inc. (address above), 1985.

Youcha, Geraldine. *Women and Alcohol: A Dangerous Pleasure.* New York: Hawthorne Books, 1986.

Youcha, Geraldine, and Judith S. Seixas. *Children of Alcoholism: A Survivor's Manual.* New York: Crown, 1985. A self-help book for adult children of alcoholics.

Over-the-Counter and Prescription Drugs

Organizations

AARP Pharmacy Service Center
7609 Energy Parkway, Suite 1003
Baltimore, MD 21226-1755
Tel. (800) 456-2226

American Association of Retired Persons (AARP) operates the largest nonprofit mail-order pharmacy service in the world. The *AARP Pharmacy Service Catalog* contains over eight-hundred generic and brand-name prescription drugs as well as vitamins and other health-care products. For the address of the pharmacy that serves AARP members in your area, contact your local office or request a catalog from the address above.

Commission on Accreditation of Rehabilitation Facilities
101 North Wilmot Rd., Suite 500
Tucson, AZ 85711
Tel. (602) 748-1212

Accredits rehabilitation and pain-control facilities.

Narcotics Anonymous
World Service Office
16155 Wyandotte St.
Van Nuys, CA 91406
Tel. (818) 780-3951

Narcotics Anonymous has a program modeled after Alcoholics Anonymous for persons addicted to any kind of drug, including tranquilizers and other prescription drugs. See your phone book or contact the national office.

Books

These basic reference books describe the ingredients and effects of many medicines.

If your local library does not have drug reference directories, request that they purchase them.

Graedon, Joe, and Teresa Graedon. *The Graedons' People's Pharmacy for Older Adults.* New York: Bantam Books, 1988. Available from Graedon Enterprises, Inc., P.O. Box 52027, Durham, NC 27717-2027. Pays special attention to how to take your medicine, drug interactions, and drugs that cause memory loss and depression and interfere with sexuality.

The Handbook of Nonprescription Drugs, 10th ed. Washington, DC: American Pharmaceutical Association, 1993.

Physicians' Desk Reference. 47th ed. Oradell, NJ: Medical Economics Co., 1993.

Physician's Desk Reference for Nonprescription Drugs. 14th ed. Oradell, NJ: Medical Economics Co., 1993.

Wolfe, Sidney M. *Worst Pills, Best Pills.* Washington, DC: Public Citizen Health Research Group, 1988.

Constipation and Other Bowel Disorders

Organizations

International Foundation of Bowel Dysfunction, Inc.
P.O. Box 17864
Milwaukee, WI 53217
Tel. (414) 964-1799

Free sample of quarterly newsletter available. $15 annual subscription. Includes information on constipation, diarrhea, irritable bowel syndrome, and fecal incontinence.

National Digestive Diseases Information Clearinghouse
Box NDDIC
9000 Rockville Pike
Bethesda, MD 20892
Tel. (301) 468-6344

This service of the National Institutes of Health answers questions, makes referrals, and provides publication lists and publications to promote understanding of digestive health and disease.

OUR LOOKS AND OUR LIVES

Books and Other Publications

Baker, Nancy C. *The Beauty Trap: Exploring Woman's Greatest Obsession.* New York: Franklin Watts, 1984. Contains chapters on women's feelings about looking older, cosmetic surgery, and weight.

Brumberg, Elaine. *Save Your Money, Save Your Face: What Every Cosmetic Buyer Needs to Know.* New York: Facts on File, 1986. Contains a detailed list of hundreds of cosmetic products, their ingredients, and possible irritants.

Chapkis, Wendy. *Beauty Secrets: Women and the Politics of Appearance*, 1986. South End Press, 116 St. Botolph St., Boston, MA 02115. Looks at the role of gender, class, race, and age in shaping images of beauty.

Cosmetic Regulation: Information on Voluntary Actions Agreed to by FDA and the Industry. 1990. This publication describes the voluntary nature of cosmetics regulation. Authority of the FDA over cosmetics is less comprehensive than its authority to regulate safety in food and drugs. Available from U.S. General Accounting Office, P.O. Box 6015, Gaithersburg, MD 20877. A single copy is free.

Freedman, Rita. *Bodylove: Learning to Like Our Looks and Ourselves.* New York: Harper & Row, 1989. Excellent resource for overcoming negative messages about your body and your age.

Goldwyn, Robert M., ed. *The Unfavorable Result in Plastic Surgery: Avoidance and Treatment.* 2nd ed. Boston: Little, Brown, 1984. Critical assessment of the field by a plastic surgeon.

Hansen, Joseph, and Evelyn Reed. *Cosmetics, Fashions, and the Exploitation of Women.* New York: Pathfinder Press, 1986. Includes reprints of classic articles from the 1950s on the relationship between the capitalist system and the oppression of women.

Hutchinson, Marsha Germaine. *Transforming Body Image: Learning to Love the Body You Have.* Trumansburg, NY: The Crossing Press, 1985. Exercises in learning to love our bodies.

Hyman, Jane Wegsheider and Esther Rome, in cooperation with the Boston Women's Health Book Collective. *Sacrificing Health for Love.* A work in progress. Includes an exhaustive critique of cosmetic surgery, breast implants, and abusive relationships and other threats to women's health.

Macdonald, Barbara, with Cynthia Rich. *Look Me in the Eye: Old Women, Aging, and Ageism.* Minneapolis: Spinsters Ink, n.d. Collection of essays and reviews. Highly recommended.

Melamed, Elissa. *Mirror, Mirror: The Terror of Not Being Young.* New York: Linden Press/Simon & Schuster, 1983.

Scheiner, Ann. "My Face-lift: A Cautionary Tale." *Ms.*, November 1986, pp. 58, 63, 81–83.

Sontag, Susan. "The Double Standard of Aging." *Saturday Review,* Vol. 95, No. 39 (Sept. 23, 1972). The ground-breaking article on this subject.

Wolf, Naomi. *The Beauty Myth: How Images of Beauty Are Used Against Women.* New York: Doubleday/Anchor, 1992. Insightful critique of the beauty mystique in social institutions from the workplace to religious life.

Audiovisual

WOMEN MAKE MOVIES (SEE PAGE 447)
This distributor offers a broad range of excellent films by and about women. A number focus on body-image issues, for example, *Mirror, Mirror,* which explores the attitudes of thirteen women of diverse ages and ethnicity toward their bodies, and *On Her Baldness,* a powerful documentary about women who have lost their hair due to illness or treatment and women who have chosen to shave their heads.

WEIGHTY ISSUES

Organizations

AMERICAN ANOREXIA/BULIMIA ASSOCIATION
418 E. 76TH ST.
NEW YORK, NY 10021
TEL. (212) 734-1114
General meetings led by professionals and recovered anorexics/bulimics are free to members and open to the public by donation. A reading list

and a newsletter are mailed to all interested persons in the United States and elsewhere.

ANOREXIA NERVOSA AND RELATED EATING DISORDERS
P.O. BOX 5102
EUGENE, OR 97405
TEL. (503) 344-1144
Collects and distributes information about eating disorders. Provides speakers, workshop and seminar leaders, trains professionals. Operates a treatment program in Eugene.

NATIONAL ANOREXIC AID SOCIETY
1925 E. DUBLIN GRANVILLE RD.
COLUMBUS, OH 43229
TEL. (614) 436-1112
Provides information and education. Publishes an international referral directory for treatment and support groups. Quarterly newsletter for members. Annual conference for professionals.

Books and Other Publications

Bordo, Susan. *Unbearable Weight: Feminism, Western Culture, and the Body.* Berkeley: University of California Press, 1993. A historical perspective tracing modern anxieties about the body back to the ancient Greek philosophers. Views eating disorders as reflecting the sickness of a culture in which women are seen as caregivers, "without need, without want, without body."

Boskind-White, Marlene, and William White. *Bulimarexia: The Binge-Purge Cycle.* New York: Norton, 1983.

Chernin, Kim. *Reflections on the Tyranny of Slenderness.* New York: Harper & Row, 1981.

Hall, Lindsey, and Leigh Cohn. *Eat Without Fear.* Santa Barbara, CA: Gurze Books, 1980. True story of Hall's recovery from bulimia.

Haskell, William, et al., eds. *Nutrition and Athletic Performance.* Palo Alto, CA: Bull Publishing Co., 1982. Proceedings of a 1981 conference including papers on consequences of rapid weight loss and advice for older athletes.

Hirschmann, Jane R., and Carol M. Munter. *Overcoming Overeating.* New York: Fawcett, 1989.

Kano, Susan. *Making Peace with Food: A Step-by-Step Guide to Freedom from Diet/Weight Conflict.* New York: Perennial, 1989. Highly recommended.

Kaplan, Jane R. *A Woman's Conflict: The Special Relationship Between Women and Food.* Englewood Cliffs, NJ: Prentice-Hall, 1980. Hard-to-find but excellent collection of articles attentive to race and ethnic cultural differences that shape women's conflicts with food. Good section on fatness.

Meadow, Rosalyn, and Lillie Weiss. *Women's Conflicts About Eating and Sexuality: The Relationship Between Food and Sex.* Binghamton, NY: Harrington Park Press, 1993.

Millman, Marcia. *Such a Pretty Face: Being Fat in America.* New York: Berkley Publishing Corp., 1981. Excellent. Explores balance of cultural and personal factors in being fat for middle-class white women.

Newman, Leslea, ed. *Eating Our Hearts Out.* Freedom, CA: The Crossing Press, 1993.

Orbach, Susie. *Fat Is a Feminist Issue. A Self-Help Guide for Compulsive Eaters.* New York: Berkley Publishing Corp., 1979. The antidiet guide to permanent weight loss. Helps distinguish between "mouth hunger" and "stomach hunger" and teaches how to enjoy food.

———. *Hunger Strike: The Anorectic's Struggle as a Metaphor of Our Age.* New York: W. W. Norton, 1986. Analyzes the structural relationship of women to food and the culture's desire to control women's bodies. Addresses issues of self-help; offers therapeutic guidelines.

Radiance: The Magazine for Large Women. P.O. Box 30246, Oakland, CA 96904. Tel. (510) 482-0680. Quarterly, $15 per year. Profiles dynamic, large women from all walks of life, with articles on health, media, fashion, and politics. Ask for the flyer describing their new T-shirt enscribed, "It's not a hot flash, it's a power surge!" Available in sizes M to 8XL.

Schoenfielder, Lisa, and Barb Wieser, eds. *Shadow on a Tightrope: Writings by Women on Fat Oppression,* 1983. Aunt Lute Book Co., P.O. Box 2568, Iowa City, IA 52244. Anthology of articles about fat oppression and fat liberation.

Schwartz, Hillel. *Never Satisfied: A Cultural History of Diets, Fantasies and Fat.* New York: Free Press, 1986. A detailed and political view of the pressures and contradictions facing women throughout history.

Voda, Ann M., Nancy S. Christy, and Julene M. Morgan. "Body Composition Changes in Menopausal Women." *Women and Therapy,* Vol. 11, No. 2 (1991), pp. 71–96.

Waterhouse, Debra. *Outsmarting the Female Fat Cell: First Weight-Control Program Designed Specifically for Women.* New York: Hyperion, 1993. Advocates weight loss through healthful eating and exercise. Raises issues too rarely covered in conventional diet books, such as the difference between male and female "types" of fat and the consequent greater difficulty of weight loss for women, and the dangers of constant on-and-off dieting for health and long-term weight loss.

Audiovisual

Size 10 by Susan Lambert and Sara Gibson. Film, 20 minutes, color, 1978. Available from Women Make Movies (General Resources, page 447). Australian film that shows how women's body image has been formed and deformed by advertising and sexism. Helps us reclaim our bodies.

EATING WELL

Organizations

AMERICAN DIETETIC ASSOCIATION
TEL. (800) 366-1655
Recorded messages in English and Spanish, and registered dietitian available to answer questions. 9 A.M. to 4 P.M. Central Time.

CENTER FOR SCIENCE IN THE PUBLIC INTEREST
1875 CONNECTICUT AVE. NW, SUITE 300
WASHINGTON, DC 20009-5728
TEL. (202) 332-9110
A nonprofit public-interest organization that advocates improved health and nutrition policies. Publishes *Nutrition Action Healthletter* with both nutrition and nutrition-policy information. Often includes analysis of chain restaurant foods, frozen and packaged foods, and how to choose and combine them into nutritious meals. The January/February 1993 issue had an excellent discussion of vitamin supplementation, options for choosing, and analysis of common brands. $20 for ten issues per year.

SOCIETY FOR NUTRITION EDUCATION
2001 KILEBREW DR., SUITE 340
MINNEAPOLIS, MN 55425-1882
TEL. (612) 854-0035
Has educational materials (some in Spanish) for lay and professional persons.

Books

Brody, Jane. *Jane Brody's Nutrition Book.* New York: Bantam, 1987. Basic nutrition book, good practical suggestions.

Gershoff, Stanley. *The Tufts University Guide to Total Nutrition.* New York: Harper Perennial, 1990. Basic nutrition information and healthy eating plan. Features menu selection in restaurants.

Keeton, Kathy. *Longevity.* New York: Viking, 1992. Upbeat discussion of normal aging and practical tips on diet and exercise to keep healthy.

Moyer, Ann. *Better Food for Public Places: A Guide for Improving Institutional Food.* Emmaus, PA: Rodale Press, 1977. Discusses strategies and recipes.

National Research Council. *Diet and Health: Implications for Reducing Chronic Disease.* Washington, DC: National Academy Press, 1989.

Roe, Daphne A. *Geriatric Nutrition.* Englewood Cliffs, NJ: Prentice-Hall, 1983. Nutrition factors that affect people over sixty-five. Written for nutritionists, but understandable by lay people.

Shapiro, Laura. *Perfection Salad: Women and Cooking at the Turn of the Century.* New York: Farrar, Straus & Giroux, 1986. Traces the history of domestic science and scientific cooking, focusing on the women who set out to modernize the American diet.

Somer, Elizabeth. *The Essential Guide to Vitamins and Minerals.* New York: HarperCollins, 1992. Basic information on vitamins and minerals essential to health; their roles in prevention and treatment of disease; how medications, alcohol, and tobacco affect nutrient status; and a vitamin/mineral rich diet.

Thomas, Sherry. *We Didn't Have Much, But We Sure Had Plenty: Stories of Rural Women.* New York: Anchor/Doubleday, 1981. Contemporary stories of twelve midlife and older women farmers.

U.S. Dept. of Agriculture. *Handbook of the Nutritional Contents of Foods.* New York: Dover Publications, 1975. Vitamin, mineral, calorie, protein, carbohydrate, and fat content of common foods. Still in print.

U.S. Dept. of Agriculture Human Nutrition Information Service. *The Food Guide Pyramid.* 1992. Home and Garden Bulletin No. 252. Order from Public Documents Distribution Center, right-hand column, this page.

Cookbooks

Brody, Jane. *Jane Brody's Good Food Gourmet.* New York: Bantam, 1990. Five hundred recipes modified to fit the dietary guidelines of the 1990s.

Fisher, Helen V. *Cookbook for the 90s.* Tucson, AZ: Fisher Books, 1990. Low-fat, -sugar, and -salt recipes, higher in fiber and complex carbohydrates. Seasons with herbs rather than salt. Includes nutrient information.

Giobbi, Edward, and Richard Wolff. *Eat Right, Eat Well—The Italian Way.* New York: Knopf, 1985. Healthy Italian cooking with emphasis on low-fat, low-salt foods.

Goor, Ron and Nancy Goor. *Eater's Choice,* 3rd Ed. Boston: Houghton Mifflin, 1992. Low-fat, -salt, and -sugar recipes, higher in complex carbohydrates and fiber.

Height, Dorothy I., and National Council of Negro Women, Inc. *The Black Family Dinner Quilt Cookbook.* Memphis, TN: The Wimmer Companies, 1993; New York: Fireside, 1994. Traditional soul food recipes featured with modifications by a nutritionist to be more healthful for today's way of eating. Includes nutrient information.

Katzen, Mollie. *Moosewood Cookbook.* Rev. Berkeley: Ten Speed Press, 1992. Vegetarian cookbook with lower-fat and lower-salt recipes.

Lakhani, Fatima. *Indian Recipes for a Healthy Heart.* Los Angeles: Fahil Publishing Company, 1992. Heart-healthy gourmet Indian dishes lower in fat, cholesterol, and salt.

Lambert-Lagacé, Louise. *The Nutrition Challenge for Women.* Palo Alto, CA: Bull Publishing Co., 1990. How to eat for health, energy, and enjoyment. Includes some recipes. Contains good ideas for older and busy women.

Lappé, Frances Moore. *Diet for a Small Planet.* New York: Ballantine, 1975. Rationale for vegetarian diet, good explanation of food combinations to increase protein content. Easy recipes.

Pritikin, Nathan. *The Pritikin Program for Diet and Exercise.* New York: Bantam, 1983. *Very* low-fat diet designed for people with diabetes and heart disease.

Robertson, Laurel, et al. *The New Laurel's Kitchen.* Petaluma, CA: Nilgeri Press, 1986. Vegetarian cookbook with lots of nutrition information, including nutrients in food. Good for ideas when you are trying to change your diet.

Wilson, J. Randy. *Non-Chew Cookbook,* 1985. Wilson Publishing Co., P.O. Box 2190, Glenwood Springs, CO 81602. Tel. (800) 523-8208. Tasty recipes for those who must be on a soft or liquid diet. $14.95 per copy plus $2 shipping.

Other Publications

FOOD AND NUTRITION INFORMATION CENTER
NATIONAL AGRICULTURAL LIBRARY
10301 BALTIMORE BLVD., ROOM 304
BELTSVILLE, MD 20705
TEL. (301) 504-5719

Reference and lending service for materials on specific nutrition topics. Publishes *Pathfinder* series of resource lists for lay and professional persons.

PUBLIC DOCUMENTS DISTRIBUTION CENTER
PUEBLO, CO 81009

Distributes government pamphlets, including many on food and general nutrition. Write for list.

Tufts University Diet & Nutrition Letter. 53 Park Place, New York, NY 10007. Monthly newsletter containing the latest research findings. $20 for twelve issues per year.

U.S. Department of Agriculture. County Extension Services. These offices exist in urban areas also. Check your local telephone book under the name of your county. Provides general nutrition information, and information on preparing and preserving food.

MOVING FOR HEALTH

Organizations

MELPOMENE INSTITUTE FOR WOMEN'S HEALTH RESEARCH
C/O JUDY MAHLE LUTTER
1010 UNIVERSITY AVE.
ST. PAUL, MN 55104
TEL. (612) 642-1951

Focuses on women, physical activity, and health through research, education, and a resource center. Annual membership of $32 includes *The Melpomene Journal,* published three times a year.

Organizations for Outdoor Activities

Regional groups such as The Appalachian Mountain Club, 5 Joy St., Boston, MA 02108, Tel. (617) 523-0636, sponsor activities and hikes. Check the community pages of your local paper.

OUTDOOR VACATIONS FOR WOMEN OVER 40
P.O. BOX 200
GROTON, MA 01450
TEL. (508) 448-3331

Provides opportunities for women over forty to learn new skills and add adventure to their lives by vacationing out-of-doors.

OUTWARD BOUND
384 FIELD POINT RD.
GREENWICH, CT 06830
TEL. (800) 243-8520 OR (203) 661-0797

Outward Bound teaches self-reliance, self-confidence, and self-esteem through challenging wilderness activities. Has courses for older women and will design them for individuals and groups with special needs or interests.

THE SALVATION ARMY
615 SLATERS LANE
P.O. BOX 269
ALEXANDRIA, VA 22313
TEL. (703) 684-5500

Inexpensive programs are available at about fifty-five rural camps throughout the country. Contact your local branch or the national headquarters above.

THE SIERRA CLUB
730 POLK ST.
SAN FRANCISCO, CA 94109
TEL. (415) 776-2211

A national environmental protection organization, with publications and local group affiliations, that combines outdoor activity with exploration and preservation of beautiful natural sites.

VACATION AND SENIOR CENTERS ASSOCIATION
275 SEVENTH AVE.
NEW YORK, NY 10001
TEL. (212) 645-6590

Has general information about summer camps for the elderly. Applications must be made directly to each camp's sponsoring agency.

Books and Other Publications

Barker, Sarah. *The Alexander Technique.* New York: Bantam, 1981.

Bender, Ruth. Several books by this experienced teacher are still in print. Check your local library or bookstore.

Birkel, Dee Ann Green, and Susan Birkel Freitag. *Forever Fit: A Step-By-Step Guide for Older Adults.* New York: Plenum, 1991.

"Body Building for the Nineties." *Nutrition Action Healthletter,* Vol. 19, No. 5 (June 1992). Published by the Center for Science in the Public Interest, 1875 Connecticut Ave. NW, Suite 300, Washington, DC 20009-5728. Includes some simple measures for measuring your strength at home.

Casper, Ursula Hodge. *Joy and Comfort Through Stretching and Relaxing for Those Who Are Unable to Exercise.* New York: Seabury Press, 1982.

Evans, William, and Irwin H. Rosenberg with Jacqueline Thompson. *Biomarkers—The 10 De-*

terminants of Aging You Can Control. New York: Simon & Schuster, 1991. Emphasis on aerobic and strength training all through the years.

Feldenkrais, M. *Awareness Through Movement.* New York: Harper & Row, 1972. An international list of Feldenkrais practitioners and information about books and tapes is available free from The Feldenkrais Guild, 706 Ellsworth St., P.O. Box 489, Albany, OR 97321. Tel. (503) 926-0981.

Flatten, Kay, Barbara Wilhite, and Eleanor Reyes-Watson. *Exercise Activities for the Elderly.* New York: Springer, 1988. Excellent book with special section on initiating a home strength-training program.

Godfrey, Charles, and Michael Feldman. *The Ageless Exercise Plan—A Complete Guide to Fitness After Fifty.* New York: McGraw-Hill, 1984. Includes tips on life-style habits and progress charts.

Hayden, Sandy, Daphne Hall, and Pat Stueck. *Women in Motion: The Basic Stuff to Get You Started and Keep You Going to Total Fitness.* Boston: Beacon Press, 1983.

Jamieson, Robert H. *Exercises for the Elderly.* Verplanck, NY: Emerson Books, 1982. Large type and easy-to-follow pictures. Includes exercises to be done in a chair or bed, and for those with special needs, such as people with partial paralysis.

Kuntzleman, Charles. *The Complete Book of Walking.* Paperback ed., Skokie, IL: Consumers Guide, 1982.

Lederach, Naomi, Nona Kauffman, and Beth Lederach. *Exercise as You Grow Older.* Intercourse, PA: Good Books, 1986. Large print, good illustrations. Contains seated, standing, and moving exercises and nutritional guidance.

Leen, Edie. *Complete Women's Weight Training Guide.* Mountain View, CA: Anderson World, Inc., 1959. Still an excellent book.

Lettvin, Maggie. *Maggie's Woman's Book.* Boston: Houghton Mifflin, 1981.

Lowen, Alexander, and Leslie Lowen. *The Way to Vibrant Health.* New York: Harper & Row, 1977. Bioenergetic exercises.

Lyons, Pat, and Debby Burgard. *Great Shape: The First Fitness Guide for Large Women.* New York: Morrow, 1990.

Maisel, Edward. *Tai Chi for Health.* New York: Holt, Rinehart & Winston, 1972.

Noble, Elizabeth. *Essential Exercises for the Childbearing Year.* 3rd ed. Boston: Houghton Mifflin, 1988. Excellent chapters for women of all ages on "The Pelvic Floor" and "The Abdominal Muscles."

Olinekova, Gayle. *Go For It.* New York: Simon & Schuster, 1982. Motivational book on fitness for women.

Rush, Anne Kent. *Getting Clear: Body Work for Women.* New York: Random House/Bookworks, 1975. This book is recommended for its variety of physical-movement techniques that incorporate a mind-body approach.

Audiovisual

The Complete Guide to Exercise Videos, 1993 Ed. Collage Video Specialties, Dept. G, 5390 Main Street, NE, Minneapolis, MN 55421. Tel. (612) 571-5840. Ordering information with very brief descriptions. Inclusion of a video in this catalog means it has received some evaluation for safety.

Tai Chi for Elders. Sixty-minute video. Terra Nova Films. See page 447.

Living with Ourselves and Others as We Age

Sexuality in the Second Half of Life

Organizations

American Association of Sex Educators, Counselors and Therapists (AASECT)
435 N. Michigan Ave.
Chicago, IL 60611
Tel. (312) 644-0828

Impotence Anonymous (I-Anon)
119 South Ruth St.
Maryville, TN 37801
Tel. (615) 983-6064

Provides informational brochures, referral to state and local chapters and appropriate professionals, and support groups.

Sex Information and Education Council of United States (SIECUS)
130 W. 42nd St., Suite 2500
New York, NY 10036-7901
Tel. (212) 819-9770

Provides information about, and advocacy of, sexuality as a healthy part of life.

Books and Other Publications

Bacon, Natalie, and Ralph Bacon. *Love Talk: A Model of Erotic Communication,* 1985. Shakti Press, P.O. Box 7581, Oakland, CA 94601. Autobiographical account of an older couple learning to communicate about sex.

Barbach, Lonnie, and David L. Geisinger. *Going the Distance: Finding and Keeping Lifelong Love.* New York: NAL Dutton, 1993.

Barbach, Lonnie, and Linda Levine. *Shared Intimacies: Women's Sexual Experiences.* New York: Bantam, 1983.

Blumstein, Phillip, and Pepper Schwartz. *American Couples.* New York: Morrow, 1983. Compares heterosexual, gay, and lesbian couples.

Boston Women's Health Book Collective. *The New Our Bodies, Ourselves.* New York: Simon & Schuster, 1992. See especially chapters on Sexuality, Women and HIV/AIDS, and Women Growing Older.

Brecher, Edward. *Love, Sex and Aging.* Boston: Little, Brown, 1984. Positive report on sex and aging. Sample is disproportionately middle-class and male.

Butler, Robert, and Myrna Lewis. *Love and Sex After 40: A Guide for Men and Women for Their Mid and Later Years.* New York: Harper & Row, 1986. Knowledgeable and insightful. Available in large-print edition.

Dackman, Linda. *Up Front: Sex and the Post-Mastectomy Woman.* New York: Viking Penguin, 1990.

Dodson, Betty. *Sex for One.* New York: Random House/Crown Publishers, 1987. Teaches self-pleasuring techniques leading to orgasm in a context of feeling good about our bodies. Highly recommended.

Edelman, Deborah. *Sex in the Golden Years.* New York: Donald I. Fine, Inc., 1992. Based on extensive research including interviews with experts in the field, and first-person narratives by older persons about their feelings and experiences.

Kehoe, Monika. *Lesbians Over 60 Speak for Themselves.* New York: Haworth Press, 1989. Includes statistical data and personal experiences about lesbians and aging.

The Kensington Ladies Erotica Society. *Ladies' Own Erotica.* New York: Pocket/Simon & Schuster, 1984. Collection of erotic writings by a group of women.

Kinsey, Alfred, et al. *Sexual Behavior in the Human Female.* New York: Pocket/Simon & Schuster, 1953.

Kitzinger, Sheila. *Woman's Experience of Sex.* New York: Putnam, 1983.

Ladas, Alice, Beverly Whipple, and John Perry. *The G Spot.* New York: Dell, 1982.

Lorde, Audre. "Scratching the Surface: Some Notes on Barriers to Women and Loving." *The Black Scholar,* Vol. 9, No. 7 (April 1978), pp. 31–35. Thoughtful article about lesbian relationships.

Loulan, JoAnn. *Lesbian Sex.* San Francisco: Spinsters Ink, 1984. Material on techniques and communication of ideas useful for all women.

O'Connor, Dagmar. *How to Make Love to the Same Person for the Rest of Your Life and Still Love It.* New York: Bantam, 1986. A reassuring guide to a committed yet adventurous sexual relationship with the person you love by the director of a hospital-based sex-therapy program.

Olds, Sally Wendkos. *The Eternal Garden: Seasons of Our Sexuality.* New York: Times Books, 1985. The experience of sexuality from childhood through old age. Highly recommended.

Rhodes, Sonya. *Second Honeymoon: A Pioneering Guide for Reviving the Midlife Marriage.* New

York: Morrow, 1992. How couples can resist the high-risk roles and behaviors that put stress on relationships and understand and grow with the normal changes of midlife.

Sevely, Josephine Lowndes. *Eve's Secrets: A New Theory of Female Sexuality.* New York: Random House, 1987. Basing her conclusions on new anatomical research, the author demonstrates similarities between women and men. For example, she reports some women ejaculate prostatic fluid during lovemaking.

Sex and the Female Ostomate. Order pamphlet from United Ostomy Association, Inc., 2001 W. Beverly Blvd., Los Angeles, CA 90057. A discussion of sexuality for the woman who has had ostomy surgery.

Sex and Heart Disease. 1990. Order from your local chapter of the American Heart Association or write to the national center (see page 494).

Taylor, Dena, and Amber Coverdale Sumrall. *The Times of Our Lives: Women Write on Sex After 40.* Freedom, CA: The Crossing Press, 1992. Stories and poems by women revealing new definitions of sexuality.

Turner, Barbara F., and Catherine Adams. "The Sexuality of Older Women." In Elizabeth Markson, ed., *Older Women.* Lexington, MA: D.C. Heath/ Lexington Books, 1983.

Zilbergeld, Bernie. *The New Male Sexuality.* New York: Bantam, 1992. Good nonsexist book on male sexuality. Highly recommended.

Audiovisual

The Heart Has No Wrinkles. The love story of two residents in a nursing home. Available from The Baxley Media Group, 110 W. Main, Urbana, IL 61801. Tel. (217) 384-4838.

Rose by Any Other Name by Judith Keller. An appealingly iconoclastic 15-minute film set in a nursing home that explores the lifelong need for affection, privacy, and sexual expression. Available for rental or sale (as film or videocassette) from Pennsylvania State University (see page 447).

Sex After Fifty, by author Lonnie Barbach. A ninety-minute videotape encouraging honest discussion of sexual feelings. Covers such topics as lack of desire, chronic illness, effects of medication, erection difficulties, and loss of a partner. Available from Focus International, Inc. 1160 E. Jericho Turnpike, Huntington, NY 11743. Tel. (516) 549-5320.

Where to Find Products Mentioned in Text

Biofilm, 3121 Scott St., Vista, CA 92083. Happy to answer questions about their product, Astroglide, an excellent lubricant. (800) 325-5695, (619) 727-9030.

Eve's Garden Ltd., 119 W. 57th St., Suite 420, New York, NY 10019. Vibrators, videos, and books in a sex-positive environment. Owned and operated by women.

Good Vibrations, 1210 Valencia St., San Francisco, CA 94110. Vibrators and books, such as Joanie Blank, *Good Vibrations: The Complete Women's Guide to Vibrators.* San Francisco: Down There Press, 1984.

The Xandria Collection. Catalog of lubricants, vibrators, and other sex aids. Order from Lawrence Research Group, 1245 16th St., San Francisco, CA 74107.

AIDS/HIV

Books and Other Publications

Center for Women Policy Studies (CWPS) and American Association of Retired Persons (AARP) in November 1993, cosponsored a meeting to examine how HIV/AIDS affects midlife and older women, both as women at risk and as caregivers of others. To order a free copy of the proceedings of this ground-breaking conference, write to AARP Fulfillment, 601 E St., N.W., Washington, DC, and request publication #D15298.

Corea, Gena. *The Invisible Epidemic: The Story of Women and AIDS.* New York: HarperCollins, 1992. The author reveals that it is at least ten times more likely that a man will transmit the virus to a woman during sex than the other way around. She lets the women tell their own stories, such as the story of the woman who transcends her heartbreaking diagnosis to become a spokesperson for women with HIV/AIDS.

National Women's Health Network. *Advice for Life: A Woman's Guide to AIDS Risks and Prevention.* New York: Pantheon, 1987. Order from NWHN, 1325 G St., NW, Washington, DC 20005.

Sack, Fleur, with Ann Street. *Romance to Die For: The Startling Truth About Women, Sex And AIDS.* 1992. Available from Health Communications, Inc. 3201 S.W. 15th St., Deerfield Beach, FL 33442-8190. A family physician/health educator confronts denial of the "equal opportunity disease," HIV/AIDS, provides explicit information, and promotes wider and more effective dissemination of AIDS education.

Solomon, Karen, and Gregory Anderson. "AIDS and Older People: Two Educational Models." *SEICUS Report,* June/July 1993, pp. 13–15. (See page 460.) Confronts the mythology that elders are asexual in order to bring HIV/AIDS prevention education to diverse communities.

BIRTH CONTROL FOR WOMEN IN MIDLIFE

Organizations

See General Health resources (pp. 482–84) for organizations working in areas of women's health and reproductive rights.

Books and Other Publications

Bell, Susan, et al. "Reclaiming Reproductive Control: A Feminist Approach to Fertility Consciousness." *Science for the People,* Vol. 12, No. 1 (1980), pp. 6–9, 30–35.

Berman, Andrea Fugh. "Should Women Over Forty Take the Pill?" *Network News* (publication of the National Women's Health Network; see page 482), Vol. 14, No. 7 (January/February 1990), p. 4.

Boston Women's Health Book Collective. *The New Our Bodies, Ourselves.* New York: Simon & Schuster, 1992. New edition of the classic women's health resource. See especially chapters on Anatomy and Physiology, Birth Control, Sexually Transmitted Diseases, HIV/AIDS, and Abortion.

Chalker, Rebecca. *The Complete Cervical Cap Guide.* New York: Harper & Row, 1987. Clear, concise information about the cap and birth control generally.

Gordon, Linda. *Woman's Body, Woman's Right: A Social History of Birth Control in America.* Rev. ed. New York: Penguin, 1990.

Harlap, Susan, Kathryn Kost, and Jacqueline D. Forrest. *Preventing Pregnancy, Protecting Health: A New Look at Birth Control Choices in the United States.* 1991. Order from the Alan Guttmacher Institute, 111 Fifth Ave., New York, NY 10003.

Hatcher, Robert A., Felicia Guest, et al. *Contraceptive Technology.* Rev. ed. New York: Irvington Publishers, 1994 (in press).

Hicks, Karen M. *Surviving the Dalkon Shield IUD: Women v. the Pharmaceutical Industry.* New York: Teachers College Press, 1994. Chronicle of a women's social protest movement against a pharmaceutical company's efforts to minimize its accountability. Includes compelling personal accounts of women harmed by the Dalkon Shield. As an advocate and social scientist, the author provides a useful analysis and model for future advocacy efforts.

Hoshiko, Sumi. *Our Choices: Women's Personal Decisions About Abortion.* Binghamton, NY: The Haworth Press, 1993. Explores women's feelings about becoming pregnant unintentionally, their circumstances, and the effect of an unplanned pregnancy and abortion on their relationships. Puts the focus of the abortion debate back on the woman who must make the decision.

Liskin, L., et al. "Condoms—Now More Than Ever." *Population Reports,* Series H, No. 8, September 1990.

Mintzes, Barbara, and Anita Hardon. *A Question of Control: Women's Perspectives on the Development and Use of Contraceptive Technologies.* Amsterdam, Netherlands: Women's Health Action Foundation, 1992.

Petchesky, Rosalind Pollack. *Abortion and Woman's Choice: The State, Sexuality and Reproductive Freedom.* Rev. ed., Boston: Northeastern University Press, 1990.

Seaman, Barbara. *The Doctor's Case Against the*

Pill. New York: Dell, 1979. And Seaman, Barbara, and Gideon Seaman. *Women and the Crisis in Sex Hormones.* New York: Bantam, 1978. Two classic early critiques of the pill and other birth control methods.

Women's Health Action Foundation. *Norplant: Under Her Skin.* Amsterdam, Netherlands, 1993. 126 pp. $15. Available in the United States from Boston Women's Health Book Collective, Box 192, Somerville, MA 02144. The design of Norplant, requiring surgical removal, makes it prone to abuse. The authors describe its use in Indonesia, Brazil, Egypt, Finland, and Thailand, and assess its impact on women's well-being. They describe disturbing examples of disregard for the health and safety of the women, particularly in Third World countries.

Childbearing in Midlife

Pregnancy and Childbirth

Organizations

For a comprehensive list of organizations concerned with all aspects of pregnancy and childbirth, see Boston Women's Health Book Collective. *The New Our Bodies, Ourselves.* New York: Simon & Schuster, 1992, pp. 472–73.

International Childbirth Education Association (ICEA)
P.O. Box 20048
Minneapolis, MN 55240
Tel. (612) 854-8660

The ICEA represents parents and professionals who share an interest in childbearing. There are regional chapters. Their ICEA Bookcenter is a comprehensive and reliable source of books and pamphlets on childbearing and related subjects. They will send their publication, *Bookmarks,* containing reviews of new books, to anyone who requests it.

Books and Other Publications

Balaskas, Janet. *Active Birth: The New Approach to Giving Birth Naturally.* Boston, MA: Harvard Common Press, 1992. An empowering approach to birth. Forewords by Sheila Kitzinger and Michel Odent.

Baldwin, Rahima. *Special Delivery: The Complete Guide to Informed Birth.* Rev. ed. Milbrae, CA: Les Femmes Publishing, 1990. Positive descriptions of normal pregnancy, labor, and birth. Useful information for planning a home birth.

Boston Women's Health Book Collective. *The New Our Bodies, Ourselves.* New York: Simon & Schuster, 1992. An essential resource for all women. See especially chapters on Pregnancy, Childbirth, Infertility, and New Reproductive Technologies.

Inch, Sally. *Birthrights.* New York: Pantheon, 1984. A clear, systematic description of the few advantages and the many disadvantages of current obstetrical practices and drugs. A valuable, factual tool for parents and childbirth educators.

Kitzinger, Sheila. *Birth Over Thirty.* London: Sheldon Press, 1982. Authoritative guide by an international pioneer in childbirth education.

———. *Your Baby, Your Way: Making Pregnancy Decisions and Birth Plans.* New York: Pantheon, 1987. Supportive guide to choosing among alternatives in pregnancy and birth.

Odent, Michel. *Birth Reborn.* New York: Random House, 1984. A positive and affirming book that encourages women to listen to their own bodies, and practitioners to demedicalize their thinking about childbirth.

Pincus, Jane. *Advice Books for Childbearing Women: Choice or Coercion.* 27 pages. Available for $5 from the author at P.O. Box 72, Roxbury, VT 05669. A critical examination of modern books about childbirth by a coauthor of the Pregnancy and Childbirth chapters of *The New Our Bodies, Ourselves* (1992). Argues that most childbirth books undermine women's strength and confidence and foster a medical mindset.

Rothman, Barbara Katz. *Giving Birth: Alternatives in Childbirth.* New York: Penguin, 1984. Contrasts the medical model of childbirth with the midwifery model.

Sagov, Stanley, Richard Feinbloom, Peggy Spindell, and Archie Brodsky. *Home Birth: A Practitioner's Guide to Birth Outside the Hospital.*

Rockville, MD: Aspen Systems Corp., 1983. A medical-practice group describes their own handling of pregnancy, labor, and birth. An essential book for prenatal care providers and a reassuring guide for prospective parents.

Simkin, Penny. *The Birth Partner: Everything You Need to Know to Help a Woman Through Childbirth.* Boston: Harvard Common Press, 1989.

EXERCISE AND NUTRITION FOR THE CHILDBEARING YEAR

Books

Balaskas, Arthur, and Janet Balaskas. *New Life.* Rev. ed. London: Sidgewick and Jackson, 1983. An exercise book that stresses relaxation, squatting, and changing positions during labor. Excellent drawings of the pelvis.

Brewer, Gail. *Pregnant Vegetarian.* New York: Penguin, 1989. Helpful nutrition advice for pregnant women who are vegetarians.

Noble, Elizabeth. *Essential Exercises for the Childbearing Year.* 3rd ed. Boston: Houghton Mifflin, 1988. Easy to understand, informative, well illustrated. Includes detailed discussions of the pelvic floor and of the physiological reasons for doing specific exercises.

Schwab, Michael, and Inke Schwab. *Start Well! A Guide to Healthy Eating for You and Your Baby.* London: Pagoda Books, 1984.

INFERTILITY

Organizations

RESOLVE, INC.
1310 BROADWAY
SOMERVILLE, MA 02144
TEL. (617) 623-0744

Information, support, and referral to specialists for men and women with infertility problems. Can review the appropriateness of medical care. Has accepted funds from Serono Labs, which markets Pergonal, an ovulatory enhancement drug.

Books

Glazer, Ellen Sarasohn, and Susan Lewis Cooper. *Without Child: Experiencing and Resolving Infertility.* Lexington, MA: D. C. Heath, 1988.

Menning, Barbara Eck. *Infertility: A Guide for the Childless Couple.* 2nd ed., Englewood Cliffs, NJ: Prentice-Hall, 1988. Author is a founder of Resolve, Inc.

NEW REPRODUCTIVE TECHNOLOGIES AND PRENATAL TESTING

Books

Arditti, Rita, Renate Duelli Klein, and Shelley Minden, eds. *Test Tube Women.* Boston: Pandora Press, Routledge and Kegan Paul, 1984. This book's many varied articles provide a strong feminist insight into new reproductive technologies and other issues, such as testing during pregnancy.

Blatt, Robin J. R. *Prenatal Tests: What They Are, Their Benefits and Risks, and How to Decide Whether to Have Them or Not.* New York: Vintage/Random House, 1988.

———. *Prenatal Genetic Testing: A Consumer Guide for Women and Couples.* New York: Bergin & Garvey, 1994.

Corea, Gena. *The Mother Machine: Reproductive Technology from Artificial Insemination to Artificial Wombs.* New York: Harper & Row, 1985.

Rothman, Barbara Katz. *Recreating Motherhood: Ideology and Technology in a Patriarchal Society.* New York: Norton, 1989.

ADOPTION

Organizations

ADOPTION SUPPORT AND NETWORKING (ADOPTNET)
P.O. BOX 50514
PALO ALTO, CA 94303-0514
TEL. (415) 949-4370

Provides support for adoptive parents. Publishes bimonthly magazine, *AdoptNet*.

ADOPTIVE FAMILIES OF AMERICA
3333 HWY. 100 NORTH, SUITE 203
MINNEAPOLIS, MN 55422
TEL. (612) 535-4829

A national organization (formerly OURS, Inc.) providing problem-solving assistance and information to adoptive and prospective adoptive families. Special groups consist of single parents, families who adopt physically or emotionally challenged children, and families who adopt children from ethnic backgrounds that differ from their own. Provides information about local groups if you send them a stamped self-addressed envelope.

CONCERNED UNITED BIRTHPARENTS
2000 WALKER ST.
DES MOINES, IA 50317
TEL. (515) 263-9558

A support organization for women who have given up babies for adoption. Lobbies for rights of adoptive children and of birth parents to information.

INTERNATIONAL CONCERNS COMMITTEE FOR CHILDREN
911 CYPRESS DR.
BOULDER, CO 80303
TEL. (303) 494-8333

Researches and provides information and support for orphan children in many countries. Publishes "The Foreign Adoption Report," an annual listing of foreign adoption resources for U.S. citizens, and also a listing of children available for adoption by U.S. adoptive families.

Books

Gay, Kathlyn. *The Rainbow Effect.* New York: Franklin Watts, 1987. The author assesses the pros and cons of interracial adoption. She finds adoptive parents and their children are adaptable. The children demonstrate high self-esteem and generally do well.

Melina, Lois Ruskai. *Making Sense of Adoption: A Parent's Guide.* New York: Harper & Row, 1989.

Plumez, Jacqueline Hornar. *Successful Adoption.* New York: Harmony Books, 1982.

PARENTING

Books

Boston Women's Health Book Collective. *Ourselves and Our Children.* New York: Random House, 1978. An exploration of the whole experience of being a parent from the decision to have a child to the time the children leave home. Extensive bibliography on all aspects of parenthood. This book is out of print, but should be available at your local library.

Cohen, Judith Blackfield. *Parenthood After 30? A Guide to Personal Choice.* Lexington, MA: Lexington Books/D. C. Heath & Co., 1985. Thoughtful and thorough. Includes extensive resource list.

Daniels, Pamela, and Kathy Weingarten. *Sooner or Later: The Timing of Parenthood in Adult Lives.* New York: Norton, 1982. Report on interview study and excellent discussion of issues around midlife parenting.

Mansfield, Phyllis Kernoff. *Pregnancy for Older Women: Assessing the Medical Risks.* New York: Praeger, 1986. Compilation of research. Highly recommended.

Rothman, Barbara Katz. *The Tentative Pregnancy: Prenatal Diagnosis and the Future of Motherhood.* New York: Viking, 1986. Provocative discussion of the effect of pregnancy testing and the consequent decision to keep or abort a pregnancy on the psychological experience of pregnancy and parenting.

SINGLE PARENTING

Books

Hall, Nancy Lee. *A True Story of a Single Mother.* Boston: South End Press, 1984. A black woman's experience of single parenting.

Robinson, Susan, and H. F. Pizer. *Having a Baby Without a Man: The Woman's Guide to Alternative Insemination.* New York: Simon & Schuster/Fireside, 1985.

LESBIAN PARENTING

Organizations

LESBIAN MOTHERS NATIONAL DEFENSE FUND
BOX 21567
SEATTLE, WA 98111
TEL. (206) 325-2643
Provides information, emotional support, and referrals to attorneys for custody disputes. Also provides information on artificial insemination.

Books

Pies, Cheri. *Considering Parenthood: A Workbook for Lesbians.* San Francisco: Spinsters Ink, 1985. Examines all aspects of the decision—social, economic, biological.

Audiovisual

Choosing Children, a charming film depicting diverse lesbian families, including such options as artificial insemination, adoption, and cooperation with gay men. Order from Cambridge Documentary Films, P.O. Box 385, Cambridge, MA 02139. Tel. (617) 354-3677.

STEPPARENTING

Organizations

STEP-FAMILY ASSOCIATION OF AMERICA
215 CENTENNIAL MALL SOUTH, SUITE 212
LINCOLN, NE 68505
TEL. (402) 477-7837
Self-help groups for parents and for children. Membership of $45 includes newsletter and attendance at local group if one exists in your community. Or you can get help to start one. Newsletter without membership, $14 per year.

Books

Getzoff, Ann, and Carolyn McClenahan. *Step Kids: A Survival Guide for Teenagers in Stepfamilies (and for Stepparents Doubtful of Their Own Survival).* New York: Walker and Co., 1985. Written from the teenager's point of view, this book can be helpful to parents and stepparents.

Keshet, Jamie. *Love and Power in the Step-Family.* New York: McGraw-Hill, 1986. Highly recommended.

Audiovisual

Stepparenting: New Families, Old Ties, a 25-minute film by Henry and Marilyn Felt. Interviews with stepparents and scenes from a stepparent support group. For stepparents and professionals. Available from Polymorph Films, 118 South St., Boston, MA 02111. Tel. (617) 542-2004.

EXPERIENCING OUR CHANGE OF LIFE: MENOPAUSE

Periodicals

For periodicals that cover other women's health issues along with menopause, see also entries under General Health starting on page 482.

A Friend Indeed: For Women in the Prime of Life. Highly recommended. Letters from midlife women reporting their experiences form the core of this excellent journal. Research reports and book reviews are also included. For a one-year subscription (ten issues) send $30 to P.O. Box 1710, Champlain, NY 12919-1710. In Canada, send $32.10 (incl. GST) to Box 515, Station Place du Parc, Montreal, Canada H2W2P1. A list of all topics covered in previous issues is available free. Just send a stamped self-addressed envelope.

Books and Other Publications

Banner, Lois W. "The Twentieth Century: Menopause and Its Meaning." In *In Full Flower: Aging Women, Power, and Sexuality.* New York: Vintage, 1993. Scholarly historical perspective on midlife and menopause.

A Book About Menopause. Montreal Health Press, Inc., C.P. 1000, Station Place du Parc, Montreal, Quebec, Canada H2W2N1. Information about health issues, sexuality, and strategies for dealing with midlife and menopause. Nonjudgmental and informative. $4 for a single copy.

Also available in French. Write to them for information on bulk rates.

Borton, Joan C. *Drawing from the Women's Well: Reflections on the Life Passage of Menopause.* San Diego, CA: LuraMedia, 1992. The change of life viewed as a time for "going inward" to discover the well of our own experience. Includes an extensive list of earlier books on menopause. Highly recommended.

Callahan, Joan, ed. *Menopause: A Midlife Passage.* Bloomington and Indianapolis: Indiana University Press, 1993. In this empowering collection of essays, women from a variety of artistic and intellectual disciplines examine the cultural, ethical, and policy issues raised by menopause.

Clay, Vidal S. *Women: Menopause and Middle Age.* Pittsburgh, PA: KNOW, Inc., 1977. One of the earlier helpful books on menopause. See especially the chart on the comparison of medical and nonmedical therapies for problems in menopause and aging, pp. 88–89.

Cobb, Janine O'Leary. *Understanding Menopause: Answers and Advice for Women in the Prime of Life.* New York: NAL Dutton/Plume, 1993. Clearly written and informative guide by the founder and editor of *A Friend Indeed* (see above).

Coney, Sandra. *The Menopause Industry: How the Medical Establishment Exploits Women.* Alameda, CA: Hunter House, 1994, in press. A uniquely compelling analysis of the medicalization of menopause by a leading women's health advocate from New Zealand. Highly recommended.

Davis, Dona Lee. *Blood and Nerves: An Ethnographic Focus on Menopause.* St. John's, Newfoundland, Canada: Institute of Social and Economic Research, Memorial University of Newfoundland, 1983. The experiences of menopause in a Newfoundland fishing village. Also contains many cross-cultural references.

Downing, Christine. *Journey Through Menopause: A Personal Rite of Passage.* New York: Crossroad, 1989. The author undertakes a trip around the world and discovers the spiritual significance of menopause in her encounters with older women and men.

Greenwood, Sadja. *Menopause Naturally: Preparing for the Second Half of Life.* San Francisco: Volcano Press, 1992. A simply written and well-balanced book by a woman physician who has gone through menopause. Has chapters on osteoporosis, exercise, nutrition, and estrogen-replacement therapy. The chart showing the types of hormones and other drugs in the commonly prescribed hormonal preparations is very useful.

Greer, Germaine. *The Change: Women, Aging and the Menopause.* New York: Knopf, 1992. Insightful, but uneven critique of literary, historic, and medical views of menopause. Though there are flashes of inspiration, the book disappoints by opting for disengagement dressed up as "spirituality."

Gullette, Margaret Morganroth. "What? Menopause Again?" *Ms.*, July/August 1993. Lively critique questions the "cultural construction" of midlife and menopause. May not be helpful to women who are coping with discomforts of menopause.

Hardin, Paula Payne. *What Are You Doing with the Rest of Your Life? Choices in Midlife.* San Rafael, CA: New World Library, 1992. Research, personal experiences, and exercises for aging well.

Lark, Susan M. *The Menopause Self-Help Book: A Woman's Guide to Feeling Wonderful for the Second Half of Her Life.* Berkeley, CA: Celestial Arts, 1990. Helpful guide to nonmedical techniques such as nutrition, exercise, acupressure, and stress reduction for managing the discomforts of menopause.

Lock, Margaret, guest ed. "Anthropological Approaches to Menopause: Questioning Received Wisdom." Special issue of *Culture, Medicine and Psychiatry,* Vol. 10, No. 1 (March 1986).

McCain, Marian Van Eyk. *Transformation Through Menopause.* New York: Bergin & Garvey, 1991. Views the change of life as an opportunity for emotional and spiritual growth. Offers "exercises" and meditations for getting in touch with your inner self.

Menopause: A Self-Care Manual. Rev. ed., 1987. Santa Fe Health Education Project, P.O. Box

577, Santa FE, NM 87504-0577. $5 plus $1.75 postage. Also available in Spanish. 51 pages.

Ojeda, Linda. *Menopause Without Medicine.* Alameda, CA: Hunter House, 1991. Advocates nutritional approaches and exercise.

Reitz, Rosetta. *Menopause: A Positive Approach.* New York: Penguin, 1979. This classic in the field broke new ground by reclaiming menopause as a natural event. Full of practical and helpful advice.

Taylor, Dena, and Amber Coverdale Sumrall. *Women of the 14th Moon: Writings on Menopause.* Freedom, CA: The Crossing Press, 1991. Rich collection of essays, short stories, and poems. Affirming and empowering.

The U.S. Congress, Office of Technology Assessment, *The Menopause, Hormone Therapy, and Women's Health*, OTA-BP-BA-88, May 1992. This invaluable document compiled by leading researchers detailing the history, safety and risks of hormone treatments is available for only $6. Order from the U.S. Government Printing Office, SSOP, Washington, DC 20402-9328. ISBN 0-16-037912-1.

Voda, Ann. *Menopause, Me and You. A Personal Handbook for Women.* Salt Lake City, UT: College of Nursing, University of Utah, 1984. Pamphlet can be ordered from: Ann M. Voda, 25 South Medical Dr., Salt Lake City, UT 84112. $4.95 for a single copy. Bulk rates available. Has a section on osteoporosis. 46 pages.

Weed, Susun. *Menopausal Years: The Wise Woman Way.* Woodstock, NY: AshTree Publishing, 1992. A thorough and knowledgeable guide to the use of herbal remedies. Covers other alternative therapies as well, such as vitamins, massage, and homeopathic remedies. Do not, however, rely on it for medical advice, which is often whimsical or just incorrect.

Wolf, Honora Lee. *Menopause: The Second Spring.* Boulder, CO: Blue Poppy Enterprises Press, 1993.

RELATIONSHIPS IN MIDDLE AND LATER LIFE

Organizations

AMERICAN ASSOCIATION FOR MARRIAGE AND FAMILY THERAPY
1100 17TH ST. NW, 10TH FLOOR
WASHINGTON, DC 20036
TEL. (800) 374-2638 OR (202) 452-0109
Write to them for referrals to counselors in your area.

GRANDPARENTS'-CHILDREN'S RIGHTS, INC.
5728 BAYONNE AVE.
HASLETT, MI 48840
TEL. (517) 339-8663
Clearinghouse of information on state laws. Provides referrals to local self-help groups whenever possible.

NATIONAL ASSOCIATION FOR WIDOWED PEOPLE
P.O. BOX 3564
SPRINGFIELD, IL 62708
Offers widowed persons and their families a better understanding of the problems in dealing with grief and loneliness.

NATIONAL COALITION AGAINST DOMESTIC VIOLENCE
P.O. BOX 18749
DENVER, CO 80218-0749
TEL. (303) 839-1852
NCADV is a national grass-roots membership organization of battered-women's-shelter and -service providers and concerned individuals. Provides information on domestic violence and referrals. Contributes to public-policy discussions and national legislation.

PARENTS AND FRIENDS OF LESBIANS AND GAYS (PFLAG)
1012 14TH ST. NW, SUITE 700
WASHINGTON, DC 20005
TEL. (202) 638-4200
Newsletter and referrals to local parents' groups. Literature includes a short, simple pamphlet translated into Chinese, Spanish, French, and Japanese.

PARENTS WITHOUT PARTNERS
8807 COLESVILLE RD.
SILVER SPRING, MD 20910
TEL. (301) 588-9354
Chapters in most large cities provide social

opportunities for single parents and their children. Newsletter and magazine cover single-parent concerns.

SENIOR ACTION IN A GAY ENVIRONMENT (SAGE)
208 W. 13TH ST.
NEW YORK, NY 10011
TEL. (212) 741-2247
Network of social services and activities for older lesbians and gay men.

THEOS FOUNDATION
1301 CLARK BLDG.
717 LIBERTY AVE.
PITTSBURGH, PA 15222
TEL. (412) 471-7779
Through meetings and one-to-one mutual aid, helps younger and middle-aged widowed persons to accept, after grieving, the death of a spouse and adjust to the change, set new goals, renew personal identity, and create a new life. Eight-issue publication: Survivors' Outreach Series.

WIDOWED PERSONS SERVICE C/O AMERICAN ASSOCIATION OF RETIRED PERSONS (SEE GENERAL RESOURCES, PAGE 441).

Books and Other Publications

Adelman, Marcy. *Long Time Passing: Lives of Older Lesbians.* Boston: Alyson Publications, 1987.

Battered Women's Directory. 1989 U.S. Supplement. Order from: Terry Mehlman, 2506 Hoot Owl Drive, Hillsboro, NC 27278. This directory includes articles with helpful information and support to battered women and their friends.

Bell, Roseann P., Bettye J. Parker, and Beverly Guy-Sheftall, eds. *Sturdy Black Bridges: Visions of Black Women in Literature.* Garden City, NY: Anchor/Doubleday, 1979. See especially Mary Burgher, "Images of Self and Race in the Autobiographies of Black Women." Issues of survival, creativity, and black womanhood.

Bell, Ruth, and Leni Zeiger Wildflower. *Talking with Your Teenager.* New York: Random House, 1983. A guide to approaching difficult topics. Parents' counterpart to *Changing Bodies, Changing Lives,* a book for teens by the same authors.

Bell-Scott, Patricia, et al. *Double Stitch: Black Women Write About Mothers and Daughters.* New York: Harper Perennial, 1991. Personal narratives, fiction, essays, and poems celebrating loving/caring relationships between black mothers and daughters.

Belovitch, Jeanne, ed. *Making Remarriage Work.* Lexington, MA: D. C. Heath/Lexington Books, 1987.

Boston Lesbian Psychologies Collective, eds. *Lesbian Psychology: Explorations and Challenges.* Urbana and Chicago: University of Illinois Press, 1987. A pioneering anthology that captures the experiences of contemporary American lesbians. The articles, which were presented at a conference, focus on identity, relationships, community, and therapy.

Brans, Jo. *Mother, I Have Something to Tell You: Understanding Your Child's Chosen Lifestyle.* New York: Doubleday, 1987. How mothers cope when their children make choices different from their own.

Caine, Lynn. *Widow.* New York: Morrow, 1974. The author shares her experience of loss and makes a new beginning.

———. *What Did I Do Wrong? Mothers, Children, Guilt.* New York: Arbor House, 1985.

Cassingham, Barbie, and Sally O'Neil. *And Then I Met This Woman.* Racine, WI: Mother Courage Press, 1993. Remarkable stories of women whose lives have been transformed by relationships with women.

Clunis, D. Merilee, and G. Dorsey Green. *Lesbian Couples.* Seattle: Seal Press, 1988. Advice on creating healthy relationships.

Cowan, Connell, and Melvin Kinder. *Smart Women, Foolish Choices: Finding the Right Men and Avoiding the Wrong Ones.* New York: Signet/New American Library, 1985.

Cutler, Winnifred B. *Searching for Courtship: The Smart Woman's Guide to Finding a Good Husband.* New York: Villard Books, 1993. Practical approach to "finding the good men," establishing mutually respectful relationships, and moving toward "courtship."

Engel, Margorie L. *Weddings for Complicated Families: For Couples with Divorced Parents, and Those Planning to Remarry.* Boston: Mt. Ivy Press, 1993. Deals with all the financial and emotional minefields.

Fairchild, Betty, and Nancy Hayward. *Now That You Know: What Every Parent Should Know About Homosexuality.* New York and San Diego: Harvest/Harcourt Brace Jovanovich, 1979. Helpful book includes personal experiences and information on how to start Parents of Gays groups by founders of PFLAG. (See page 468.)

Flanner, Janet. *Darlinghissima: Letters to a Friend.* New York: Random House, 1985. Personal account of a long-standing lesbian relationship.

Getzoff, Ann, and Carolyn McClenahan. *Stepkids: A Survival Guide for Teenagers in Stepfamilies (and for Stepparents Doubtful of Their Own Survival).* New York: Walker & Co., 1985. Written from the teenager's point of view, this book can be helpful to parents and stepparents.

Gross, Zenith Henkin. *And You Thought It Was Over: Mothers and Their Adult Children.* New York: St. Martin's, 1985. Based on questionnaires sent to five hundred midlife women and interviews with a smaller number, the author describes the continuing importance of the relationship between mothers and their grown children.

Hull, Gloria T., Patricia Bell Scott, and Barbara Smith, eds. *All the Women Are White, All the Blacks Are Men. But Some of Us Are Brave.* Old Westbury, NY: Feminist Press, 1982. Collection of articles on black women, especially lesbian relationships, politics, and work.

Imber-Black, Evan, and Janine Roberts. *Rituals for Our Times: Celebrating, Healing, and Changing Our Lives and Our Relationships.* New York: HarperCollins, 1992.

Johnson, Barbara L. *Brothers and Sisters: Getting Back Together with Your Adult Siblings.* Buffalo, NY: Prometheus Books, 1991.

Jolly, Constance. "Purple Balloons on Market Street." *Broomstick,* Vol. 8, No. 6 (January–February 1986), pp. 3–8 (see page 446). Inspiring story by a mother about a lesbian daughter's coming out. Includes suggested readings.

Kimball, Gayle. *The Fifty-Fifty Marriage.* Boston: Beacon Press, 1983. Ways to achieve egalitarian relationships illustrated through stories of married couples.

Kornhaber, Arthur. *Between Parents and Grandparents.* New York: St. Martin's, 1986.

Kornhaber, Arthur, and Kenneth Woodward. *Grandparents, Grandchildren: The Vital Connection.* Garden City, NY: Anchor/Doubleday, 1981.

Lenz, Elinor. *Once My Child, Now My Friend.* New York: Warner, 1982.

Lerner, Harriet Goldhor. *The Dance of Intimacy: A Woman's Guide to Courageous Acts of Change in Key Relationships.* New York: Harper & Row, 1989; *The Dance of Deception: Pretending and Truth-Telling in Women's Lives,* 1993. In this and two earlier works, the author continues her compassionate yet respectful and empowering exploration of issues in women's lives. All are highly recommended.

Lightner, Candy, and Nancy Hathaway. *Giving Sorrow Words: How to Cope with Grief and Get On with Your Life.* New York: Warner, 1990.

Mairs, Nancy. *Ordinary Times: Cycles in Marriage, Faith and Renewal.* Boston: Beacon Press, 1993. Story of a woman coping with illness and disability as she struggles for relationship and self-definition.

Minkler, Meredith, and Kathleen M. Roe. *Grandmothers as Caregivers: Raising Children of the Crack Cocaine Epidemic.* Newbury Park, CA: Sage Publications, 1993. Moving exploration of older black women raising children whose parents are casualties of the crack epidemic. Advocates for social policy needs.

Morrison, Toni. *Sula.* New York: Knopf, 1974. Novel about a lifelong friendship between two black women.

Nicarthy, Ginny. *Getting Free: A Handbook for Women in Abusive Relationships.* Seattle: Seal Press, 1982. Includes exercises to help women examine their options and make decisions with more objectivity.

Pogrebin, Letty Cottin. *Among Friends: Who We*

Like, Why We Like Them, and What We Do with Them. New York: McGraw-Hill, 1986.

Polikoff, Nancy. *The Custody Handbook: A Woman's Guide to Child Custody Disputes,* 1984. Women's Legal Defense Fund, 2000 P St. NW, Suite 400, Washington, DC 20036. $4.00.

Powell, Barbara. *Overcoming Shyness: Practical Scripts for Everyday Encounters.* New York: McGraw-Hill, 1979. Beginning new relationships.

Rafkin, Louise, ed. *Different Daughters: A Book by Mothers of Lesbians.* Pittsburgh: Cleis Press, 1987. Twenty-five mothers raise the essential questions mothers of lesbians confront.

———, ed. *Different Mothers: Sons and Daughters of Lesbians Talk About Their Lives.* Pittsburgh: Cleis Press, 1990. Portrays the richness and diversity of lesbian parenting and the resiliency of their children.

Raymond, Janice G. *A Passion for Friends: Towards a Philosophy of Female Affection.* Boston: Beacon Press, 1986.

Reese, Lyn, Jean Wilkinson, and Phyllis Koppelman, eds. *I'm On My Way Running: Women Speak of Coming of Age.* New York: Avon, 1983. Primarily about younger women. See Chapter 4 on mother-daughter relationships.

Robertson, Christina. *A Woman's Guide to Divorce and Decision-Making: A Supportive Workbook for Women Facing the Process of Divorce.* New York: Simon & Schuster, 1988.

Rodgers-Rose, La Frances, ed. *The Black Woman.* Beverly Hills, CA: Sage Publications Inc., 1980. Articles on work, marriage, family roles, attitudes, and relationships.

Rubin, Lillian. *Just Friends: The Role of Friendship in Our Lives.* New York: Harper & Row, 1985. Engaging report on the importance of friendship, a frequently undervalued relationship.

Sarton, May. *The Magnificent Spinster.* New York: Norton, 1985. About a fifty-year-long friendship between women.

Schneider, Nina. *The Woman Who Lived in a Prologue.* Boston: Houghton Mifflin, 1980. Portrait over time of a woman in many roles—wife, mother, lover, grandmother.

Silverman, Phyllis. *Widow-to-Widow.* New York: Springer, 1985. Reports on self-help groups for widows.

Simon, Barbara Levy. *Never Married Women.* Philadelphia: Temple University Press, 1987.

Switzer, David K., and Shirley Switzer. *Parents of the Homosexual.* Philadelphia: Westminster Press, 1980. Enlightening and compassionate from a religious perspective.

Triere, Lynette, with Richard Peacock. *Learning to Leave: A Woman's Guide.* New York: Warner, 1982.

Walker, Alice. *In Search of Our Mothers' Gardens.* New York: Harcourt Brace Jovanovich, 1983. See especially the title article and "Brothers and Sisters."

Witkin, Mildred Hope, with Burton Lehrenbaum. *45 and Single Again.* New York: Dembner Books, 1985. Addressed to women who face the trauma of losing a valued mate through divorce or death. Coping with issues such as love, sex, finances, and grown children, and with the process of starting a new life.

The Women's Initiative of AARP. Older Battered Woman Report. Proceedings of a dialogue between advocates from the fields of elder abuse and domestic violence. A free copy is available from AARP Fulfillment. 601 E St., N.W., Washington, DC. Ask for publication #D15218.

Audiovisual

Widows. Film portrays a group of women of diverse ages venting their anger and frustration at being left alone, and expressing optimism, humor, and coping skills. Useful for anyone wishing to start a widows support group. Available from Terra Nova Films, Inc. (See p. 447.)

HOUSING ALTERNATIVES AND LIVING ARRANGEMENTS

Organizations

See other organizations listed throughout Resources section. Many other organizations concerned with issues of older people also have materials on housing.

ADAPTIVE ENVIRONMENTS CENTER
374 CONGRESS ST., SUITE 301
BOSTON, MA 02210
TEL. (617) 695-1225 VOICE OR TDD
Provides consultation and educational programs on home modification, accessibility legislation, and universal design. Publications include the *Consumers Guide to Home Modification,* and *Achieving Physical and Communications Accessibility.* Write for publications list.

AMERICAN ASSOCIATION OF RETIRED PERSONS (AARP)
(See page 441.) Free booklets include *Housing Options for Older Americans,* 1984, 42 pp., large type; and *Your Home, Your Choice: A Workbook for Older People and Their Families,* 1991. (Requests should be addressed to AARP, Attention: Housing.)

CENTER FOR ACCESSIBLE HOUSING
NORTH CAROLINA STATE UNIVERSITY
P.O. BOX 8613
RALEIGH, NC 27695
TEL. (919) 515-3082 OR VOICE OR TDD
Telephone technical assistance and information packages on a wide range of housing needs. Publications include *Fact Sheets on Financing Home Modifications, Fair Housing Amendments Act,* and *Housemate Agreements.* Call or write to Jan Reagan, Information Specialist.

NATIONAL LOW INCOME HOUSING COALITION
1012 14TH ST. NW, SUITE 1200
WASHINGTON, DC 20005
TEL. (202) 662-1530
A national membership organization that lobbies for the housing needs of low-income people.

WOMEN'S INSTITUTE FOR HOUSING AND ECONOMIC DEVELOPMENT, INC.
179 SOUTH ST.
BOSTON, MA 02111
TEL. (617) 423-2296
A national nonprofit corporation that assists groups with housing and business development through information referrals as well as intensive project assistance. Publications include *Making It Ourselves: A Primer on Women's Housing and Business Development* and *More Than Shelter: A Manual on Transitional Housing.* $15 each.

Books and Other Publications

Baum, Alice S., and Donald W. Burnes. *A Nation in Denial: The Truth About Homelessness.* Boulder, CO: Westview Press, 1993.

Hyde, Joan, and Susan Lanspery, eds. *Staying Put: Adapting the Places Instead of the People.* Amityville, NY: Baywood Publishing, 1994, in press. Highly recommended

Phillips, Alice H., and Caryl K. Roman. *A Practical Guide to Independent Living for Older People.* Seattle: Pacific Search Press, 1984. Written by two active older women. Specific and clear, with extensive resources. Large type.

Polniaszek, Susan. *Long Term Living: How to Live Independently as Long as You Can and Plan for the Time When You Can't.* United Seniors Health Cooperative, 1990.

Porcino, Jane. *Living Longer, Living Better: Adventures in Community Housing for Those in the Second Half of Life.* New York: Crossroad Continuum, 1991. Highly recommended.

Room for Improvement: The Lack of Affordable, Adaptable and Accessible Housing for Midlife and Older Women. Mother's Day Report, May 6, 1993, Older Women's League (see pages 443–44).

Safety for Older Consumers. A home-safety checklist available from the U.S. Consumer Product Safety Commission. Washington, DC 20207. Tel. (800) 638-2772.

Somers, Anne R., and Nancy L. Spears. *The Continuing Care Retirement Community.* New York: Springer, 1992.

Tone, Teona, and D. Sclar. *Housemates: A Practical Guide to Living with Other People.* New York: Ballantine, 1985.

SPECIAL HOUSING PROGRAMS FOR WOMEN

THE SUSAN B. ANTHONY MEMORIAL UNREST HOME. For more information write to the home at Rte. 1, Box 215, Millfield, OH 45761. Residents are involved in social activism, conservation, and recreation. Campgrounds are available to individuals and groups of women by advance reservation only. Feminists interested in a visit or in residential community are invited to write or send tape cassettes.

QUEST, Box 31, Montreal, WI 54550. The Midwest's and perhaps the nation's first shared housing program for gay and lesbian senior citizens and retirees. Write to them for current information.

HOME EQUITY CONVERSION INFORMATION

Organizations

AMERICAN BAR ASSOCIATION
COMMISSION ON LEGAL PROBLEMS OF THE ELDERLY
1800 M ST. NW
WASHINGTON, DC 20036
TEL. (202) 331-2200

Publications

Consumer's Guide to Home Equity Conversion: Man-Made Money. Rev. ed., 1991. Pub. No. D12894. AARP, see page 441.

SHARED LIVING

THE COHOUSING COMPANY
1250 ADDISON ST., #113
BERKELEY, CA 94702
TEL. (510) 549-9980
An architectural and consulting firm assisting groups and individuals in creating their cohousing community. Offers free information by phone or mail, and referrals to cohousing groups in your local community.

Publications

Franck, Karen A., and Sherry Ahrentzen, eds., *New Households, New Housing.* New York: Van Nostrand Reinhold, 1991.

Is Homesharing for You? A Self-Help Guide for Homeowners & Renters. 1983. National Shared Housing Resource Center, Inc., 431 Pine St., Burlington, VT 05401. Tel. (802) 862-2727. $3. For individuals who have no access to match-up programs or prefer to seek a home-sharing arrangement independently.

Living with Tenants—How to Happily Share Your House with Renters for Profit and Security. The Housing Connection, P.O. Box 5536, Arlington, VA 22205. $7.

McCaman, Kathryn, and Charles Durrett. *Cohousing: A Contemporary Approach to Housing Ourselves.* Rev. ed. Berkeley, CA: Ten Speed Press, 1994. Begun in Denmark in the 1970s, cohousing is a type of "resident-developed group housing" in which residents build and own their own homes on cooperatively owned land with the purpose of creating an intentional community. This approach combines individual and family privacy with community.

Shared Living: What Is It? Would I Like It? $3; *Shared Living: An Individual Planning Guide.* $4. *Shared Living: A Community Planning Guide,* $4; *Planning and Developing a Shared Living Project: A Guide for Community Groups*, $6; and *The Planning Game* (community planning for all kinds of elder housing in game form). Action for Boston Community Development, Inc. (ABCD), Community Services Dept., 178 Tremont St., Boston, MA 02111, Tel. (617) 357-6000. Takes readers through a step-by-step process in establishing their own shared-living arrangements.

Audiovisual

Open House, film or video. Shows living alternatives for older persons and explores crucial issues for sharing housing. Action for Boston Community Development, Inc. See Publications—Shared Living, above.

CONDOS AND CO-OPS

NATIONAL ASSOCIATION OF HOUSING COOPERATIVES
1614 KING ST.
ALEXANDRIA, VA 22314
TEL. (703) 549-5201

Questions and Answers About Condominiums.

U.S. Department of Housing and Urban Development. 53-page booklet from the U.S. Consumer Information Center, Pueblo, CO 81002.

ACCESSORY APARTMENTS AND ECHO HOUSING

Hare, Patrick H. *Accessory Apartments: Using Surplus Space in Single Family Housing.* 1981. American Planning Association, 1313 E. 60th St., Chicago, IL 60637. Xerox copy available for $20 plus $5 shipping. Relevant zoning issues and sample language for a zoning amendment to permit accessory apartments.

———. *ECHO Housing.* Available from AARP (see pages 441–42).

CONTINUING CARE AND RETIREMENT COMMUNITIES

A Consumer Guide to Life Care Communities. National Consumers League, 815 15th St. NW, Suite 928, Washington, DC 20005. Tel. (202) 639-8140. $4.

The Continuing Care Retirement Community: A Guidebook for Consumers. American Association of Homes for the Aging, 901 E St. NW, Suite 500, Washington, DC 20004. Tel. (202) 783-2242. $5.Checklist of facts and examples of contracts for CCRCs.

National Directory of Retirement Facilities. Phoenix, AZ: Oryx Press, 1992. This listing is in many public libraries.

INDEPENDENT LIVING RESEARCH UTILIZATION (ILRU)
INSTITUTE FOR REHABILITATION AND RESEARCH
OF THE TEXAS MEDICAL CENTER
P.O. BOX 20095
HOUSTON, TX 77225
ILRU is a national center for information, training, and technical assistance in the field of independent living. Write for a publication list. Every state has one or more independent-living centers. Call your State Department of Rehabilitation.

HOME CARE

See Resources—Caregiving, page 481.

WORK AND RETIREMENT

Organizations

AMERICAN ASSOCIATION OF RETIRED PERSONS (AARP) (see page 441). The AARP offers a do-it-yourself booklet, *Returning to the Job Market: A Woman's Guide to Employment Planning,* that takes you step-by-step through the job-search process with exercises for assessing skills and goals, filling out applications, building a résumé, and putting together a job-search plan. AARP also publishes an informative guidebook to assist women who are planning for retirement, *Focus Your Future: A Woman's Guide to Retirement Planning.* Other AARP publications that feature issues relevant to women's work are *Women's Initiative Fact Sheets* and the magazine *Working Age.*

AMERICAN CIVIL LIBERTIES UNION (see page 477). The ACLU publishes a series of useful inexpensive books on workers' rights, such as *The Rights of Women* and *The Rights of Employees.* Ask for their list of titles.

AMERICAN FEDERATION OF STATE, COUNTY AND MUNICIPAL EMPLOYEES (AFSCME)
1625 L ST. NW
WASHINGTON, DC 20036
This union has provided leadership in the fight for pay equity and is a good source of information and support for women workers.

COALITION OF LABOR UNION WOMEN
15 W. UNION SQUARE
NEW YORK, NY 10003
TEL. (212) 242-0700
Offers programs and resources for employed women, including a committee for older and retired women workers. Ask for their pamphlet on organizing women workers.

ELDERHOSTEL
75 FEDERAL ST.
BOSTON, MA 02110
TEL. (617) 426-8056
Short-term campus-based educational experiences for older adults. Seven catalogs per year.

GRAY PANTHERS (see page 442) has done excellent work toward abolishing mandatory retirement.

National Commission on Working Women
1325 G St. NW
Washington, DC 20005
Tel. (202) 737-5764

Committed to promoting the rights of working women, they are especially concerned with ageism, and provide information about employment rights as well as facts about older working women.

National Committee on Pay Equity
1126 16th St. NW, Room 411
Washington, DC 20036
Tel. (202) 331-7343

Offers information and fact sheets on pay equity, particularly concerning women and people of color.

National Displaced Homemakers Network
1625 K St. NW, Suite 300
Washington, DC 20006
Tel. (202) 467-6346

Over twelve hundred programs serving displaced homemakers nationwide. The national network will put you in touch with the services nearest you. Their programs include job clubs specifically designed to make job hunting a group project instead of the lonely and frustrating burden that it usually is. In such activities as peer counseling (one person acting as a sounding board for the other), women draw on their life experience to help someone else with similar problems.

9 to 5 National Association of Working Women
614 Superior Ave. NW
Cleveland, OH 44113
Tel. (216) 566-9308

A national association of women office workers. Membership dues include a bimonthly newsletter and discounts on publications such as books and pamphlets on automation, stress, and occupational health and hazards.

Older Women's League (OWL) (see pages 443–44) has a Task Force on Women and Work and publishes Gray Papers on a variety of topics, including women and work. Their pamphlet *Older Women and Job Discrimination: A Primer* (1984) is indispensable to women fighting unfair treatment at work ($5). The pamphlet discusses kinds of discrimination and contains a list of Equal Employment Opportunity Commission (EEOC) field offices.

Retired Senior Volunteer Program (RSVP), jointly funded by the federal government and local communities, enables older persons to use their time, experience, and skills to benefit their communities. Look in your phone book under Elder Services—Volunteer Opportunities, or check with your area Agency on Aging.

U.S. Department of Labor
Bureau of Labor Statistics
441 G St. NW
Washington, DC 20212
Tel. (202) 606-5886

An excellent source of general statistical information on working women.

A Working Woman's Guide to Her Job Rights, 1993. The Women's Bureau, U.S. Department of Labor, Frances Perkins Bldg., 200 Constitution Ave. NW, Washington, DC 20210. Information about laws that affect our work experiences. Includes procedures for fighting back, such as the EEOC complaint process for sex, age, race, and disability discrimination, and Social Security, pension, and Medicare issues. Contains an extensive list of federal and regionally based sources of assistance.

Books and Other Publications

Allen, Jeffry G., and Jess Gorkin. *Finding the Right Job at Midlife.* New York: Simon & Schuster, 1985. For women and men coping with fear of younger competitors. Layoff survival kit and how to recognize signs of a coming layoff.

Anzalone, Joan, ed. *Good Works: A Guide to Careers in Social Change.* New York: Dembner Books, 1985. Lists six hundred organizations in the United States, their starting salaries, and contact persons. Regional and topical index.

Balser, Diane. *Sisterhood and Solidarity: Feminism and Labor in Modern Times.* Boston: South End Press, 1987. Brings to life the histories of three working-women's organizations. Examines the problems of organizing around gender and work.

Bepko, Claudia, and Jo-Ann Krestan. *Singing at the Top of Our Lungs: Women, Love and Creativ-*

ity. New York: HarperCollins, 1993. A bold and original exploration of how women deal with the conflicts between their passions for work and relationships. Highly recommended.

Beyer, Cathy, et al. *Surviving Unemployment: A Family Handbook for Weathering Hard Times.* New York: Henry Holt, 1993. This book may be more useful for women who still have children at home. It does not address the problems of women who are unemployed and alone.

Bird, Caroline. *Second Careers: New Ways to Work After 50.* Boston: Little, Brown, 1992. Reports on the second careers of AARP members. Provides self-help tips for those considering career change.

Bolles, Richard Nelson. *The New Quick Job-Hunting Map;* and *The 1993 What Color Is Your Parachute.* Berkeley, CA: Ten Speed Press, 1993. Job-hunting and career-changing guidebooks. Detailed and cheerful advice. Both are updated annually.

Brudney, Juliet F., and Hilda Scott. *Forced Out: Why Veteran Employees Are Driven from Their Careers—and What They Can Do.* New York: Simon & Schuster/Fireside, 1987. Interviews with 150 women and men about the growing difficulties faced by older workers.

Chastain, Sherry. *Winning the Salary Game.* New York: Wiley, 1980. Indispensable tool for demystifying salary negotiations. Out of print. Check your public library.

Committee on an Aging Society, Institute of Medicine and National Research Council. *America's Aging: Productive Roles in an Older Society.* Washington, DC: National Academy Press, 1986. Research and analysis of the role of older volunteers.

Cort-Van Arsdale, Diana, and Phyllis Newman. *Transitions: A Woman's Guide to Successful Retirement.* New York: HarperPerennial, 1992. Through questionnaires, helps women examine the importance of work and social networks in their lives, identify personal needs, and make positive choices.

Fillmore, Mary D. *A Foot in the Door: Women MBAs in the Eighties.* Boston: G. K. Hall, 1987. Provocative assessment of the pros and cons of the value of an MBA degree for women's chances for advancement in organizations. Includes an excellent chapter on starting one's own business.

Groneman, Carol, and Mary Beth Norton, eds. *To Toil the Livelong Day: America's Women at Work, 1780–1980.* Ithaca, NY: Cornell University Press, 1987.

How to Get College Credit for What You Learned as a Homemaker or Volunteer. Princeton, NJ: Educational Testing Service, 1988.

Kenan, Regina, Susan Klitzman, and Lin Nelson. *Resource Guide on Women's Occupational and Environmental Health.* 1987. National Women's Health Network (see page 482).

Koltnow, Emily, and Lynne S. Dumas. *Congratulations! You've Been Fired: Sound Advice for Women Who've Been Terminated, Downsized or Otherwise Unemployed.* New York: Fawcett Columbine, 1990. Practical advice about coping with job loss, job search, salary and benefit negotiation, and self-employment alternatives.

Mendelsohn, Pam. *Happier by Degrees—The Most Complete Sourcebook for Women Who Are Considering Going Back to School.* New York: Dutton, 1980.

Moore, Lynda L., ed. *Not as Far as You Think: The Realities of Working Women.* Lexington, MA: D. C. Heath/Lexington Books, 1986. Articles on such issues as women as bosses, and older women working for younger women.

Scollard, Jeannette B. *The Self-Employed Woman: How to Start Your Own Business and Gain Control of Your Life.* New York: Simon & Schuster, 1985. A step-by-step guide to starting and managing one's own business, with attention to problems and issues that women are likely to face.

Shea, Beverly. "Late Bloomers: They Got Their First Jobs at 50." *Ms.,* November 1985.

Sher, Barbara, with Anne Gottlieb. *Wishcraft: How to Get What You Really Want.* New York: Ballantine, 1979. How to learn about yourself and what you want. How to get help for brainstorming, networking, and support.

Shields, Laurie. *Displaced Homemakers: Fighting for a New Life.* New York: McGraw-Hill, 1981. An exciting account of women's struggles to win recognition for displaced homemakers and to establish new lives. Available from Older Women's League (see pages 443–44). $7.

Shuman, Nancy, and William Lewis. *Back to Work: How to Re-enter the Working World.* New York: Barron's, 1985. Practical basic advice. Includes descriptions of new automated equipment a woman reentering the busines world might encounter for the first time.

Smith, Maggie. *Changing Course: A Positive Approach to a New Job or Lifestyle.* San Diego: Pfeiffer & Co., 1993. This book offers values-clarification exercises to help the reader make individually appropriate choices.

Wilkinson, Carroll Wetzel. "Work: Challengers to Occupational Segregation." In Mary McFeely, ed., *The Woman's Annual,* No. 5. Boston: G. K. Hall, 1986, pp. 149–67. Article focuses on female pioneers in nontraditional jobs, especially blue-collar jobs. Includes an extensive bibliography.

Money Matters: The Economics of Aging for Women

Organizations

American Association of Retired Persons publishes a variety of books and pamphlets on older persons and money matters, including *Divorce After Fifty—Challenges and Choices.* Write to AARP Program Dept. (see pages 441–42).

American Civil Liberties Union
132 W. 43rd St.
New York, NY 10036
Tel. (212) 944-9800
Publishes a series of helpful books on legal and financial issues such as *The Rights of Single People; The Rights of Gay People;* and *The Rights of Crime Victims.* Write for their literature list.

Center for Popular Economics
P.O. Box 785
Amherst, MA 01004
Tel. (413) 545-0743
Conducts week-long intensive workshops for activists to help them understand how the economy works. Scholarships available.

Developmental Disabilities State Protection and Advocacy Agencies. These agencies, in each state, help protect your legal rights if you should become disabled. They will advocate for you with the Social Security system and in cases of job discrimination. A social-service agency can put you in touch with the office in your state.

Funding Exchange
666 Broadway, 5th Floor
New York, NY 10012
Tel. (212) 529-5300
Raises money from individual donors, including donor-advised accounts. Distributes funds to grass-roots organizations working for social change nationally and internationally.

Gray Panthers (see page 442). The Panthers publish useful material on older women's economic and financial problems, and chapters often organize around economic issues affecting older women.

National Association of Community Action Agencies
1826 18th St. NW
Washington, DC 20009
Tel. (202) 265-7546
Community Action Program (CAP) agencies are antipoverty programs. They often provide services for low-income elders and can help you find out if you are eligible for public assistance. The national office can help you find the CAP agency nearest you.

National Foundation for Consumer Credit
8611 2nd Ave., Suite 100
Silver Spring, MD 20910
Tel. (800) 388-2227 or (301) 589-5600
Provides education and counseling on budgeting and appropriate use of credit. Local branches are listed as Consumer Credit Counseling Service.

The National Network of Women's Funds
1821 University Ave., Suite 409 N.
St. Paul, MN 55104
Tel. (612) 641-0742
Provides information on women's funds nationally and locally.

Nolo Press
950 Parker St.
Berkeley, CA 94710
Tel. (510) 549-1976
Publishes a newsletter that helps the lay reader deal with legal issues such as sexual harassment in the workplace. Also publishes sourcebooks, workbooks, and computer software about benefits, entitlements, wills, and other financial and legal matters. Write for their list.

Older Women's League (see pages 443–44). OWL publishes pamphlets on various economic issues such as no-fault divorce and women and pensions.

Organization for the Enforcement of Child Support
1712 Deer Park Rd.
Finksburg, MD 21048
Tel. (410) 876-1826
Makes people aware of their rights and obligations under current child-support laws. Works with all branches and levels of government to improve the child-support enforcement system. Educates legislators, courts, and the public on the problems involved in collecting child support. Send stamped, self-addressed business envelope for literature packet.

Pension Rights Center
1346 Connecticut Ave. NW
Washington, DC 20036
Publishes "A Guide to Understanding Your Pension Plan."

Social Investment Forum
430 First Ave. N., Suite 290
Minneapolis, MN 55401
Tel. (612) 333-8338
Ask for their directory, *Social Investment Services: A Guide to Forum Members*. Socially responsible investment opportunities, advisers, mutual funds, community investments, and other socially responsible investment vehicles.

Women for Economic Justice
32 Rutland St.
Boston, MA 02118
Tel. (617) 266-1215
Their newsletter, "Talk Back," reports on their activities and provides general information about the economy and its effects on low-income women. Ask for their occasional publication *PROGRESS*, which covers economic issues of concern to women, such as pay equity, welfare, and economic literacy.

The Women's Fund
3543 18th St.
San Francisco, CA 94110
Tel. (415) 431-1290
Raises money to fund womens' and girls' projects in Northern California. Special focus on women over forty and women over sixty.

Periodicals

Dollars & Sense. 1 Summer St., Somerville, MA 02143. Tel. (617) 628-8411 or 8433. Explains in everyday language current economic issues and trends from an activist's perspective. Covers women's issues often, but not exclusively.

Goodmoney. 28 Main St., Montpelier, VT 05602. Looks at traditional and alternative investments. A newsletter for social investing that uses a minimum of technical language.

Insight. 711 Atlantic Ave., 5th Floor, Boston, MA 02111. Tel. (617) 423-6655. Analyzes the impact of social issues on the financial and economic environment. An advisory letter for social investing.

Money. Box 2519, Boulder, CO 80322. Overview of current financial problems facing individuals and families. Written in understandable language; often includes a case study.

Books and Other Publications

Barsness, Anita O. *Money Matters in Second Marriages*. University of Wisconsin Center for Consumer Affairs, 1986.

Domini, Amy L., and Peter D. Kinder. *Ethical Investing: How to Make Profitable Investments Without Sacrificing Your Principles*. Reading, MA: Addison-Wesley, 1986. Highly recommended.

Eisenberg, Ronni. *Organize Yourself!* New York: Collier Books, 1986.

Engel, Margorie L. *Divorce Help and Sourcebook: Resources and References*. Detroit, MI: Gail Research (in press). Lists organizations available to help divorcing women in areas such as financial, legal, child care, etc. Provides overview of the process including a history of divorce in the United States.

Engel, Margorie L., and Diana Gould. *The Divorce Decisions Workbook: A Planning and Action Guide with FORMulas to Help You in Four Key Decision Areas—Financial, Legal, Practical and Emotional.* New York: McGraw-Hill, 1992. Includes checklist for hiring an attorney.

Kingson, Eric R., Barbara A. Hirshorn, and Linda K. Harootyan. *The Common Stake: The Interdependence of Generations.* A report of The Gerontological Society of America debunking the myth of competition between generations for public funds. Available from Seven Locks Press, P.O. Box 27, Cabin John, MD 20818.

Leonard, Frances. *Money and the Mature Woman.* New York: Addison-Wesley, 1993. Highly recommended.

Leonard, Robin. *Money Troubles: Legal Strategies to Cope with Your Debts.* Berkeley, CA: Nolo Press, 1991. (See p. 478 for more on Nolo Press.)

Martin, Don, and Renee Martin, with Joan Scobey, ed. *A Survival Kit for Wives: How to Avoid Financial Chaos Before Tragedy Strikes.* New York: Villard Books, 1986.

Quinn, Jane Bryant. *Making the Most of Your Money.* New York: Simon & Schuster, 1991.

Rix, Sara E. *Older Women: The Economics of Aging.* This and other excellent publications are available from Women's Research and Educational Institute, 1700 18th St. NW, Suite 400, Washington, DC 20009. Tel. (202) 328-7070. Packed with data on the financial situation of older women. $5.00.

Siverd, Bonnie. *A Woman's Guide to Sudden Financial Change.* New York: Putnam, 1983.

Supplemental Social Security Income: The Promise and the Performance. SOS Education Fund, 1201 16th St. NW, Suite 222, Washington, DC 21136. Single free copy; bulk rates available.

Warschaw, Tessa Albert. *Rich Is Better.* New York: Doubleday, 1985. Takes a brisk approach to the intersection of money and psychological issues in women's lives, with good sections on divorce and using financial experts effectively.

Wilson, Carol Ann. *The Survival Manual for Women in Divorce.* Boulder, CO: Quantum, 1990.

Audiovisual

Women: The New Poor. A videotape by Bea Milwe. Looks at the consequences of job discrimination and the changing economy on the lives of four women. Realistic and empowering. Available from Women Make Movies. (See p. 447.)

CAREGIVING

Organizations

CHILDREN OF AGING PARENTS (CAPS)
1609 WOODBOURNE RD., SUITE 302A
LEVITTOWN, PA 19057
TEL. (215) 945-6900

CAPS is a nonprofit organization that offers information, referral, support, and guidance nationally to caregivers, professionals, and agencies dealing with elders and their families. CAPS actively helps start support groups, publishes a bimonthly newsletter, fact sheets, directory, and manuals for starting support groups.

ELDERCARE LOCATOR
TEL. (800) 677-1116

Collaborative project of the U.S. Agencies on Aging and related state agencies. Provides information on local resources for elders and their caregivers.

FAMILY SERVICE OF AMERICA INC.
(COUNSELING AND REFERRALS)
11700 WEST LAKE PARK DR.
MILWAUKEE, WI 53224
TEL. (414) 359-1040

Agencies in forty states provide counseling for families of the elderly and make referrals to other services.

NATIONAL ASSOCIATION OF PRIVATE GERIATRIC CARE MANAGERS
655 N. ALVERNON WAY, SUITE 108
TUCSON, AZ 85711
TEL. (602) 881-8008

The National Council on the Aging (see page 443) has a Family Caregivers Program that provides literature and other resources.

National Women's Law Center
1616 P St. NW
Washington, DC 20036
Tel. (202) 328-5160
If you provide care for a dependent member of your household at home, you may be eligible for tax relief. The NWLC gathers and provides information on the Dependent Care Tax Credit for federal and state taxes.

Older Women's League (OWL) (see pages 443–44) has task forces on caregiving issues in many local chapters. Tish Sommers and Laurie Shields are coauthors of *Women Take Care.* Gainesville, FL: Triad, 1987. Available from OWL for $9.95, this landmark book documents the plight of caregivers and urges women to take appropriate action.

Well Spouse Foundation
P.O. Box 28876
San Diego, CA 92198-0876
Membership is open to partners of chronically ill people and includes newsletter and local support groups.

Books

Bayless, Pamela J., ed. *Caring for Dependent Parents.* Research Institute of America, 90 Fifth Ave., New York, NY 10011. Well-written 58-page pamphlet covering long-term care of aging parents, including financial, legal, emotional, and psychological issues.

Caston, Don. *Eighty-eight Easy to Make Aids for Older People and for Special Needs.* Point Roberts, WA: Hartley & Marks, 1988. Illustrations and step-by-step instructions for creating practical aids to make living more comfortable, safe, and independent using household tools and inexpensive materials.

Greenberg, Vivian. *Your Best Is Good Enough.* New York: Lexington, 1989. Scenarios help caregivers identify with relationship and communication issues.

Hooyman, Nancy R., and Wendy Lustbader. *Taking Care: Supporting Older Women and Their Families.* New York: Free Press, 1986. An excellent book of strategies for coping. Reports on the various lifestyles of caregivers from nuclear families to gay and lesbian couples.

Koch, Tom. *Mirrored Lives: Aging Children and Elderly Parents.* New York: Praeger, 1990. Explores the emotional issues of a son caring for his father over a period of years as their roles change. The afterword is a primer on planning, finding help, and coping.

Lester, Andrew D., and Judith L. Lester. *Understanding Aging Parents.* Christian Care Books #8. Philadelphia: Westminster Press, 1980. Strong Christian viewpoint, but provides sound guidance for all readers.

Levin, Nora Jean. *How to Care for Your Parents: A Handbook for Adult Children.* Washington, DC: Storm King Press, 1993. New information on Medicare, Medicaid, and housing options plus a manual for finding your community's resource networks.

Lowe, Paula C. *CarePooling: How to Get the Help You Need to Care for the Ones You Love.* San Francisco: Berrett-Koehler Publishers, 1993. Encourages interdependence through forming support networks for child care and elder care. Provides clear guidelines for mobilizing potential helpers.

McGurn, Sheelagh. *Under One Roof: Caring for an Aging Parent.* Park Ridge, IL: Parkside Publishing, 1992. Caregivers' fears, expectations, and practical solutions taken from interviews with other caregivers. How to maintain a manageable life as caregiver, spouse, mother, employee.

Niebuhr, Sheryl, and Jane Royse. *Take Care! A Guide for Caregivers on How to Improve Their Self-Care.* St. Paul, MN: Amherst H. Wilder Foundation, 1989. 30-page pamphlet advises caregivers on how to manage their own stress and negative feelings, learn how to relax, and ask for help.

Portnow, Jay, and Martha Houtman. *Home Care for the Elderly: The First Guide for the Millions of Americans Caring for Elderly Loved Ones.* New York: McGraw-Hill, 1987. A doctor and nurse help home caregivers improve the quality of life of the ill or bedfast person. Includes nutrition and exercise, adaptive gadgets, personal hygiene, signs of illness, care for the bedfast, resources, and specialized help.

Rob, Caroline. *The Caregiver's Guide.* Boston: Houghton-Mifflin, 1991. Useful health information for caregivers in a readable style.

Shapiro, Barbara A., et al. *The Big Squeeze: Balancing the Needs of Aging Parents, Dependent Children and You.* Bedford, MA: Mills & Sanderson, 1991. An eight-step survival plan for dealing with conflicting responsibilities. Highly recommended.

Silverstone, Barbara, and Helene K. Hyman. *You and Your Aging Parent: The Modern Family's Guide to Emotional, Physical and Financial Problems.* 3rd ed. New York: Pantheon, 1989. Comprehensive, well-written guide for anyone who is a caregiver or expects to be one.

Smith, Kerri S. *Caring for Your Aging Parents: A Sourcebook of Timesaving Techniques and Tips.* Lakewood, CO: American Source Books, 1992. Each chapter focuses on a specific caregiving concern and includes a timesavers page of "Things to Do This Week."

Periodicals

Parent Care Advisor. American Health Consultants, P.O. Box 71266, Chicago, IL 60691-9986. Tel. (800) 688-2421. Expert-oriented but practical monthly newsletter. $39 per year. First issue is free.

Parent Care: Resources to Assist Family Caregivers. Gerontology Center, 316 Strong Hall, University of Kansas, Lawrence, KS 66045. An excellent newsletter of articles, book reviews, and other up-to-date information equally useful to family caregivers and professionals.

HOME CARE

Organizations

NATIONAL HOME CARE COUNCIL, INC.
A DIVISION OF FOUNDATION FOR HOSPICE AND HOME CARE, INC.
519 C ST. NE
WASHINGTON, DC 20002
TEL. (202) 547-6586

Has many publications including *All About Home Care: A Consumer's Guide,* which was published with the Better Business Bureau. $2 plus stamped self-addressed envelope.

Publications

How to Hire Helpers: A Guide for Helpers and Their Families. Task Force on Aging, Church Council of Greater Seattle, 4759 15th Ave. NE, Seattle, WA 98105. $3; bulk rates available. Discounts for quantity purchases. Emphasizes the importance of developing a job description for the care provider and offers a sample contract form and a checklist to use in interviews.

Mail-Order Catalogs for Home Health Aids

Medical supply stores can help you get equipment and are aware of what Medicare and Medicaid will or will not pay for. Their catalogs offer ideas for helpful adaptive devices and their rental and purchase prices. Catalogs may also be available at rehabilitation hospitals and pharmacies that deal in home health equipment. These catalogs offer many practical items that make it easier for someone disabled, for example, by crippling arthritis, to feed her/himself, pull up zippers, open bottles, and perform many other daily chores that are otherwise difficult. (See section on adapting housing, page 163, and Resources, page 472.)

Audiovisual

My Father, My Mother, an award-winning documentary, presents four examples of families dealing with the aging of a parent. *My Father, My Mother: Seven Years Later.* Sequel as effective and stimulating as original brings the viewer up-to-date on current issues in caregiving and care receiving. Unusually candid film and videotape spark identification and helpful discussion. Order from Terra Nova Films, Inc. See Resources, page 447.

Understanding, Preventing, and Managing Medical Problems

General Health

Organizations

Agency for Health Care Policy and Research (AHCPR)
U.S. Dept. of Health and Human Services, Public Health Service
Executive Office Center
2101 East Jefferson St., Suite 501
Rockville, MD 20852
Tel. (800) 358-9295

AHCPR produces clinical guidelines and patient education brochures on various procedures, conditions, and diseases. Available free to the public as well as to professionals. Call for list of subjects for which guidelines have been developed.

Center for Medical Consumers and Health Care Information
237 Thompson St.
New York, NY 10012
Tel. (212) 674-7105

Free medical library for the lay public with a strong women's health section. Visit the library when you are in New York. It does not have a phone service. The center publishes a monthly newsletter, *HealthFacts,* $21.00 per year.

Exceptional Cancer Patients
1302 Chapel st.
New Haven, CT 06511
Tel. (203) 865-8392

Started for people with cancer but now assists people with any catastrophic illness, integrating self-healing with standard medical treatment. Offers counseling and support groups in New Haven. Has catalog of audio- and videotapes and books based on the work of Bernie Siegel. (See his book under Books, following this section.)

Health/PAC (Health Policy Advisory Center)
853 Broadway, #1607
New York, NY 10003
Tel. (212) 614-1660

A progressive health activist organization. Membership provides a discount on its publications and *Health PACKETS,* a newsletter, *Inside Friends,* and a bimonthly magazine, *Health/PAC Bulletin.*

National Black Women's Health Project
1237 Ralph David Abernathy Blvd. SW
Atlanta, GA 30310
Tel. (404) 758-9590

Programs for education and advocacy on black women's health issues. Membership organization with local self-help groups.

National Council on Patient Information and Education
666 Eleventh St. NW, Suite 810
Washington, DC 20001
Tel. (202) 347-6711

Produces useful booklets and guides, including information for women about prescription-drug use.

National Health Information Center
P.O. Box 1133
Washington, DC 20013-1133
Tel. (800) 336-4797

Operated by the Public Health Service. It publishes *Healthfinder* and other publications on a variety of health topics, has a list of some one hundred hot lines on various subjects, and a database of over eleven hundred health-information resources.

National Latina Health Organization
P.O. Box 7567
Oakland, CA 94601

Publishes bilingual materials for advocacy and education projects.

National Organization for Rare Disorders
P.O. Box 8923
New Fairfield, CT 06812-1783
Tel. (800) 999-NORD

Founded by a woman after she experienced how hard it was to get information on her three children's rare condition. Has reports on the symptoms, therapies, and current research on 950 rare diseases. The first two requests are free; subsequent reports cost $3.75 each.

National Women's Health Network
1325 G St. NW
Washington, DC 20005
Tel. (202) 347-1140

The only national membership organization devoted exclusively to women and health; publishes bimonthly newsletter, *The Network News,* and monitors federal health policy affecting women. Provides information and referrals on seventy-five topics.

NATIVE AMERICAN WOMEN'S HEALTH EDUCATION RESOURCE CENTER
P.O. BOX 572
LAKE ANDES, SD 57356

Publishes newsletter and other information on women's health from Native American women's perspectives. Advocacy and education projects.

PEOPLE'S MEDICAL SOCIETY
462 WALNUT ST.
ALLENTOWN, PA 18102
TEL. (215) 770-1670

A nonprofit citizens' action group committed to better, more responsive, and less expensive medical care. For a $20.00 yearly donation, members receive a bimonthly newsletter plus discounts on publications such as *Take This Book to the Hospital with You.*

PUBLIC CITIZEN HEALTH RESEARCH GROUP
2000 P ST. NW
WASHINGTON, DC 20036
TEL. (202) 833-3000

Works to change the political and social problems in the health field by monitoring government agencies and initiating legal action and legislative change. Publishes a bimonthly newsletter, *Health Letter,* $9.00 per year. Publication list of excellent books and pamphlets such as *Worst Pills, Best Pills.* Membership: $20 per year.

WOMEN'S HEALTH INFORMATION CENTER
BOSTON WOMEN'S HEALTH BOOK COLLECTIVE
240 ELM ST.
SOMERVILLE, MA 02144
TEL. (617) 625-0271

Materials used in writing this and the 1987 edition are in the WHIC and are available for public use. The Center's collection of books, periodicals, and clippings includes extensive materials on birth control, abortion, and reproductive rights. Information requests by mail or phone are answered for a nominal fee or donation to cover costs. Call for current hours of operation before visiting the center.

Books

Braithwaite, Ronald L., and Sandra E. Taylor, eds. *Health Issues in the Black Community.* San Francisco: Jossey-Bass, 1992. Includes an overview plus chapters on women's health, elderly issues, and specific diseases.

Butler, Robert N., and Myrna I. Lewis. *Aging & Mental Health.* St. Louis, MO: C.V. Mosby, 1983.

Corea, Gena. *The Hidden Malpractice: How American Medicine Mistreats Women.* Rev. ed. New York: Harper & Row, 1985. Remains the most stunning investigative report on American medicine's shameful history with regard to women.

Feltin, Marie. *A Woman's Guide to Good Health After 50.* An AARP Book. Glenview, IL: Scott, Foresman, 1987.

Haug, Marie R., Amasa B. Ford, and Marian Sheafor. *The Physical and Mental Health of Aged Women.* New York: Springer, 1985.

Hubbard, Ruth. *The Politics of Women's Biology.* New Brunswick, NJ: Rutgers University Press, 1990. A feminist critique of major distortions in scientific thinking about women and why we need to know how our bodies really function.

Hubbard, Ruth, and Elijah Wald. *Exploding the Gene Myth: How Genetic Information Is Produced and Manipulated by Scientists, Physicians, Employers, Insurance Companies, Educators, and Law Enforcers.* Boston: Beacon Press, 1993. A readable book about the dangers of explaining so much in biology and medicine by genetic determination.

Kaptchuk, Ted. *The Web That Has No Weaver.* New York: Congdon and Weed, 1984. Explains the differences between Western and Eastern medicine and contains an excellent explanation of acupuncture.

Lettvin, Maggie. *Maggie's Women's Book.* Boston: Houghton Mifflin, 1980. See especially the warmups for early-morning stiffness, pp. 54–58.

Lewin, Ellen, and Virgina Oleson, eds. *Women, Health and Healing.* New York: Methuen, 1985.

Payer, Lynn. *Disease-Mongers.* New York: John Wiley, 1992. Takes aim at conventional and some alternative doctors for exaggerating the severity of diseases and minimizing the effects of treatment.

Pitzele, Sefra Kobrin. *We Are Not Alone: Learning to Live with Chronic Illness.* New York: Workman, 1986. A useful handbook on chronic illness that includes chapters on pain, health care and rights, finding help, and other important subjects. The chapter on adaptive living strategies contains photos of useful gadgets.

Siegel, Bernie. *Love, Medicine, and Miracles: Lessons Learned About Self-healing from a Surgeon's Experience with Exceptional Patients.* New York: Harper & Row, 1986; and *How to Live Between Office Visits.* New York: HarperCollins, 1993. Helpful for anyone facing a life-threatening disease, especially cancer or AIDS.

Table Manners: A Guide to the Pelvic Examination for Disabled Women and Health Care Providers. Planned Parenthood, Education Dept., 815 Eddy St., Suite 300, San Francisco, CA 94109. Tel. (415) 441-7858 (TTY). $1.00. Bulk rate available. How to provide sensitive care to women with physical, visual, and hearing disabilities. Includes alternative positioning, transfers to the examining table, and other considerations.

White, Evelyn C., ed. *The Black Women's Health Book: Speaking for Ourselves.* Seattle: Seal Press, 1990. Selected issues from the viewpoint of black women.

Wolfe, Sidney M. *Women's Health Alert.* Reading, MA: Addison-Wesley, 1991. Good exposé of problems.

Other Publications

Consumer Reports on Health. Consumers Union of the U.S., Subscription Dept., Box 56356, Boulder, CO 80322-6356. Tel. (800) 234-2188. Monthly newsletter, $24 per year. Also publishes *Consumer Reports,* which contains longer articles on health issues, the drug industry, and system reform.

Golub, Sharon, and Rita J. Freedman, eds. "Health Needs of Women as They Age." Special issue of *Women and Health,* Vol. 10, Nos. 2 and 3 (Summer/Fall 1985).

"Health Care of the Older Woman." *Geriatrics,* Vol. 48, Suppl. 1 (June 1993), entire issue.

Healthsharing. 14 Skey Lane, Toronto, Ontario M6J 3S4, Canada. Tel. (416) 532-0812. A quarterly newsletter covering a wide range of women's health concerns. $15 per year.

Hopper, Susan V. "The Influence of Ethnicity on the Health of Older Women." *Clinics in Geriatric Medicine,* Vol. 9, No. 1 (February 1993), pp. 231–59.

Off Our Backs, 2423 18th St. NW, Washington, DC 20009. an excellent feminist newspaper with regular coverage of women's health issues. Monthly, $21 per year.

WomenWise, New Hampshire Feminist Health Center, 38 S. Main St., Concord, NH 03301. Tel. (603) 225-2739. An excellent publication that covers a wide variety of topics on women and health. Quarterly, $10.00 per year.

WOMEN'S HEALTH AND REFORMING THE MEDICAL CARE SYSTEM

Organizations

Many of the organizations listed in the General Resources pages and in the General Health resource pages such as AARP (especially its Women's Initiative), Families USA Foundation (including A.S.A.P. program), Gray Panthers, Health/PAC, Older Women's League, and others have positions and materials on health-system issues. See also organizations listed under other chapters such as Center for Science in the Public Interest (page 456).

THE CAMPAIGN FOR WOMEN'S HEALTH
C/O OWL
666 ELEVENTH ST. NW, SUITE 700
WASHINGTON, DC 20001
TEL. (202) 783-6686

The major coalition of women's organizations on health issues including church groups and labor unions. Offers brochures summarizing problems in women's health and criteria for evaluating national-health-plan proposals such as "Model Benefits Package for Women in Health Care Reform." Welcomes memberships and contributions to support the work of the coalition.

CHURCH WOMEN UNITED (CWU)
110 MARYLAND AVE. NE
WASHINGTON, DC 20002
TEL. (202) 544-8747

National ecumenical women's group offers a workshop on "Ethical Choices: Reforming the Health Care System."

COALITION OF LABOR UNION WOMEN (CLUW)
15 UNION SQUARE
NEW YORK, NY 10003
Produces fact booklets especially for working women.

HEALTH CARE: WE GOTTA HAVE IT!
121 W. 27TH ST., #1202A
NEW YORK, NY 10001
TEL. (212) 366-6700
Has fact sheets and a flyer on how to organize a community town meeting, plus a short video on women and health care reform.

HUMAN RIGHTS ACTION FOR HEALTH CARE
2111 FLORIDA AVE. NW
WASHINGTON, DC 20004
TEL. (202) 347-8800
Lesbian and gay groups united in support of single-payer reform.

LONG TERM CARE CAMPAIGN
P.O. BOX 27394
WASHINGTON, DC 20038
TEL. (202) 393-2092
Coalition of national groups working to ensure progressively financed, comprehensive long-term-care legislation.

NATIONAL ASSOCIATION FOR PUBLIC HEALTH POLICY
208 MEADOWOOD DR.
SOUTH BURLINGTON, VT 05403
TEL. (802) 658-0136
Publishes *Journal of Public Health Policy* and maintains an informal network of progressive health-reform activists.

NATIONAL HEALTH LAW PROGRAM
2639 SOUTH LA CIENEGA BLVD.
LOS ANGELES, CA 90034
TEL. (310) 204-6010
Provides technical assistance and training to lawyers and advocates from all over the country focused on issues concerning access to health care for low-income people. Publishes a newsletter, *Health Advocate,* eight times each year. Publication list is available.

NURSES FOR NATIONAL HEALTH CARE
TEL. (708) 983-0886
Supports single-payer system. Provides speakers, slides, fact sheets, and updated information on legislation. Organized regionally. This Chicago region office can help you contact the chapter in your region.

PHYSICIANS FOR A NATIONAL HEALTH PROGRAM (PNHP)
332 S. MICHIGAN AVE., SUITE 500
CHICAGO, IL 60604
TEL. (312) 554-0382
Organized for a single-payer system, PNHP has chapters nationwide and provides speakers and slides on all aspects of health systems here and in other countries.

UNIVERSAL HEALTH CARE ACTION NETWORK
1800 EUCLID AVE., SUITE 318
CLEVELAND, OH 44115
TEL. (216) 566-8100/241-8422
Publishes *Action for Universal Health Care.* This national coalition works for single-payer reform of the U.S. system.

Books and Other Publications

Annas, George, and the American Civil Liberties Union. *The Basic ACLU Guide to Patient Rights.* 2nd ed. Carbondale, IL: Southern Illinois University Press, 1989.

Brundin, Jennifer. "How the U.S. Press Covers the Canadian Health Care System." *International Journal of Health Services,* Vol. 23, No. 2 (1993), pp. 275–77.

Burgess, Ann W., and Carol R. Hartman, eds. *Sexual Medicine,* Vol. 4: *Sexual Exploitation of Patients by Health Professionals.* New York: Praeger, 1986. Crucial information unavailable elsewhere.

Bursztajn, Harold, Robert M. Hann, and Archie Brodsky. *Medical Choices, Medical Chances: How Patients, Families and Physicians Can Cope with Uncertainty.* New York: Routledge, 1990. Important new approach to medical decision making.

Committee on an Aging Society. Institute of Medicine and National Research Council. *America's Aging: Health in an Older Society.* Washington, DC: National Academy Press, 1986.

"The Drug Manufacturing Industry: A Prescription for Profits." Staff Report of the Special Committee on Aging, U. S. Senate. Washington, DC:

U.S. Government Printing Office, September 1991, Serial No. 102-F.

Ehrenreich, Barbara, and Dierdre English. *For Her Own Good: 150 Years of the Experts' Advice to Women.* New York: Doubleday/Anchor, 1978. Classic analysis.

Gorman, John. Office of Rep. John Conyers. "Expanding Primary Care and Promoting Prevention." *Public Health Comments,* Vol. 6, No. 11/12 (November/December 1992), pp. 5–8.

Grumbach, Kevin, Thomas Bodenheimer, David U. Himmelstein, and Steffie Woolhandler. "Liberal Benefits, Conservative Spending: The Physicians for a National Health Program Proposal." *Journal of the American Medical Association,* Vol. 265, No. 19 (May 15, 1991), pp. 2549–54.

"Health Care Emergency." *Dollars & Sense,* Special Issue, May 1993. One Summer St., Somerville, MA 02143. $3.50 for a back copy.

Himmelstein, David U., and Steffie Woolhandler. "A National Health Program for the United States." *The New England Journal of Medicine,* Vol. 320, No. 2 (Jan. 12, 1989), pp. 102–8.

Inlander, Charles, and Ed Weiner. *Take This Book to the Hospital with You: A Consumer's Guide to Surviving Your Hospital Stay.* Emmaus, PA: Rodale Press, 1983.

Isaacs, Stephen L., and Ava C. Swartz. *The Consumer's Legal Guide to Today's Health Care: Your Medical Rights and How to Assert Them.* Boston: Houghton Mifflin, 1992. Several chapters of special interest to the elderly.

Lubitz, James D., and Gerald Riley. "Trends in Medicare Payments in the Last Year of Life." *The New England Journal of Medicine,* Vol. 328, No. 15 (Apr. 15, 1993), pp. 1092–96.

"Managed Competition: Reform or Retreat?" (Analysis, Critique, Alternatives) *Health/PAC Bulletin,* Special Report, Vol. 23, No. 1 (Spring 1993).

Mechanic, David. *From Advocacy to Allocation.* New York: Free Press, 1986. Examines the problems of increased medical expenditures in the United States and argues for the greater involvement of people in their own care and prevention, and other ways to prevent abuses. Contains a chapter on older people.

Minkler, Meredith, and Carroll L. Estes, eds. *Readings in the Political Economy of Aging.* Farmingdale, NY: Baywood Publishing, 1984.

Naierman, Naomi, et al. "Critical Condition: Midlife and Older Women in America's Health Care System." *Mother's Day Report,* Older Women's League, May 1992. Outstanding report, a must for every health-reform activist.

Norsigian, Judy. "Women and National Health Reform: A Progressive Feminist Agenda." *Journal of Women's Health,* Vol. 2, No. 1 (1993), pp. 91–94.

Public Citizen Health Research Group. *Medical Records: Getting Yours,* 1992, $10.00. See General Health resources under Organizations.

"Pushing Drugs to Doctors" and "Miracle Drugs or Media Drugs." Two-part series, *Consumer Reports,* Vol. 57, No. 2 (February 1992), pp. 87–94, and Vol. 57, No. 3 (March 1992), pp. 142–46.

Ratcliff, Kathryn J., ed. *Healing Technology: Feminist Perspectives.* Ann Arbor, MI: University of Michigan Press, 1989. Excellent framework for examining women's health issues.

Todd, Alexandra D. *Intimate Adversaries: Cultural Conflict Between Doctors and Women Patients.* Philadelphia: University of Pennsylvania Press, 1989. Useful insights into why women are so often dissatisfied with medical encounters.

"Unhealthy Money, Part III: The Health and Insurance Industries' Long-term Investment in Congress—Campaign Contributions Since 1989." Citizen Action, 1120 19th Street NW, #630, Washington, DC 20036. Tel. (202) 628-3030.

Wellstone, Paul, and Ellen Shaffer. "The American Health Security Act: A Single-Payer Proposal." *The New England Journal of Medicine,* Vol. 328, No. 20 (May 20, 1993), pp. 1489–93.

Women Without Health Insurance. Special Report, National Women's Law Center, April 1993. Available free from the center at 1616 P St. NW, Washington, DC 20036. Tel. (202) 328-5160.

NURSING HOMES

Organizations

AMERICAN ASSOCIATION OF HOMES FOR THE AGING
901 E ST. NW, SUITE 500
WASHINGTON, DC 20004-2837
TEL. (202) 783-2242 OR FAX (202) 783-2255

The national organization of nonprofit long-term care facilities offers numerous publications and other information. They support resident empowerment and have often sided with consumers on quality-care issues.

THE GRAY PANTHERS (see page 442) have over one hundred local chapters; many of these advocate on behalf of, or in conjunction with, nursing-home residents and their allies.

NATIONAL ASSOCIATION OF STATE UNITS ON AGING
1225 I ST. NW, SUITE 725
WASHINGTON, DC 20005
TEL. (202) 898-2578

Organization of all state offices or departments on aging. Has information about ombudsprograms, activities, and materials on long-term care.

NATIONAL CITIZENS' COALITION FOR NURSING HOME REFORM (NCCNHR)
1224 M ST. NW, SUITE 301
WASHINGTON, DC 20005-5183
TEL. (202) 393-2018 OR FAX (202) 393-4122

This nonprofit, consumer-based organization of over 250 groups, and 300 individual members is the best source of information, publications, and analyses from an advocacy point of view. NCCHNR's goal is to improve long-term health care and quality of life for residents. They coordinate many special projects and respond to proposed new or revised laws and regulations. *Quality Care Advocate,* their bimonthly newsletter, is available to nonmembers for $45 annually. Ask for a sample newsletter, their list of publications, and for referral to advocacy groups in your area.

State Consumer Organizations

COALITION OF INSTITUTIONALIZED AGED AND DISABLED
C/O BROOKDALE CENTER ON AGING
425 E. 25TH ST., ROOM 818
NEW YORK, NY 10010
TEL. (212) 481-4348

The New York State coalition of residents' councils provides assistance, training, and materials for organizing residents' councils. Coordinates advocacy activities on behalf of members.

L.I.F.E. (LIVING IS FOR THE ELDERLY)
27 MAPLE ST.
ARLINGTON, MA 02174
TEL. (617) 666-1000, EXT. 4733

The Massachusetts nursing home residents' organization. Organizes residents to advocate on their own behalf, individually and in groups, in their own facilities and communities as well as with policymakers. Meetings, conferences, and other events educate residents, families, and staff, and encourage resident autonomy.

MINNESOTA ALLIANCE FOR HEALTH CARE CONSUMERS
5609 LYNDALE AVE. S.
MINNEAPOLIS, MN 55419
TEL. (612) 866-4373

Advocacy group offers consumer-oriented materials and assistance. Recognizes outstanding achievements of resident and family councils and nursing assistants.

Books and Other Publications

Bausell, R. Barker, and Michael A. Rooney. *How to Evaluate and Select a Nursing Home.* Emmaus, PA: People's Medical Society, 1984.

Bove, Alexander, Jr. *Medicaid Planning Handbook.* Boston: Little, Brown, 1992.

Guide to Choosing a Nursing Home. Order from U.S. Dept. of Health and Human Services, Health Care Financing Administration, 6325 Security Blvd., Baltimore, MD 21207. Free 18-page guidebook includes information and checklists covering quality of life, legal rights of residents, the families' role, and financing issues. Ask for a list of their other publications; most are free to consumers. Their toll-free number, (800) 638-6833, provides a range of information on insurance and financing issues for elders.

Horner, Joyce. *That Time of Year: A Chronicle of Life in a Nursing Home.* Amherst, MA: The University of Massachusetts Press, 1982. Journal of a retired English professor's last years in a nursing home demonstrates her resilience of spirit as she struggles with the routines and inertia of nursing-home life.

Institute of Medicine, *Improving the Quality of Care in Nursing Homes.* Washington, DC: National Academy Press, 1987. Useful for citizens' groups striving for higher standards in nursing homes.

Kane, Rosalie, and Robert L. Kane. *A Will and a Way: What the US Can Learn from Canada About Caring for the Elderly.* New York: Columbia University Press, 1988.

Karr, Katherine. *Promises to Keep: The Family's Role in Nursing Home Care.* New York: Prometheus Books, 1991.

Kautzer, Kathleen. "Empowering Nursing Home Residents: A Case Study of the LIFE Organization." In Shulamit Reinharz and Graham Rowles, eds., *Qualitative Gerontology.* New York: Springer, 1987. An in-depth study of the Massachusetts nursing-home residents' organization.

Mendelson, Mary Adelaide. *Tender Loving Greed.* New York: Vintage, 1975. The original investigation into profit-taking excesses in the nursing-home industry. Written before the growth of consumer and resident advocacy groups in the mid- to late seventies, some of the problems described have since been addressed by new laws and regulations. Still very useful for anyone interested in reform.

Nursing Home Life: A Guide for Residents and Families. Publication No. 13063 and *Fact Sheet on Nursing Homes.* Write to AARP Fulfillment (see page 441).

Pieper, Hanns G. *The Nursing Home Primer: A Comprehensive Guide to Nursing Homes and Other Long-Term Care Options.* White Hall, VA: Betterway Publications, 1989.

Planning for Long-Term Health Care. An 86-page guidebook that includes information about financing long-term care and selecting a nursing home. Available free from Evensky and Brown, Attn: Deena Katz, 241 Sevilla Ave., Suite 902, Coral Gables, FL 33134-6622.

Quinn, Mary Jo. *Elder Abuse and Neglect.* New York: Springer, 1986.

Savishinsky, Joel. *The Ends of Time: Life and Work in a Nursing Home.* New York: Bergin & Garvey, 1991. Anthropological study examines interactions among nursing-home residents, staff, families, volunteers, and visiting pets. Well written and moving, it offers insight into the complex world of nursing homes and the individuality of those who are part of that world.

Audiovisual

Rose by Any Other Name, by Judith Keller, an appealingly iconoclastic film that explores the lifelong need for affection, privacy, and sexual expression in the context of relationships among nursing-home residents. Available from Pennsylvania State University, see page 447.

Agencies and Services

Many of the agencies and services that can help you with problems ranging from discrimination at admission to residents' rights violations are hard to find. Following is a list of potential sources of help and suggestions for finding them in your area.

Nursing-home ombudsprograms investigate complaints related to residents' rights or resident care. Look for the state agency with a name such as Aging, Elder Affairs, or Elder Services. Local ombudsprograms can be found through the state agency or through your area agency on aging, or legal services office.

Legal services. See National Health Law Program on page 485 and General Resources under Organizations.

Licensing agencies are generally responsible for promulgating and enforcing regulations, inspecting facilities, and investigating complaints, including abuse. They are usually located in agencies for health, public health, health and human services, etc.

Area agencies on aging. See page •••

Consumer protection may be covered through your state's attorney general's office and/or a department or office of consumer affairs.

Medicaid is usually administered through a state welfare, public assistance, or social-services agency. A Medicaid fraud unit often is part of the Medicaid division, and suspicions of fraud and discrimination should be reported to them.

State nursing-home associations, or provider groups, exist in most states and can provide varied information. They are usually affiliates of the National Association of State Units of Aging and the American Association of Homes for the Aging (see above under Organizations).

JOINT AND MUSCLE PAIN, ARTHRITIS AND RHEUMATIC DISORDERS

Organizations

ARTHRITIS FOUNDATION
1314 SPRING ST. NW
ATLANTA, GA 30309
TEL. (800) 283-7800 OR (404) 872-7100

Publishes many booklets including *Arthritis, The Basic Facts, Living and Loving with Arthritis, The Self-Help Manual for Patients with Arthritis,* and a bimonthly magazine, *Arthritis Today. The Self-Help Manual* has useful material on wrist problems. Offers aquatic-exercise programs in cooperation with the YMCA. Has prescription-discount service for members. Check your phone book for local chapters, which may have additional pamphlets.

ARTHRITIS INFORMATION CLEARINGHOUSE
NAMSC, BOX AMS
9000 ROCKVILLE PIKE
BETHESDA, MD 20892
TEL. (301) 495-4484

Offers materials and bibliographies. Funded by the National Institute of Arthritis, Musculoskeletal, and Skin Disease (see below).

FIBROMYALGIA NETWORK
5700 STOCKDALE HWY, SUITE 100
BAKERSFIELD, CA 93309
TEL. (805) 631-1950

Publishes *Fibromyalgia Network,* a quarterly newsletter, and provides health-care and support-group listings by state.

NATIONAL INSTITUTE OF ARTHRITIS, MUSCULOSKELETAL, AND SKIN DISEASE (NIAMS)
INFORMATION OFFICER
BUILDING 31, ROOM 4C05
9000 ROCKVILLE PIKE
BETHESDA, MD 20892
TEL. (301) 496-8188

Write them for their publications and for the address of the federally funded research and treatment center for arthritis nearest you.

Books and Other Publications

American Medical Association. *Guide to Back Care.* Rev. ed. New York: Random House, 1984.

Berson, Dvera, with Sander Roy. *Pain-Free Arthritis.* New York: Simon & Schuster, 1978. At age sixty-five, Berson demonstrated the value of persistent exercise in water.

Carr, Rachel. *Arthritis: Relief Beyond Drugs.* New York: Harper & Row, 1981. Contains yoga techniques.

Fernandez-Madrid, Felix. *Treating Arthritis: Medicine, Myth, and Magic.* New York: Plenum Press, 1989.

Fries, James F. *A Comprehensive Guide to Arthritis.* 3rd ed. Reading, MA: Addison-Wesley, 1990. Includes excellent brief descriptions of arthritis in nontechnical language.

Gordon, Neil F. *Arthritis: Your Complete Exercise Guide.* Dallas, TX: Human Kinetics Publishers, 1993. Shows the small steps that make a big difference such as walking ten minutes three times a week. Graphic detail on stretching.

Kantrowitz, Fred G. *Taking Control of Arthritis.* New York: HarperCollins, 1990. A user-friendly book in question-and-answer format.

Klein, Arthur C., and Dava Sobel. *Backache Relief.* New York: Random House/Times Books, 1985. Read this one first if you have back pain. Lists twenty-five often-mentioned ways to free yourself from back pain.

Krewer, Semyon, with Ann Edgar. *The Arthritis Exercise Book.* New York: Simon & Schuster/Cornerstone Library, 1981. Offers preventive exercises for everyone and corrective exercises for those with arthritis.

Kushner, Irving, et al., eds. *Understanding Arthritis.* Published for the Arthritis Foundation by Consumers Union, Mount Vernon, NY 1984. Especially good section on fibrositis.

Lettvin, Maggie. *Maggie's Back Book.* Boston: Houghton Mifflin, 1987. Useful when your back hurts. The author tells you how the exercise will ultimately be done, and then takes you through the steps to get there.

Lorig, Kate, and James F. Fries, *The Arthritis Helpbook.* Reading, MA: Addison-Wesley, 1992. Developed with participants of arthritis self-management classes, this book explains what the doctor may not have explained.

Root, Leon, and Thomas Kiernan. *Oh, My Aching Back.* New York: New American Library, 1985. Recommended by people who regularly do the exercises.

White, Augustus A., III. *Your Aching Back. A Doctor's Guide to Relief.* New York: Bantam, 1983.

Temporomandibular Joints

Organizations

Jaw Joints & Allied Musculo-Skeletal Disorders Foundation, Inc. (JJAMD)
Forsyth Research Institute
140 Fenway
Boston, MA 02115
Tel. (617) 262-5200, ext. 360, or (617) 266-2550

Membership, pamphlets, support groups, lectures, and seminars. Starting state chapters. *Jaw Joints* booklet available for $5.

Books

American Dental Association. *Temporomandibular Disorders.* 211 E. Chicago Ave., Chicago, IL 60611. Single copy available free. Tel. (312) 440-2500.

Lupus

Organizations

American Lupus Society
3914 Del Amo Blvd.
Torrance, CA 90503
Tel. (800) 331-1802 or (310) 542-8891

Literature, media awareness, and fund-raising for research.

Lupus Foundation of America
4 Research Place, Suite 180
Rockland, MD 20850-3226
Tel. (800) 558-0121 or (301) 670-9292

A membership organization. Chapters offer medical referrals, educational materials, and counseling.

Books

Aladjem, Henrietta. *Understanding Lupus.* Rev. ed. New York: Scribner, 1985.

Osteoporosis and Fracture Prevention

Organizations

National Osteoporosis Foundation
1150 17th St. NW, Suite 500
Washington, DC 20036-4603

Publishes pamphlets and a quarterly newsletter, *The Osteoporosis Report,* $10 per year. Includes information on injury prevention, exercise, nutrition, and rehabilitation as well as on bone scanning and medical treatment.

Books and Other Publications

Publications such as *A Friend Indeed: For Women in the Prime of Life,* Vol. 7, No. 2 (May 1991) (see page 466), and *HealthFacts,* Vol. 18, No. 164 (January 1993) (see page 482), are excellent sources of current information about osteoporosis.

Greenwood, Sadja. *Menopause, Naturally.* San Francisco: Volcano Press, 1992. A simply written and well-balanced book by a woman physician. Has chapters on osteoporosis, exercise, nutrition, and estrogen-replacement therapy.

Goulart, Frances S. *Nutritional Self Defense.* New York: Dodd Mead, 1984. A common-sense, helpful approach to nutrition.

Kamen, Betty, and Si Kamen. *Osteoporosis: What It Is, How to Prevent It, How to Stop It.* New York: Pinnacle Books, 1984. This is an extremely valuable aid to understanding the connection between nutrition and osteoporosis. Easy to read.

Notelovitz, Morris, Marsha Ware, and Diane Tonnessen. *Stand Tall: The Informed Woman's Guide to Preventing Osteoporosis.* 2nd ed., 1994. Triad Publishing, P.O. Drawer 13355, Gainesville, FL 32604. An easy-to-understand explanation of the complex problem of osteoporosis.

"Osteoporosis. Part One: Screening Tests plus Prescription Drugs Blamed for Falls and Fractures." *Health Letter,* Vol. 3, No. 5 (May 1987), pp. 1–4; and "Part Two: Prevention and Treatment." *Health Letter,* Vol. 3, No. 6 (June 1987), pp. 1–6. Excellent articles. The June issue contains information on the disintegration and dissolution times of various commercial calcium supplements. Public Citizen Health Research Group (see page 483).

"Osteoporosis." Part 3 in Sandra Coney, *The Menopause Industry: A Guide to Medicine's 'Discovery' of the Mid-Life Woman.* Alameda, CA: Hunter House, 1994, in press. Excellent section in a highly recommended book.

Porcino, Jane. *Growing Older, Getting Better: A Handbook for Women in the Second Half of Life.* New York: Crossroad Continuum, 1991. Chapter on osteoporosis takes a strong stand against both estrogen and fluoride therapy.

Seaman, Barbara, and Gideon Seaman. *Women and the Crisis in Sex Hormones.* New York: Bantam, 1977. Has a chapter on osteoporosis containing an important history of the estrogen therapy debates.

DENTAL HEALTH

Organizations

AMERICAN DENTAL ASSOCIATION
DEPARTMENT OF PUBLIC INFORMATION AND EDUCATION
211 E. CHICAGO AVE.
CHICAGO, IL 60611
TEL. (312) 440-2593

Many pamphlets available including *Periodontal Disease* and *Tips for Older Adults.* Send business-size self-addressed stamped envelope.

INTERNATIONAL DENTAL HEALTH FOUNDATION, INC.
11484 WASHINGTON PLAZA WEST
RESTON, VA 22090
TEL. (703) 471-8349

Send $3.00 and a business size self-addressed stamped envelope for information about the Keyes technique and referral to a dentist in your area trained in the technique.

NATIONAL INSTITUTE OF DENTAL RESEARCH
P.O. BOX 547-93
WASHINGTON, DC 20032
TEL. (301) 594-7654

Send for free pamphlets: No. 91-3174, *Dry Mouth (Xerostomia),* and No. 87-2946, *Periodontal Disease and Diabetes: A Guide for Patients.* (Also available in Spanish.)

Books and Other Publications

American Academy of Periodontology. 737 N. Michigan Ave., Suite 800, Chicago, IL 60611. Sample packet of information on periodontal disease available.

American Dental Hygienists' Association. *A Beautiful Smile Is Ageless.* 444 N. Michigan Ave., Suite 3400, Chicago, IL 60611.

Denholtz, Melvin, and Elaine Denholtz. *How to Save Your Teeth and Your Money (A Consumers' Guide to Better, Less Costly Dental Care).* New York: Van Nostrand Reinhold, 1980.

Finkelman, Ellen S., and Sharon Compton. "The Keyes Method of Alternative Periodontal Therapy: A Critical Review." *Dental Hygiene,* July 1985, pp. 302–5.

Mellberg, James R., et al. *Fluoride in Preventive Dentistry: Theory and Clinical Applications.* Chicago: Quintessence Publishing, 1983. Section on remineralization, pp. 51–9.

Wilson, J. Randy. *Non-Chew Cookbook.* See Eating Well resources, under Cookbooks (page 457) if you must eat soft foods.

URINARY INCONTINENCE

Organizations

CONTINENCE RESTORED, INC.
785 PARK AVE.
NEW YORK, NY 10021

Forming support groups with medically trained leaders. For information, send stamped self-addressed business-size envelope.

HELP FOR INCONTINENT PEOPLE (HIP)
P.O. BOX 544
UNION, SC 29379
TEL. (800) BLADDER OR (803) 579-7900

An international clearinghouse of information among lay people, medical professionals, industry, and social workers on services, treatments, and products available for people with incontinence. Publishes *The HIP Report,* a quarterly newsletter (annual subscription $7.00). A sample copy is available for $1.00 plus a stamped self-addressed business-size envelope. Also publishes *Resource Guide of Continent Aids and Services* for $10.00.

INTERSTITIAL CYSTITIS ASSOCIATION
P.O. BOX 1553
MADISON SQUARE STATION
NEW YORK, NY 10159
TEL. (212) 979-6057

Free brochure on how to get diagnosis and treatment. Has some local support groups. Quarterly newsletter and other materials available for donation or sale.

THE SIMON FOUNDATION
P.O. BOX 815
WILMETTE, IL 60091
TEL. (800) 23-SIMON

For a sample copy of *The Informer,* an informative and supportive quarterly newsletter, send a stamped self-addressed business-size envelope. Also publishes a list of urinary incontinence treatment centers and helpful letters from readers.

Books and Other Publications

Agency for Health Care Policy and Research (see page 482). Call or write for free copies of these guidelines for yourself and to give to your physicians: *Urinary Incontinence in Adults: Clinical Practice Guideline,* AHCPR Pub. No. 92-0038, March 1992; *Urinary Incontinence in Adults: A Patient's Guide,* AHCPR Pub. No. 92-0040, available in English and Spanish; *Urinary Incontinence in Adults: Quick Reference Guide for Clinicians,* AHCPR Pub. No. 92-0041.

Burgio, Kathleen, et al. *Staying Dry: A Practical Guide to Bladder Control.* Baltimore: Johns Hopkins University Press, 1989. A practical book with a simple five-step program for more effective management of urinary incontinence. Order from (800) 537-JHUP.

Chalker, Rebecca, and Kristene E. Whitmore. *Overcoming Bladder Disorders: Compassionate, Authoritative Medical and Self-help Solutions for Incontinence, Cystitis, Interstitial Cystitis, Prostate Problems, Bladder Cancer.* New York: HarperCollins, 1991. Contains excellent self-help and medical material for women and men.

Fugh-Berman, Adriane. "Standard Bladder Infection Treatment May Bring On Interstitial Cystitis." *The Network News,* May/June 1985, pp. 4–5.

Gartley, Cheryle B., ed. *Managing Incontinence.* Ottawa, IL: Jameson Books, 1985. A pioneering book by the founder of The Simon Foundation offers experiences, advice, practical help, and encouragement for all those who live with or manage incontinence in themselves or others. Available from the foundation, see left-hand column, this page.

Journal of the American Geriatrics Society, Vol. 38, No. 3 (March 1990). Issue devoted to papers from the National Institutes of Health Consensus Development Conference on Urinary Incontinence, Bethesda, MD, October 3–5, 1988.

Kilmartin, Angela. *Cystitis: The Complete Self-Help Guide.* New York: Warner, 1980.

Rose, Molly A., et al. "Behavioral Management of Urinary Incontinence in Homebound Older Adults." *Home HealthCare Nurse,* Vol. 8, No. 5 (1990), pp. 10–15.

Products

For products to aid bladder control, look in drug stores, medical-supply stores, in novelty mail-order catalogs, and in catalogs such as Sears, Roebuck and Company's *Home Health Care Products.* Watch the ads for new products.

A small "urinary director" was developed for the American Women's North Pole Expedition through which a woman can urinate without squatting or undressing. Several designs with or without disposal bags are available from novelty mail-order catalogs, camping equipment stores, or call Campmor (800) 526-4784.

HYSTERECTOMY AND OOPHORECTOMY

Organizations

HERS (HYSTERECTOMY EDUCATIONAL RESOURCES AND SERVICES)
422 BRYN MAWR AVE.
BALA CYNWYD, PA 19004
TEL. (215) 667-7757

Provides information and telephone counseling for women who have had hysterectomies and for those to whom hysterectomy has been recommended. Sponsors conferences in other cities and has a physician referral list. Quarterly newsletter, $20.00 per year. Telephone counseling by appointment, 9–5 EST, weekdays.

Books and Other Publications

Cutler, Winnifred Berg. *Hysterectomy: Before & After.* New York: Harper & Row, 1988. Describes vital role of the uterus and ovaries and contains many suggestions for promoting health after a hysterectomy. Lists almost one thousand references.

Goldfarb, Herbert A., with Judith Grief. *The No Hysterectomy Option.* New York: John Wiley, 1990. Read as much as you can about alternatives to hysterectomies. Author is a proponent of laser ablation and dismisses posthysterectomy depression.

Lauersen, Nils, and Eileen Stulcane. *Listen to Your Body: A Gynecologist Answers Women's Most Intimate Questions.* New York: Berkley, 1983.

Malesky, Gale, and Charles B. Inlander. *Take This Book to the Gynecologist with You.* Reading, MA: Addison-Wesley, 1991. A critical look at hysterectomies, ovary removal, and hormone therapy. Helps women take charge of their medical care, has key to medical terms, and explains how to make changes on a consent form.

Mendelsohn, Robert. *Malpractice—How Doctors Manipulate Women.* Chicago: Contemporary Books, 1981. In the chapter "What Do You Need Your Uterus for Anyway?" The author blasts medicine's condescending attitude toward women.

Morgan, Susanne. *Coping with a Hysterectomy.* New York: Dial, 1982. A highly recommended pioneer work that gives good suggestions for avoiding unnecessary surgery. Author is a sociologist who herself had a hysterectomy.

Payer, Lynn. *How to Avoid a Hysterectomy: An Indispensable Guide to Exploring All Your Options Before You Consent to a Hysterectomy.* New York: Pantheon, 1987. Highly recommended. The author struggled to get a myomectomy for fibroids.

Stokes, Naomi Miller. *The Castrated Woman: What Your Doctor Won't Tell You About Hysterectomy.* New York: Franklin Watts, 1986.

Strausz, Ivan K. *You Don't Need a Hysterectomy: New and Effective Ways of Avoiding Major Surgery.* Reading, MA: Addison-Wesley, 1993. Excellent but less questioning about hormones than about surgery and still relates posthysterectomy sexual and psychological problems to prior conditions.

Wolfe, Sidney M., Public Citizen Health Research Group, with Rhoda Donkin Jones. *Women's Health Alert.* Reading, MA: Addison-Wesley, 1991. Good concise chapter on hysterectomy.

Audiovisual

Sudden Changes. The Cinema Guild, 1697 Broadway, New York, NY 10019. Tel. (212) 246-5522. Rental or purchase. Emphasis in myomectomy discussion is on younger women.

Hypertension, Heart Disease, and Stroke

Organizations

American Heart Association
National Center
7320 Greenville Ave.
Dallas, TX 75231
Tel. (800) 242-8721 or (214) 373-6300
Publications available from local chapters include *An Older Person's Guide to Cardiovascular Health, Sex and Heart Disease* (a short, nonsexist treatment of a sometimes sensitive topic), *How Stroke Affects Behavior* (a short description of possible behavior traits of a stroke victim; helpful to family and patient).

National Rehabilitation Information Center
Tel. (800) 346-2742
Database service that provides information about programs to cope with disabilities, including recovering from strokes.

The Stroke Connection
7272 Greenville Ave.
Dallas, TX 75231
Tel. (800) 553-6321
Complimentary membership for stroke survivors who cannot afford the $8 annual fee. Provides bimonthly newsletter, publications, telephone consultation, referral to local support groups and care.

Books and Other Publications

Brody, Jane. "Personal Health: Early Action is Crucial in Combating Heart Failure." *The New York Times,* Sept. 29, 1993, p. C12.

Cousins, Norman. *The Healing Heart: Antidotes to Panic and Helplessness.* New York: Norton, 1983. A personal account combining information about the technology of coronary care with the power of positive thinking.

Ornish, Dean. *Dr. Dean Ornish's Program for Reversing Heart Disease.* New York: Ballantine, 1992. How we can prevent heart disease through exercise, diet, and stress management.

Weisfeldt, Myron. *The Aging Heart.* New York: Raven Press, 1980.

Cancer

For alternative therapies, see John M. Fink, *Third Opinion: An International Directory to Alternative Therapy Centers for the Treatment and Prevention of Cancers.* Garden City Park, NY: Avery Publishing Group, 1992. See also the Boston Women's Health Book Collective, *The New Our Bodies, Ourselves.* New York: Simon & Schuster, 1992, pp. 614–16.

Organizations

American Cancer Society (ACS)
1599 Clifton Road NE
Atlanta, GA 30329
Tel. (404) 320-3333
See the telephone directory for your local and state chapters. Chapters have lists of local community resources, home-care items for loan, transportation services, and public education programs including literature, films, and speakers. ACS offers two short-term programs of one-to-one visits by a person with the same kind of cancer: *Reach to Recovery* for women with breast cancer, and *CanSurmount* for people with any other kind of cancer. Also has two group rehabilitation and support programs: one for people who have had a laryngectomy (removal of the voice box) and the second for people with ostomies, in cooperation with the United Ostomy Association. Offers a support group for people with cancer: *I Can Cope.*

American Institute for Cancer Research
1759 R St. NW
Washington, DC 20009
Tel. (202) 328-7744
Booklets on fiber, fat, and dietary guidelines to lower cancer risk are available free. Publication list available.

Cancer Information Service (CIS)
Tel. (800) 4-CANCER
CIS is a program of the National Cancer Institute (NCI), which provides information, referral, and free publications about cancer. Also operates PDQ (Physician Data Query), a computerized information base developed by NCI that provides information on standard and experimental treatments for more than eighty types of cancer.

DES Action USA
1615 Broadway, Suite 510
Oakland, CA 94612.
Also has an affiliate, DES Cancer Network, with information about clear-cell cancer and providing education and patient-to-patient support.

Encore support and exercise groups for women who have had mastectomies. Contact your local YWCA.

Exceptional Cancer Patients (see page 482).

Greenpeace
1017 W. Jackson Blvd.
Chicago, IL 60607
An environmental organization concerned about organochlorines, among other environmental pollutants. Publishers of *Breast Cancer and the Environment—The Chlorine Connection.*

Make Today Count
P.O. Box 222
Osage Beach, MO 65065
Tel. (314) 346-6644
Sponsors support groups in many communities for people with cancer.

National Breast Cancer Coalition
P.O. Box 66373
Washington, DC 20035
Tel. (800) 935-0434 or (202) 296-7477
A coalition of more than 160 groups. Contact them to learn more about their advocacy efforts and about groups in your area.

National Coalition for Cancer Survivorship
1010 Wayne Ave., 5th Floor
Silver Spring, MD 20910
Tel. (301) 650-8868
A coalition of individual members, cancer-support organizations, and treatment centers. Clearinghouse for information on cancer survivorship concerns, and advocate on behalf of cancer survivors on state and national level.

National Coalition of Feminist and Lesbian Cancer Projects
P.O. Box 90437
Washington, DC 20090
Tel. (202) 332-5536
A coalition of grass-roots women's cancer groups that supports advocacy, networking, and education around cancer issues.

National Lymphedema Network
Tel. (800) 541-3259
Information and resource center for lymphedema and other venous disorders. Leave request for literature or specific question on tape and your call will be returned.

Ovarian Cancer Prevention and Early Detection Foundation
P.O. Box 447
Paauilo, HI 96776-0447
Write for information and send $25 for newsletter subscription.

United Ostomy Association, Inc.
36 Executive Park, Suite 120
Irvine, CA 92714
Tel. (714) 660-8624
Quarterly newsletter, $25.00 per year. Over six hundred chapters in North America. Local dues average $15 per year, which entitle members to the national quarterly, local bulletin, other literature, and meeting notices.

Y-ME
18220 Harwood Ave.
Homewood, IL 60430
Tel. (800) 221-2141 hot line Monday–Friday, 10 a.m. to 6 p.m. EST or
(708) 799-8228 24-hour answering service
National organization that provides counseling, support, and self-help meetings for people with breast cancer, their families, and friends.

Books and Other Publications

American Academy of Dermatology. *Melanoma/Skin Cancer: You Can Recognize the Signs.* Includes information on prevention. Send a stamped self-addressed envelope to the Academy at P.O. Box 681069, Schaumburg, IL 60168-1069.

American Cancer Society. *Cancer Facts and Figures.* Published annually. Available from your local chapter or the National Office (see page 494).

Bailer, John C., III, and Elaine M. Smith. "Progress Against Cancer?" *The New England Journal of Medicine*, Vol. 314, No. 19 (May 8, 1986), pp. 1226–32. An important article that presents data showing we are losing the war against cancer and arguing for more emphasis on research for prevention than for treatment.

Boyle, Robert H. *Malignant Neglect: Known or Suspected Cancer-Causing Agents in Our Environment and How by Controlling Them We Can Control the Spread of Cancer Itself.* New York: Random House, 1980.

Brady, Judith, ed. *One in Three Women Confront the Cancer Epidemic.* Pittsburgh: Cleis Press, 1991.

Dreher, Henry. *Your Defense Against Cancer: The Complete Guide to Cancer Prevention.* New York: Harper & Row, 1989.

Epstein, Samuel. *The Politics of Cancer.* New York: Anchor/Doubleday, 1979.

Fiore, Neil. *The Road Back to Health: Coping with the Emotional Aspects of Cancer.* Berkeley, CA: Celestial Arts, 1991.

Gorbach, Sherwood L., et al. *The Doctors' Anti–Breast Cancer Diet.* New York: Dial, 1983. Ra-tionale and recipes for a low-fat diet.

Greenwald, Howard P. *Who Survives Cancer?* San Francisco: University of California Press, 1992.

Henderson, I. Craig, and Jay R. Harris. "Breast Cancer: Current Trends in Diagnosis and Treatment." In R. G. Petersdorf, et al., eds. *Harrison's Principles of Internal Medicine. Update VII.* New York: McGraw-Hill, 1986, pp. 181–208.

Hubbard, Ruth, and Elijah Wald. *Exploding the Gene Myth.* See page 483.

Kelly, Patricia T. *Understanding Breast Cancer Risk.* Philadelphia: Temple University Press, 1991. An important book for understanding what risk does and does not mean.

Kemeny, Margaret M. *Breast Cancer and Ovarian Cancer: Beating the Odds.* Reading, MA: Addison-Wesley, 1992.

LeShan, Lawrence. *Cancer as a Turning Point: A Handbook for People with Cancer, Their Families, and Health Professionals.* New York: Dutton, 1989.

Lettvin, Maggie. *Maggie's Woman's Book.* Boston: Houghton Mifflin, 1980. Contains section on exercises for lymphedema of the arms.

Lorde, Audre. *Cancer Journals.* Minneapolis, MN: Spinsters Ink, 1980. And *A Burst of Light.* Ithaca, NY: Firebrand Books, 1988. A black lesbian feminist poet's personal experiences with breast cancer and mastectomy.

Love, Susan M., with Karen Lindsey. *Dr. Susan Love's Breast Book.* Reading, MA: Addison-Wesley, 1990. Excellent book though not cautious enough on the subject of breast implants.

Morra, Marion, and Eve Potts. *Choices: Realistic Alternatives in Cancer Treatment.* Rev. ed. New York: Avon, 1987. Thorough and clearly written overview of conventional medical procedures involved in diagnosis and treatment of cancer.

Moss, Ralph W. *The Cancer Industry: Unraveling the Politics.* New York: Paragon House, 1989.

———. *Cancer Therapy: The Independent Consumer's Guide to Non-Toxic Treatment and Prevention.* New York: Equinox Press, 1992.

Mullan, Fitzhugh, Barbara Hoffman, and the Editors of Consumer Reports Books, eds. *An Almanac of Practical Resources for Cancer Survivors: Charting the Journey.* Mt. Vernon, NY: Consumers Union, 1990.

Mullen, Barbara D., and Kerry A. McGinn. *The Ostomy Book.* Palo Alto, CA: Bull Publishing Co., 1980. A vivid personal experience that includes much practical information.

National Research Council. *Diet, Nutrition and Cancer.* Washington, DC: National Academy Press, 1982.

"The Politics of Breast Cancer." *Ms.*, Vol. 3, No. 6 (May/June 1993), pp. 38–60. Excellent special insert covering all the current controversies. Includes additional resources and bibliography.

Rinzler, Carol Ann. *Estrogen and Breast Cancer: A Warning to Women.* New York: Macmillan, 1993.

Sarton, May. *A Reckoning.* New York: Norton, 1978. And *Recovering,* New York: Norton, 1980. A superb writer's personal accounts of coping with cancer.

Siegel, Bernie. *Love, Medicine, and Miracles.* (See page 484.)

Simonton, Carl, et al. *Getting Well Again: A Step-by-Step Self-Help Guide to Overcoming Cancer for Patients and Their Families.* New York: Bantam, 1978. A discussion of methods by which the mind can influence the body.

Stocker, Midge. *Cancer as a Woman's Issue.* Chicago: Third Side Press, 1991.

Stocker, Midge, ed. *Confronting Cancer, Creating Change.* Chicago: Third Side Press, 1993. Second volume in a series. Essays by women confronting myths about cancer, releasing fear, and taking power.

Temoshok, Lydia, and Henry Draker. *The Type C Connection.* New York: Random House, 1992. Deals with the behavioral links to cancer without blaming anyone for becoming ill. Describes ways to strengthen one's resistance to cancer.

United Ostomy Association. *Sex and the Female Ostomate,* 1982. (See page 495.)

DIABETES

Organizations

AMERICAN ASSOCIATION OF DIABETES EDUCATORS
444 N. MICHIGAN AVE., SUITE 1240
CHICAGO, IL 60611
TEL. (312) 644-AADE

AADE maintains a membership list of health professionals who are active in diabetes care. Contact them if you need assistance in locating a diabetes educator in your area.

AMERICAN DIABETES ASSOCIATION (ADA)
NATIONAL SERVICE CENTER
1660 DUKE ST.
ALEXANDRIA, VA 22314
TEL. (800) 232-3472

ADA offers information at all levels from self-care to research and practice. For membership and a list of publications, contact your local ADA affiliate or the national service center. You will receive *Diabetes Forecast,* a monthly magazine with articles on topics such as cookery, insurance, pregnancy, menopause, and aging. Publications include *Type II Diabetes: Your Healthy Living Guide,* 1992; *ADA Guide to Exercise,* 1993; and *Right From the Start,* 1994.

INTERNATIONAL DIABETES CENTER (IDC)
5000 WEST 39TH ST.
MINNEAPOLIS, MN 55416
TEL. (612) 927-3393

IDC offers a wide range of material for self-care, including *Fast Food Facts: Nutritive Values for Fast Food Restaurants, Gestational Diabetes, A Guide to Healthy Eating,* and a free quarterly, *Living Well with Diabetes.*

INTERNATIONAL DIABETIC ATHLETES ASSOCIATION
P.O. BOX 10010
PHOENIX, AZ 85064
TEL. (602) 230-8155

This organization promotes athletics for all persons with diabetes. Its annual meetings provide opportunities for competition, training, and shared enthusiasm at international sites.

JOSLIN DIABETES CENTER
ONE JOSLIN PLACE
BOSTON, MA 02215
TEL. (617) 732-2695

Joslin is the oldest diabetes center in the nation. It offers outpatient education services and publications, including the *Self-Manager Series* (short booklets on subjects such as foot care) and *Guide for Women with Diabetes Who Are Pregnant or Plan to Be.*

Books and Other Publications

American Diabetes Association. *Month of Meals.* Four volumes, 1989–1993. Each meal planner offers twenty-eight days' worth of meals that may be mixed and matched to your taste. Includes recipes, calories, and exchanges.

American Diabetes Association. *1993 Buyer's Guide to Diabetes Products.* A guide for comparing features from different manufacturers for test strips, blood glucose monitors, insulin, syringes, jet injectors, insulin pumps, and other products.

Curtis, Judy. *Living with Diabetic Complications: A Survival Guide for Patients by a Patient.* Shippensburg, PA: Companion Press, 1993.

Joslin Diabetes Center. *Diabetes Treated Without Insulin: A Short Guide, 1988* and *Diabetes Treated With Insulin: A Short Guide, 1989.* (See above.)

Jovanovic, Lois, June Bierman, and Barbara Toohey. *The Diabetic Woman.* Los Angeles: J. P. Tarcher, 1987.

Krall, Leo, ed. *Joslin's Diabetes Manual.* Philadelphia: Lea Febiger, 1985.

Sims, Dorothea F., and Ethan A. H. Sims. *The Other Diabetes.* Rev. ed. Alexandria, VA: American Diabetes Association, 1987. A paperback on Type II diabetes describing causes, treatment, and psychosocial aspects of self-care.

Valentine, Virginia, June Biermann, and Barbara Toohey. *Diabetes: Type II and You and What to Do.* Los Angeles: Lowell House, 1993. Contains personal and professional experiences with easy-to-understand explanations.

Warshaw, Hope. *The Restaurant Companion: A Guide to Healthier Eating Out.* Chicago: Surrey Books Inc., 1990. How to savor restaurant meals while counting calories, fat, cholesterol, and sodium. Includes sample menus, ordering models, and diabetic exchanges.

Gallstones and Gallbladder Disease

Organizations

National Digestive Diseases Information Clearinghouse
P.O. Box NDDIC
9000 Rockville Pike
Bethesda, MD 20892
Tel. (301) 468-6344
Part of the National Institutes of Health. Provides fact sheets, resource lists, directories of lay and professional groups, and an annotated listing of educational materials on a variety of subjects related to gallbladder function, digestion, and related subjects. Free packet of materials available, including a brochure called *Gallbladder.*

Books and Other Publications

"Gallstones and Laparoscopic Cholecystectomy." *NIH Consensus Statement,* Vol. 10, No. 3 (Sept. 14–16, 1992). Available from the Office of Medical Applications of Research, NIH, Federal Building, Room 816, Bethesda, MD 20892.

Vision, Hearing, and Other Sensory Loss Associated with Aging

Vision

Organizations

American Foundation for the Blind
15 W. 16th St.
New York, NY 10011
Tel. (212) 620-2000
National private organization with five regional offices. Provides information and services. Catalog of special products.

Commission for the Blind. In each state.

National Association for Visually Handicapped
22 W. 21st St., 6th Floor
New York, NY 10010
Tel. (212) 889-3141
Western states, Alaska, and Hawaii:
3201 Balboa St.
San Francisco, CA 94121
Tel. (415) 221-8753
Serves the partially sighted (not totally blind), their families, and professionals with counsel, information, and referral. Offers large-print loan library free of charge through the mail, literature, and adult discussion groups in New York City and San Francisco. Dues $40.00 per year.

National Eye Care Project
P.O. Box 429098
San Francisco, CA 94142-9098
Tel. (800) 222-EYES
Sponsored by The Foundation of the American Academy of Ophthalmology and state societies, the project provides medical and surgical eye care for disadvantaged elders. Callers who meet eligibility requirements are referred to volunteer eye doctors in the community.

National Library Services for the Blind and Physically Handicapped
Library of Congress
Washington, DC 20542

Publishes *The Directory of Library Resources for the Blind and Physically Handicapped.* Anyone who is unable to read or use standard printed materials as a result of a temporary or permanent visual or other limitation may receive services, such as talking books, magnifiers, Braille materials, Kurzweil reading machines, large print and Braille typewriters, etc. Check first to see what is available at your library. For more information, call (800) 424-8567. When you apply, bring a brief written description of your limitation from a professional, such as a physician, nurse, or optometrist. Ask your librarian to help you.

Vision Foundation, Inc.
818 Mt. Auburn St.
Watertown, MA 02172
Tel. (617) 926-4232 or
(800) 852-3029, Massachusetts only

Provides information and support for people with low vision, newly blind people, and those with progressive eye conditions. $20 membership ($10 for seniors) includes newsletter. Support groups for mixed ages and for elders; telephone buddies for the homebound. Produces *The Vision Resource List* in large print and on cassette.

Books and Other Publications

Caffery, Barbara. "The Problem of Dry Eyes." *A Friend Indeed,* Vol. 10, No. 9 (February 1994), pp. 1–4. (See page 466.)

Clay, Rebecca A. *Resource List for the Blind & Visually Impaired.* Washington, DC: AARP Disability Initiative, 1992. See pages 441–42. Ask also for fact sheet, "Facts About Vision Loss."

Dickman, Irving. *Making Life More Livable: Simple Adaptations for the Homes of Blind and Visually Impaired Older People.* New York: American Foundation for the Blind, 1983. Large print. $16.95.

Independent Living Aids, 27 East Mall, Plainview, NY 11803. Tel. (516) 752-8080. Ask for catalog of low vision products available by mail order.

Living with Low Vision. Resources for Rehabilitation, 33 Bedford St., Suite 19A, Lexington, MA 02173. Large print guide. $35.

Rosenbloom, Alfred, Jr., and Meredith W. Morgan, eds. *Vision and Aging: General and Clinical Perspectives.* New York: Professional Press/Fairchild Publications, 1986.

Schaeffer, Susan Fromberg. *Mainland.* New York: Linden Press/Simon & Schuster, 1985. A novel about a woman struggling with vision loss along with midlife issues.

Smith, Margaret M. *If Blindness Strikes: Don't Strike Out—A Lively Look at Living with a Visual Impairment.* 1984. Charles C. Thomas, Publisher, 2600 S. First St., Springfield, IL 62794–9265. $44. Concentrates on the common problems that confront a person who is losing his or her sight. Offers practical solutions and shows how the reader can take control of his or her own life. Includes a chapter for family members and a resource list. Available on tape from Readings for the Blind, Inc., 29451 Greenfield, Suite 116, Southfield, MI 48076. Four-track (five cassettes) $7.50, two-track (nine cassettes) $13.50. Available on loan from The National Library Service for the Blind and Physically Handicapped. Cassette (RC 21060); Braille (BR 5858).

Hearing

Organizations

American Association of Retired Persons (AARP) (see pages 441–42). Ask for their pamphlets, "Have You Heard? Hearing Loss and Aging," and "Product Report: Hearing Aids."

American Speech-Language-Hearing Association (ASHA)
10801 Rockville Pike
Rockville, MD 20852
Tel. (301) 897-5700

ASHA is the professional, scientific, and accrediting organization representing 60,000 speech-language pathologists and audiologists. A consumer affiliate of ASHA, (800) 638-8255, is set up to handle specific questions about communication problems and how to find professional assistance. Publishes literature on communication disorders. Provides information on insurance coverage for consumers and a directory of sites, such as libraries, community centers, and religious centers around the country equipped with assistive devices for the hearing-impaired.

AMERICAN TINNITUS ASSOCIATION
P.O. BOX 5
PORTLAND, OR 97207
TEL. (503) 248-9985
Information and referral to worldwide network of clinics and self-help groups. Research and education.

BETTER HEARING INSTITUTE
5021 BLACKLICK ROAD
ANNANDALE, VA 22003
TEL: (800) EAR-WELL
Educational organization providing free information on a variety of issues related to hearing.

NATIONAL LIBRARY SERVICES FOR THE BLIND AND PHYSICALLY HANDICAPPED
LIBRARY OF CONGRESS
WASHINGTON, DC 20542
Publishes *The Directory of Library Resources for the Blind and Physically Handicapped.* Anyone who needs special help because of a physical limitation, including hearing impairment, may apply for use of such aids as amplifiers and telecommunications devices for the deaf, including teletypewriters that enable deaf persons to make or receive telephone calls, and TV decoders that provide close-captioned access to TV programs. Not every library provides these services, so check first to see what is available at yours. For more information, call (800) 424-8567. When you apply, bring a brief written description of the limitation from a professional, such as a physician, nurse, or audiologist. Or a professional librarian may recommend these services.

OFFICE OF SCIENTIFIC AND HEALTH REPORTS
NATIONAL INSTITUTE OF DEAFNESS AND OTHER COMMUNICATION DISORDERS
9000 ROCKVILLE PIKE
BUILDING 31, ROOM 3C35
BETHESDA, MD 20892
TEL. (301) 496-7243
Ask for their pamphlet, "Hearing Loss: Hope Through Research," and other publications.

SHHH (SELF-HELP FOR HARD-OF-HEARING PEOPLE, INC.)
7800 WISCONSIN AVE.
BETHESDA, MD 20814
TEL. (301) 657-2248
A self-help organization for hard-of-hearing people and their families. Local groups meet regularly, offering understanding, information, and self-help strategies for people of all ages. $20 annual dues include a bimonthly magazine, discounts on other publications and participating providers. Send for catalog. Publications include, "Can Medications Affect My Hearing?" and "Sexuality and Intimacy with Hearing Loss."

Books and Other Publications

Becker, Gaylene. *Growing Old in Silence: Deaf People in Old Age.* Berkeley and Los Angeles: University of California Press, 1980. An anthropological study of aging among the lifelong deaf provides a positive view of social support through interdependence.

"How to Buy a Hearing Aid." *Consumer Reports,* Vol. 57, No. 11 (November 1992), pp. 716–21.

Shimon, Debra A. *Coping with Hearing Loss and Hearing Aids.* San Diego, CA: Singular Publishing, 1991.

HYPOTHERMIA

Articles

"Hypothermia." In the American Medical Association, *Family Medical Guide.* New York: Random House, 1987. See also "First Aid" which warns: **Do not give alcohol.**

Siwolop, Sana. "Why Women Get Cold." *Savvy,* June 1985, pp. 70–1.

Products

A regular mercury thermometer may detect a low temperature only if it has been shaken down to its lowest point. Usually the occurrence and severity of the hypothermia can be determined only by using a low-reading or subnormal thermometer, or a rectal probe.

SMELL AND TASTE

Fact Sheet: Smell and Taste Disorders. NIH Pub. No. 86-2655, December 1985.

MEMORY LAPSE AND MEMORY LOSS

Organizations

ALZHEIMER'S DISEASE AND RELATED DISORDERS ASSOCIATION (ADRDA)
919 N. MICHIGAN AVE., SUITE 1000
CHICAGO, IL 60611
TEL. (800) 272-3900

Newsletter contains informative articles. Also has pamphlets, books, and state and local chapters that sponsor support groups and lists of community resources.

AMERICAN ACADEMY OF NEUROLOGY
2221 UNIVERSITY AVE. SE, SUITE 335
MINNEAPOLIS, MN 55414
TEL. (612) 623-8115

AMERICAN ASSOCIATION FOR GERIATRIC PSYCHIATRY
P.O. BOX 376-A
GREENBELT, MD 20768
TEL. (301) 220-0952

AMERICAN GERIATRICS SOCIETY
770 LEXINGTON AVE., SUITE 300
NEW YORK, NY 10021
TEL. (212) 308-1414

GERONTOLOGICAL SOCIETY OF AMERICA
1275 K ST. NW, SUITE 350
WASHINGTON, DC 20005-4006
TEL. (202) 842-1275

NATIONAL COUNCIL ON THE AGING
409 THIRD ST. SW, SUITE 200
WASHINGTON, DC 20024
TEL. (202) 479-1200

NATIONAL INSTITUTE ON AGING
TEL. (800) 438-4380

Information on Alzheimer's disease, lists of research centers and projects.

Books and Other Publications

The American Journal of Alzheimer's Care and Related Disorders. 470 Boston Post Road, Weston, MA 02193. Tel. (617) 899-2702. Quarterly covering major areas of interest to caregivers and professionals.

Cohen, Donna, and Carl Eisdorfer. *The Loss of Self: A Family Resource for the Care of Alzheimer's Disease and Related Disorders.* New York: Norton, 1986. Contains many personal accounts by persons with Alzheimer's disease and their relatives. Practical and readable without being simplistic.

Heston, Leonard L., and June A. White. *The Vanishing Mind: A Practical Guide to Alzheimer's Disease and Other Dementias.* New York: Freeman & Co., 1991.

Hoffman, Stephanie B., and Constance A. Platt. *Comforting the Confused: Strategies for Managing Dementia.* Owings Mills, MD: National Health Publication, 1991.

Inoue, Yasushi. *Chronicle of My Mother.* New York: Kodansha International Ltd., 1982. Moving account of a family coping with a woman's gradual mental decline.

Mace, Nancy L., and Peter V. Rabins. *The 36-Hour Day: A Family Guide to Caring for Persons with Alzheimer's Disease, Related Dementing Illnesses, and Memory Loss in Later Life.* Rev. ed. Baltimore: Johns Hopkins University Press, 1991. Excellent guide for anyone caring for an older person with memory loss, disorientation, and/or increased dependence.

McGowin, Diana Friel. *Living in the Labyrinth: A Personal Journal Through the Maze of Alzheimer's.* San Francisco: Elder Books, 1993. Available from ADRDA, see left-hand column, this page.

Noyes, Lin E. *What's Wrong with My Grandma?* Distributed by ADRDA, Northern Virginia Chapter, 8316 Arlington Blvd., Suite 401, Fairfax, VA 22031. $3.10. Tel. (703) 207-7044. Illustrated booklet to help children understand Alzheimer's disease.

Powell, Lenore S., and Katie Courtice. *Alzheimer's Disease: A Guide for Families.* Reading, MA: Addison-Wesley, 1983.

Safford, Florence. *Caring for the Mentally Impaired Elderly.* New York: Henry Holt, 1986. Sound, innovative, and informative.

Sheridan, Carmel. *Failure-Free Activities for the Alzheimer's Patient.* San Francisco: Cottage Books, 1987.

West, Robin. *Memory Fitness Over 40.* Gainesville, FL: Triad Publishing, 1985. Includes practical ways to improve memory.

Dying and Death

Organizations

Choice in Dying, Inc.
200 Varick St.
New York, NY 10014
Tel. (212) 366-5540
Advocates for recognition and protection of individual rights at the end of life. Literature available on legislation concerning dying and death. Free copies of state-specific advance directives, including living wills and forms for appointing health-care agents are provided upon request. Membership is $15 annually and includes *Choice in Dying Newsletter,* published quarterly. Write for their list of publications, including pamphlets on such topics as pain management; advance directives at $1.50 each.

Compassionate Friends
P.O. Box 3696
Oak Brook, IL 60522-3696
Tel. (708) 990-0010
Self-help organization offering friendship and understanding to bereaved parents and siblings—to support and aid them in the resolution of their grief, and to foster the physical and emotional health of the bereaved parents and their other children.

Continental Association of Funeral and Memorial Societies, Inc.
6900 Lost Lake Road
Egg Harbor, WI 54029
Tel. (800) 458-5563 or (414) 868-3136
Federation of nonprofit consumer organizations fostering freedom of choice in funeral arrangements. Checklists, pamphlets, directories, and other publications. Write for addresses of local memorial societies that can help with preplanning of a simple, dignified, affordable funeral.

Hemlock Society
P.O. Box 11830
Eugene, OR 97440-3900
Tel. (800) 247-7421
Books and articles on euthanasia and self-deliverance. Will provide a durable power of attorney for health-care form. Newsletter available.

Hospice Association of America
519 C St. NE
Washington, DC 20002
Tel. (202) 546-4759
Organized to be a voice for the grass-roots hospice movement and to advocate for legislative changes that would permit more community-based hospices to participate in Medicare.

National Hospice Organization
1901 North Moore St., Suite 901
Arlington, VA 22209
Tel. (703) 243-5900
Advocate for the terminally ill. Provides membership services for community-based hospice programs. Publishes *The Hospice Journal, Hospice Magazine,* and *NHO Newsline.*

Older Women's League (OWL) (see pages 443–44) offers a variety of resources on dying and death, such as their *Living Will Packet* (send $1.00), which includes a sample living will and durable power of attorney, flyer on wills and trusts, and a compilation of practical information on memorial services and burial. Other publications include *Taking Charge of the End of Your Life: Proceedings of a Forum on Living Wills and Other Advance Directives,* July 1985; and *Death and Dying: Staying in Control to the End of Our Lives,* Gray Paper, 1986. $3.00

Suicide Prevention

Check your phone directory's community services section or listings for local hot lines run by the Samaritans or local mental-health agencies. Or write to either of the following:

American Association of Suicidology
2459 S. Ash St.
Denver, CO 80222
Tel. (303) 692-0985
Provides referrals to suicide-prevention services throughout the United States.

The Samaritans
500 Commonwealth Ave.
Boston, MA 02215
Tel. (617) 536-2460
Provides referrals on the East Coast of the United States and in some countries abroad.

WIDOWHOOD

See Relationships in Middle and Later Life resources, pages 468–71, for books and organizations.

Books and Other Publications

Ainley, Rosa, ed. *Dreams and Deathblows: Surviving Your Mother's Death.* New York: Sheba Feminist Press/Sheba Books International, in press. Letters, poetry, and personal accounts of women whose mothers died recently or long ago, whose relationships were close or difficult. Includes foster and adoptive mothers and varied cultural and economic backgrounds.

Becker, Ernest. *The Denial of Death.* New York: Free Press, 1973. The thesis of this book is that the fear and denial of death is the mainspring of all human activity—activity largely designed to overcome our fear by denying in some way that death is our final destiny.

"Funerals." *Modern Maturity,* December 1984/January 1985, p. 16.

Kübler-Ross, Elisabeth. *On Death and Dying.* New York: Macmillan, 1969. Classic presentation of the theory that dying persons move through stages from denial to acceptance.

———. *Death: The Final Stage of Growth.* Englewood Cliffs, NJ: Prentice-Hall, 1975. Essays chiefly centered on what the dying teach about the value of life.

Levine, Steven. *Meetings at the Edge: Dialogues with the Grieving and the Dying, the Healing and the Healed.* New York: Doubleday, 1984.

———. *Who Dies? An Investigation of Conscious Living and Dying.* New York: Doubleday, 1982.

Little, Deborah. *Home Care for the Dying.* New York: Doubleday, 1985. Highly recommended.

Mitford, Jessica. *The American Way of Death.* New York: Fawcett, 1979. Classic exposé of the burial and funeral businesses. Has sparked some reforms.

Morgan, Ernest. *Dealing Creatively with Death: A Manual of Death Education and Simple Burial.* Burnsville, NC: Celo Press, 1984.

Munley, Ann. *The Hospice Alternative: A New Context for Death and Dying.* New York: Basic Books, 1983. This book is strongest in those sections in which the author empathically describes the inner struggles of dying persons and their loved ones. It is unfortunately too uncritical of the policies and politics that have hampered the hospice movement from accomplishing its purposes.

Nearing, Helen. *Loving and Leaving the Good Life.* Post Mills, VT: Chelsea Green Publishers, 1992.

Nelson, Thomas C. *It's Your Choice: The Practical Guide to Planning a Funeral,* 1982. $5.00, from AARP Books, Dept. CATA, 400 S. Edward St., Mount Prospect, IL 60056.

Rollin, Betty. *Last Wish.* New York: Linden Press/Simon & Schuster, 1985. Author tells of her terminally ill mother's decision to stop treatment. Though quite ill, her mother remained in charge until her death.

Sankar, Andrea. *Dying at Home: A Family Guide for Caregiving.* Baltimore: Johns Hopkins University Press, 1991.

Sarton, May. *A Reckoning.* New York: W. W. Norton, 1981. A novel that celebrates caring and connection, and honors the process of dying itself, which the protagonist experiences as "ripening."

Saunders, Dame Cicely, and Mary Baines. *Living with Dying: The Management of Terminal Diseases.* New York: Oxford University Press, 1983. Home health care for the dying.

Silverman, Phyllis. *Helping Women Cope with Grief.* Beverly Hills, CA: Sage Publications, 1981. Highly recommended.

Slagle, Kate Walsh. *Live with Loss.* Englewood Cliffs, NJ: Prentice-Hall, 1982. Practical, compassionate techniques for coping with many kinds of loss and moving through grief to growth.

Special Committee on Biomedical Ethics. *Values in Conflict: Ethical Issues in Hospital Care.* Chicago: American Hospital Association, 1985.

Vozenilek, Helen, ed. *Loss of the Ground-Note: Women Writing About the Loss of Their Mothers.* Los Angeles: Clothespin Fever Press, 1992.

Wanzer, Sidney H., et al. "The Physician's Responsibility Toward Hopelessly Ill Patients." *The New England Journal of Medicine,* Vol. 310, No. 15 (Apr. 12, 1984), pp. 955–99.

Weizman, Savine G., and Phyllis Kamm. *About Mourning: Support and Guidance for the Bereaved.* New York: Human Sciences Press, 1985. Written for mental-health workers, but contains helpful, sensitively written information for the general reader.

Wentzel, Kenneth. *To Those Who Need It Most—Hospice Means Hope.* Boston: Charles River Books, 1981. A general introduction to the philosophy of hospice care.

CHANGING SOCIETY AND OURSELVES

See General Resources for organizations that advocate for women and elders. See also organizations listed under specific chapters.

Books and Other Publications

Building Self-Advocacy in the Community. This manual and other materials that would be useful for all people, including those with disabilities, are available from Association for Retarded Citizens (ARC) of the U.S., 500 E. Border St., Suite 30, Arlington, TX 76010. Tel. (817) 261-6003.

Cheatham, Annie, and Mary Clare Powell. *This Way Daybreak Comes.* Philadelphia: New Society Publishers, 1985. The authors traveled thirty thousand miles to talk with American women in all walks of life about creating new institutions and changing old ones by valuing nurturance and cooperation, and living as one with others and with the natural world.

DuBois, Ellen C., and Vicki L. Ruiz, eds. *Unequal Sisters: A Multi-Cultural Reader in U.S. Women's History.* New York: Routledge, 1990. Culturally and ethnically inclusive collection of articles on work, family, and political activism.

Durr, Virginia Foster. *Outside the Magic Circle.* Birmingham, AL: University of Alabama Press, 1985. Memoirs, beginning in the 1930s, of a "proper Alabama lady" who stepped outside the privileged circle into which she was born to challenge the cruelty of racial segregation.

Flexner, Eleanor. *Century of Struggle: The Woman's Rights Movement in the United States.* New York: Atheneum, 1973. A history of women's fight for equality in education, work, and voting rights.

Giddings, Paula. *When and Where I Enter.* New York: Morrow, 1984. Historical account of black women in social-reform movements in the United States.

Goodman, Ellen. *Value Judgments.* New York: Farrar, Straus, & Giroux, 1993. Thoughtful essays on changing sex roles and social values by a nationally syndicated columnist.

Huckle, Patricia. *Tish Sommers, Activist, and the Founding of the Older Women's League.* Knoxville, TN: University of Tennessee Press, 1991.

Jacobs, Ruth Harriet, ed. *We Speak for Peace: An Anthology.* 1993. Order from Kit Publishers, 1131-0 Tolland Turnpike, Suite 175, Manchester, CT 06040. Voices of young, old, women, men, children, and war veterans on the plight of a world in need of an alternative to war for resolving conflict.

Kuhn, Maggie. *No Stone Unturned: The Life and Times of Maggie Kuhn.* New York: Ballantine, 1991.

Lykes, M. Brinton, et al., eds. *Unmasking Social Inequalities: Victims, Voice and Resistance.* Philadelphia: Temple University Press, in Press. Collection of critical articles on inequities in health, mental health, housing, and employment. Documents instances of community resistance to oppressive conditions; advocates community empowerment and social change.

McAllister, Pam, ed. *Reweaving the Web of Life: Feminism and Nonviolence.* Philadelphia: New Society Publishers, 1982. Explores women's commitment to nonviolent means of change.

"Older, Wiser, Stronger: Southern Elders." Special Issue of *Southern Exposure,* Vol. 13, No. 2–3

(March–June, 1985). Order from Southern Exposure, P.O. Box 531, Durham, NC 27702. Tel. (919) 419-8310. Fascinating and original compilation of elder activism in the South.

Philbin, Marianne, ed. *The Ribbon: Celebration of Life: The Remarkable Ribbon Around the Pentagon, A Unique Worldwide Plea for Peace.* 1985. Lark Books, 50 College St., Asheville, NC 28801.

Reinharz, Shulamit. "Women as Competent Community Builders." In Annette U. Rickel, et al., eds., *Social and Psychological Problems of Women: Prevention and Crisis Intervention.* Washington, DC: Hemisphere Publishing Corporation, 1984. Article focuses on women's strengths, especially as active agents in their communities.

Steinem, Gloria. *Moving Beyond Words.* New York: Simon & Schuster, 1994, in press. Celebrates "brave women . . . exploring the outer edge of human possibility, with no history to guide them."

Presses

New Society Publishers
4527 Springfield Ave.
Philadelphia, PA 19143
Tel. (215) 382-6543

Publishes a variety of self-help manuals for social-change activists on such subjects as working collectively, feminist leadership, empowering ourselves in the nuclear age, and consensus decision making. Their publications include Virginia Coover, Ellen Deacon, et al., *Resource Manual for a Living Revolution,* 1985, which includes innovative decision-making techniques; Joanna Rogers Macy, *Despair and Personal Power in the Nuclear Age,* 1983; and Jean McLaren and Heide Brown, *Raging Grannies Songbook,* 1993, antiwar lyrics to familiar songs.

INDEX

✦

In this index, a boldface page number is used to indicate the major discussion of the topic. An italic *r* refers to the Resources section; an italic *n* refers to a footnote.

B

C

E

N

O

T

U

Paula B. Doress-Worters is coauthor of *Our Bodies, Ourselves, Ourselves and Our Children,* and a series of articles on sex education and censorship. She is a founding member of the Boston Women's Health Book Collective and has lectured on a variety of women's health issues. As coordinator of the "Women Growing Older" chapter in *The New Our Bodies, Ourselves,* Paula became aware of the need for more information by and about older women and conceived the idea for *Ourselves, Growing Older.* Paula was among the first to develop a curriculum for and teach women's studies courses at the college level. She holds a master's degree in Women's Studies and a Ph.D. in Social Psychology.

Diana Laskin Siegal holds a master's degree in Public Administration and has worked for health departments and programs in Kansas and Massachusetts. A pioneer member of the first class to graduate from Brandeis University, she has never had a job that someone else held before. She has been involved in starting many health planning and public health programs. Always a consumer advocate and an activist, she has served on many committees, boards, and political campaigns. Currently she is at the Massachusetts Department of Public Health, directing a project to reduce urinary incontinence among the elderly. For this project, she wrote and produced her first video.

The first edition of *Ourselves, Growing Older* has been adapted and published in Great Britain, Germany, and Spain. For information, contact Paramount Publishing, New York, New York.

The Boston Women's Health Book Collective is a nonprofit organization devoted to education about women and health. Their many projects include a Women's Health Information Center, open to the public; extensive distribution of materials to women and organizations in the United States and other countries; the publication and distribution of a Spanish-language edition of *Our Bodies, Ourselves (Nuestros Cuerpos, Nuestras Vidas);* and distribution of a videotape about teenage pregnancy. The Collective is the repository of books and files from *Ourselves, Growing Older* and has added the area of women and aging to the considerable list of topics on which it can provide information to the public. Tax-deductible donations (made payable to BWHBC) are welcome to help support the work of the Collective. Send to BWHBC, Box 192, Somerville, MA 02144.

Other books by the Boston Women's Health Book Collective:

Our Bodies, Ourselves
Ourselves and Our Children
The New Our Bodies, Ourselves